JN235067

プロメテウス
解剖学アトラス
コンパクト版

PROMETHEUS
Anatomy Flash Cards
−Anatomy on the Go

PROMETHEUS
Anatomy Flash Cards
—Anatomy on the Go

Edited by
Anne M. Gilroy

Consulting Editors
Jonas Broman, Anna Josephson

Based on the work of
Michael Schünke, Erik Schulte, Udo Schumacher

Illustrations by
Markus Voll, Karl Wesker

プロメテウス
解剖学アトラス
コンパクト版

監訳
坂井 建雄　順天堂大学医学部 教授

訳
市村 浩一郎　順天堂大学医学部 准教授
澤井 直　順天堂大学医学部

医学書院

編集
Anne M. Gilroy

編集顧問
Jonas Broman
Anna Josephson

執筆協力
Michael Schünke
Erik Schulte
Udo Schumacher

イラスト
Markus Voll
Karl Wesker

Copyright © 2008 of the original English language edition by Thieme Medical Publishers, Inc., New York, USA. Original title: "Anatomy Flash Cards-Anatomy on the Go", edited by Anne M. Gilroy.
Consulting Editors: Jonas Broman, Anna Josephson.
Based on the work of Michael Schünke, Erik Schulte, Udo Schumacher.
Illustrations by Markus Voll, Karl Wesker.
© First Japanese edition 2011 by Igaku-Shoin Ltd., Tokyo

Printed and bound in Japan

プロメテウス解剖学アトラス
コンパクト版

発　行　2011年3月1日　第1版第1刷
　　　　2017年12月1日　第1版第5刷
監訳者　坂井建雄
発行者　株式会社　医学書院
　　　　代表取締役　金原　優
　　　　〒113-8719　東京都文京区本郷1-28-23
　　　　電話 03-3817-5600(社内案内)

印刷・製本　横山印刷

本書の複製権・翻訳権・上映権・譲渡権・貸与権・公衆送信権(送信可能化権を含む)は株式会社医学書院が保有します．

ISBN978-4-260-01126-6

本書を無断で複製する行為(複写，スキャン，デジタルデータ化など)は，「私的使用のための複製」など著作権法上の限られた例外を除き禁じられています．大学，病院，診療所，企業などにおいて，業務上使用する目的(診療，研究活動を含む)で上記の行為を行うことは，その使用範囲が内部的であっても，私的使用には該当せず，違法です．また私的使用に該当する場合であっても，代行業者等の第三者に依頼して上記の行為を行うことは違法となります．

JCOPY 〈出版者著作権管理機構 委託出版物〉
本書の無断複製は著作権法上での例外を除き禁じられています．複製される場合は，そのつど事前に，出版者著作権管理機構(電話 03-3513-6969，FAX 03-3513-6979，info@jcopy.or.jp)の許諾を得てください．

監訳者序

　『プロメテウス解剖学アトラス』は，21世紀を代表する解剖学アトラスである．オリジナルの3冊本は2005～2006年に出版され，その精細で迫真の解剖図は世界中の人々に強烈な印象を与え，数多くの国々で翻訳・出版されている．その日本語版も2007～2009年に出版され，わが国の医療関係者と学生に広く迎え入れられた．1冊本の『プロメテウス解剖学コア アトラス』も，オリジナルが2008年に出版され，日本語版が2010年に出版されて多くの読者に支持されている．

　本書『プロメテウス解剖学アトラス コンパクト版』は，このように広がり続ける「プロメテウス」シリーズから生み出された，きらりと輝く小品である．「プロメテウス」のすばらしい解剖図が，解剖学の学習に手軽に利用してもらうために編まれている．原書は箱入りの367枚のカードという形式で出版されたが，日本語版の製作にあたっては読者の便を考えてポケット版の冊子体を採用した．

　本書には，解剖学の学習に役立つさまざまな工夫が凝らされている．見開きの左に解剖図，右に用語解説という構成にしているが，これにより必要な情報をひと目で見つけ出し，的確に理解することができる．さらに，原書にはない巻末の索引を利用することにより，必要なときに必要な図をすばやく探し出すことができる．また，臨床的なコメントや，理解を深めるためのQ＆Aが随所に挿入されている．より深い学習への足がかりにしていただけるとありがたい．さらに人体のさまざまな構造について詳しい情報を得たい人には，見開きの右頁下部に記した『プロメテウス解剖学コア アトラス』の頁と図の番号を手がかりにし，同書を参照してより幅広い情報を引き出していただきたい．

翻訳にあたっては，若手の優秀な解剖学者である市村と澤井が日本語訳の作業を行い，坂井が全体に目を通して監訳を担当した．特に『プロメテウス解剖学コア アトラス』および解剖学用語との内容および用語の整合性に配慮した．日本語訳にあたっては瑕疵がないように細心の注意をしたつもりではあるが，至らぬところは監訳者の責である．

本書『プロメテウス解剖学アトラス コンパクト版』が，解剖学の学習の場で多くの学生たちに役立てていただけることを願うものである．

2010年12月5日
八王子の寓居にて

坂井建雄

目次

背部

脊柱 1 ……………………………………… 2
脊柱 2 ……………………………………… 4
脊柱 3 ……………………………………… 6
椎骨の構成要素 …………………………… 8
頸椎 1 ……………………………………… 10
頸椎 2 ……………………………………… 12
頸椎 3 ……………………………………… 14
頸椎 4 ……………………………………… 16
胸椎 ………………………………………… 18
腰椎 ………………………………………… 20
仙骨と尾骨 1 ……………………………… 22
仙骨と尾骨 2 ……………………………… 24
脊柱の関節 ………………………………… 26
頸部脊柱の靱帯 1 ………………………… 28
頸部脊柱の靱帯 2 ………………………… 30
胸腰部脊柱の靱帯 1 ……………………… 32
胸腰部脊柱の靱帯 2 ……………………… 34
胸腰部脊柱の靱帯 3 ……………………… 36
背部浅層の筋 ……………………………… 38
項部の固有筋 ……………………………… 40
固有背筋 1 ………………………………… 42
固有背筋 2 ………………………………… 44
背部の動脈 ………………………………… 46
背部の静脈 ………………………………… 48
背部の神経 ………………………………… 50
項部の神経・血管(局所解剖) …………… 52
背部の神経・血管(局所解剖) …………… 54
背部の体表解剖 …………………………… 56

胸部

胸部の骨格 ………………………………… 60
胸部の構造 ………………………………… 62
胸骨 ………………………………………… 64
胸壁の筋肉 ………………………………… 66
原位置の横隔膜 1 ………………………… 68
原位置の横隔膜 2 ………………………… 70
横隔膜の開口部 …………………………… 72
胸壁の動脈 ………………………………… 74
胸壁の静脈 ………………………………… 76
胸壁の神経 ………………………………… 78
肋間神経の経路 …………………………… 80
横隔膜の神経・血管 ……………………… 82
女性の乳房への栄養血管 ………………… 84
女性の乳房のリンパ管 …………………… 86
女性の乳房の構造 ………………………… 88
縦隔の区分 ………………………………… 90
胸部のCTスキャン ……………………… 92
胸大動脈 …………………………………… 94
奇静脈系 …………………………………… 96
胸腔のリンパ管 …………………………… 98
胸腔の神経 ………………………………… 100
縦隔 1 ……………………………………… 102
縦隔 2 ……………………………………… 104
縦隔 3 ……………………………………… 106
縦隔 4 ……………………………………… 108
心膜の折れ返り 1 ………………………… 110
心膜の折れ返り 2 ………………………… 112
原位置の心臓 ……………………………… 114
心臓の胸肋面 ……………………………… 116
心臓の底面 ………………………………… 118
心臓の室 1 ………………………………… 120
心臓の室 2 ………………………………… 122
心臓の室 3 ………………………………… 124
心臓弁 ……………………………………… 126
心臓の動脈と静脈 1 ……………………… 128
心臓の動脈と静脈 2 ……………………… 130
心臓刺激伝導系 …………………………… 132
心臓の自律神経 …………………………… 134
心臓のX線像 1 …………………………… 136
心臓のX線像 2 …………………………… 138
水平断面での心臓 ………………………… 140
出生前の循環 ……………………………… 142

出生後の循環	144
壁側胸膜	146
原位置の肺	148
右肺	150
左肺	152
気管	154
気管支樹の区分	156
気管支樹の呼吸部	158
肺動脈と肺静脈	160
胸膜腔のリンパ節	162
胸部の体表解剖	164

腹部・骨盤

寛骨	168
下肢帯	170
骨盤の靱帯 1	172
骨盤の靱帯 2	174
腹壁の筋 1	176
腹壁の筋 2	178
腹壁の筋 3	180
鼡径部 1	182
鼡径部 2	184
男性の骨盤底	186
女性の骨盤底 1	188
女性の骨盤底 2	190
腹腔：骨盤腔	192
腹膜腔	194
網嚢	196
腸間膜と臓器	198
腹膜腔の後壁	200
男性骨盤の内容	202
女性骨盤の内容	204
腹部の水平断面	206
原位置の胃	208
十二指腸	210
大腸	212
原位置の直腸	214
直腸と肛門管	216
肝臓の表面 1	218
肝臓の表面 2	220
肝外胆管	222

原位置の胆路	224
膵臓	226
原位置の腎臓と尿管	228
女性の膀胱と尿道	230
膀胱三角	232
子宮と卵管 1	234
子宮と卵管 2	236
女性の外生殖器	238
女性の勃起組織	240
女性会陰の神経・血管	242
陰茎の横断面	244
陰茎	246
精巣と精巣上体	248
精巣の被膜	250
男性の付属生殖腺	252
原位置の前立腺	254
男性会陰の神経・血管	256
腹大動脈	258
腎動脈	260
腹腔動脈 1	262
腹腔動脈 2	264
上腸間膜動脈	266
下腸間膜動脈	268
下大静脈の支脈	270
腎動脈・静脈	272
門脈の分布	274
原位置の門脈	276
女性骨盤の血管	278
直腸の血管	280
男性生殖器の血管	282
壁側リンパ節	284
自律神経叢	286
女性骨盤の神経支配	288
男性骨盤の神経支配	290
腹部・骨盤の体表解剖	292

上肢

上肢の骨格	296
鎖骨	298
肩甲骨 1	300
肩甲骨 2	302

項目	ページ
上腕骨 1	304
上腕骨 2	306
上肢帯の関節	308
胸鎖関節	310
肩関節(肩甲上腕関節) 1	312
肩関節(肩甲上腕関節) 2	314
肩の前額断面	316
肩と上腕の筋(前面) 1	318
肩と上腕の筋(前面) 2	320
肩と上腕の筋(前面) 3	322
肩と上腕の筋(前面) 4	324
肩と上腕の筋(後面) 1	326
肩と上腕の筋(後面) 2	328
肩と上腕の筋(後面) 3	330
橈骨と尺骨	332
肘関節 1	334
肘関節 2	336
前腕の筋(前面) 1	338
前腕の筋(前面) 2	340
前腕の筋(前面) 3	342
前腕の筋(後面) 1	344
前腕の筋(後面) 2	346
手首と手の骨格 1	348
手首と手の骨格 2	350
手首と手の関節	352
手の筋 1	354
手の筋 2	356
手の筋 3	358
手の筋 4	360
手背	362
上肢の動脈	364
上肢の皮静脈	366
腕神経叢の構造	368
腕神経叢の走行	370
腕神経叢からの神経 1 (腋窩神経)	372
腕神経叢からの神経 2 (橈骨神経)	374
腕神経叢からの神経 3 (筋皮神経)	376
腕神経叢からの神経 4 (正中神経)	378
腕神経叢からの神経 5 (尺骨神経)	380
肩の後部における神経・血管 1	382
肩の後部における神経・血管 2	384
腋窩の神経・血管 1	386
腋窩の神経・血管 2	388
腋窩の神経・血管 3	390
上腕の神経・血管	392
前腕の神経・血管	394
手根管	396
浅掌動脈弓	398
深掌動脈弓	400
解剖学的嗅ぎタバコ入れ	402
手における感覚神経の分布 1	404
手における感覚神経の分布 2	406
上腕の横断面	408
前腕の横断面	410
手の体表解剖	412

下肢

項目	ページ
下肢の骨格	416
寛骨の構成	418
大腿骨	420
股関節 1	422
股関節 2	424
股関節の靱帯 1	426
股関節の靱帯 2	428
骨盤と大腿の筋(前面) 1	430
骨盤と大腿の筋(前面) 2	432
骨盤と大腿の筋(前面) 3	434
骨盤と大腿の筋(内側面)	436
骨盤と大腿の筋(後面) 1	438
骨盤と大腿の筋(後面) 2	440
骨盤と大腿の筋(後面) 3	442
骨盤と大腿の筋(外側面)	444
脛骨と腓骨	446
膝関節 1	448
膝関節 2	450
膝関節の靱帯 1	452
膝関節の靱帯 2	454
膝関節の靱帯 3	456
下腿の筋(前面)	458
下腿の筋(外側面)	460
下腿の筋(後面) 1	462
下腿の筋(後面) 2	464
下腿の筋(後面) 3	466
足の骨格 1	468
足の骨格 2	470

足首と足の関節 1 ················ 472
足首と足の関節 2 ················ 474
足首と足の関節 3 ················ 476
足首と足の靱帯 1 ················ 478
足首と足の靱帯 2 ················ 480
足首と足の靱帯 3 ················ 482
足底の筋 1 ························ 484
足底の筋 2 ························ 486
足底の筋 3 ························ 488
足底の筋 4 ························ 490
足首と足 ···························· 492
下肢の動脈 1 ····················· 494
下肢の動脈 2 ····················· 496
腰仙骨神経叢 1 ·················· 498
腰仙骨神経叢 2 ·················· 500
腰神経叢からの神経 1 ········· 502
腰神経叢からの神経 2 ········· 504
仙骨神経叢からの神経 1 ····· 506
仙骨神経叢からの神経 2 ····· 508
皮静脈と皮神経 ·················· 510
鼡径部 ······························ 512
坐骨孔 ······························ 514
大腿前面の神経・血管 ········ 516
大腿後面の神経・血管 ········ 518
下腿後面の神経・血管 ········ 520
足根管 ······························ 522
下腿外側の神経・血管 ········ 524
下腿前面の神経・血管 ········ 526
足背の神経・血管 ··············· 528
足底の神経・血管 ··············· 530
大腿の横断面 ····················· 532
下腿の横断面 ····················· 534
下肢の体表解剖 ·················· 536

頭頸部

頭蓋の骨 1 ························ 540
頭蓋の骨 2 ························ 542
頭蓋の骨 3 ························ 544
頭蓋底 1 ···························· 546
頭蓋底 2 ···························· 548
頭蓋底 3 ···························· 550

表情筋 ······························ 552
脳神経 1 ···························· 554
脳神経 2 ···························· 556
脳神経 3 ···························· 558
脳神経 4 ···························· 560
脳神経 5 ···························· 562
脳神経 6 ···························· 564
脳神経 7 ···························· 566
脳神経 8 ···························· 568
脳神経 9 ···························· 570
脳神経 10 ·························· 572
感覚神経支配 ····················· 574
頭蓋と顔面の動脈 1 ············ 576
頭蓋と顔面の動脈 2 ············ 578
頭頸部の静脈 1 ·················· 580
頭頸部の静脈 2 ·················· 582
顔面浅層の神経・血管 1 ····· 584
顔面浅層の神経・血管 2 ····· 586
耳下腺咬筋部 1 ·················· 588
耳下腺咬筋部 2 ·················· 590
側頭下窩 1 ························ 592
側頭下窩 2 ························ 594
側頭下窩 3 ························ 596
翼口蓋窩 ···························· 598
眼窩の骨 ···························· 600
眼窩の筋 ···························· 602
眼窩の神経 1 ····················· 604
眼窩の神経 2 ····················· 606
眼窩の局所解剖 1 ··············· 608
眼窩の局所解剖 2 ··············· 610
眼瞼と結膜 ························ 612
涙器 ·································· 614
眼球の構造 ························ 616
鼻腔の骨 1 ························ 618
鼻腔の骨 2 ························ 620
鼻腔の骨 3 ························ 622
鼻腔の神経・血管 1 ············ 624
鼻腔の神経・血管 2 ············ 626
外耳 ·································· 628
耳介の構造 ························ 630
鼓室 ·································· 632
耳小骨連鎖 ························ 634
内耳 ·································· 636
下顎骨 ······························ 638

口腔の三叉神経	640
舌背	642
舌の筋肉	644
舌の感覚性神経支配	646
舌の神経と血管	648
口腔の区分 1	650
口腔の区分 2	652
唾液腺 1	654
唾液腺 2	656
咽頭筋 1	658
咽頭筋 2	660
咽頭の神経・血管	662
頸部の筋	664
頸部の動脈	666
頸部の神経	668
甲状腺	670
甲状腺の関係	672
喉頭の構造	674
喉頭腔	676
喉頭の神経・血管 1	678
喉頭の神経・血管 2	680
頸部の部位	682
胸郭上口 1	684
胸郭上口 2	686
外側頸三角部の局所解剖 1	688
外側頸三角部の局所解剖 2	690
頭頸部の体表解剖	692

神経解剖

成人の脳 1	696
成人の脳 2	698
大脳白質	700
海馬とその関連構造	702
間脳	704
脳の内部構造 1	706
脳の内部構造 2	708
脳の内部構造 3	710
脳幹 1	712
脳幹 2	714
脊髄	716
脊髄の横断面	718
髄膜 1	720
髄膜 2	722
硬膜中隔	724
脳脊髄液の循環	726
脳室系	728
静脈洞交会	730
頭蓋底にある硬膜静脈洞	732
脳の動脈	734
脊髄の動脈	736
感覚系と運動系	738
脊髄の上行路	740
脊髄の下行路	742
視覚系	744
自律神経系	746

索引 749

アイコン一覧

本文中のアイコンは，それぞれ下記を意味しています。

Q クエスチョン　　**解説**

A アンサー　　**臨床**

また，本文中の見開き右頁下部に記した①，②の頁と図の番号は，それぞれ「プロメテウス解剖学コア アトラス」の初版，第 2 版における掲載頁と図の番号を示しています。

背部 Back

- 脊柱 1 ……………………………………… 2
- 脊柱 2 ……………………………………… 4
- 脊柱 3 ……………………………………… 6
- 椎骨の構成要素 …………………………… 8
- 頸椎 1 ……………………………………… 10
- 頸椎 2 ……………………………………… 12
- 頸椎 3 ……………………………………… 14
- 頸椎 4 ……………………………………… 16
- 胸椎 ………………………………………… 18
- 腰椎 ………………………………………… 20
- 仙骨と尾骨 1 ……………………………… 22
- 仙骨と尾骨 2 ……………………………… 24
- 脊柱の関節 ………………………………… 26
- 頸部脊柱の靱帯 1 ………………………… 28
- 頸部脊柱の靱帯 2 ………………………… 30
- 胸腰部脊柱の靱帯 1 ……………………… 32
- 胸腰部脊柱の靱帯 2 ……………………… 34
- 胸腰部脊柱の靱帯 3 ……………………… 36
- 背部浅層の筋 ……………………………… 38
- 項部の固有筋 ……………………………… 40
- 固有背筋 1 ………………………………… 42
- 固有背筋 2 ………………………………… 44
- 背部の動脈 ………………………………… 46
- 背部の静脈 ………………………………… 48
- 背部の神経 ………………………………… 50
- 項部の神経・血管(局所解剖) …………… 52
- 背部の神経・血管(局所解剖) …………… 54
- 背部の体表解剖 …………………………… 56

Vertebral Column I

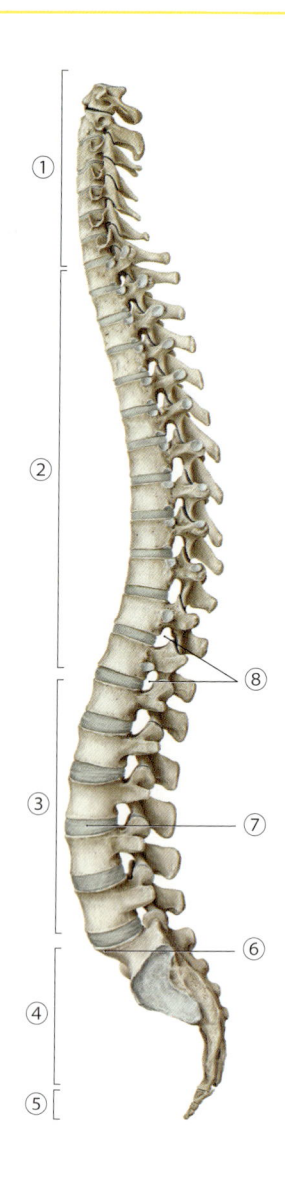

脊柱 1

左外側面

① □ 第 1-7 頸椎　　　　　　　□ C1-C7 vertebrae

② □ 第 1-12 胸椎　　　　　　□ T1-T12 vertebrae

③ □ 第 1-5 腰椎　　　　　　　□ L1-L5 vertebrae

④ □ 仙骨（第 1-5 仙椎）　　　□ Sacrum (S1-S5 vertebrae)

⑤ □ 尾骨　　　　　　　　　　□ Coccyx

⑥ □ 岬角　　　　　　　　　　□ Promontory

⑦ □ 椎間円板　　　　　　　　□ Intervertebral disk

⑧ □ 椎間孔　　　　　　　　　□ Intervertebral foramina

解説

成人では脊柱に特徴的な弯曲（4 ヵ所）が見られる．この弯曲は生後の発達過程で形成される．新生児では胸部脊柱の後弯のみが見られる．腰部脊柱の前弯は生後に発達し，思春期に安定化する．

1 図 1.1B, p.2　2 図 2.1B, p.4

Vertebral Column II

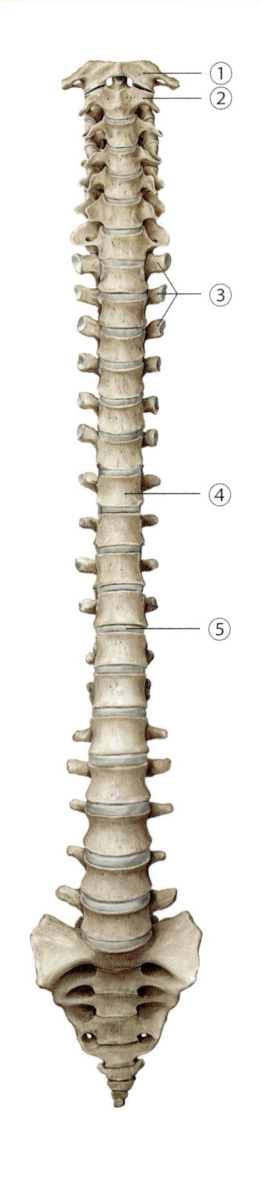

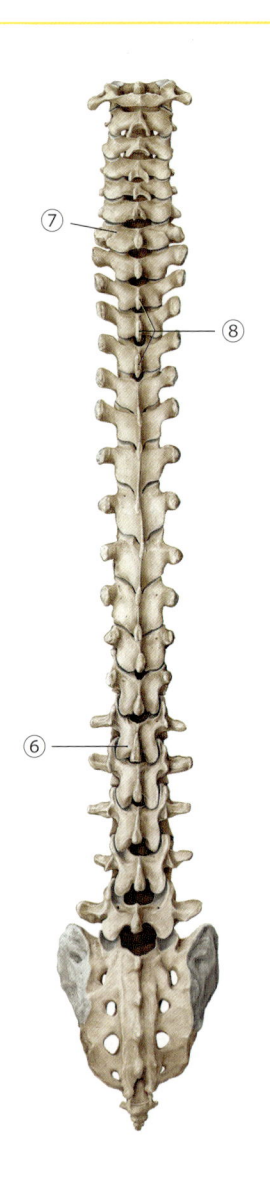

脊柱 2

左：前面，右：後面

① ☐ 環椎（第1頸椎） ☐ Atlas (C1 vertebra)

② ☐ 軸椎（第2頸椎） ☐ Axis (C2 vertebra)

③ ☐ 横突起 ☐ Transverse processes

④ ☐ 椎体 ☐ Vertebral body

⑤ ☐ 椎間円板 ☐ Intervertebral disk

⑥ ☐ 第1腰椎 ☐ L1 vertebra

⑦ ☐ 隆椎（第7頸椎） ☐ Vertebra prominens (C7 vertebra)

⑧ ☐ 棘突起 ☐ Spinous processes

臨床

脊柱は骨格の退行性疾患（例えば，変形性関節症や骨粗鬆症）によって最も侵されやすい部位である．骨粗鬆症では，骨吸収が骨形成を上回り，骨量が減少する．この疾患では椎体の圧迫骨折により背部痛を生じる場合がある．

1 図 1.3A, B. p.4　2 図 2.3A, B. p.6

6 Back

Vertebral Column III

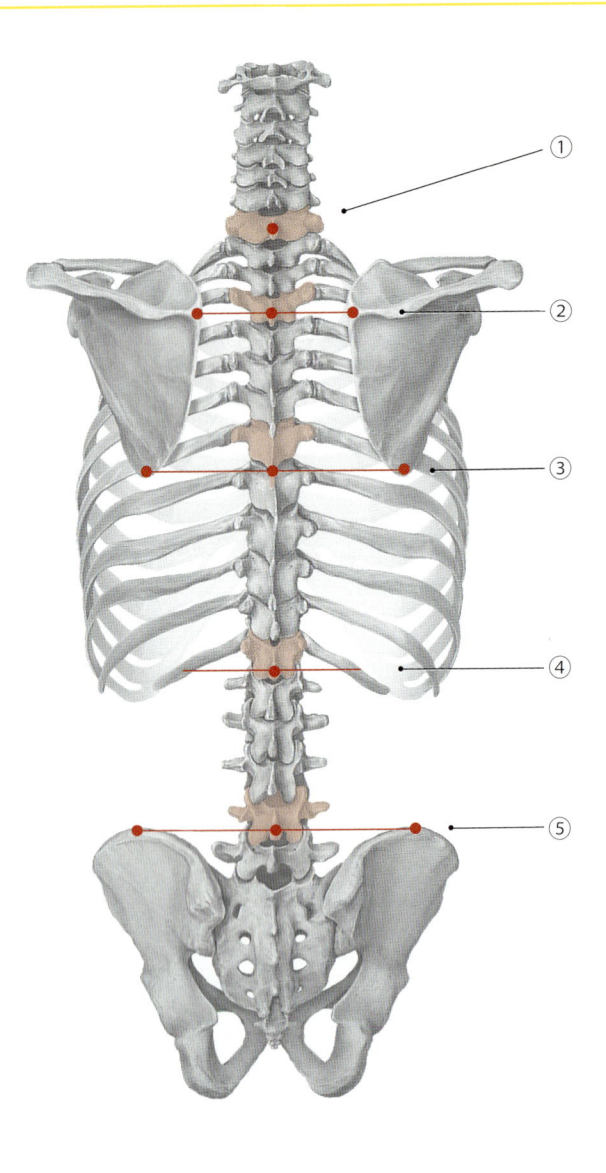

①
②
③
④
⑤

脊柱 3

指標としての棘突起 Spinous processes，後面

① ☐ 頸椎と胸椎の移行部 （第7頸椎）　　☐ Cervicothoracic junction (C7 vertebra)

② ☐ 肩甲棘（第3胸椎）　　☐ Scapular spine (T3 vertebra)

③ ☐ 肩甲骨の下角（第7胸椎）　　☐ Inferior scapular angle (T7 vertebra)

④ ☐ 第12肋骨　　☐ 12th rib (T12 vertebra)

⑤ ☐ 腸骨稜（第4腰椎）　　☐ Iliac crest (L4 vertebra)

臨床

棘突起は体表から容易に触知することができ，理学的診察の際に特定の位置を表す指標として役立つ．

1 図 1.4. p.4

Structural Elements of a Vertebra

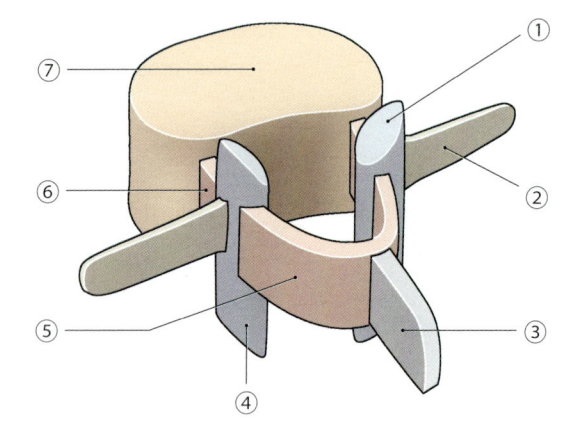

椎骨の構成要素

左後上面

① □ 上関節突起　　　　　□ Superior articular process

② □ 横突起　　　　　　　□ Transverse process

③ □ 棘突起　　　　　　　□ Spinous process

④ □ 下関節突起　　　　　□ Inferior articular process

⑤ □ 椎弓板　　　　　　　□ Lamina of vertebral arch

⑥ □ 椎弓根　　　　　　　□ Pedicle of vertebral arch

⑦ □ 椎体　　　　　　　　□ Vertebral body

解説

環椎(C1)と軸椎(C2)以外の椎骨は，共通した構成要素(椎弓，椎体，棘突起，横突起，関節突起)からなる．椎弓は椎弓根と椎弓板からなり，椎体とともに椎孔を形成する．すべての椎骨の椎孔が縦に連なり，脊柱管が形成される．

1 図1.5, p.5　2 図2.4, p.7

Cervical Vertebrae I

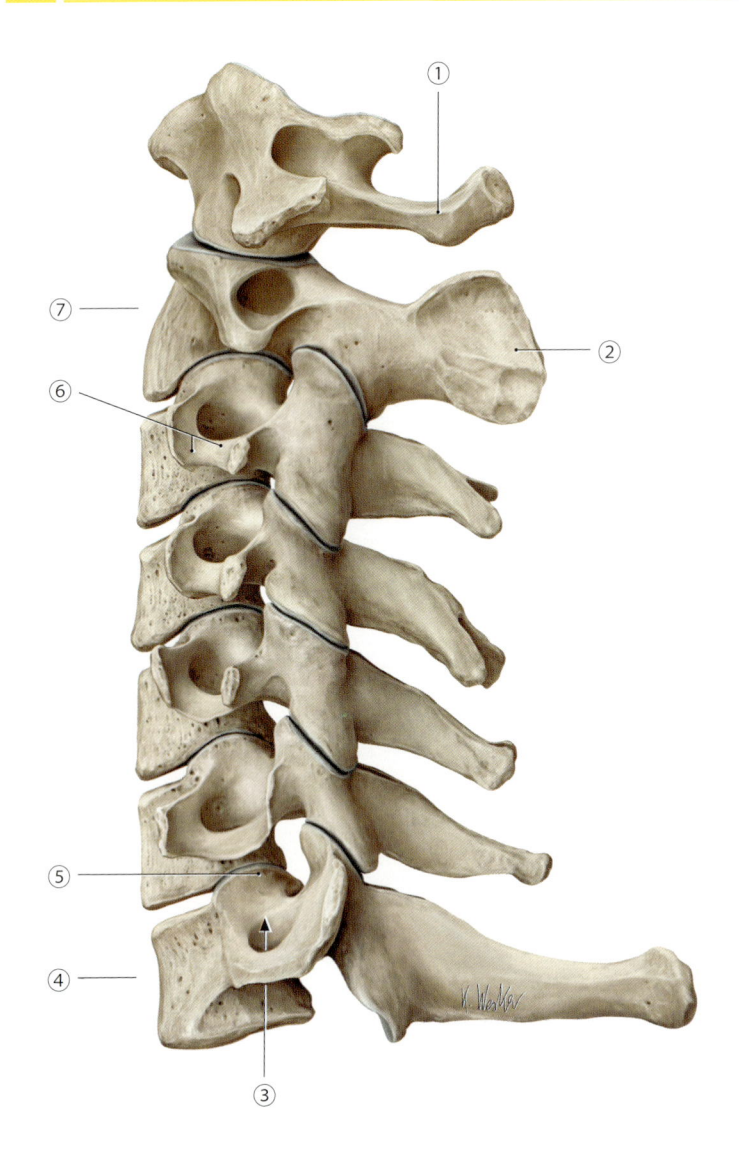

頸椎 1

左外側面

① ☐ 環椎後弓 ☐ Posterior arch of atlas
② ☐ 棘突起 ☐ Spinous process
③ ☐ 横突起 ☐ Transverse foramen
④ ☐ 第 7 頸椎（隆椎） ☐ C7 vertebra（vertebra prominens）
⑤ ☐ 鉤状突起 ☐ Uncinate process
⑥ ☐ 脊髄神経溝 ☐ Sulcus for spinal nerve
⑦ ☐ 第 2 頸椎（軸椎） ☐ C2 vertebra（axis）

臨床

頸部脊柱は過伸展による損傷（いわゆる"むち打ち症"）を受けやすい部位であり，頭部が通常の可動域を大きく超えて後方に伸展した場合に生じる．頸部脊柱で見られる最も多い外傷は，歯突起骨折，外傷性脊椎すべり症（椎体の前方への偏位），環椎骨折である．これらの患者の予後は，損傷を受けた脊髄の高さにほぼ依存する．

1 図 1.7A. p.6　2 図 2.6A. p.8

Cervical Vertebrae II

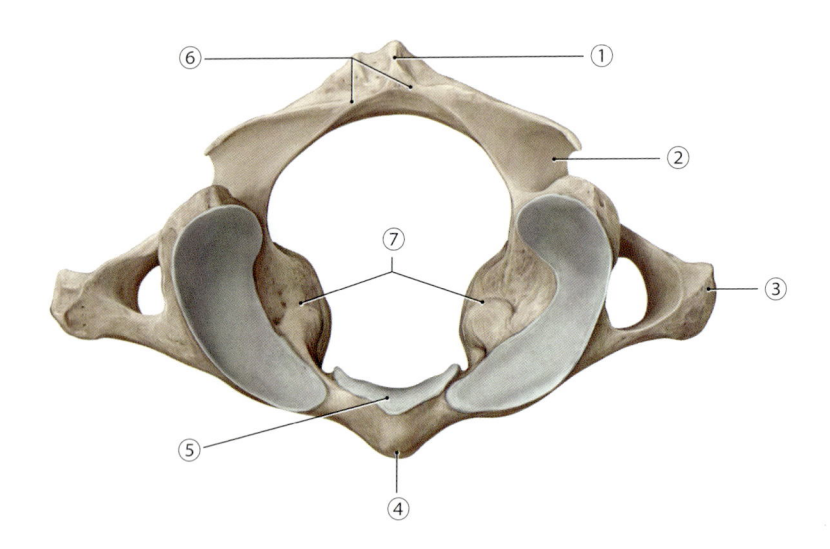

環椎（C1）の基本構造は，典型的な頸椎（C3-C7）とどのように異なるか？

頸椎 2

環椎(C1) Atlas(C1),上面

① □ 後結節 □ Posterior tubercle
② □ 椎骨動脈溝 □ Groove for vertebral artery
③ □ 横突起 □ Transverse process
④ □ 前結節 □ Anterior tubercle
⑤ □ 歯突起窩 □ Facet for dens
⑥ □ 後弓 □ Posterior arch
⑦ □ 外側塊 □ Lateral masses

> **A** 環椎は典型的な頸椎(C3-C7)で見られるような椎体と棘突起を欠く．環椎は上方では頭蓋(後頭骨)の後頭顆と関節をなす．

[1] 図 1.8C. p.7　[2] 図 2.7C. p.9

Cervical Vertebrae III

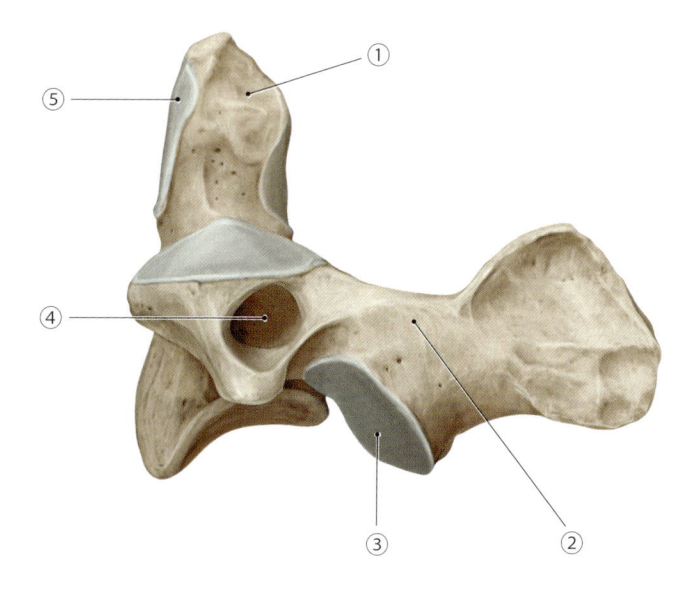

頸椎 3

軸椎(C2) Axis(C2),左外側面

① □ 歯突起　　　　　　　□ Dens
② □ 椎弓　　　　　　　　□ Vertebral arch
③ □ 下関節面　　　　　　□ Inferior articular facet
④ □ 横突孔　　　　　　　□ Transverse foramen
⑤ □ 前関節面　　　　　　□ Anterior articular facet

解説

軸椎は上方に突出する特有の突起(歯突起)を有する．歯突起は環椎の前弓と関節をなす．

1 図 1.9A. p.6　2 図 2.8A. p.8

16 Back

Cervical Vertebrae IV

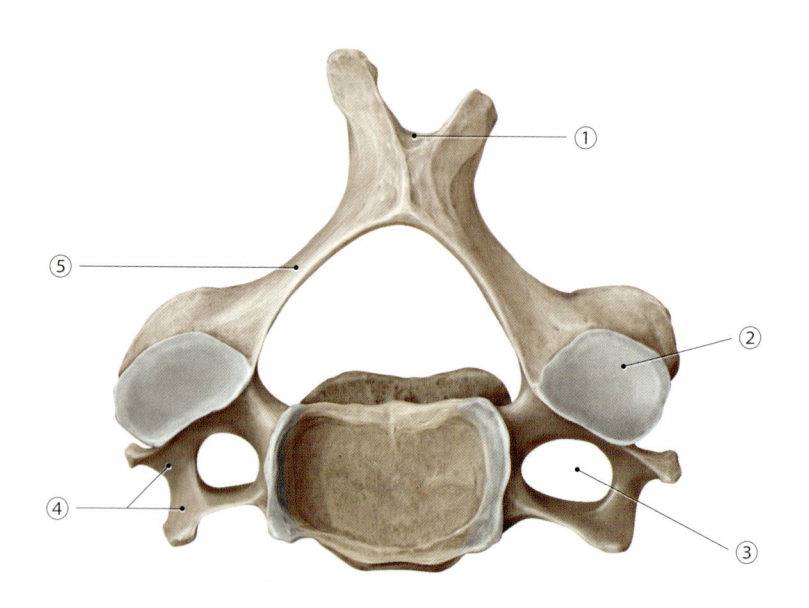

①
⑤
②
④
③

Q 頸椎の横突孔を通る構造は何か？

頸椎 4

頸椎（C4） Cervical vertebra（C4），上面

① □ 棘突起　　　　　　　　□ Spinous process
② □ 上関節面　　　　　　　□ Superior articular facet
③ □ 横突孔　　　　　　　　□ Transverse foramen
④ □ 横突起，脊髄神経溝　　□ Transverse process with sulcus for spinal nerve
⑤ □ 椎弓板　　　　　　　　□ Lamina of vertebral arch

A 椎骨動脈が C1-C6 の横突孔を通る．

① 図 1.6A. p.5　② 図 2.5A. p.7

Thoracic Vertebrae

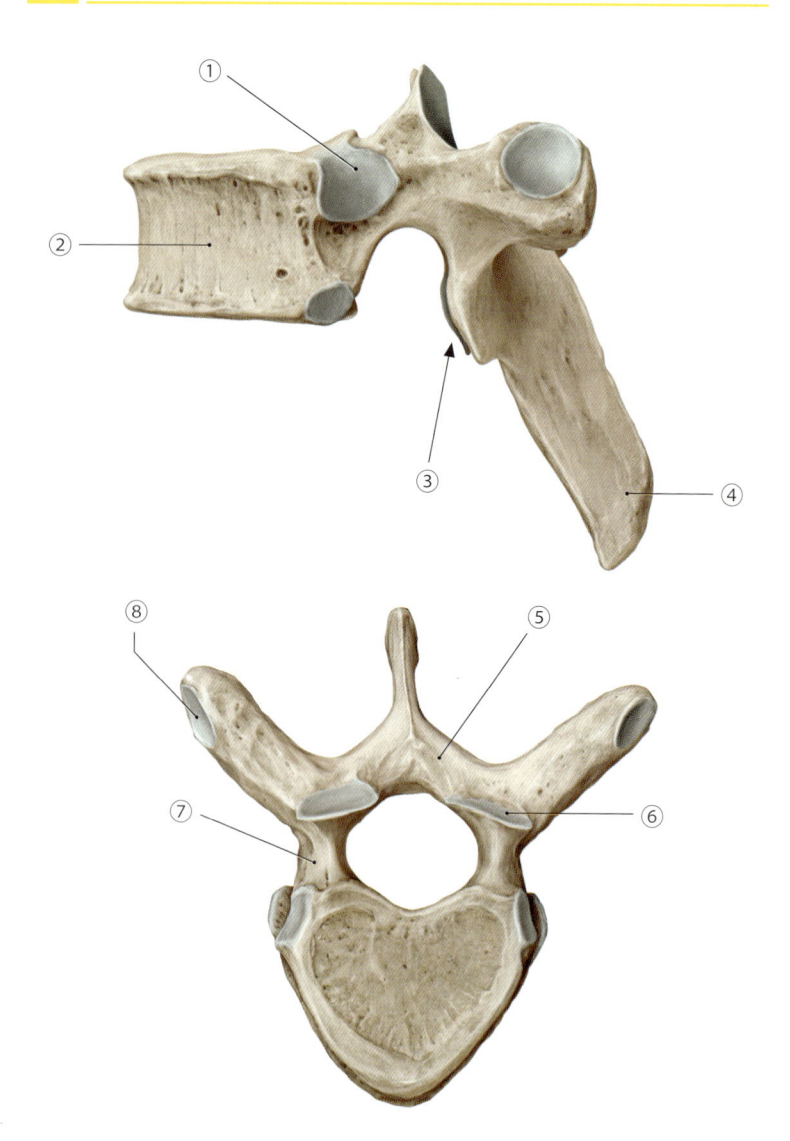

背部 **19**

胸椎

**典型的な胸椎(T6) Thoracic vertebra(T6),
上:左外側面,下:上面**

① ☐ 上肋骨窩　　　　　　　　☐ Superior costal facet

② ☐ 椎体　　　　　　　　　　☐ Vertebral body

③ ☐ 下関節面　　　　　　　　☐ Inferior articular facet

④ ☐ 棘突起　　　　　　　　　☐ Spinous process

⑤ ☐ 椎弓板　　　　　　　　　☐ Lamina of vertebral arch

⑥ ☐ 上関節面　　　　　　　　☐ Superior articular facet

⑦ ☐ 椎弓根　　　　　　　　　☐ Pedicle of vertebral arch

⑧ ☐ 横突肋骨窩　　　　　　　☐ Costal facet on transverse process

1 図 1.12A, C. p.8　　2 図 2.11A, C. p.10

Lumbar Vertebrae

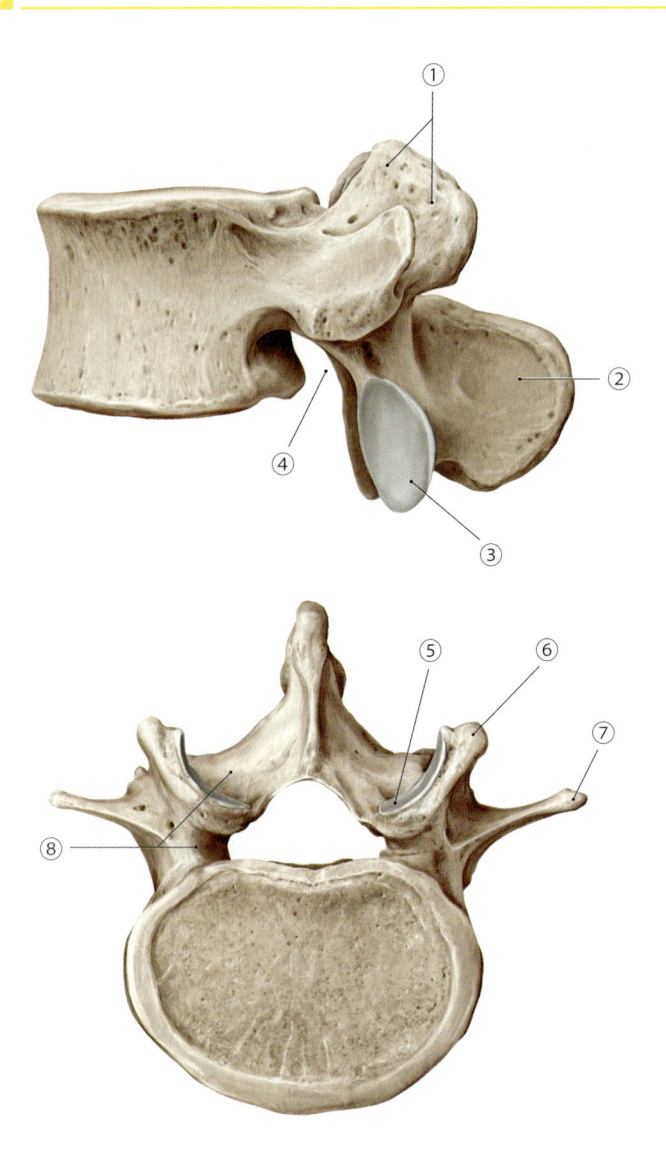

腰椎

腰椎（L4） Lumbar vertebra (L4),
上：左外側面，下：上面

① □ 上関節突起　　　　　□ Superior articular process

② □ 棘突起　　　　　　　□ Spinous process

③ □ 下関節面　　　　　　□ Inferior articular facet

④ □ 下椎切痕　　　　　　□ Inferior vertebral notch

⑤ □ 上関節面　　　　　　□ Superior articular facet

⑥ □ 乳頭突起　　　　　　□ Mammillary process

⑦ □ 横突起　　　　　　　□ Transverse process

⑧ □ 椎弓　　　　　　　　□ Vertebral arch

Sacrum & Coccyx I

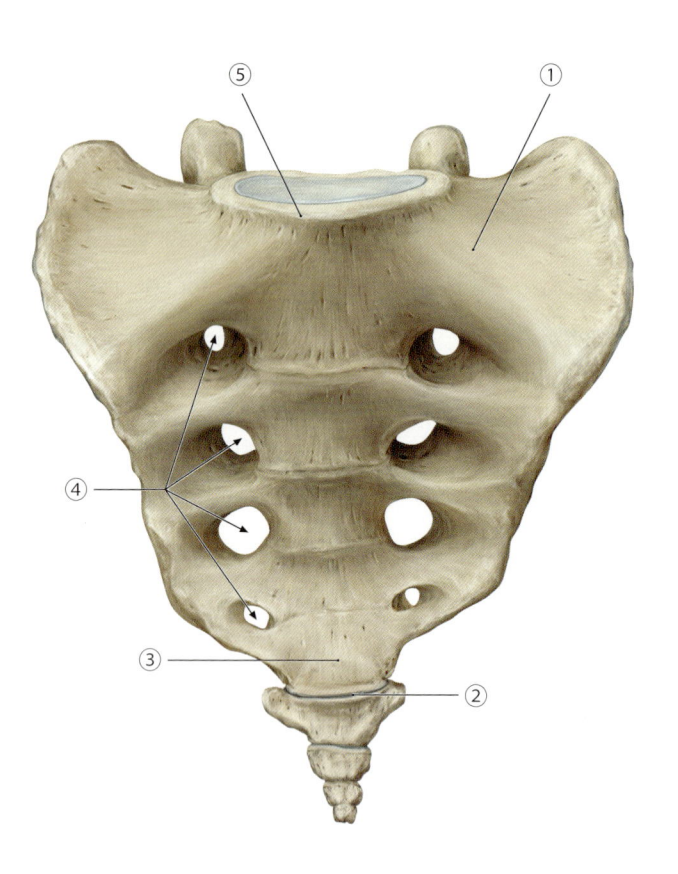

Q 前仙骨孔を通る構造は何か？

仙骨と尾骨 1

前面

① □ 仙骨翼　　　　　□ Wing of sacrum
② □ 仙尾関節　　　　□ Sacrococcygeal joint
③ □ 仙骨尖　　　　　□ Apex of sacrum
④ □ 前仙骨孔　　　　□ Anterior sacral foramina
⑤ □ 岬角　　　　　　□ Promontory

仙骨神経の前枝が前仙骨孔を通過し，仙骨神経叢を形成する．

Sacrum & Coccyx II

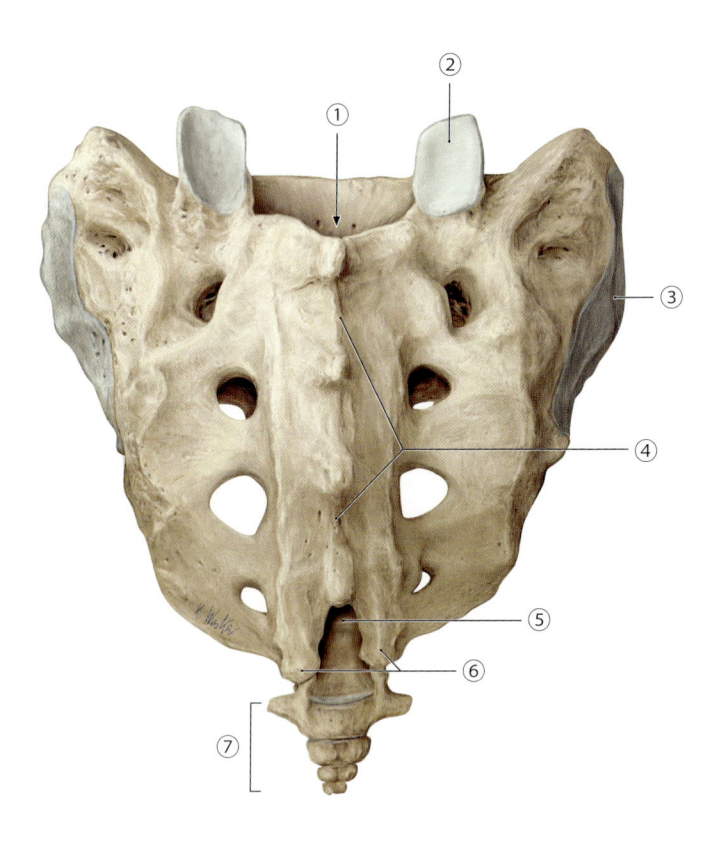

仙骨と尾骨 2

後面

① □ 仙骨管　　　　　　□ Sacral canal
② □ 上関節面　　　　　□ Superior articular facet
③ □ 耳状面　　　　　　□ Auricular surface
④ □ 正中仙骨稜　　　　□ Median sacral crest
⑤ □ 仙骨裂孔　　　　　□ Sacral hiatus
⑥ □ 仙骨角　　　　　　□ Sacral cornua
⑦ □ 尾骨　　　　　　　□ Coccyx

解説

　仙骨は生後に癒合した5つの仙椎からなる．仙骨底はL5と，仙骨尖は尾骨と，それぞれ関節をなす．仙骨裂孔は仙骨角の間にできる裂隙であり，仙骨管内に麻酔薬を投与する経路として利用される．

1 図 1.15B．p.10　2 図 2.14B．p.12

Joints of the Vertebral Column

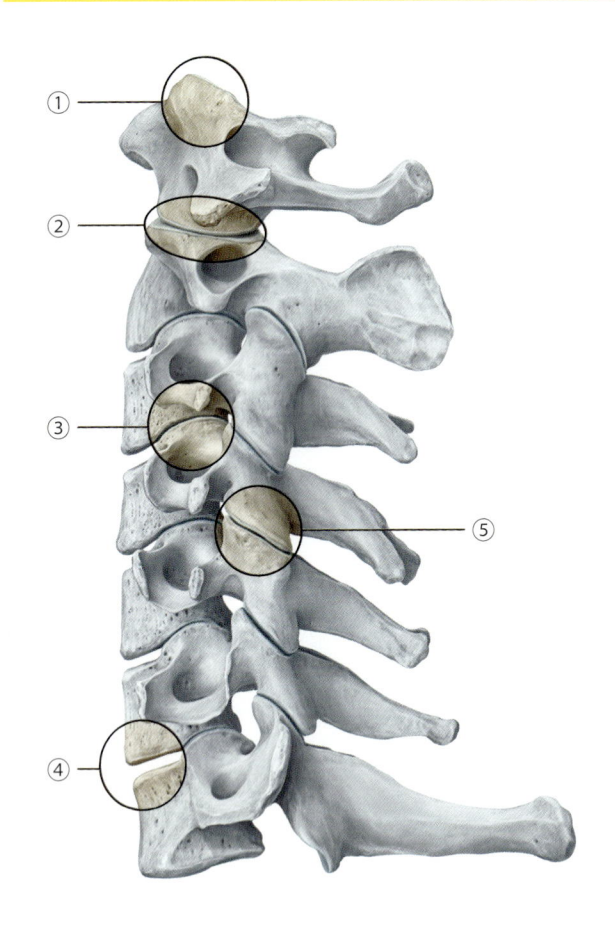

①
②
③
④
⑤

Q 頸部脊柱に特有の関節はどれか？

脊柱の関節

左外側面

① □ 環椎後頭関節　　　　　　□ Atlanto-occipital joint

② □ 環軸関節　　　　　　　　□ Atlantoaxial joint

③ □ 鉤椎関節　　　　　　　　□ Uncovertebral joint

④ □ 椎体間関節　　　　　　　□ Intervertebral joint

⑤ □ 椎間関節　　　　　　　　□ Zygapophyseal joint

A 環椎後頭関節（頭蓋とC1），環軸関節（C1とC2），鉤椎関節（C3-C6）が頸部脊柱に特有の関節である．椎間関節はすべての椎骨間で見られる．椎体間関節（椎間円板を伴う）はC1-C2間を除くすべての椎骨間で見られる．

① 図1.21. p.14　② 表2.2. p.16

Cervical Spine Ligaments I

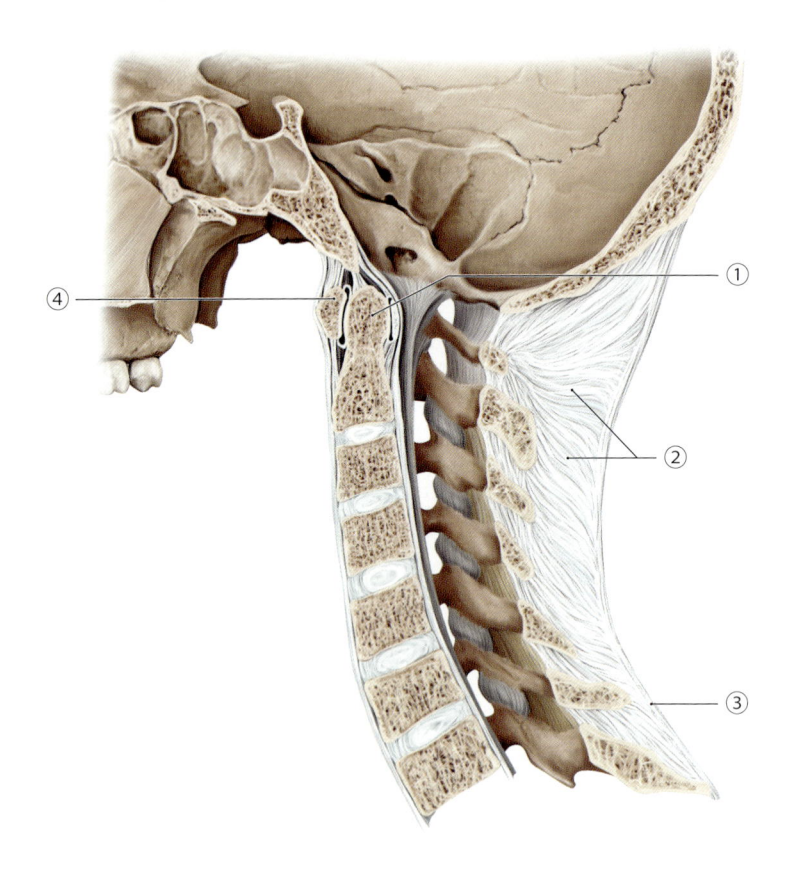

頸部脊柱の靱帯 1

正中矢状断面，左外側面

① □ 軸椎の歯突起（第 2 頸椎）　　□ Dens of axis（C2 vertebra）

② □ 項靱帯　　□ Nuchal ligament

③ □ 棘上靱帯　　□ Supraspinous ligament

④ □ 環椎の前弓（第 1 頸椎）　　□ Anterior arch of atlas（C1 vertebra）

臨床

項靱帯は棘上靱帯が矢状方向に広がったものであり，隆椎（C7）の棘突起と後頭骨の外後頭隆起の間に存在する．

1 図 1.30A. p.19　2 図 2.28A. p.21

Cervical Spine Ligaments II

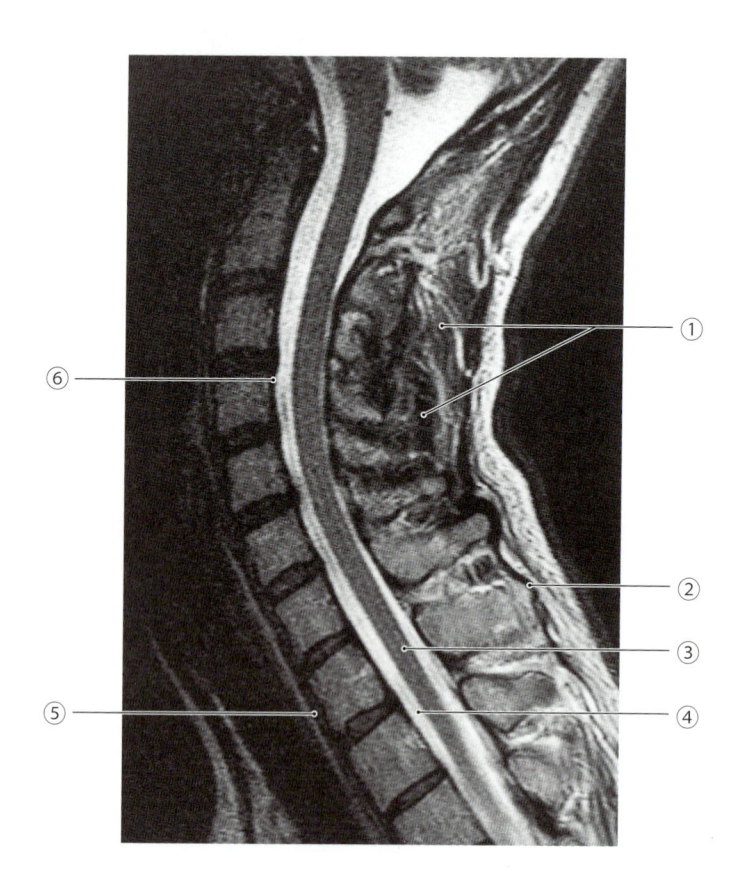

頸部脊柱の靭帯 2

T2 強調 MR 像(正中矢状断面), 左外側面

① □ 項靭帯 □ Nuchal ligament
② □ 棘上靭帯 □ Supraspinous ligament
③ □ 脊髄 □ Spinal cord
④ □ クモ膜下腔 □ Subarachnoid space
⑤ □ 前縦靭帯 □ Anterior longitudinal ligament
⑥ □ 後縦靭帯 □ Posterior longitudinal ligament

1 図 1.30B. p.19 2 図 2.28B. p.21

Thoracolumbar Spine Ligaments I

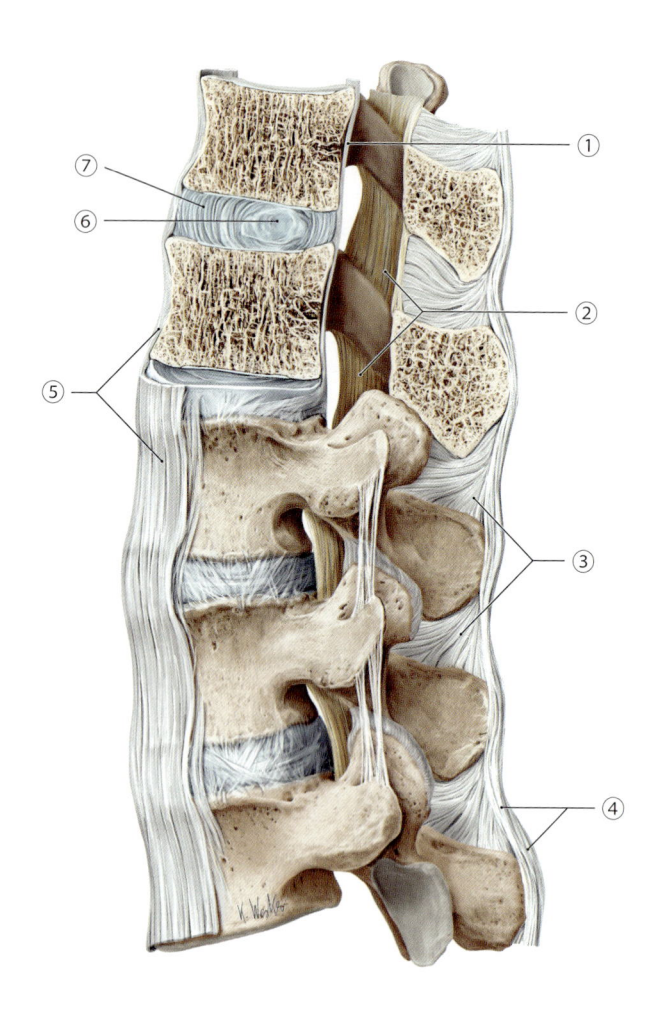

胸腰部脊柱の靱帯 1

胸腰部の連結 Thoracolumbar junction
T11-L3 の左外側面．T11-T12 は正中矢状断面が見えている

① ☐ 後縦靱帯　　　　　　　☐ Posterior longitudinal ligament

② ☐ 黄色靱帯　　　　　　　☐ Ligamenta flava

③ ☐ 棘間靱帯　　　　　　　☐ Interspinous ligaments

④ ☐ 棘上靱帯　　　　　　　☐ Supraspinous ligament

⑤ ☐ 前縦靱帯　　　　　　　☐ Anterior longitudinal ligament

⑥ ☐ 椎間円板の髄核　　　　☐ Nucleus pulposus of intervertebral disk

⑦ ☐ 椎間円板の線維輪　　　☐ Anulus fibrosus of intervertebral disk

解説

脊椎の靱帯は椎骨どうしをしっかりと連結し，大きな荷重やせん断ストレスから脊柱を保護している．

[1] 図 1.31, p.20　[2] 図 2.29, p.22

Thoracolumbar Spine Ligaments II

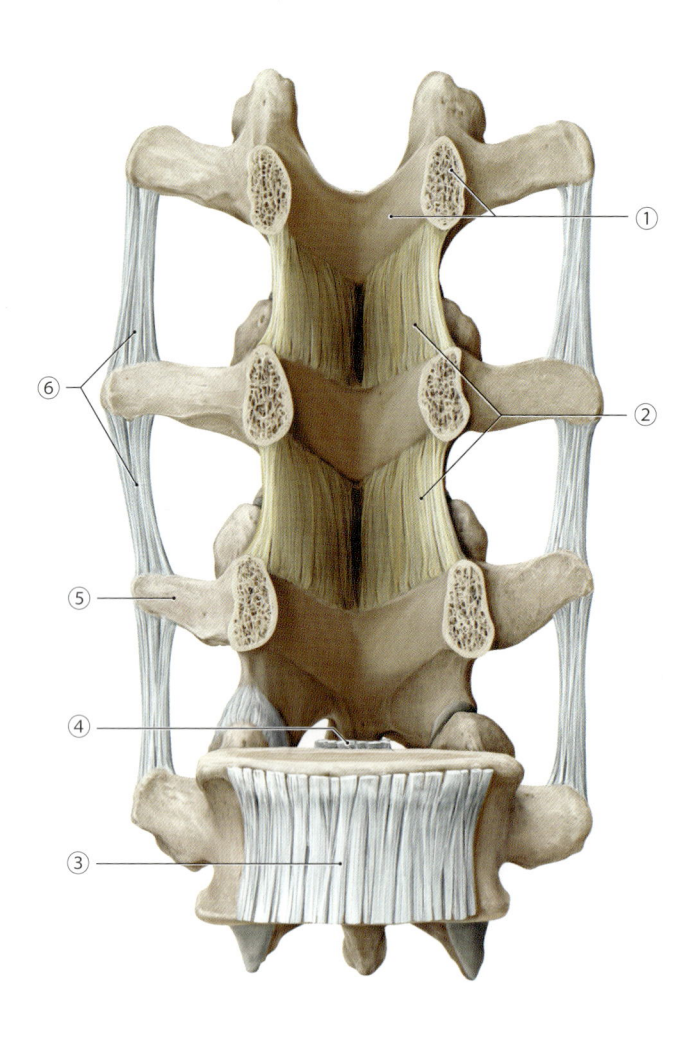

胸腰部脊柱の靭帯 2

脊柱管を開放したところ，前面

① ☐ 椎弓板 ☐ Lamina of vertebral arch
② ☐ 黄色靭帯 ☐ Ligamenta flava
③ ☐ 前縦靭帯 ☐ Anterior longitudinal ligament
④ ☐ 後縦靭帯 ☐ Posterior longitudinal ligament
⑤ ☐ 横突起 ☐ Transverse process
⑥ ☐ 横突間靭帯 ☐ Intertransverse ligaments

解説

黄色靭帯は主に弾性線維からなる．この靭帯は特有の色（黄色）をしており，これは弾性線維を豊富に含むためである．

1 図 1.33. p.21　2 図 2.31. p.23

Thoracolumbar Spine Ligaments III

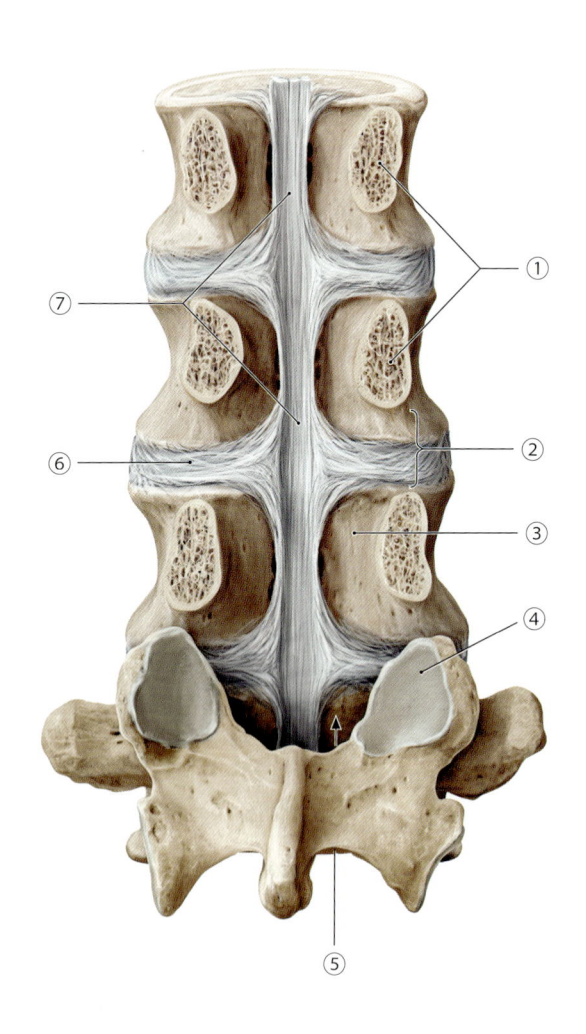

胸腰部脊柱の靱帯 3

脊柱管を開放したところ，後面

① □ 椎弓根 □ Pedicles of vertebral arches
② □ 椎間孔 □ Intervertebral foramen
③ □ 椎体 □ Vertebral body
④ □ 上関節面 □ Superior articular facet
⑤ □ 脊柱管 □ Vertebral canal
⑥ □ 椎間円板 □ Intervertebral disk
⑦ □ 後縦靱帯 □ Posterior longitudinal ligament

1 図 1.34. p.21 2 図 2.32. p.23

Superficial Muscles of the Back

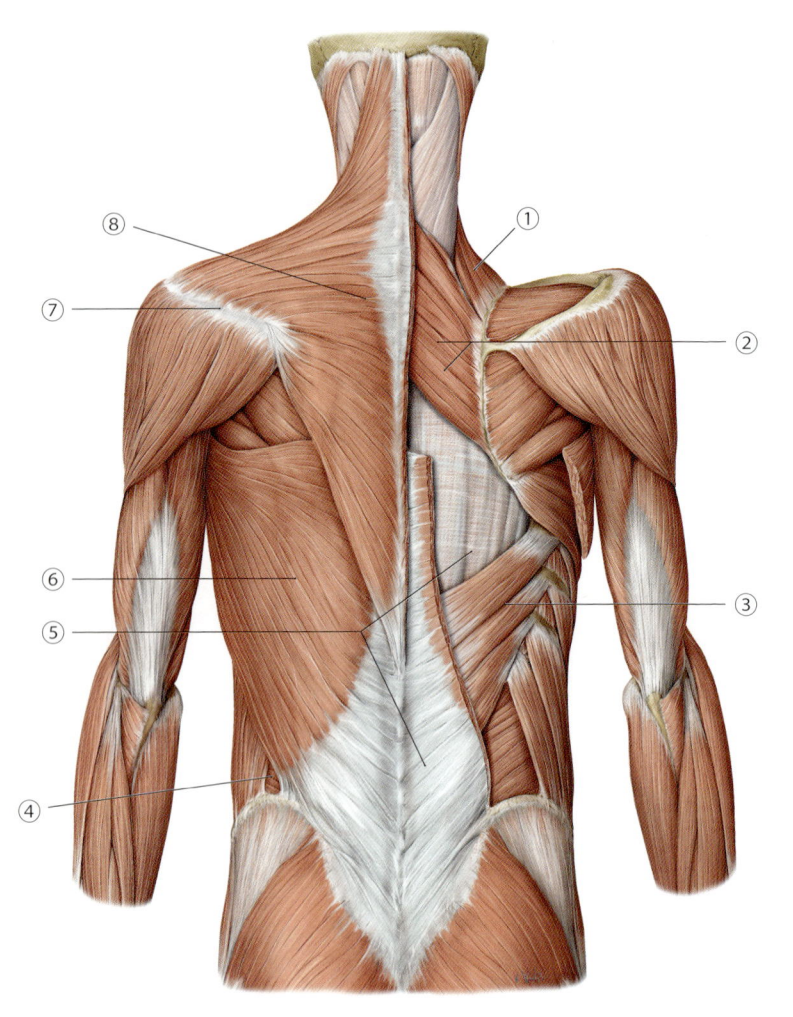

Q 背部浅層の筋(数字が付けられた筋)のうち，固有背筋に含まれるのはどれか？

背部浅層の筋

後面

① ☐ 肩甲挙筋 　　　　　　　　☐ Levator scapulae

② ☐ 大菱形筋 　　　　　　　　☐ Rhomboideus major

③ ☐ 下後鋸筋 　　　　　　　　☐ Serratus posterior inferior

④ ☐ 腰三角, 内腹斜筋 　　　　☐ Lumbar triangle, internal oblique

⑤ ☐ 胸腰筋膜, 浅葉 　　　　　☐ Thoracolumbar fascia, superficial layer

⑥ ☐ 広背筋 　　　　　　　　　☐ Latissimus dorsi

⑦ ☐ 肩甲棘 　　　　　　　　　☐ Scapular spine

⑧ ☐ 僧帽筋, 横行部 　　　　　☐ Trapezius, transverse part

A 　背部浅層の筋のうち, 上・下後鋸筋だけが固有背筋に含まれる. 僧帽筋, 広背筋, 肩甲挙筋, 大・小菱形筋は, 肩もしくは上腕の運動に関与し, 上肢の筋(外来背筋)として扱われる.

1 図 2.1, p.22　 2 図 3.1, p.24

Intrinsic Muscles of the Nuchal Region

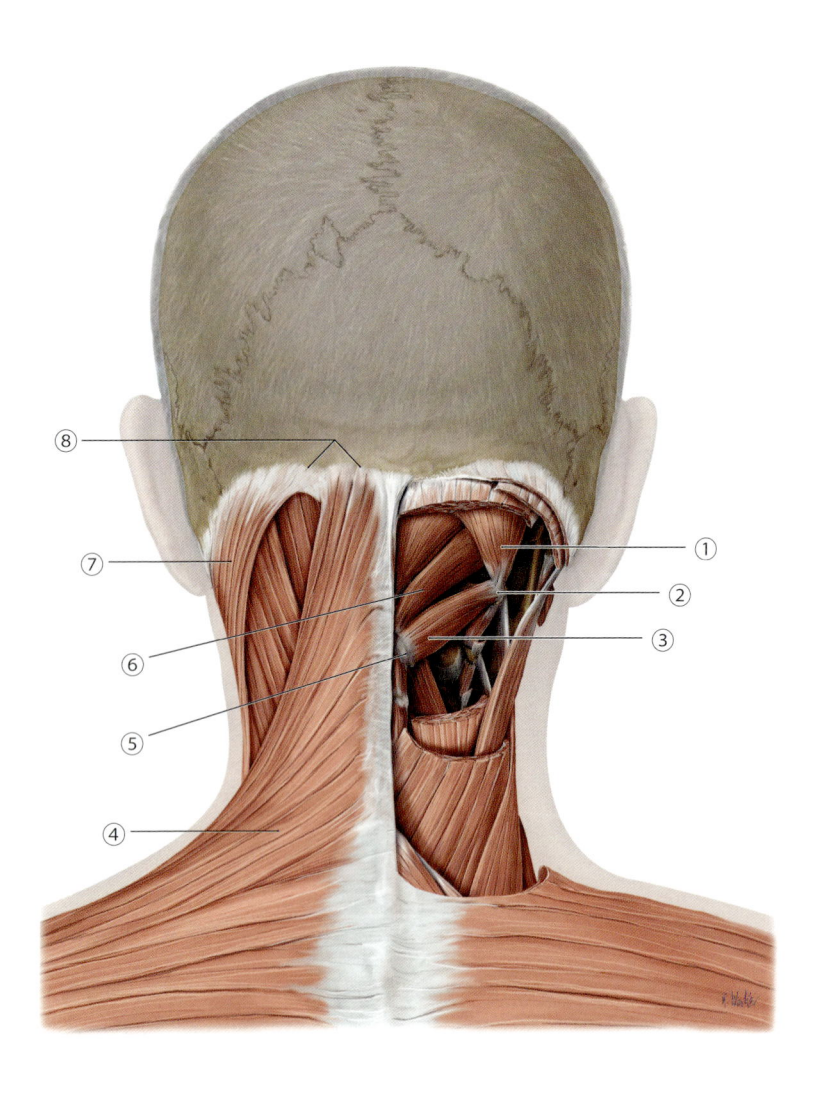

項部の固有筋

後面

① ☐ 上頭斜筋　　　　　　　　　☐ Obliquus capitis superior
② ☐ 環椎（第1頸椎），横突起　　☐ Atlas (C1 vertebra), transverse process
③ ☐ 下頭斜筋　　　　　　　　　☐ Obliquus capitis inferior
④ ☐ 僧帽筋　　　　　　　　　　☐ Trapezius
⑤ ☐ 軸椎（第2頸椎），棘突起　　☐ Axis (C2 vertebra), spinous process
⑥ ☐ 大後頭直筋　　　　　　　　☐ Rectus capitis posterior major
⑦ ☐ 胸鎖乳突筋　　　　　　　　☐ Sternocleidomastoid
⑧ ☐ 上項線　　　　　　　　　　☐ Superior nuchal line

1 図 2.3. p.24　2 図 3.3. p.26

Intrinsic Muscles of the Back I

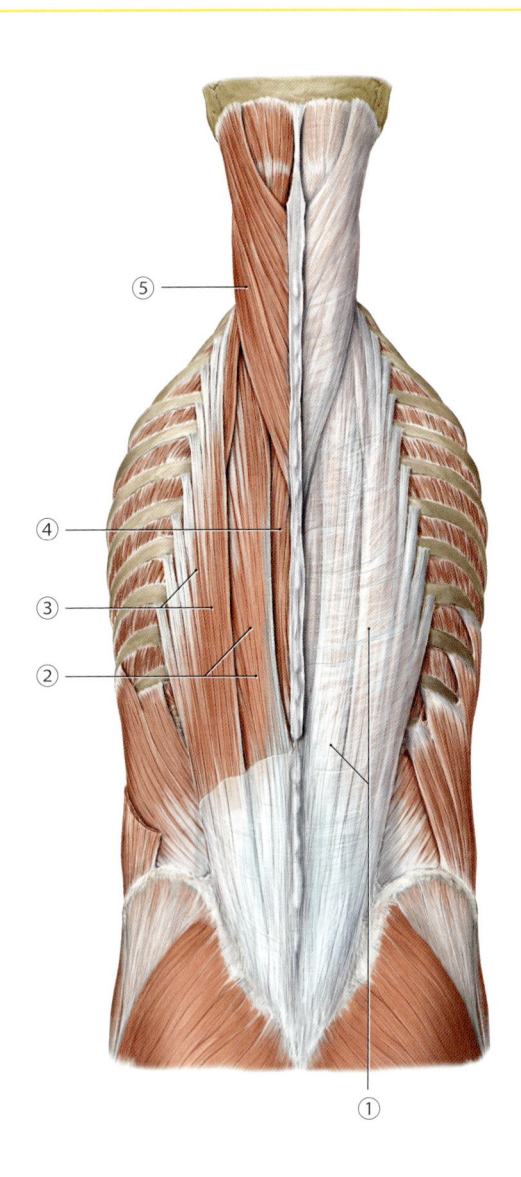

固有背筋 1

固有背筋の浅層と中間層，後面

① □ 胸腰筋膜，浅葉　　□ Thoracolumbar fascia, superficial layer
② □ 最長筋　　□ Longissimus
③ □ 腸肋筋　　□ Iliocostalis
④ □ 棘筋　　□ Spinalis
⑤ □ 頸板状筋　　□ Splenius cervicis

解説

　固有背筋は骨と筋膜によって囲まれる空間に納まっている．この空間は胸腰筋膜の深葉と浅葉，椎弓，肋骨などにより形成される．固有背筋の一部である脊柱起立筋が両側で収縮すると，脊柱が伸展する．固有背筋は脊髄神経の後枝によって支配される．

1 図 2.5B. p.26　2 図 3.5B. p.28

Intrinsic Muscles of the Back II

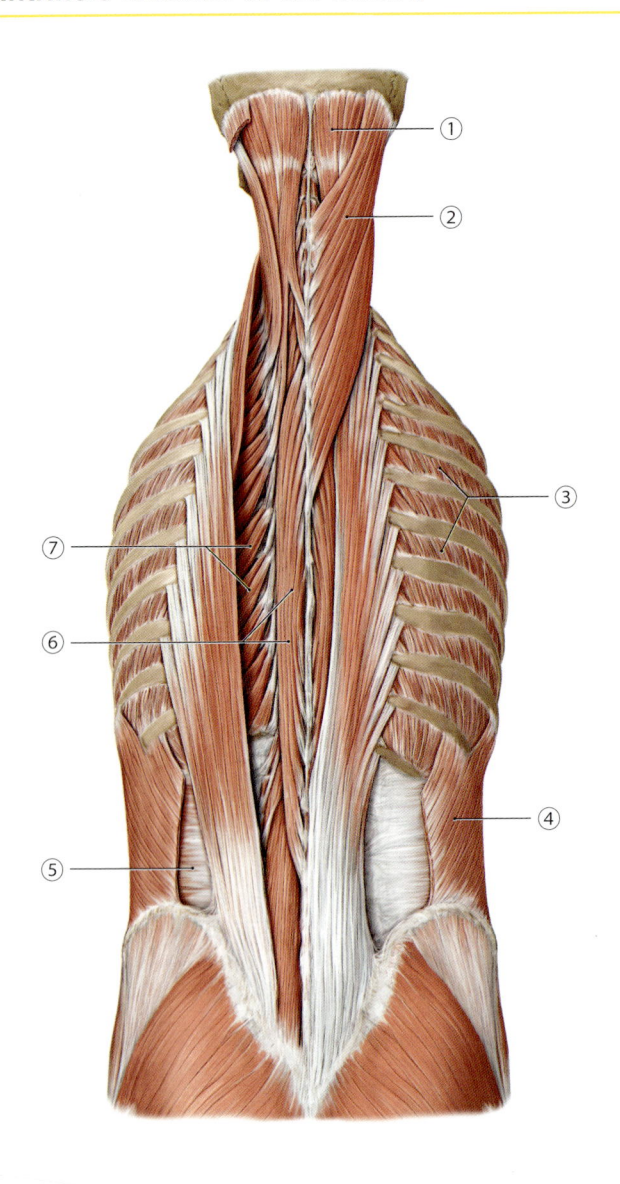

固有背筋 2

固有背筋の中間層と深層，後面

① ☐ 頭半棘筋　　　　　　　　☐ Semispinalis capitis

② ☐ 頭板状筋　　　　　　　　☐ Splenius capitis

③ ☐ 外肋間筋　　　　　　　　☐ External intercostal muscles

④ ☐ 内腹斜筋　　　　　　　　☐ Internal oblique

⑤ ☐ 腹横筋　　　　　　　　　☐ Transversus abdominis

⑥ ☐ 棘筋　　　　　　　　　　☐ Spinalis

⑦ ☐ 肋骨挙筋　　　　　　　　☐ Levatores costarum

1 図 2.5C. p.27　　2 図 3.5C. p.29

Arteries of the Back

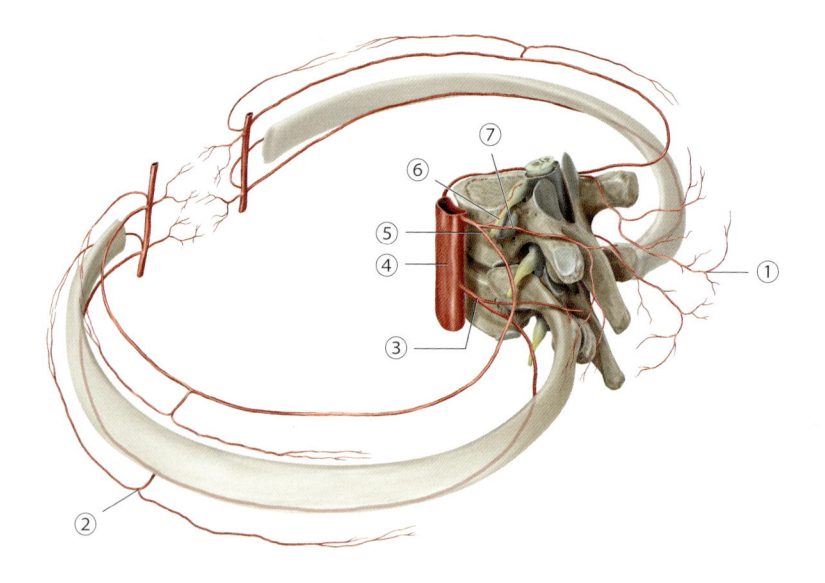

背部の動脈

左後上面

① □ 内側皮枝　　　　□ Medial cutaneous branch
② □ 外側皮枝　　　　□ Lateral cutaneous branch
③ □ 肋間動脈　　　　□ Posterior intercostal artery
④ □ 胸大動脈　　　　□ Thoracic aorta
⑤ □ 前枝　　　　　　□ Anterior ramus
⑥ □ 脊髄枝　　　　　□ Spinal branch
⑦ □ 後枝　　　　　　□ Posterior ramus

解説

背部の構造には肋間動脈の後枝が分布する．肋間動脈は胸大動脈もしくは鎖骨下動脈から起こる．肋間動脈の後枝は，皮枝，筋枝，脊髄枝に分かれる．

1 図 3.1C, p.34　2 図 4.1C, p.36

Veins of the Back

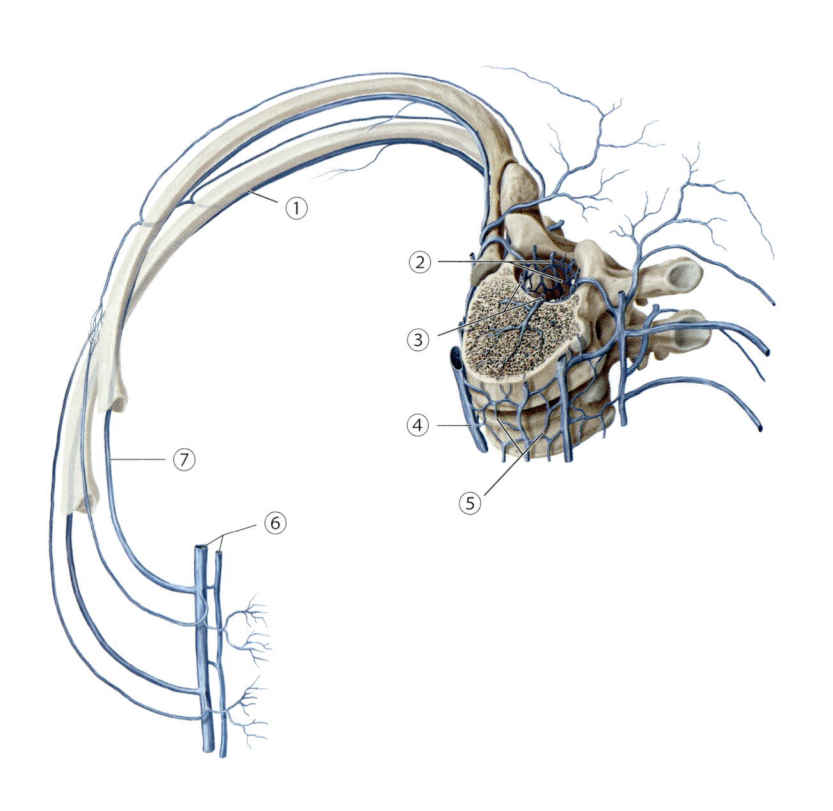

背部の静脈

肋間静脈と椎骨静脈叢 Intercostal veins and vertebral venous plexus, 右前上面

① ☐ 肋間静脈　　　　　　　☐ Posterior intercostal vein

② ☐ 後内椎骨静脈叢　　　　☐ Posterior internal vertebral venous plexus

③ ☐ 前内椎骨静脈叢　　　　☐ Anterior internal vertebral venous plexus

④ ☐ 奇静脈　　　　　　　　☐ Azygos vein

⑤ ☐ 前外椎骨静脈叢　　　　☐ Anterior external vertebral venous plexus

⑥ ☐ 内胸静脈　　　　　　　☐ Internal thoracic veins

⑦ ☐ 前肋間静脈　　　　　　☐ Anterior intercostal vein

解説

背部の静脈は，半奇静脈，副半奇静脈，上行腰静脈を介して奇静脈に流入する．脊柱の内部からの静脈は，脊柱に沿って存在する椎骨静脈叢を介して流出する．

[1] 図 3.2C. p.35　[2] 図 4.2C. p.37

Nerves of the Back

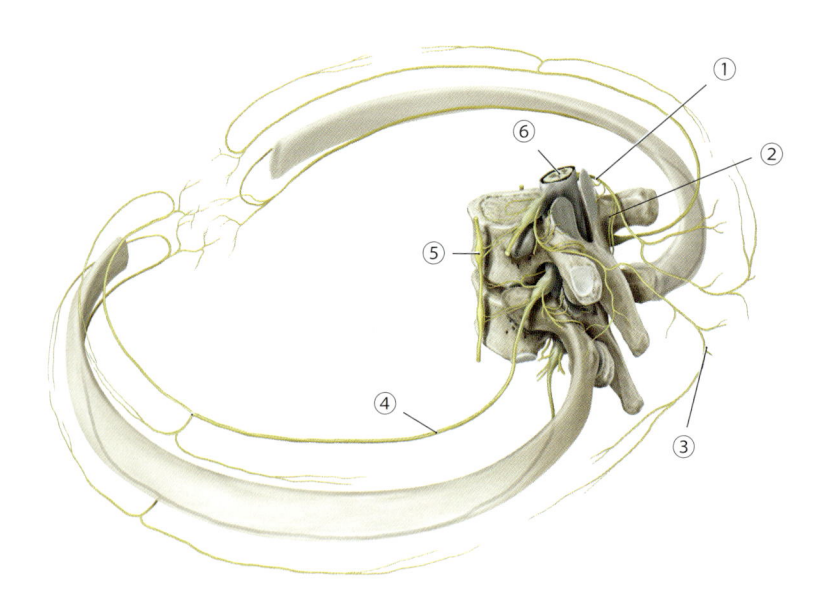

背部の神経

脊髄神経の枝 Spinal nerve branches，左後上面

① □ 後枝　　　　　　　　□ Posterior ramus

② □ 関節枝　　　　　　　□ Articular branch

③ □ 内側枝　　　　　　　□ Medial branch

④ □ 前枝　　　　　　　　□ Anterior ramus

⑤ □ 交感神経幹神経節　　□ Sympathetic ganglion

⑥ □ 脊髄　　　　　　　　□ Spinal cord

解説

　背部の構造には脊髄神経の後枝が分布する．脊髄神経の後枝は皮枝，筋枝，関節枝（椎間関節に分布する）に分かれる．後枝からの筋枝は固有背筋に分布する．外来背筋には脊髄神経の前枝が分布する．

1 図 3.3B. p.36　　2 図 4.14A. p.43

Neurovascular Topography of the Nuchal Region

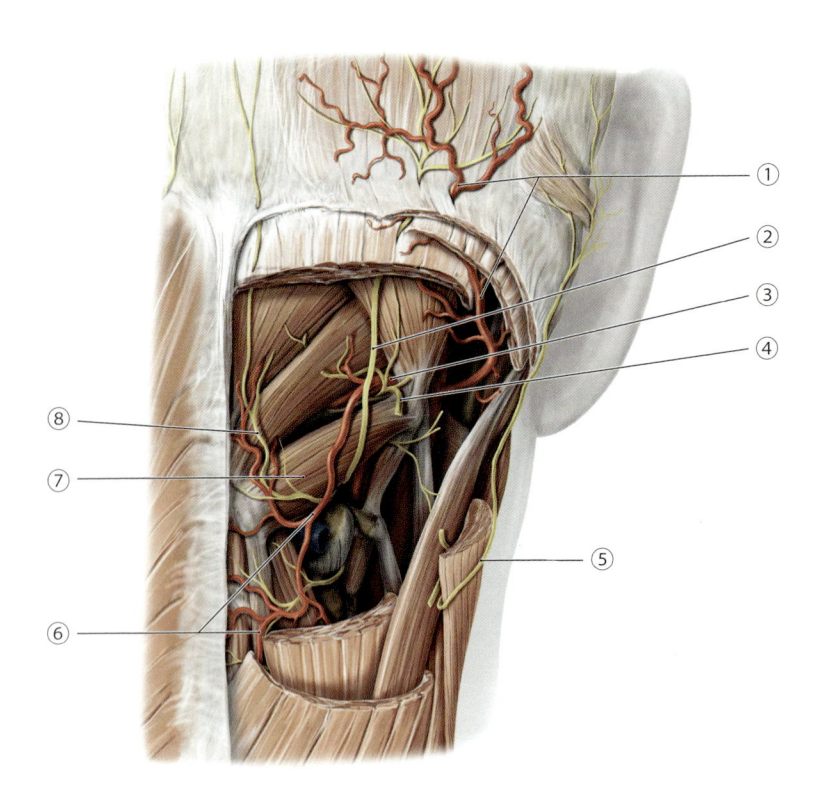

項部の神経・血管（局所解剖）

項部の神経と動脈 Neurovasculature of the nuchal region, 後面

① ☐ 後頭動脈　　　　　☐ Occipital artery

② ☐ 大後頭神経　　　　☐ Greater occipital nerve（C2）

③ ☐ 椎骨動脈　　　　　☐ Vertebral artery

④ ☐ 後頭下神経　　　　☐ Suboccipital nerve（C1）

⑤ ☐ 大耳介神経　　　　☐ Great auricular nerve

⑥ ☐ 深頸動脈　　　　　☐ Deep cervical artery

⑦ ☐ 下頭斜筋　　　　　☐ Obliquus capitis inferior

⑧ ☐ 第3後頭神経　　　☐ 3rd occipital nerve（C3）

解説

項部の構造には脊髄神経の後枝が分布する．C1-C3の後枝には特に名称が付けられている：後頭下神経（C1），大後頭神経（C2），第3後頭神経（C3）．小後頭神経と大耳介神経は脊髄神経の前枝（C1-C4）から起こり，頭頸部の前外側の皮膚に分布する．

1 図 3.6. p.38　　2 図 4.17. p.46

Neurovascular Topography of the Back

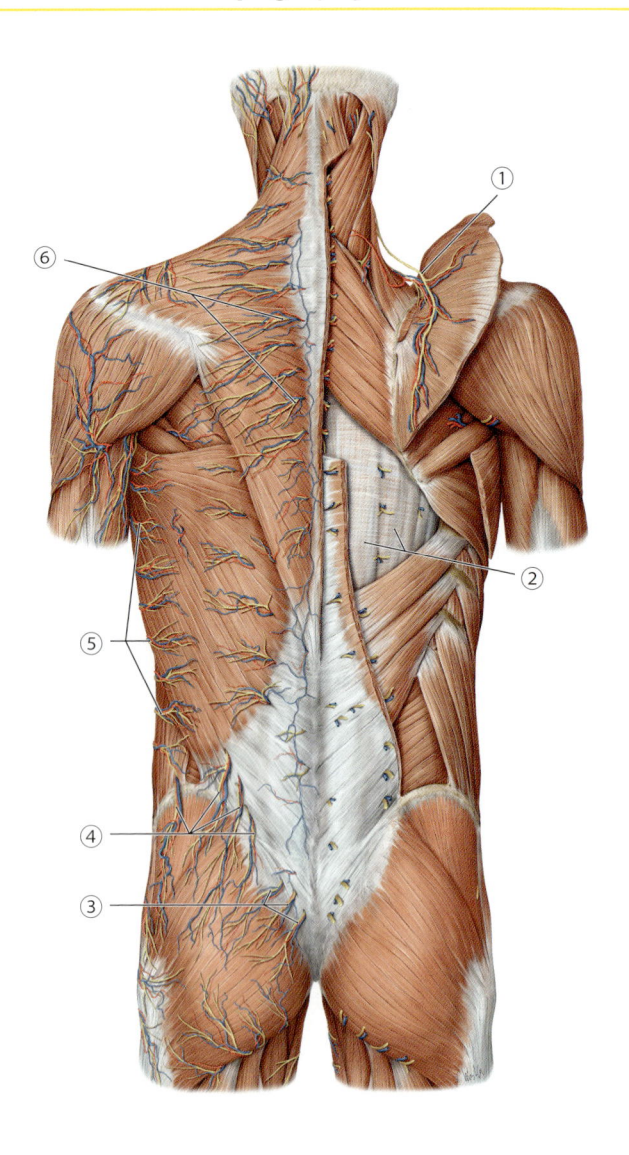

背部の神経・血管（局所解剖）

後面

① □ 副神経 □ Accessory nerve

② □ 胸腰筋膜 □ Thoracolumbar fascia

③ □ 中殿皮神経 □ Middle cluneal nerves

④ □ 上殿皮神経 □ Superior cluneal nerves

⑤ □ 肋間神経と肋間動脈・静脈，それぞれの外側皮枝 □ Intercostal nerves and posterior intercostal arteries and veins, lateral cutaneous branches

⑥ □ 脊髄神経，後枝（内側皮枝） □ Spinal nerves, posterior rami (medial cutaneous branches)

1 図 3.7, p.39　2 図 4.18, p.47

Surface Anatomy

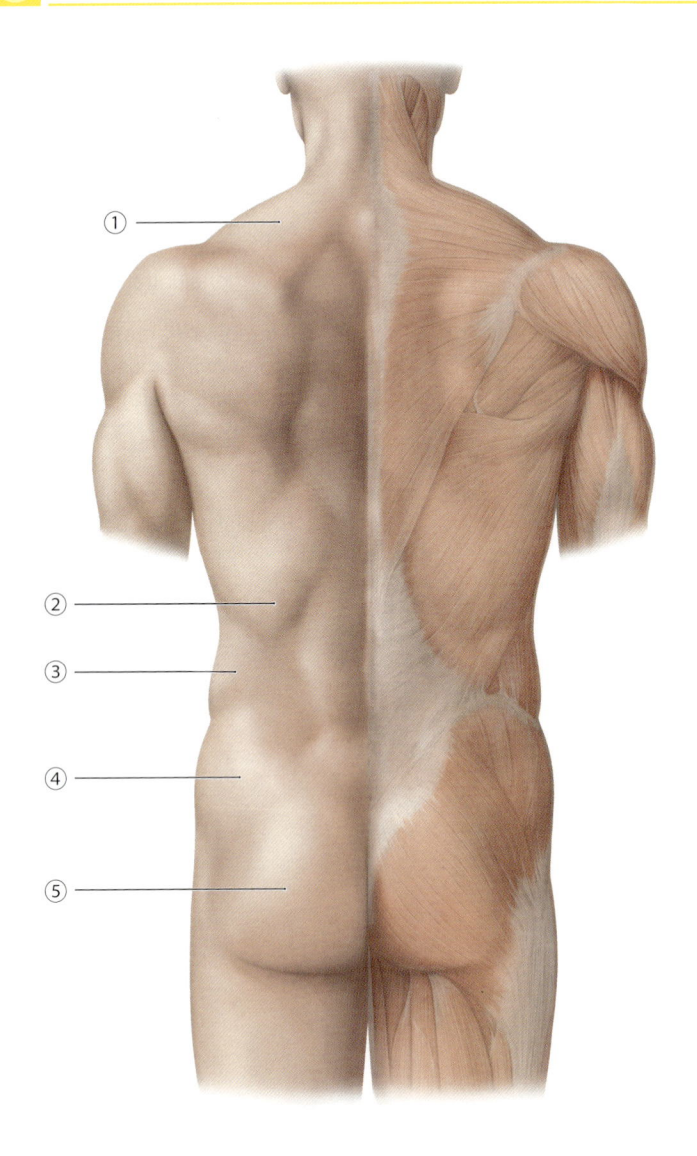

①
②
③
④
⑤

背部の体表解剖

背部の浅層の筋 Musculature of the back, 後面

① □ 僧帽筋　　　　　□ Trapezius
② □ 広背筋　　　　　□ Latissimus dorsi
③ □ 外腹斜筋　　　　□ External oblique
④ □ 中殿筋　　　　　□ Gluteus medius
⑤ □ 大殿筋　　　　　□ Gluteus maximus

1 図 4.1B. p.40　2 図 1.1B. p.2

胸部 Thorax

胸部の骨格 …………………………… 60
胸部の構造 …………………………… 62
胸骨 …………………………………… 64
胸壁の筋肉 …………………………… 66
原位置の横隔膜 1 …………………… 68
原位置の横隔膜 2 …………………… 70
横隔膜の開口部 ……………………… 72
胸壁の動脈 …………………………… 74
胸壁の静脈 …………………………… 76
胸壁の神経 …………………………… 78
肋間神経の経路 ……………………… 80
横隔膜の神経・血管 ………………… 82
女性の乳房への栄養血管 …………… 84
女性の乳房のリンパ管 ……………… 86
女性の乳房の構造 …………………… 88
縦隔の区分 …………………………… 90
胸部の CT スキャン ………………… 92
胸大動脈 ……………………………… 94
奇静脈系 ……………………………… 96
胸腔のリンパ管 ……………………… 98
胸腔の神経 …………………………… 100
縦隔 1 ………………………………… 102
縦隔 2 ………………………………… 104
縦隔 3 ………………………………… 106
縦隔 4 ………………………………… 108
心膜の折れ返り 1 …………………… 110
心膜の折れ返り 2 …………………… 112

原位置の心臓 ………………………… 114
心臓の胸肋面 ………………………… 116
心臓の底面 …………………………… 118
心臓の室 1 …………………………… 120
心臓の室 2 …………………………… 122
心臓の室 3 …………………………… 124
心臓弁 ………………………………… 126
心臓の動脈と静脈 1 ………………… 128
心臓の動脈と静脈 2 ………………… 130
心臓刺激伝導系 ……………………… 132
心臓の自律神経 ……………………… 134
心臓の X 線像 1 ……………………… 136
心臓の X 線像 2 ……………………… 138
水平断面での心臓 …………………… 140
出生前の循環 ………………………… 142
出生後の循環 ………………………… 144
壁側胸膜 ……………………………… 146
原位置の肺 …………………………… 148
右肺 …………………………………… 150
左肺 …………………………………… 152
気管 …………………………………… 154
気管支樹の区分 ……………………… 156
気管支樹の呼吸部 …………………… 158
肺動脈と肺静脈 ……………………… 160
胸膜腔のリンパ節 …………………… 162
胸部の体表解剖 ……………………… 164

60　Thorax

Thoracic Skeleton

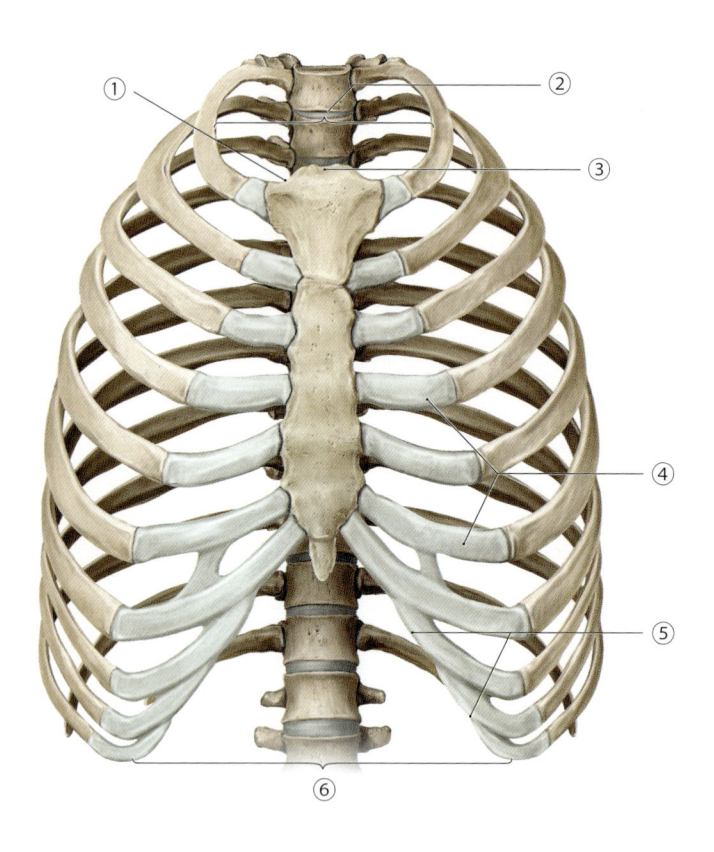

①
②
③
④
⑤
⑥

Q 肋軟骨を介して胸骨に連結する真肋は何番目から何番目の肋骨か？

胸部の骨格

前面

① □ 鎖骨切痕　　　　　　　□ Clavicular notch

② □ 胸郭上口　　　　　　　□ Superior thoracic aperture

③ □ 頸切痕　　　　　　　　□ Jugular notch

④ □ 肋軟骨　　　　　　　　□ Costal cartilage

⑤ □ 肋骨弓　　　　　　　　□ Costal margin (arch)

⑥ □ 胸郭下口　　　　　　　□ Inferior thoracic aperture

A 第1-7肋骨の肋軟骨は直接胸骨と連結する．第8-10肋骨は胸骨に間接的に連結し，仮肋と呼ばれる。第11・12肋骨は胸骨に連結せず，浮遊肋と呼ばれる．

1 図 5.1A. p.44　2 図 6.1A. p.52

62 Thorax

Structure of a Thoracic Segment

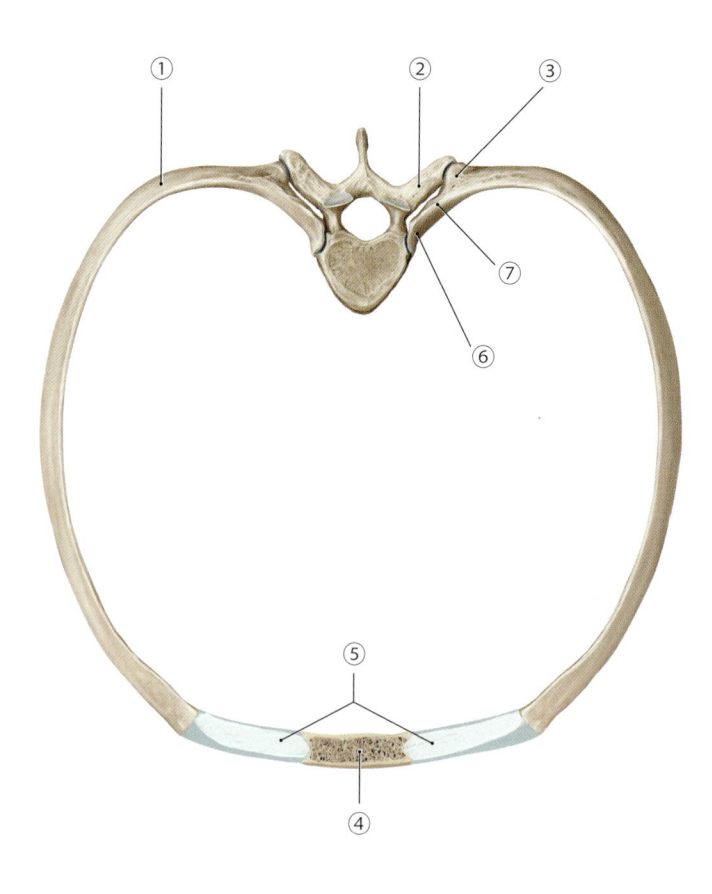

胸部の構造

第6肋骨 6th rib pair, 上面

① ☐ 肋骨角　　　　　　　　　☐ Costal angle

② ☐ 横突起　　　　　　　　　☐ Transverse process

③ ☐ 肋骨結節　　　　　　　　☐ Costal tubercle

④ ☐ 胸骨　　　　　　　　　　☐ Sternum

⑤ ☐ 肋軟骨　　　　　　　　　☐ Costal cartilage

⑥ ☐ 肋骨頭　　　　　　　　　☐ Head of rib

⑦ ☐ 肋骨頸　　　　　　　　　☐ Neck of rib

1 図 5.2. p.45　2 図 6.2. p.53

Sternum

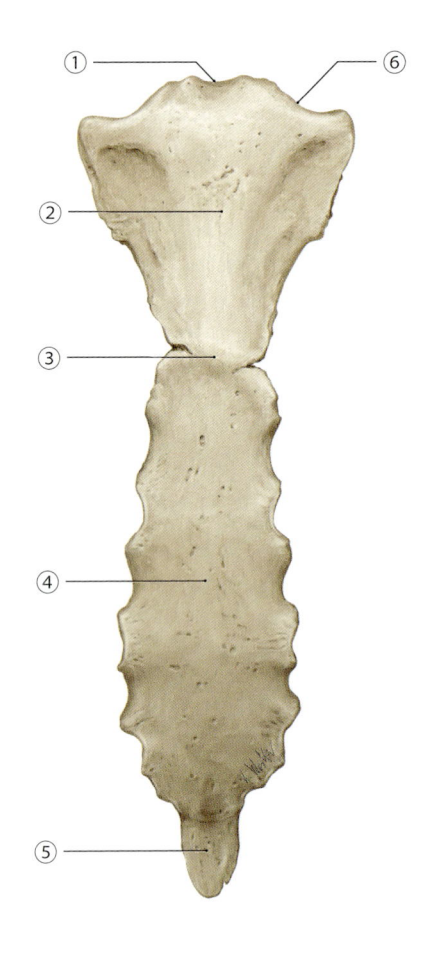

①
②
③
④
⑤
⑥

胸骨角で胸骨に連結するのは通常どの肋骨か？

胸骨

前面

① ☐ 頸切痕 ☐ Jugular notch
② ☐ 胸骨柄 ☐ Manubrium sterni
③ ☐ 胸骨角 ☐ Sternal angle
④ ☐ 胸骨体 ☐ Body
⑤ ☐ 剣状突起 ☐ Xiphoid process
⑥ ☐ 鎖骨切痕 ☐ Clavicular notch

A 胸骨角は第2肋骨の高さにある．

1 図5.4A. p.46   2 図6.4A. p.54

Thoracic Wall Muscles

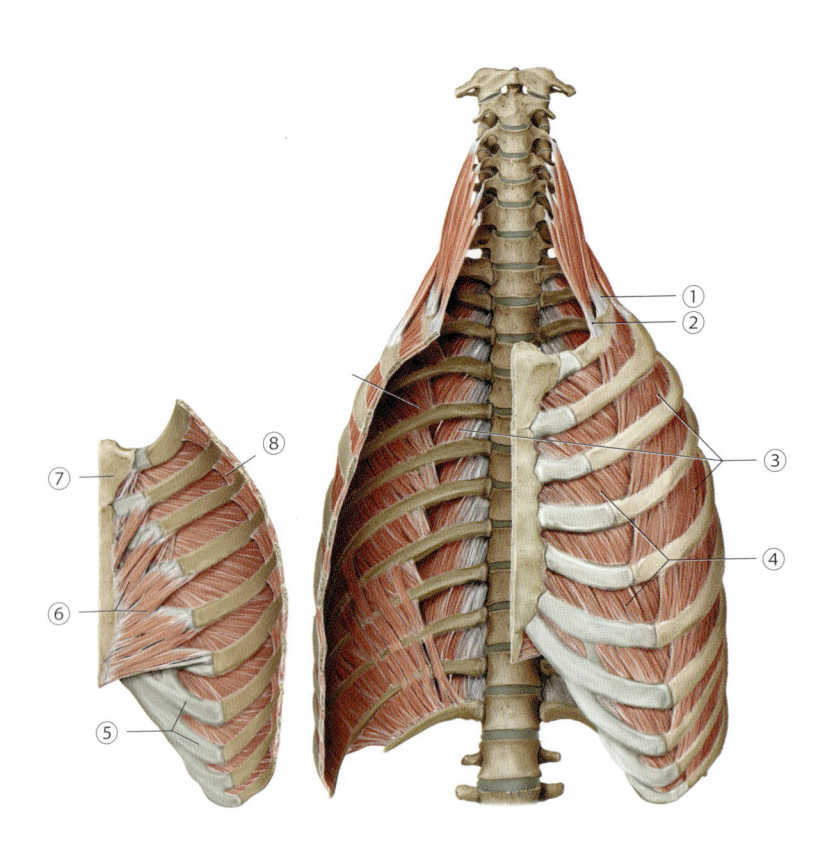

胸壁の筋肉

前面，胸郭を開き，前壁の後面を見せる

① □ 中斜角筋　　　　　　　　□ Middle scalene

② □ 前斜角筋　　　　　　　　□ Anterior scalene

③ □ 外肋間筋　　　　　　　　□ External intercostals

④ □ 内肋間筋　　　　　　　　□ Internal intercostals

⑤ □ 肋軟骨　　　　　　　　　□ Costal cartilage

⑥ □ 胸横筋　　　　　　　　　□ Transversus thoracis

⑦ □ 胸骨柄　　　　　　　　　□ Manubrium sterni

⑧ □ 最内肋間筋　　　　　　　□ Innermost intercostals

解説

　胸壁の筋肉は胸式呼吸の主要筋である．努力呼吸時には他の筋肉も働く．肋間筋は肋骨の挙上・下制および胸壁の安定に働く．

1 図 5.11, p.51　　2 図 6.11, p.59

Diaphragm in Situ I

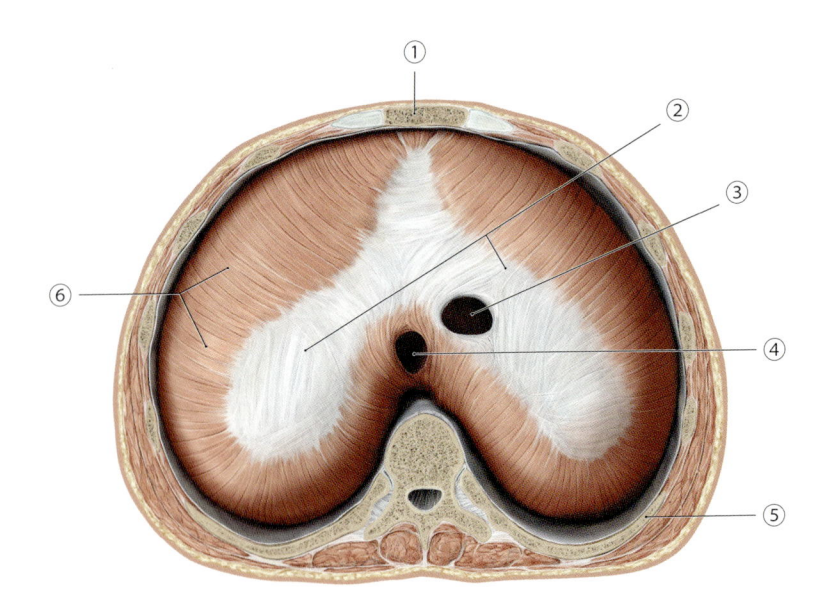

原位置の横隔膜 1

上面

① □ 胸骨　　　　　　　　　□ Sternum

② □ 腱中心　　　　　　　　□ Central tendon

③ □ 大静脈孔　　　　　　　□ Caval aperture

④ □ 食道裂孔　　　　　　　□ Esophageal aperture

⑤ □ 肋骨　　　　　　　　　□ Rib

⑥ □ 横隔膜（肋骨部）　　　□ Diaphragm (costal part)

解説

　横隔膜は，呼吸の主要筋であり，胸腔と腹腔を隔てている．肋間縁と腰椎から起始するが，中心腱は T8 の高さまで盛り上がったドームになっている．

1 図 5.13A. p.53　　2 図 6.13A. p.61

Diaphragm in Situ II

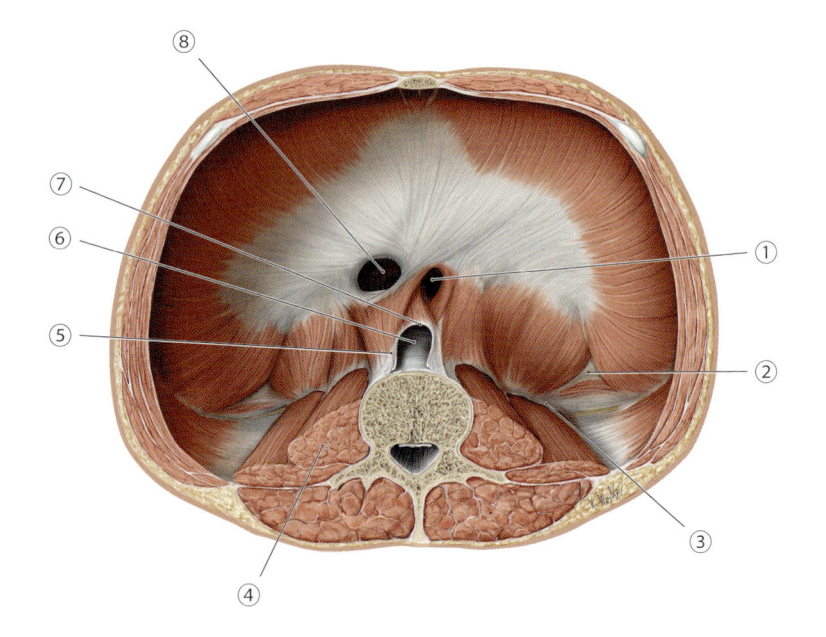

原位置の横隔膜 2

下面

① □ 食道裂孔　　　　　　　　□ Esophageal aperture

② □ 腰肋三角（ボクダレク三角）　□ Lumbocostal triangle (Bochdalek's triangle)

③ □ 外側弓状靱帯　　　　　　□ Lateral arcuate ligament

④ □ 大腰筋　　　　　　　　　□ Psoas major

⑤ □ 右脚　　　　　　　　　　□ Right crus

⑥ □ 大動脈裂孔　　　　　　　□ Aortic aperture

⑦ □ 正中弓状靱帯　　　　　　□ Median arcuate ligament

⑧ □ 大静脈孔　　　　　　　　□ Caval aperture

臨床

胸腔出口は横隔膜によって閉ざされているが，通常横隔膜の開口部が胸部と腹部の間にある構造の通路となっている．この開口部は臨床的に重要であり，穴が拡張して腹部の構造が胸腔に脱出することもある．脱出は食道裂孔においてよく起こる（裂孔ヘルニア）．

1 図 5.13B. p.53　　2 図 6.13B. p.61

Diaphragmatic Apertures

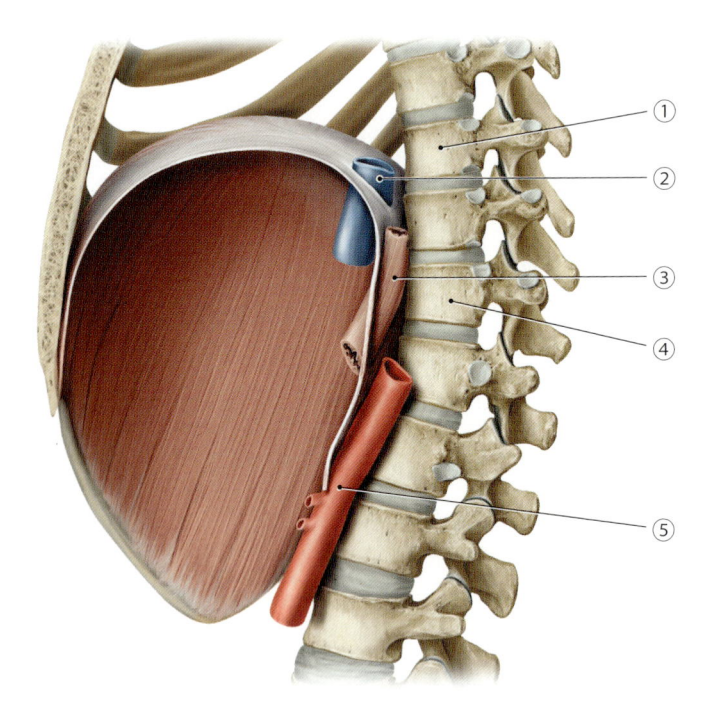

横隔膜の開口部

左外側面

① ☐ 第8胸椎　　　　　☐ T8 vertebra

② ☐ 下大静脈　　　　　☐ Inferior vena cava

③ ☐ 食道　　　　　　　☐ Esophagus

④ ☐ 第10胸椎　　　　☐ T10 vertebra

⑤ ☐ 大動脈　　　　　　☐ Aorta

74 Thorax

Arteries of the Thoracic Wall

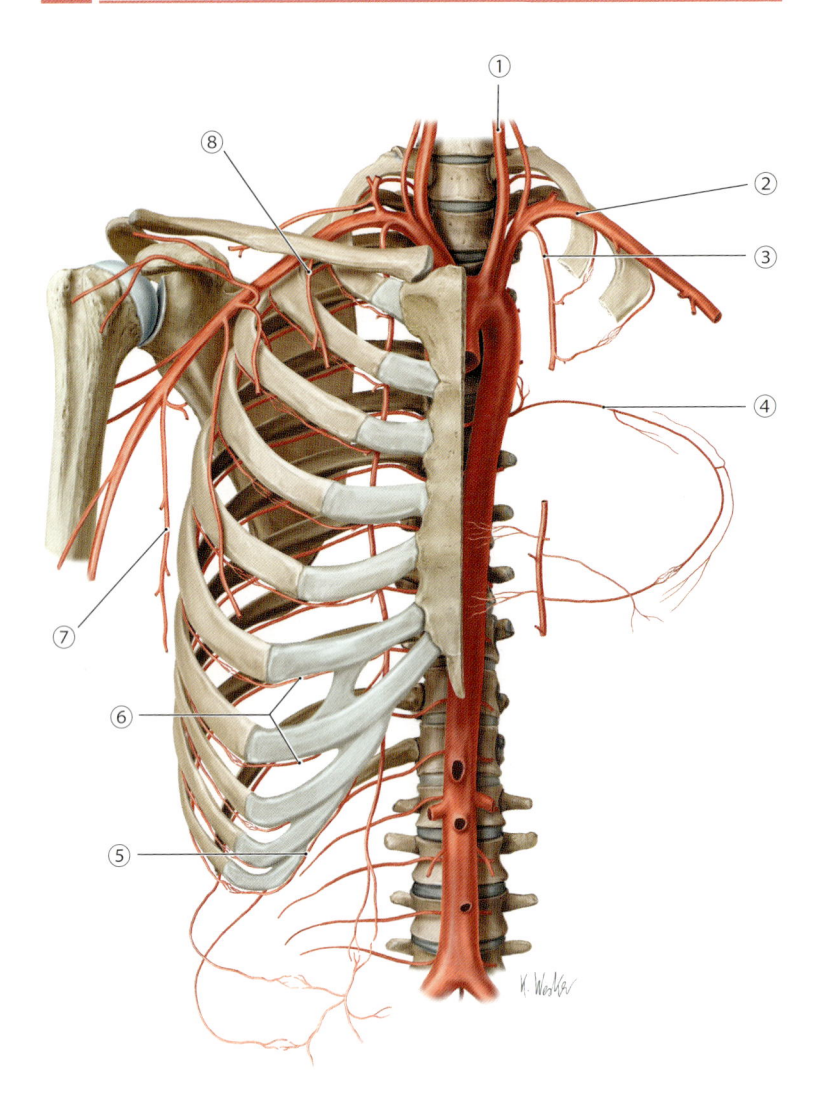

胸壁の動脈

前面

① □ 総頸動脈　　　　　　　□ Common carotid artery

② □ 鎖骨下動脈　　　　　　□ Subclavian artery

③ □ 内胸動脈　　　　　　　□ Internal thoracic artery

④ □ 肋間動脈　　　　　　　□ Posterior intercostal artery

⑤ □ 筋横隔動脈　　　　　　□ Musculophrenic artery

⑥ □ 内胸動脈の前肋間枝　　□ Anterior intercostal arteries

⑦ □ 外側胸動脈　　　　　　□ Lateral thoracic artery

⑧ □ 最上胸動脈　　　　　　□ Superior thoracic artery

解説

肋間動脈は内胸動脈の前肋間枝と吻合し，胸壁の構造を栄養する．肋間動脈は胸大動脈から分岐するが，第1および第2肋間動脈は肋頸動脈の枝の最上肋間動脈から起こる．

1 図5.17, p.56　2 図6.17, p.64

Veins of the Thoracic Wall

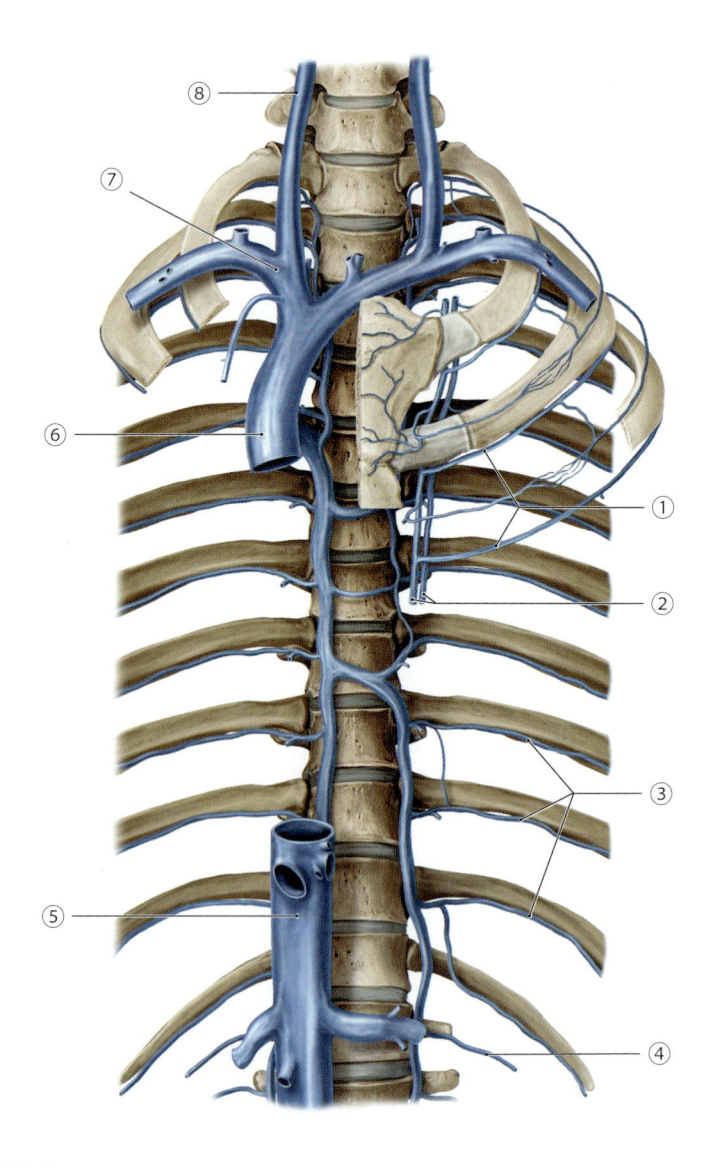

胸壁の静脈

前面

① □ 前肋間静脈　　　　　　　□ Anterior intercostal veins

② □ 内胸静脈　　　　　　　　□ Internal thoracic veins

③ □ 肋間静脈　　　　　　　　□ Posterior intercostal veins

④ □ 第1腰静脈　　　　　　　□ 1st lumbar vein

⑤ □ 下大静脈　　　　　　　　□ Inferior vena cava

⑥ □ 上大静脈　　　　　　　　□ Superior vena cava

⑦ □ 右腕頭静脈　　　　　　　□ Right brachiocephalic vein

⑧ □ 内頸静脈　　　　　　　　□ Internal jugular vein

解説

　肋間静脈は主に奇静脈系へと連絡するが，内胸静脈にも注ぐ．血液は最終的には上大静脈を介して心臓に戻る．肋間静脈は肋間動脈と同様の位置に分布するが，脊柱の静脈は脊椎を全長にわたって横切る前・後外椎骨静脈叢を作る．

1 図 5.19A. p.57　　2 図 6.19A. p.65

Nerves of the Thoracic Wall

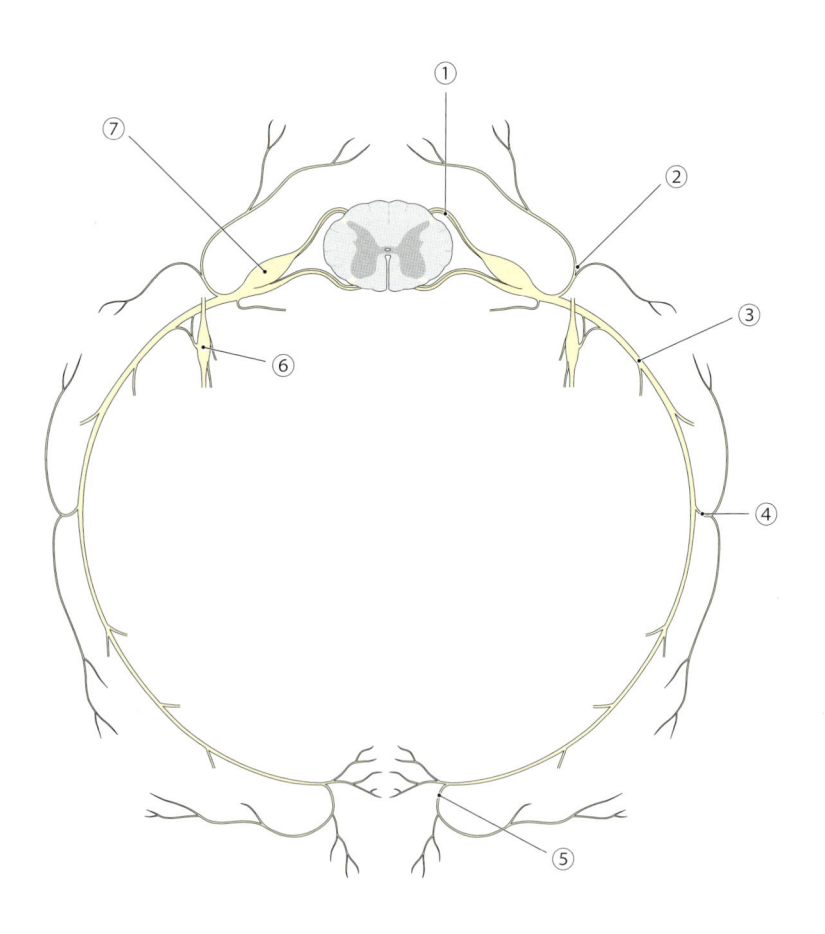

胸壁の神経

脊髄神経の枝 Spinal nerve branches, 上面

① □ 後根　　　　　　　　　□ Dorsal root

② □ 後枝　　　　　　　　　□ Posterior (dorsal) ramus

③ □ 前枝（肋間神経）　　　　□ Anterior (ventral) ramus (intercostal nerve)

④ □ 外側皮枝　　　　　　　□ Lateral cutaneous branch

⑤ □ 前皮枝　　　　　　　　□ Anterior cutaneous branch

⑥ □ 交感神経幹神経節　　　□ Sympathetic ganglion

⑦ □ 脊髄神経節　　　　　　□ Spinal ganglion

解説

　後根（感覚性）と前根（運動性）からなる1cm足らずの脊髄神経が椎間孔を通過し，脊柱管の外に出る．脊髄神経の後枝は背部の皮膚と固有背筋を支配し，前枝は肋間神経をなす．

①図 5.23, p.59　②図 6.23, p.67

Course of the Intercostal Nerves

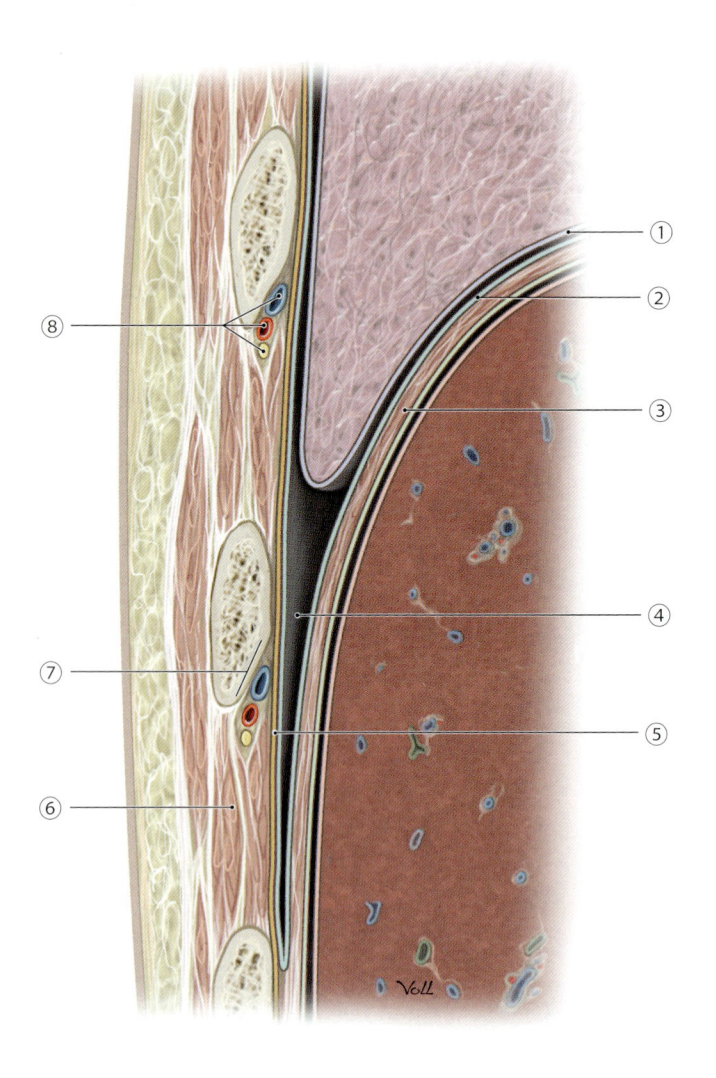

肋間神経の経路

冠状断面，前面

① ☐ 臓側胸膜（肺胸膜）　　　　　☐ Visceral pleura

② ☐ 壁側胸膜，横隔部　　　　　　☐ Parietal pleura,
　　　（横隔胸膜）　　　　　　　　　　diaphragmatic part

③ ☐ 横隔膜　　　　　　　　　　　☐ Diaphragm

④ ☐ 肋骨横隔洞　　　　　　　　　☐ Costodiaphragmatic recess

⑤ ☐ 胸内筋膜　　　　　　　　　　☐ Endothoracic fascia

⑥ ☐ 外肋間筋　　　　　　　　　　☐ External intercostal

⑦ ☐ 肋骨溝　　　　　　　　　　　☐ Costal groove

⑧ ☐ 肋間静脈・動脈・神経　　　　☐ Intercostal vein, artery, and nerve

臨床

気管支癌に起因する胸水のような，胸膜腔に貯留する過剰な滲出液には胸腔チューブが必要である．一般に，座位で最も有効な穿刺部位は後腋窩線沿いの第7-8肋間だとされる．チューブは肋骨上縁で挿入される．これは肋間動脈・静脈・神経を傷つけないためである．

1 図 5.24. p.59　2 図 6.24. p.67

Neurovasculature of the Diaphragm

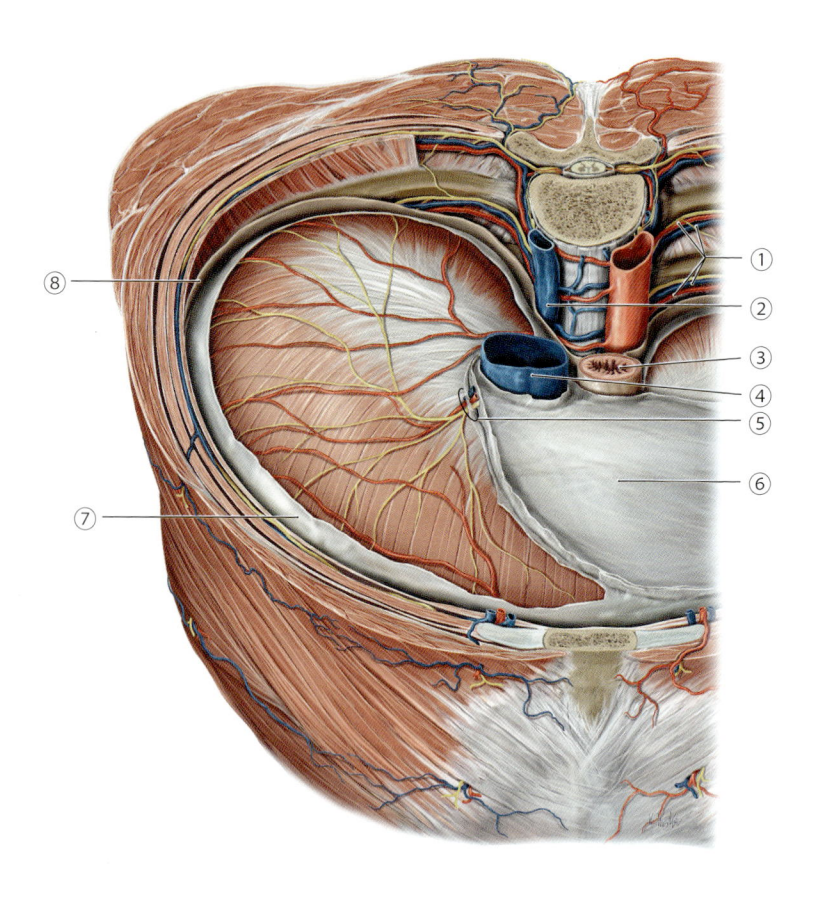

横隔膜の支配神経はどの高さの脊髄から起こるか？

横隔膜の神経・血管

横断面, 前上面

① □ 肋間動脈・静脈　　　　　　□ Posterior intercostal arteries and veins

② □ 奇静脈　　　　　　　　　　□ Azygos vein

③ □ 食道　　　　　　　　　　　□ Esophagus

④ □ 下大静脈　　　　　　　　　□ Inferior vena cava

⑤ □ 横隔神経, 心膜横隔動脈・静脈　□ Phrenic nerve, pericardiacophrenic artery and vein

⑥ □ 心膜　　　　　　　　　　　□ Pericardium

⑦ □ 壁側胸膜, 肋骨部（肋骨胸膜）　□ Parietal pleura, costal part

⑧ □ 胸内筋膜　　　　　　　　　□ Endothoracic fascia

A 横隔神経は C3-C5 の前枝から起こる.

1 図 5.27, p.61　　2 図 6.27, p.69

Blood Supply to the Female Breast

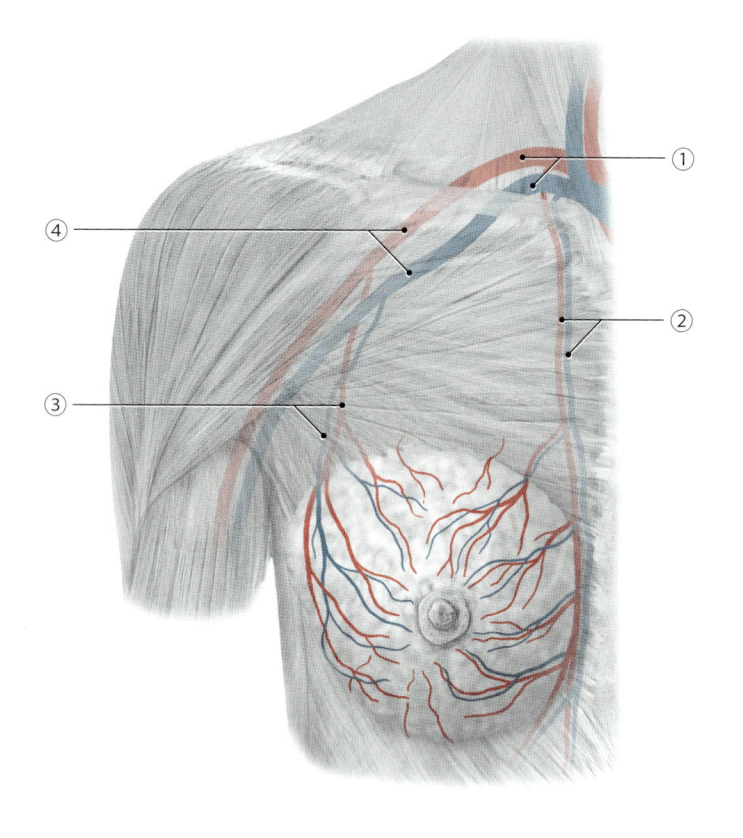

女性の乳房への栄養血管

前面

① □ 鎖骨下動脈・静脈　　　　　□ Subclavian artery and vein

② □ 内胸動脈・静脈　　　　　　□ Internal thoracic artery and vein

③ □ 外側胸動脈・静脈　　　　　□ Lateral thoracic artery and vein

④ □ 腋窩動脈・静脈　　　　　　□ Axillary artery and vein

1 図 5.30. p.62　2 図 6.30. p.70

Lymphatics of the Female Breast

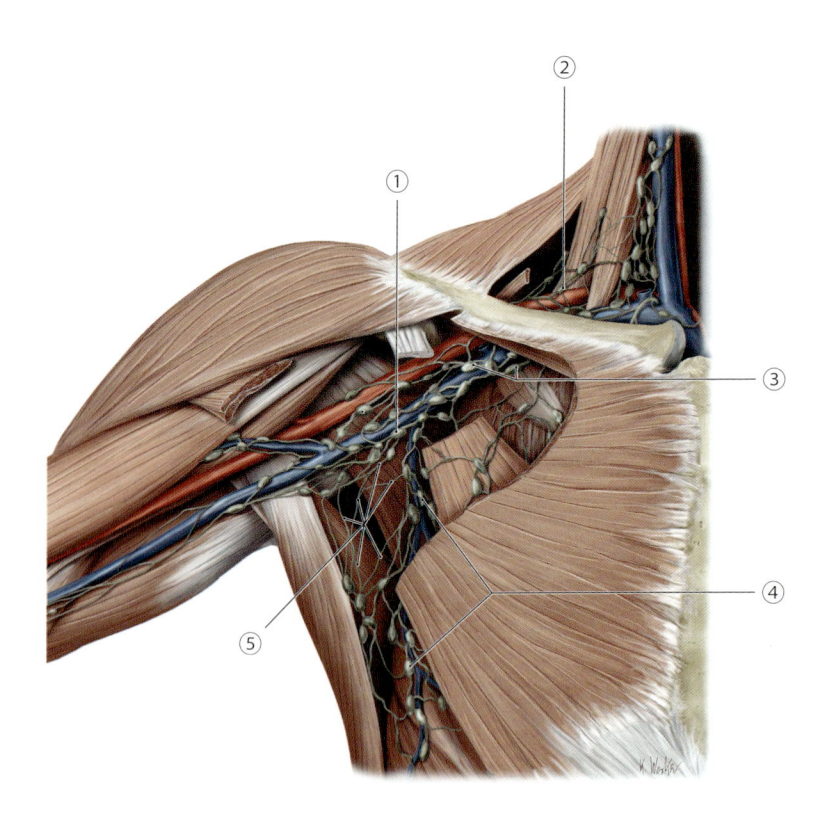

女性の乳房のリンパ管

前面

① □ 中心腋窩リンパ節　　　　　　□ Central axillary lymph node

② □ 鎖骨上リンパ節　　　　　　　□ Supraclavicular lymph node

③ □ 上腋窩リンパ節　　　　　　　□ Apical axillary lymph node

④ □ 胸筋腋窩リンパ節　　　　　　□ Pectoral axillary lymph node

⑤ □ 腋窩リンパ叢　　　　　　　　□ Axillary lymphatic plexus

> **臨床**
>
> 乳房腫瘍はリンパ管を通して広がる．胸骨傍リンパ節を経て正中線を越えて反対側に広がることもあるが，深リンパ管系（レベルⅢ）が特に重要である．乳癌の生存率は，腋窩リンパ節各レベルの転移したリンパ節の数と強く相関している．

[1] 図 5.33B, p.64　　[2] 図 6.33B, p.72

Structures of the Female Breast

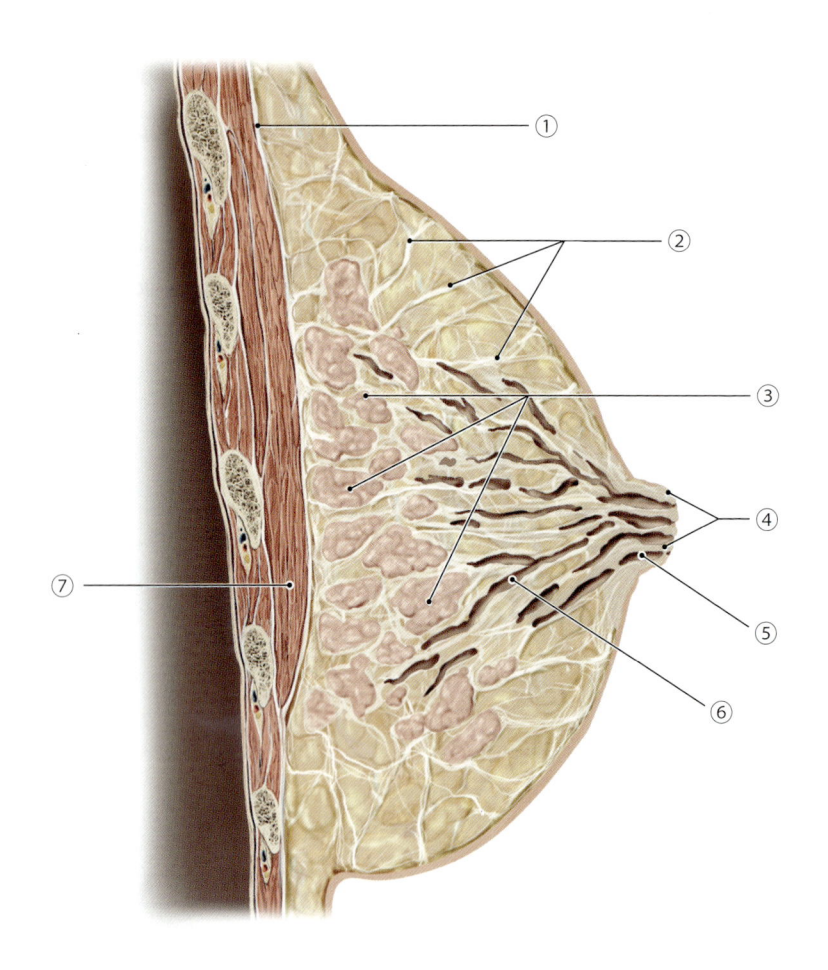

Q 乳房のリンパ管は主にどのリンパ管系に注ぐか？

女性の乳房の構造

矢状断面

① □ 胸筋筋膜　　　　　　　　　□ Pectoral fascia

② □ 乳房提靱帯（クーパー靱帯）　□ Suspensory (Cooper's) ligaments

③ □ 乳腺葉　　　　　　　　　　□ Mammary lobes

④ □ 乳頭　　　　　　　　　　　□ Nipple

⑤ □ 乳管洞　　　　　　　　　　□ Lactiferous sinus

⑥ □ 乳管　　　　　　　　　　　□ Lactiferous duct

⑦ □ 大胸筋　　　　　　　　　　□ Pectoralis major

A 乳房のリンパ管は 75% が腋窩リンパ節に注ぐ．

① 図 5.32A. p.63　② 図 6.32A. p.71

Divisions of the Mediastinum

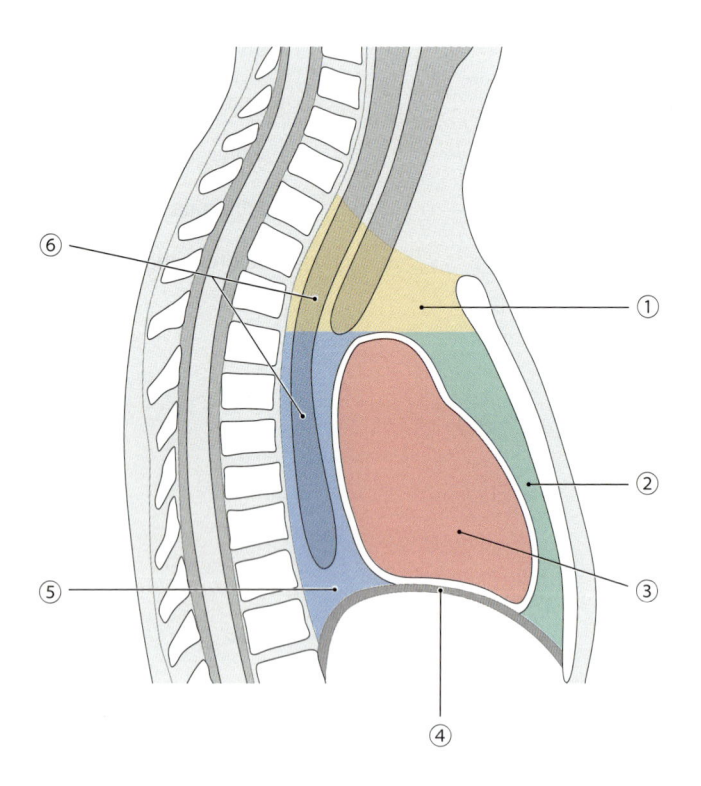

縦隔の区分

外側面

① ☐ 上縦隔　　　　　　　　　☐ Superior mediastinum

② ☐ 前縦隔　　　　　　　　　☐ Anterior mediastinum

③ ☐ 中縦隔　　　　　　　　　☐ Middle mediastinum

④ ☐ 横隔膜　　　　　　　　　☐ Diaphragm

⑤ ☐ 後縦隔　　　　　　　　　☐ Posterior mediastinum

⑥ ☐ 食道，胸部　　　　　　　☐ Esophagus, thoracic part

解説

縦隔は両肺の胸膜嚢の間に挟まれた胸部の空間で，上縦隔と下縦隔に分けられる．下縦隔はさらに前縦隔，中縦隔，後縦隔に分けられる．

[1] 図 6.2B. p.67　[2] 図 7.2B. p.75

CT Scan of the Thorax

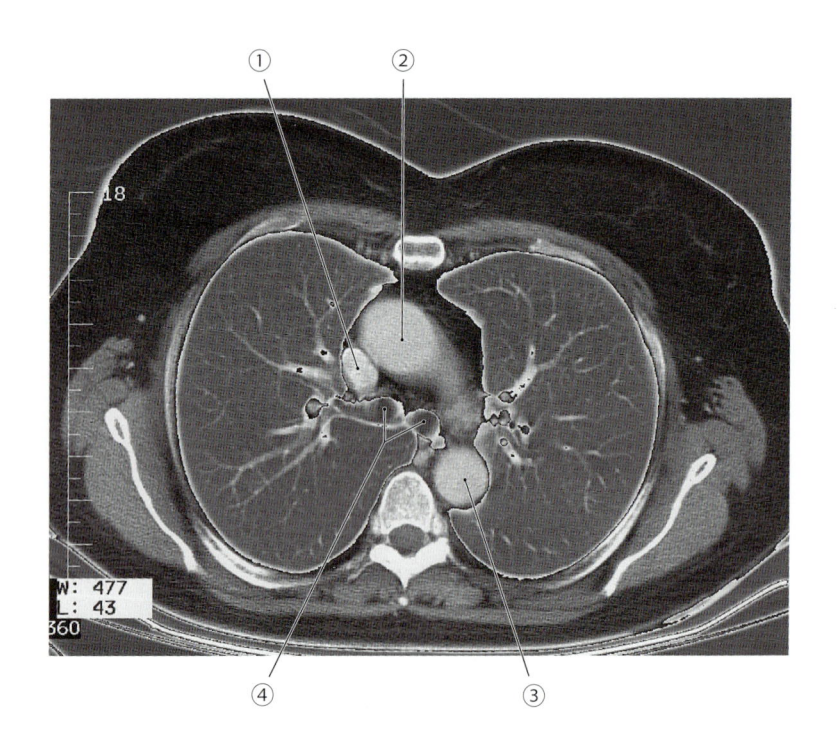

胸部のCTスキャン

水平断面, 下面

① ☐ 上大静脈　　　　　　　☐ Superior vena cava

② ☐ 上行大動脈　　　　　　☐ Ascending aorta

③ ☐ 下行大動脈　　　　　　☐ Descending aorta

④ ☐ 右・左主気管支　　　　☐ Right and left main bronchii

臨床

　大動脈の内膜裂傷によって血液が大動脈壁の層を分離させることで偽腔が生じ,潜在的に生死に関わる大動脈破裂につながる.急性動脈解離は上行大動脈でよく起こり,一般的に外科手術が必要である.これより遠位の動脈解離は合併症がない場合は,保存的に治療される.冠状動脈分岐部での大動脈解離は心筋梗塞を引き起こす.

1 図 6.3A. p.67　2 図 7.3A. p.75

Thoracic Aorta

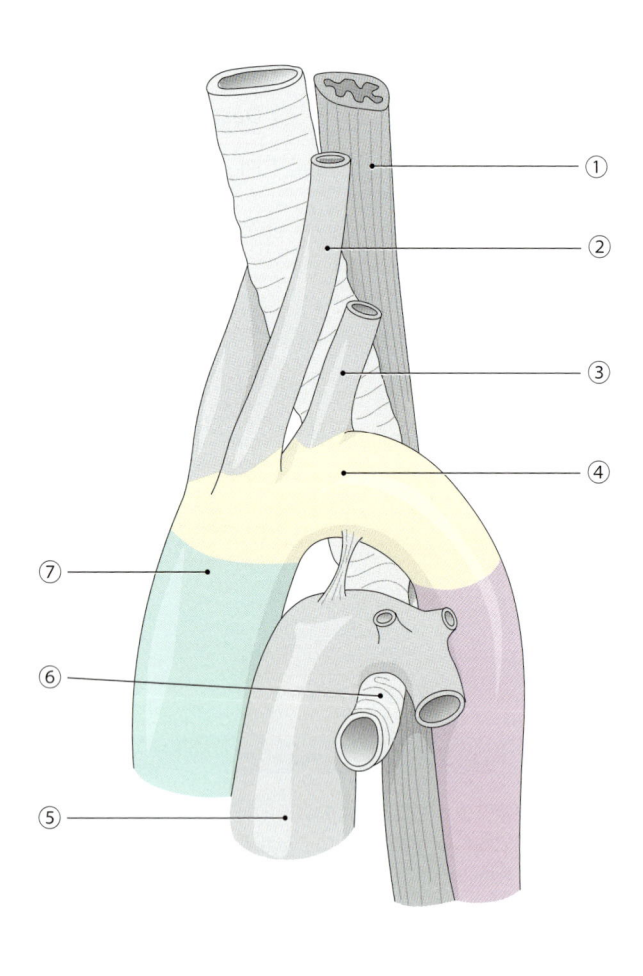

胸大動脈

左外側面

① ☐ 食道 　　　　　　　　☐ Esophagus
② ☐ 左総頸動脈 　　　　　☐ Left common carotid artery
③ ☐ 左鎖骨下動脈 　　　　☐ Left subclavian artery
④ ☐ 大動脈弓 　　　　　　☐ Aortic arch
⑤ ☐ 肺動脈幹 　　　　　　☐ Pulmonary trunk
⑥ ☐ 左主気管支 　　　　　☐ Left main bronchus
⑦ ☐ 上行大動脈 　　　　　☐ Ascending aorta

解説

　大動脈弓からは，腕頭動脈，左総頸動脈，左鎖骨下動脈の3つの大きな枝が分かれる．大動脈弓を経て大動脈は下行し，胸骨角の高さで胸大動脈となり，横隔膜の大動脈裂孔を通過後に腹大動脈となる．

[1] 図 6.4A. p.68　[2] 図 7.4B. p.77

Azygos System

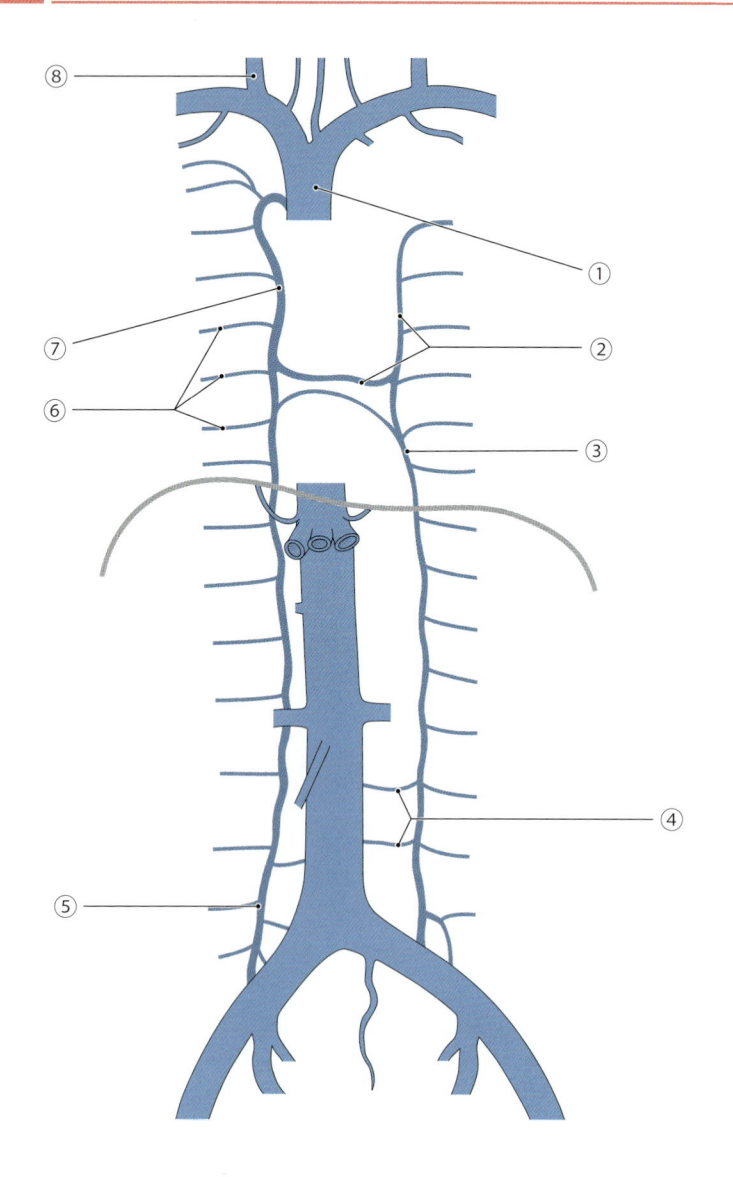

奇静脈系

前面

① □ 上大静脈 □ Superior vena cava
② □ 副半奇静脈 □ Accessory hemiazygos vein
③ □ 半奇静脈 □ Hemiazygos vein
④ □ 腰静脈 □ Lumbar veins
⑤ □ 右上行腰静脈 □ Right ascending lumbar vein
⑥ □ 肋間静脈 □ Posterior intercostal veins
⑦ □ 奇静脈 □ Azygos vein
⑧ □ 右内頸静脈 □ Right internal jugular vein

解説

奇静脈系は頭部・頸部・上肢の静脈系と上大静脈によって連絡し，腹部・下肢の静脈系と下大静脈によって連絡する．

Lymphatics of the Thoracic Cavity

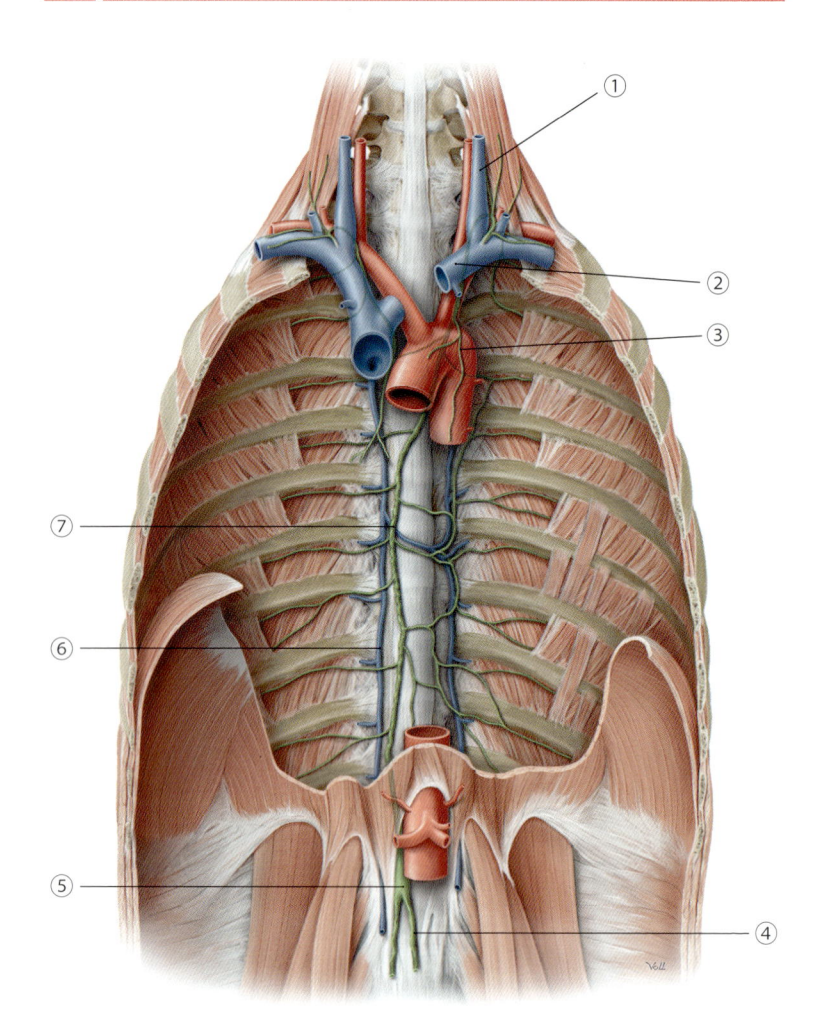

どの領域のリンパ管が胸管に注ぐか？

胸腔のリンパ管

前面

① □ 内頸静脈　　　　　　　　　□ Internal jugular vein

② □ 左腕頭静脈　　　　　　　　□ Left brachiocephalic vein

③ □ 気管支縦隔リンパ本幹　　　□ Bronchomediastinal trunk

④ □ 左腰リンパ本幹　　　　　　□ Left lumbar trunk

⑤ □ 乳ビ槽　　　　　　　　　　□ Cisterna chyli

⑥ □ 奇静脈　　　　　　　　　　□ Azygos vein

⑦ □ 胸管　　　　　　　　　　　□ Thoracic duct

A 人体の主要なリンパ管は胸管である．胸管は，腹部の乳ビ槽から始まり，横隔膜より下の両側のリンパ，および左側の頭部・頸部・左肺下葉を除く胸部・上肢からのリンパが注ぐ．これ以外の領域では右リンパ本幹に注ぐ．

1 図 6.7. p.72　2 図 7.7. p.80

Nerves of the Thoracic Cavity

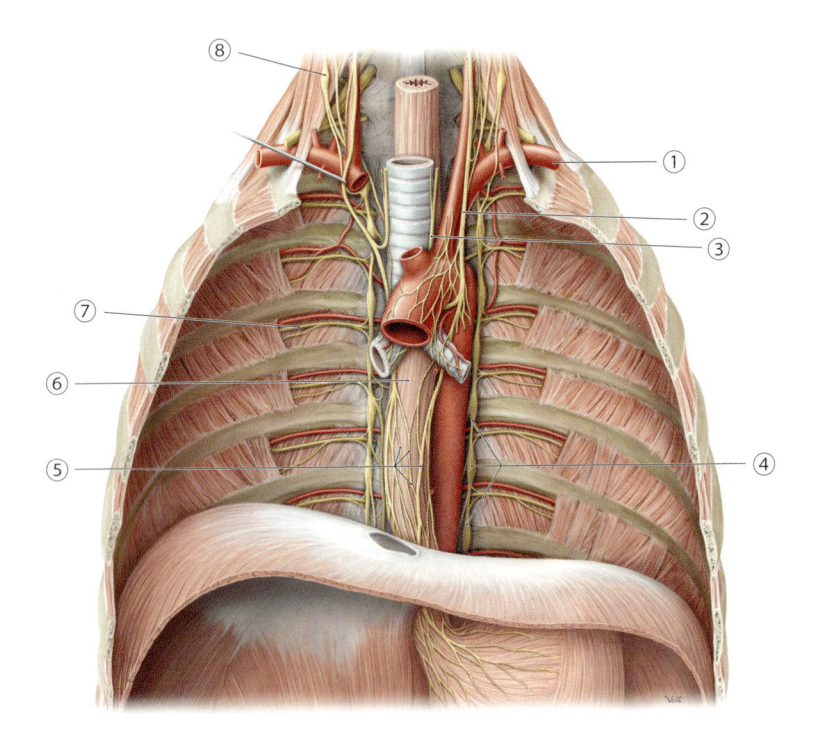

胸腔の神経

前面

① ☐ 左鎖骨下動脈　　　　　　　　☐ Left subclavian artery

② ☐ 左迷走神経　　　　　　　　　☐ Left vagus nerve

③ ☐ 左反回神経　　　　　　　　　☐ Left recurrent laryngeal nerve

④ ☐ 交感神経幹　　　　　　　　　☐ Sympathetic trunk

⑤ ☐ 前迷走神経幹と食道神経叢　　☐ Anterior vagal trunk (with esophageal plexus)

⑥ ☐ 食道，胸部　　　　　　　　　☐ Esophagus, thoracic part

⑦ ☐ 肋間神経　　　　　　　　　　☐ Intercostal nerve

⑧ ☐ 交感神経幹，中頸神経節　　　☐ Sympathetic trunk, middle cervical ganglion

解説

胸部の神経支配はほとんどが自律神経で，交感神経幹と副交感性の迷走神経に由来する．例外は，心膜と横隔膜を支配する横隔神経と胸壁を支配する肋間神経の2つである．

１ 図 6.11B. p.74　　２ 図 7.11B. p.82

Mediastinum I

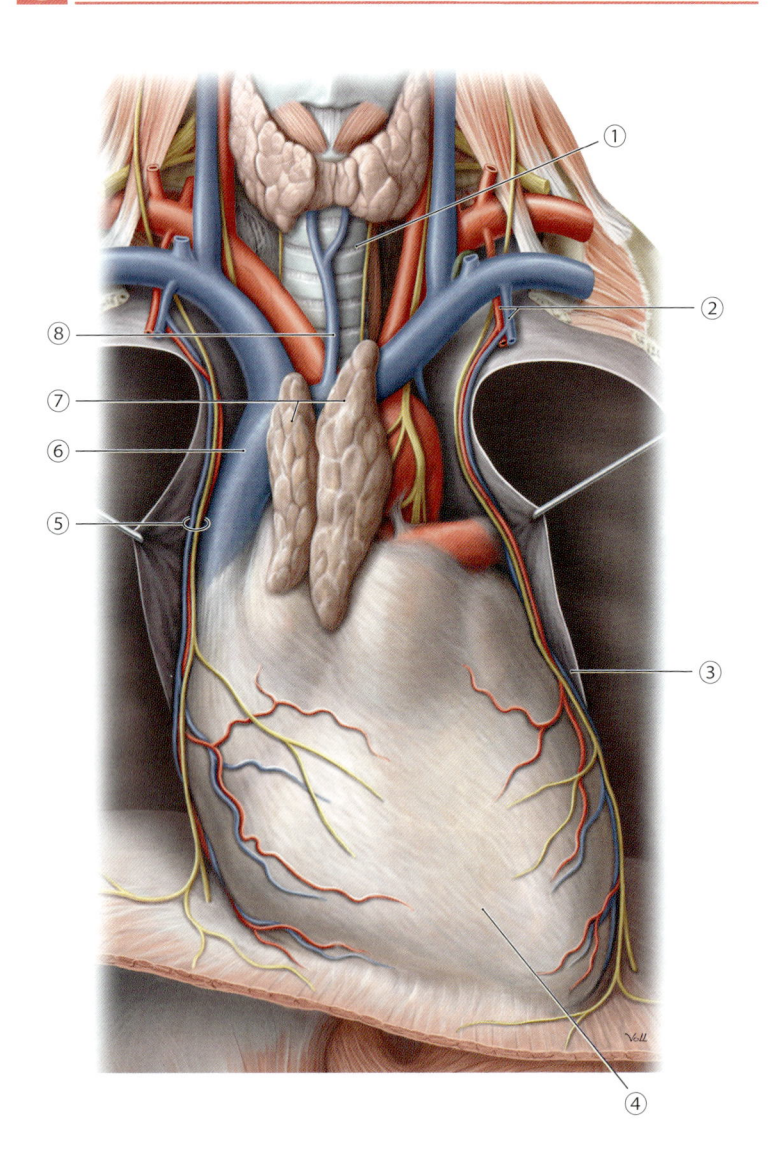

縦隔 1

前面

① □ 気管 — □ Trachea
② □ 内胸動脈・静脈 — □ Internal thoracic artery and vein
③ □ 壁側胸膜, 縦隔部（縦隔胸膜） — □ Parietal pleura, mediastinal part
④ □ 線維性心膜 — □ Fibrous pericardium
⑤ □ 心膜横隔動脈・静脈, 横隔神経 — □ Pericardiacophrenic artery and vein, phrenic nerve
⑥ □ 上大静脈 — □ Superior vena cava
⑦ □ 胸腺 — □ Thymus
⑧ □ 下甲状腺静脈 — □ Inferior thyroid vein

Mediastinum II

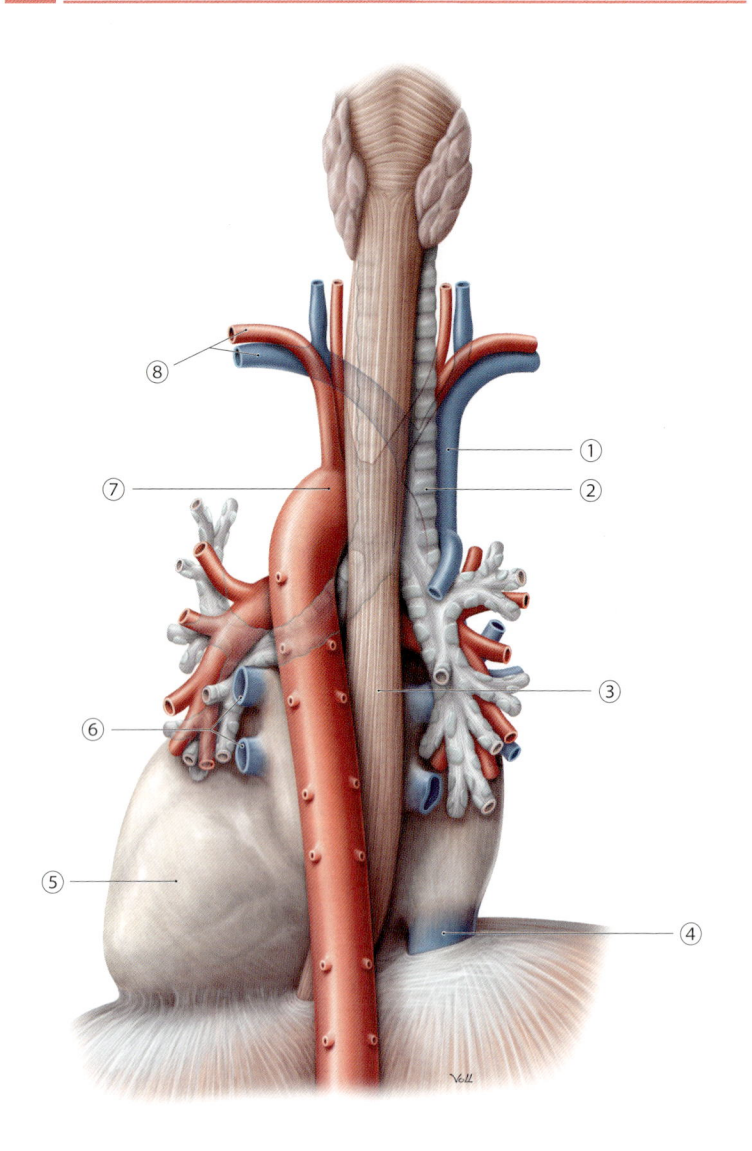

縦隔 2

縦隔の内容，後面

① □ 上大静脈　　　　　　　　　　□ Superior vena cava
② □ 気管　　　　　　　　　　　　□ Trachea
③ □ 食道，胸部　　　　　　　　　□ Esophagus, thoracic part
④ □ 下大静脈（大静脈孔の中の）　□ Inferior vena cava (in caval aperture)
⑤ □ 線維性心膜，左心室　　　　　□ Fibrous pericardium, left ventricle
⑥ □ 左肺静脈　　　　　　　　　　□ Left pulmonary veins
⑦ □ 大動脈弓　　　　　　　　　　□ Aortic arch
⑧ □ 左鎖骨下動脈・静脈　　　　　□ Left subclavian artery and vein

106 Thorax

Mediastinum III

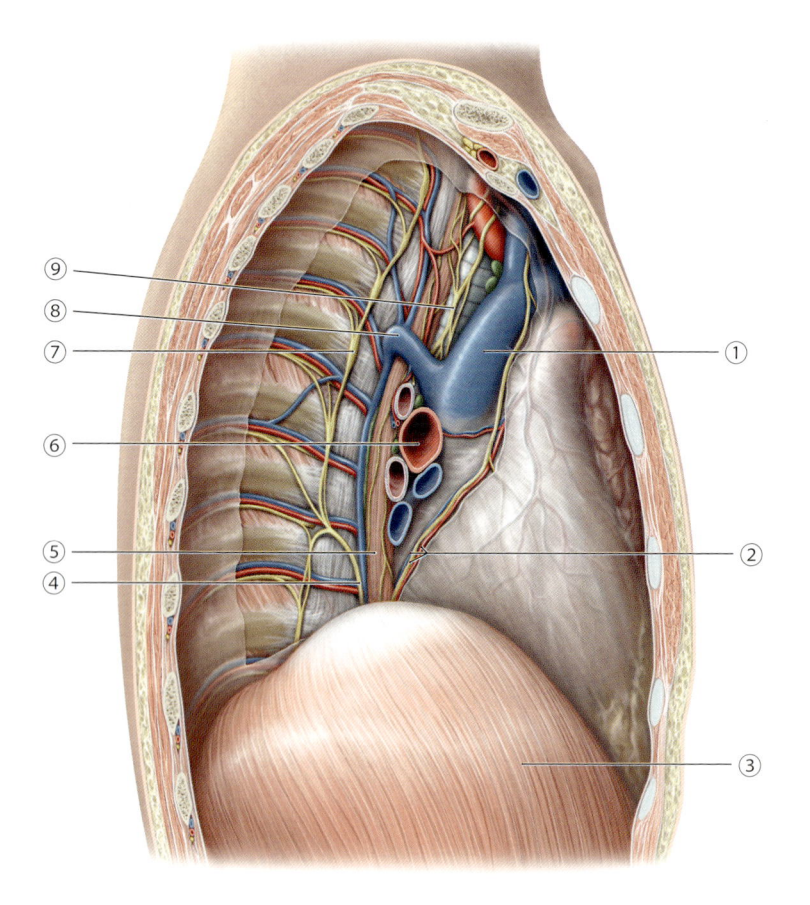

縦隔 3

傍矢状断面，右側面

① □ 上大静脈　　　　　　　　　　□ Superior vena cava
② □ 横隔神経，心膜横隔動脈・　　□ Phrenic nerve,
　　　静脈　　　　　　　　　　　　　 pericardiacophrenic artery
　　　　　　　　　　　　　　　　　　 and vein
③ □ 横隔膜　　　　　　　　　　　□ Diaphragm
④ □ 大内臓神経　　　　　　　　　□ Greater splanchnic nerve
⑤ □ 食道　　　　　　　　　　　　□ Esophagus
⑥ □ 右肺動脈　　　　　　　　　　□ Right pulmonary artery
⑦ □ 交感神経幹，胸神経節　　　　□ Sympathetic trunk, thoracic
　　　　　　　　　　　　　　　　　　 ganglion
⑧ □ 奇静脈　　　　　　　　　　　□ Azygos vein
⑨ □ 右迷走神経　　　　　　　　　□ Right vagus nerve

1 図 7.3A, p.78　 2 図 8.3A, p.86

108 Thorax

Mediastinum IV

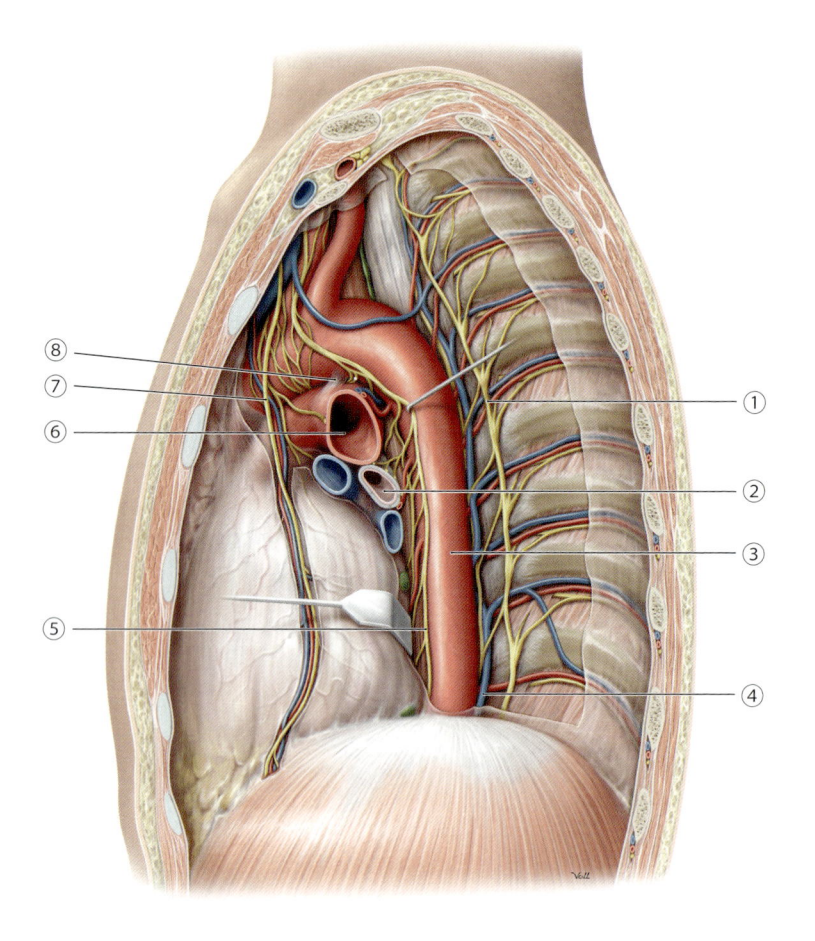

縦隔 4

傍矢状断面, 左外側面

① ☐ 交感神経幹 ☐ Sympathetic trunk
② ☐ 左主気管支 ☐ Left main bronchus
③ ☐ 胸大動脈(下行大動脈) ☐ Thoracic aorta (descending aorta)
④ ☐ 半奇静脈 ☐ Hemiazygos vein
⑤ ☐ 左迷走神経 ☐ Left vagus nerve
⑥ ☐ 左肺動脈 ☐ Left pulmonary artery
⑦ ☐ 左横隔神経 ☐ Left phrenic nerve
⑧ ☐ 動脈管索 ☐ Ligamentum arteriosum

1 図 7.3B. p.79 2 図 8.3B. p.87

Pericardial Reflections I

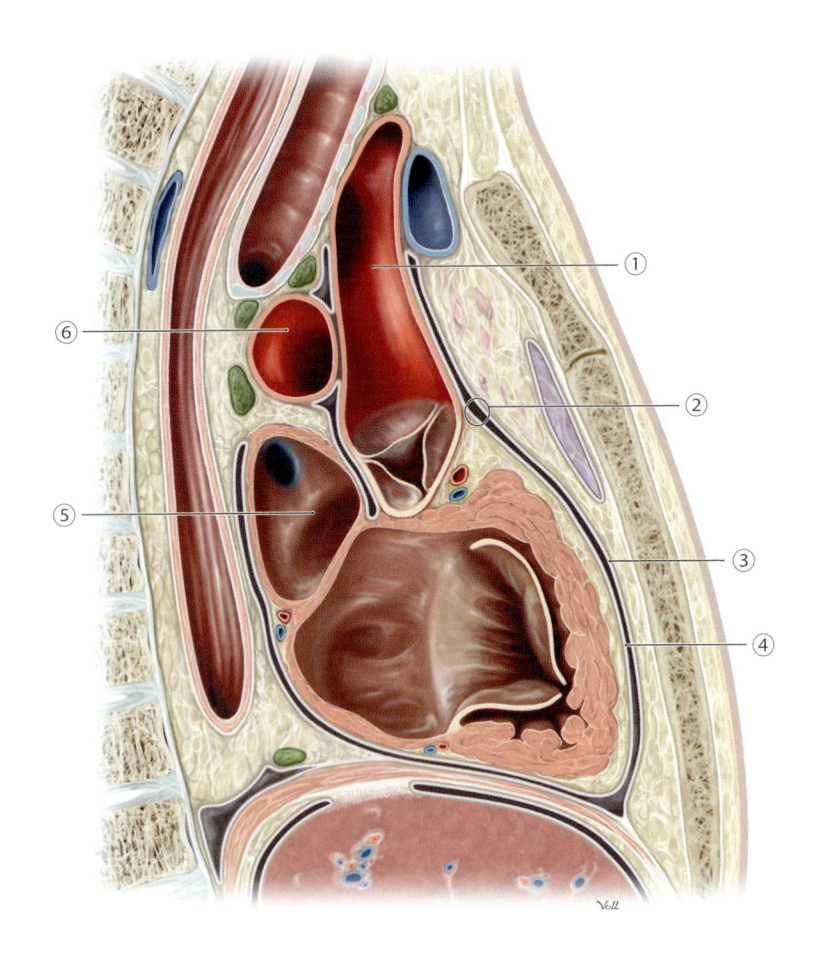

心膜の折れ返り 1

縦隔の矢状断面

① □ 上行大動脈　　　　　□ Ascending aorta

② □ 心膜腔　　　　　　　□ Pericardial cavity

③ □ 漿膜性心膜壁側板　　□ Parietal layer of the serous pericardium

④ □ 漿膜性心膜臓側板　　□ Visceral layer of the serous pericardium

⑤ □ 左心房　　　　　　　□ Left atrium

⑥ □ 右肺動脈　　　　　　□ Right pulmonary artery

解説

漿膜性心膜の臓側板と壁側板は心臓の大血管周囲で連続している．動脈の折れ返り部と静脈の折れ返り部の間にある空洞が心膜横洞である．

[1] 図 7.7A. p.81　[2] 図 8.10. p.91

Pericardial Reflections II

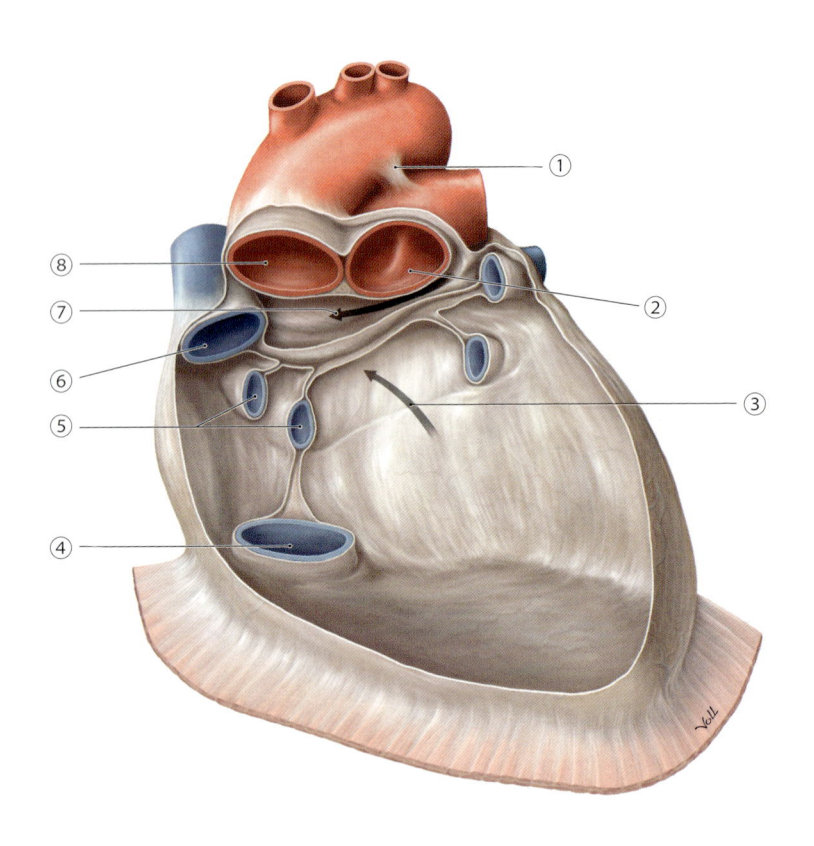

心膜横洞とは何か？

心膜の折れ返り 2

心臓を取り除いた心膜，前面

① □ 動脈管索　　　　　　　□ Ligamentum arteriosum

② □ 肺動脈幹　　　　　　　□ Pulmonary trunk

③ □ 心膜斜洞　　　　　　　□ Oblique pericardial sinus

④ □ 下大静脈　　　　　　　□ Inferior vena cava

⑤ □ 右肺静脈　　　　　　　□ Right pulmonary veins

⑥ □ 上大静脈　　　　　　　□ Superior vena cava

⑦ □ 心膜横洞　　　　　　　□ Transverse pericardial sinus

⑧ □ 上行大動脈　　　　　　□ Ascending aorta

A 　心膜横洞は心臓の流入路（上・下大静脈と肺静脈）と流出路（大動脈と肺動脈幹）を隔てている．

1 図 7.7B. p.81

Heart in Situ

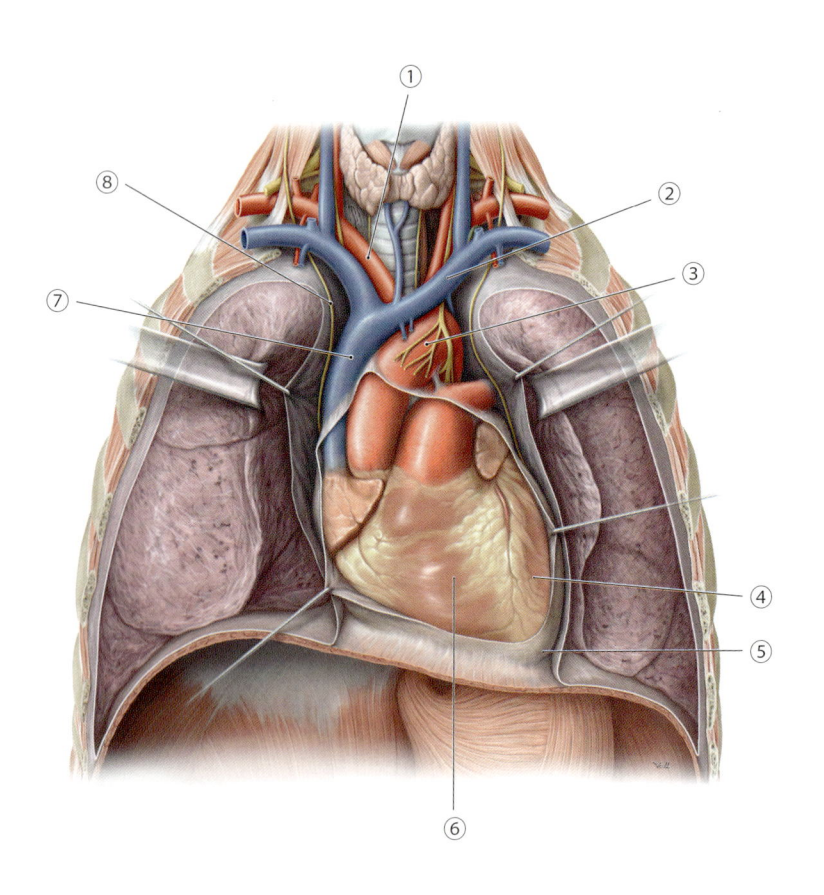

Q 胸郭の骨に対する心臓の位置はどこか？

原位置の心臓

前面

① □ 腕頭動脈　　　　　□ Brachiocephalic trunk
② □ 左腕頭静脈　　　　□ Left brachiocephalic vein
③ □ 大動脈弓　　　　　□ Aortic arch
④ □ 左心室　　　　　　□ Left ventricle
⑤ □ 心尖　　　　　　　□ Cardiac apex
⑥ □ 右心室　　　　　　□ Right ventricle
⑦ □ 上大静脈　　　　　□ Superior vena cava
⑧ □ 右横隔神経　　　　□ Right phrenic nerve

A 心臓は胸骨体の後方で第2-6肋軟骨の間にある．心臓は下縦隔の中縦隔にあり，胸腔左側に投影される．

1 図7.10. p.83　2 図8.6B. p.89

Sternocostal Surface of the Heart

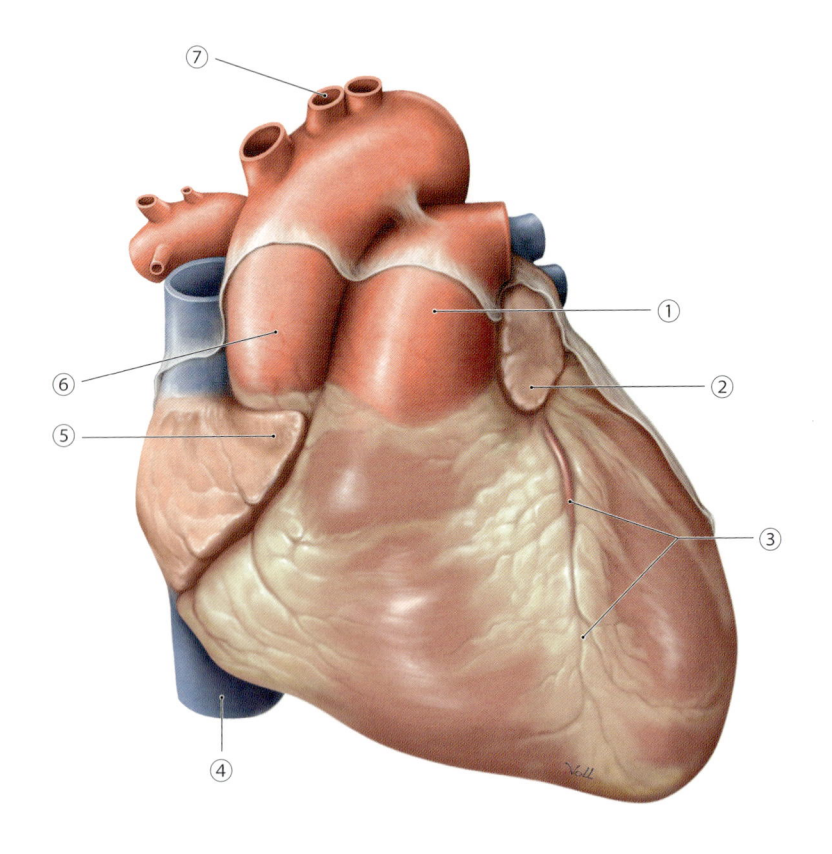

心臓の胸肋面

前面

① ☐ 肺動脈幹　　　　　☐ Pulmonary trunk
② ☐ 左心耳　　　　　　☐ Left auricle
③ ☐ 前室間溝　　　　　☐ Anterior interventricular sulcus
④ ☐ 下大静脈　　　　　☐ Inferior vena cava
⑤ ☐ 右心耳　　　　　　☐ Right auricle
⑥ ☐ 上行大動脈　　　　☐ Ascending aorta
⑦ ☐ 左総頸動脈　　　　☐ Left common carotid artery

Base of the Heart

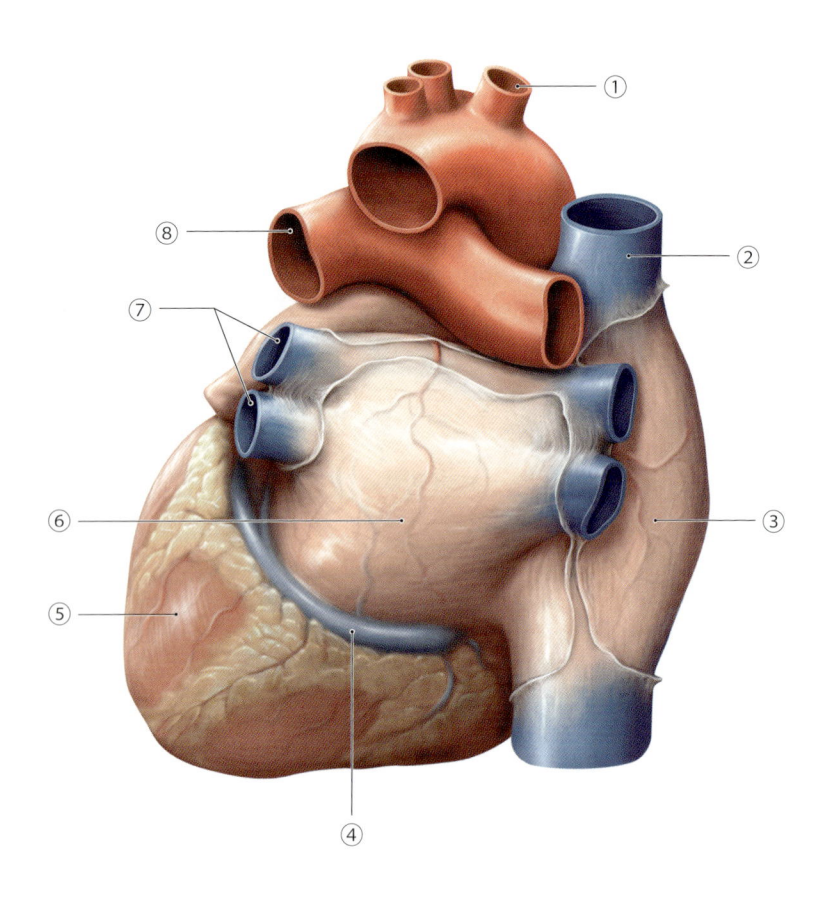

心臓の底面

後面

① ☐ 腕頭動脈 　　　　　　　☐ Brachiocephalic trunk

② ☐ 上大静脈 　　　　　　　☐ Superior vena cava

③ ☐ 右心房 　　　　　　　　☐ Right atrium

④ ☐ 冠状静脈洞 　　　　　　☐ Coronary sinus

⑤ ☐ 左心室 　　　　　　　　☐ Left ventricle

⑥ ☐ 左心房 　　　　　　　　☐ Left atrium

⑦ ☐ 左肺静脈 　　　　　　　☐ Left pulmonary veins

⑧ ☐ 左肺動脈 　　　　　　　☐ Left pulmonary artery

1 図 7.11B. p.84　2 図 8.11B. p.92

Chambers of the Heart I

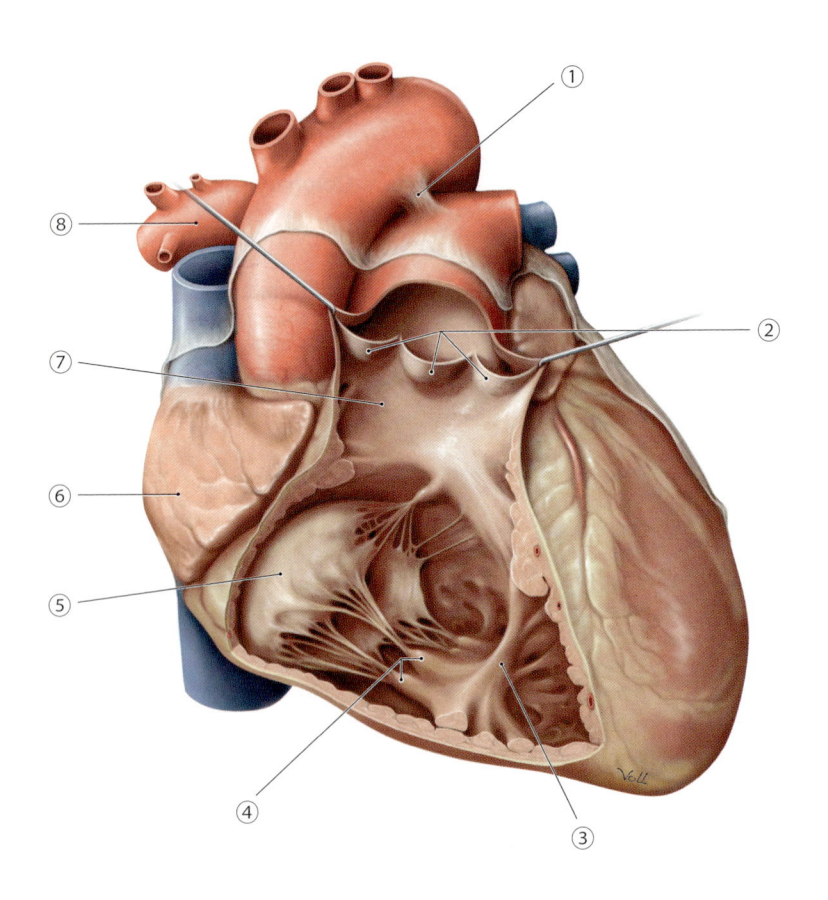

Q 肺動脈弁と大動脈弁が閉じるのは心周期のどのときか？

心臓の室 1

前面

① ☐ 動脈管索　　　　　　　　☐ Ligamentum arteriosum

② ☐ 肺動脈弁　　　　　　　　☐ Valve of pulmonary trunk

③ ☐ 中隔縁柱　　　　　　　　☐ Septomarginal trabecula

④ ☐ 前乳頭筋　　　　　　　　☐ Anterior papillary muscle

⑤ ☐ 右房室弁，前尖　　　　　☐ Right atrioventricular valve, anterior cusp

⑥ ☐ 右心房　　　　　　　　　☐ Right atrium

⑦ ☐ 動脈円錐　　　　　　　　☐ Conus arteriosus

⑧ ☐ 右肺動脈　　　　　　　　☐ Right pulmonary artery

A 動脈弁は拡張期（心室弛緩期）に閉じる．

[1] 図 7.12A. p.85　[2] 図 8.12A. p.93

Chambers of the Heart II

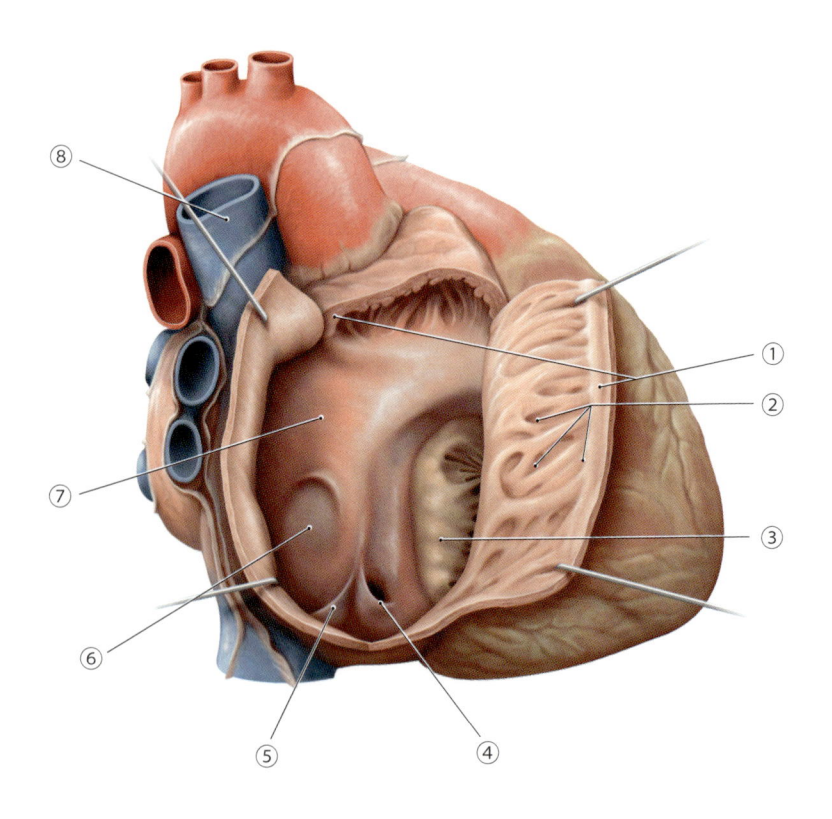

Q 右心房において胎児期に右心房と左心房を連絡していた構造の遺残物はどれか？

心臓の室 2

右外側面

① ☐ 分界稜　　　　　　　　　☐ Crista terminalis
② ☐ 櫛状筋　　　　　　　　　☐ Pectinate muscles
③ ☐ 右房室口と右房室弁　　　☐ Right atrioventricular orifice with atrioventricular valve
④ ☐ 冠状静脈口と冠状静脈弁　☐ Valved orifice of coronary sinus
⑤ ☐ 下大静脈口と下大静脈弁　☐ Valved orifice of inferior vena cava
⑥ ☐ 卵円窩　　　　　　　　　☐ Fossa ovalis
⑦ ☐ 心房中隔　　　　　　　　☐ Interatrial septum
⑧ ☐ 上大静脈　　　　　　　　☐ Superior vena cava

A 　心房壁の浅い陥凹である卵円窩は，胎児期の心臓の卵円孔の遺残物である．

1 図 7.12B. p.85　2 図 8.12B. p.93

124 Thorax

Chambers of the Heart III

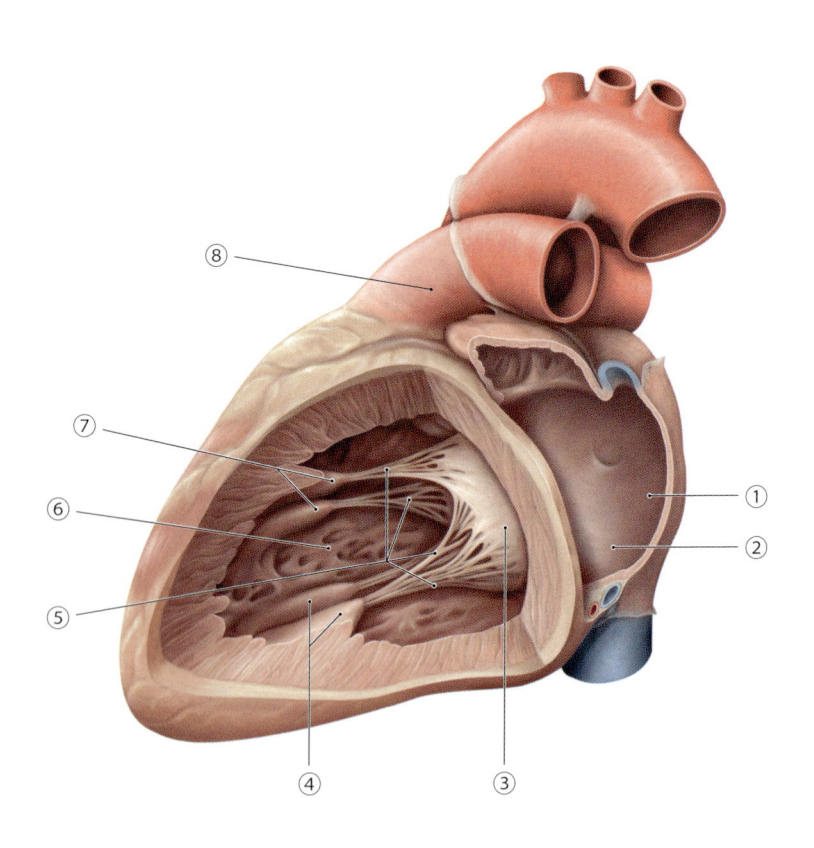

Q この絵は心周期のどのときの心臓か？

心臓の室 3

左外側面

① ☐ 左心房 ☐ Left atrium
② ☐ 心房中隔 ☐ Interatrial septum
③ ☐ 左房室弁 ☐ Left atrioventricular valve
④ ☐ 後乳頭筋 ☐ Posterior papillary muscle
⑤ ☐ 腱索 ☐ Chordae tendineae
⑥ ☐ 心室中隔の肉柱 ☐ Trabeculae carneae of interventricular septum
⑦ ☐ 前乳頭筋 ☐ Anterior papillary muscle
⑧ ☐ 肺動脈幹 ☐ Pulmonary trunk

A 収縮期（心室収縮期）．

1 図 7.12C. p.85　2 図 8.12C. p.93

Heart Valves

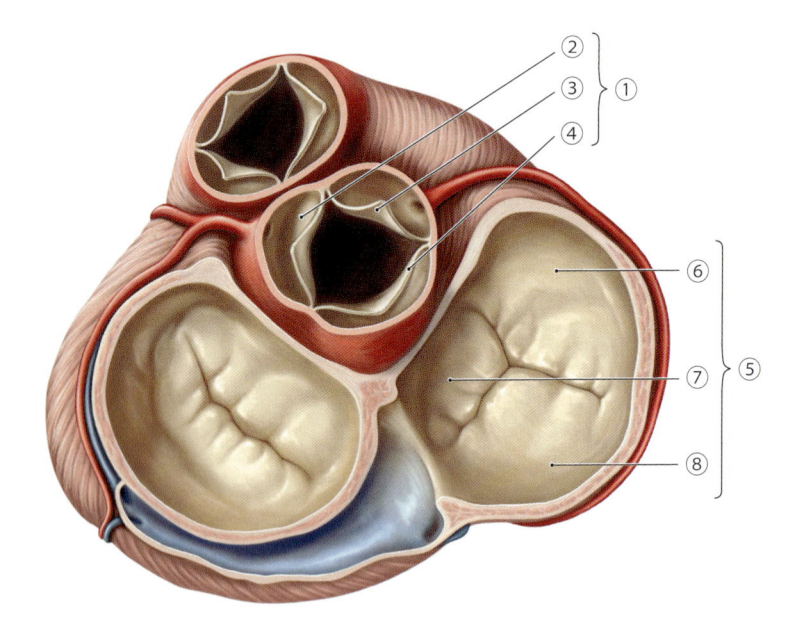

心臓弁

心室収縮期 Ventricular systole (contraction of the ventricles), 上面

① ☐ 大動脈弁　　　　　　　　　☐ Aortic valve

② ☐ 左半月弁　　　　　　　　　☐ Left cusp

③ ☐ 右半月弁　　　　　　　　　☐ Right cusp

④ ☐ 後半月弁　　　　　　　　　☐ Posterior cusp

⑤ ☐ 右房室弁　　　　　　　　　☐ Right atrioventricular valve

⑥ ☐ 前尖　　　　　　　　　　　☐ Anterior cusp

⑦ ☐ 中隔尖　　　　　　　　　　☐ Septal cusp

⑧ ☐ 後尖　　　　　　　　　　　☐ Posterior cusp

解説

心臓弁は半月弁と房室弁の2種類に分類される．半月弁には大動脈弁と肺動脈弁の2つがあり，心臓の2本の大血管基部で心室から大動脈と肺動脈幹への血流を調節する．2つの房室弁（左房室弁と右房室弁）は心房と心室の境界にある．

1 図7.13B．p.86　2 図8.13B．p.94

Arteries & Veins of the Heart I

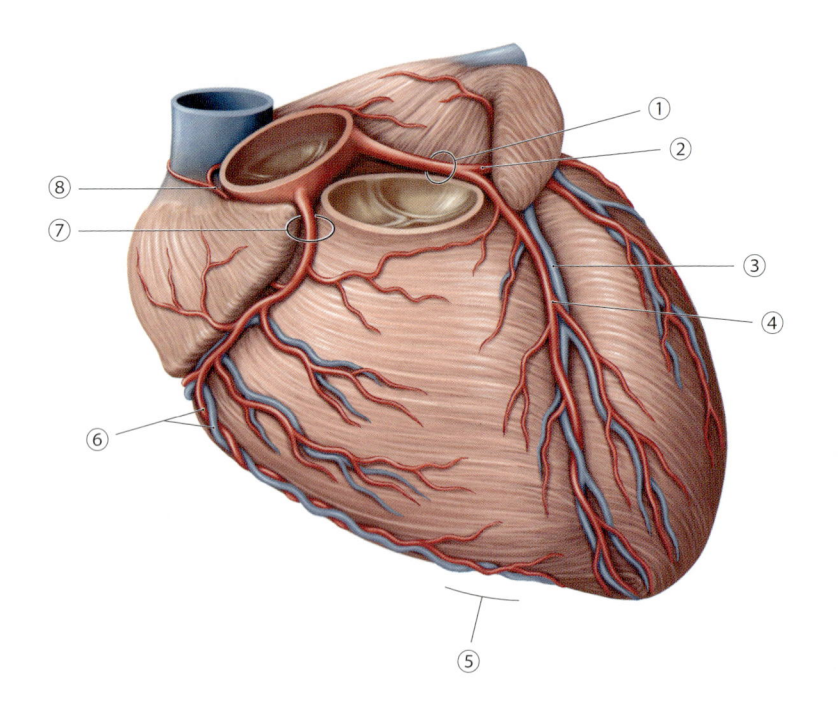

心臓の動脈と静脈 1

前面

① □ 左冠状動脈　　　　　　　□ Left coronary artery

② □ 回旋枝　　　　　　　　　□ Circumflex artery

③ □ 大心臓静脈　　　　　　　□ Great cardiac vein

④ □ 前室間枝（前下行枝）　　　□ Anterior interventricular (left anterior descending) artery

⑤ □ 右心室　　　　　　　　　□ Right ventricle

⑥ □ 右縁枝（鋭角縁枝）と右辺縁静脈　□ Right marginal artery and vein

⑦ □ 右冠状動脈　　　　　　　□ Right coronary artery

⑧ □ 洞房結節枝　　　　　　　□ Branch to sinoatrial node

臨床

冠状動脈は吻合によって互いに連絡しているが，機能の面では終動脈である．血流不足の原因として最も多いのはアテローム性動脈硬化症であり，血管壁に斑点が沈着して血管腔が狭くなる．血管狭窄が亢進した場合には，冠血流が阻害される．心筋梗塞は血流不足によって心筋組織が壊死して起こる．梗塞の部位と広がりは障害された血管によって決まる．

1 図 7.16A．p.88　2 図 8.16A．p.96

Arteries & Veins of the Heart II

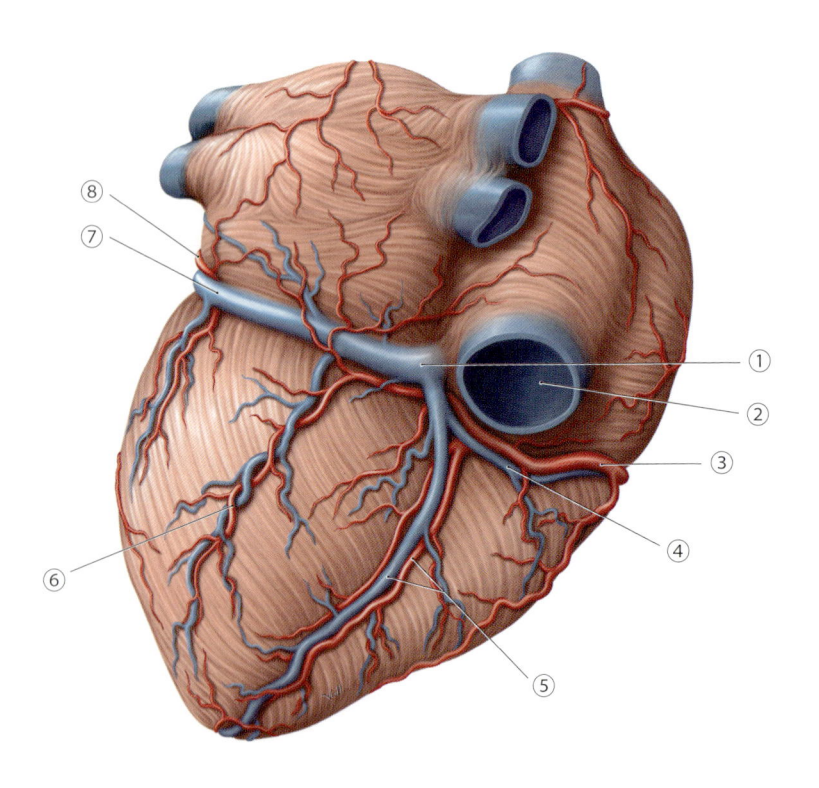

心臓の動脈と静脈 2

後下面

① □ 冠状静脈洞　　　　　　　　　□ Coronary sinus

② □ 下大静脈　　　　　　　　　　□ Inferior vena cava

③ □ 右冠状動脈　　　　　　　　　□ Right coronary artery

④ □ 小心臓静脈　　　　　　　　　□ Small cardiac vein

⑤ □ 後室間枝(後下行枝)と　　　　□ Posterior interventricular
　　後室間静脈(中心臓静脈)　　　　(descending) artery and vein

⑥ □ 右後側壁枝　　　　　　　　　□ Right posterolateral artery

⑦ □ 大心臓静脈　　　　　　　　　□ Great cardiac vein

⑧ □ 回旋枝　　　　　　　　　　　□ Circumflex artery

解説

右冠状動脈と左冠状動脈は，一般には左心房と左心室の後方で吻合する．

Cardiac Conduction System

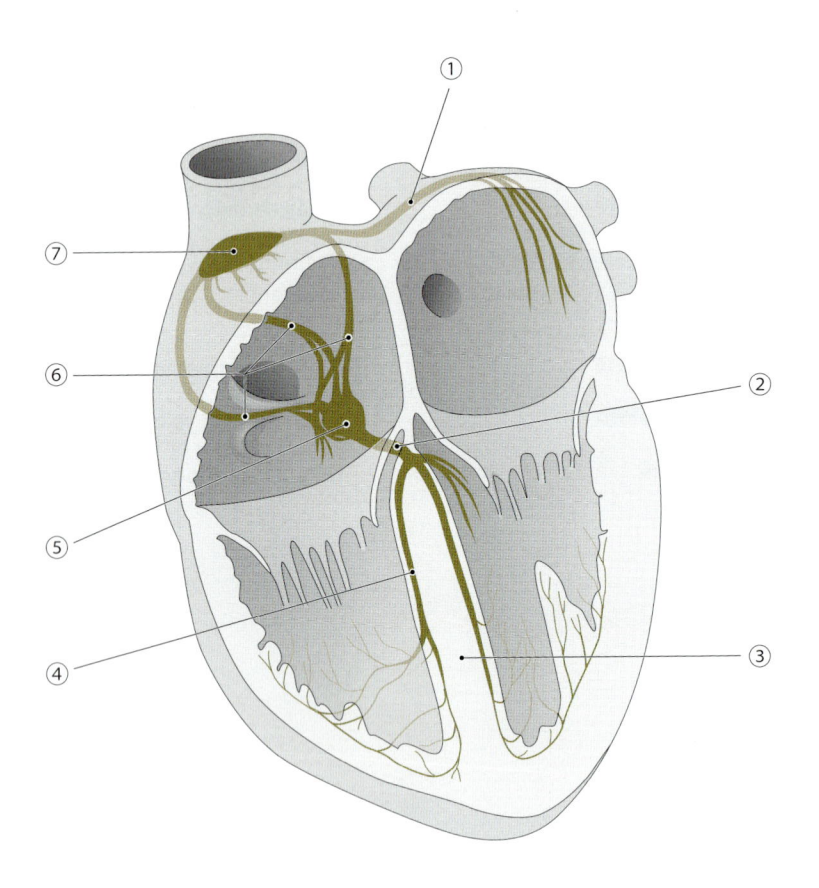

Q 洞房結節に血液を供給するのはどの血管か？

心臓刺激伝導系

前面

① ☐ 心房間束　　　　　　　☐ Interatrial bundle

② ☐ 房室束（ヒス束）　　　　☐ Atrioventricular bundle (of His)

③ ☐ 心室中隔　　　　　　　☐ Interventricular septum

④ ☐ 右脚　　　　　　　　　☐ Right bundle branch

⑤ ☐ 房室結節　　　　　　　☐ Atrioventricular (AV) node

⑥ ☐ 前・中・後結節間束　　　☐ Anterior, middle, and posterior internodal bundles

⑦ ☐ 洞房結節　　　　　　　☐ Sinoatrial (SA) node

A 通常は右冠状動脈から洞房結節へ動脈が向かう．

1 図 7.18A, p.90

Autonomic Nerves of the Heart

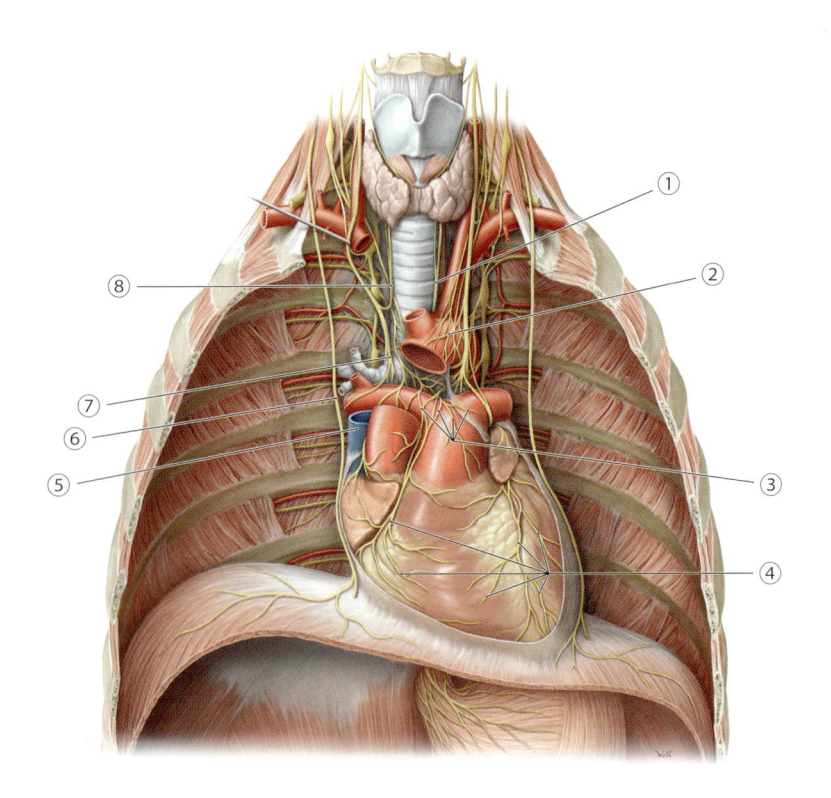

心臓の自律神経

前面，胸郭を開く

① □ 左反回神経　　　　□ Left recurrent laryngeal nerve

② □ 胸大動脈神経叢　　□ Thoracic aortic plexus

③ □ 肺神経叢　　　　　□ Pulmonary plexus

④ □ 心臓神経叢　　　　□ Cardiac plexus

⑤ □ 上大静脈　　　　　□ Superior vena cava

⑥ □ 右横隔神経　　　　□ Right phrenic nerve

⑦ □ 右迷走神経　　　　□ Right vagus nerve

⑧ □ 右反回神経　　　　□ Right recurrent laryngeal nerve

解説

心臓に分布する交感神経は，3本の頸心臓神経とT1-T6の胸神経節からの胸心臓枝である．副交感神経は迷走神経からの頸心臓枝と胸心臓枝である．交感神経と副交感神経はどちらも心臓神経叢，大動脈神経叢，肺神経叢に枝を出す．

[1] 図7.19C. p.91　[2] 図8.19C. p.99

Radiographic Appearance of the Heart I

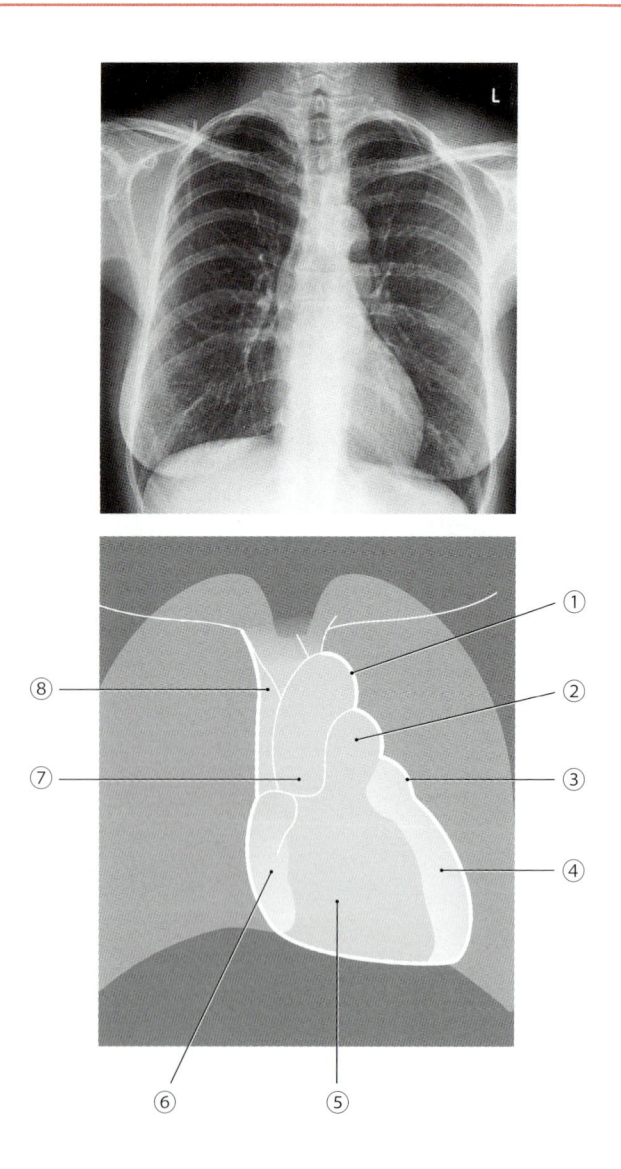

心臓の X 線像 1

上：胸部 X 線前後像，下：前面

① □ 大動脈弓（"大動脈隆起"）　　□ Aortic arch ("aortic knob")

② □ 肺動脈幹　　□ Pulmonary trunk

③ □ 左心房　　□ Left atrium

④ □ 左心室　　□ Left ventricle

⑤ □ 右心室　　□ Right ventricle

⑥ □ 右心房　　□ Right atrium

⑦ □ 上行大動脈　　□ Aorta, ascending part

⑧ □ 上大静脈　　□ Superior vena cava

1 図 7.21A, B. p.92　　2 図 8.21A, B. p.100

Radiographic Appearance of the Heart II

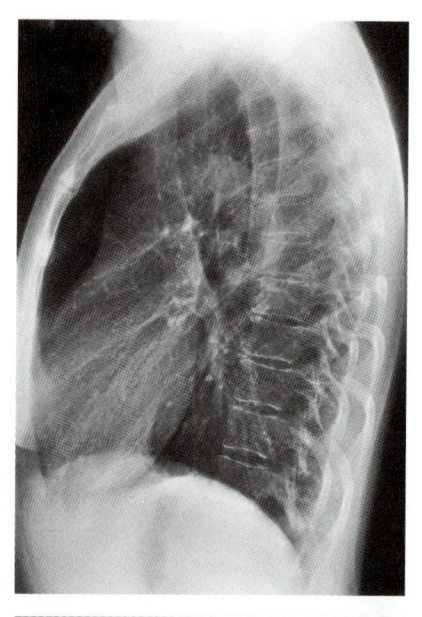

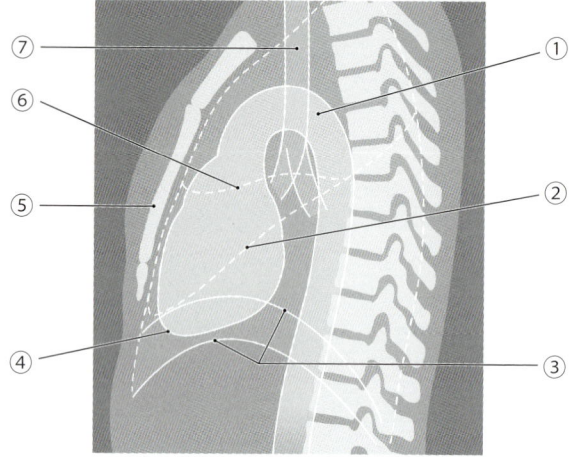

心臓の X 線像 2

上：胸部 X 線左側面像，下：外側面

① ☐ 大動脈弓 　　　　　　　　　☐ Aortic arch

② ☐ 右肺の斜裂 　　　　　　　　☐ Right lung, oblique fissure

③ ☐ 左・右の横隔膜円蓋 　　　　☐ Left and right diaphragm leaflets

④ ☐ 心尖 　　　　　　　　　　　☐ Cardiac apex

⑤ ☐ 胸骨体 　　　　　　　　　　☐ Sternum (body)

⑥ ☐ 右肺の水平裂 　　　　　　　☐ Right lung, horizontal fissure

⑦ ☐ 気管 　　　　　　　　　　　☐ Trachea

Heart in Transverse Section

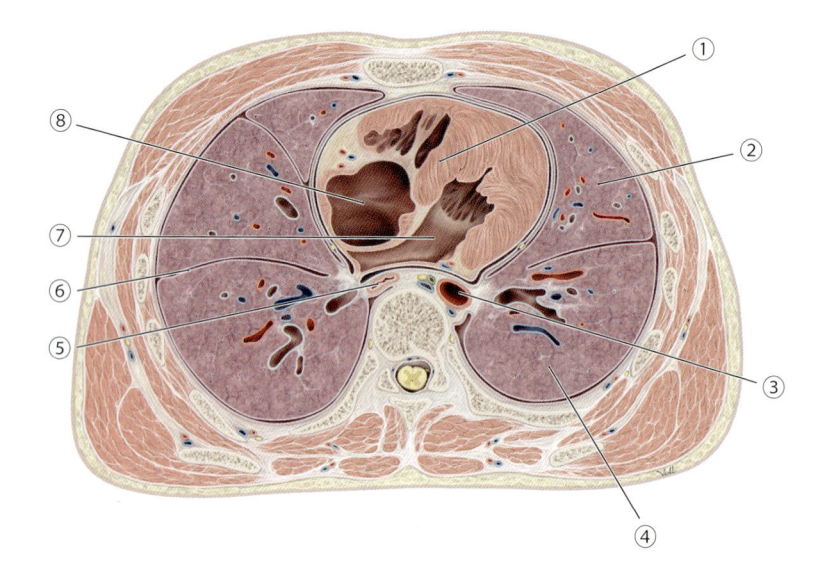

水平断面での心臓

第8胸椎(T8)の高さにおける水平断面，上面

① ☐ 心室中隔 　　　　　　　　☐ Interventricular septum
② ☐ 左肺の上葉 　　　　　　　☐ Left lung, superior lobe
③ ☐ 胸大動脈（下行大動脈） 　☐ Thoracic (descending) aorta
④ ☐ 左肺の下葉 　　　　　　　☐ Left lung, inferior lobe
⑤ ☐ 食道 　　　　　　　　　　☐ Esophagus
⑥ ☐ 右肺の斜裂 　　　　　　　☐ Oblique fissure of right lung
⑦ ☐ 左心房 　　　　　　　　　☐ Left atrium
⑧ ☐ 右心房 　　　　　　　　　☐ Right atrium

1 図 7.22B, p.93　2 図 8.22B, p.101

Prenatal Circulation

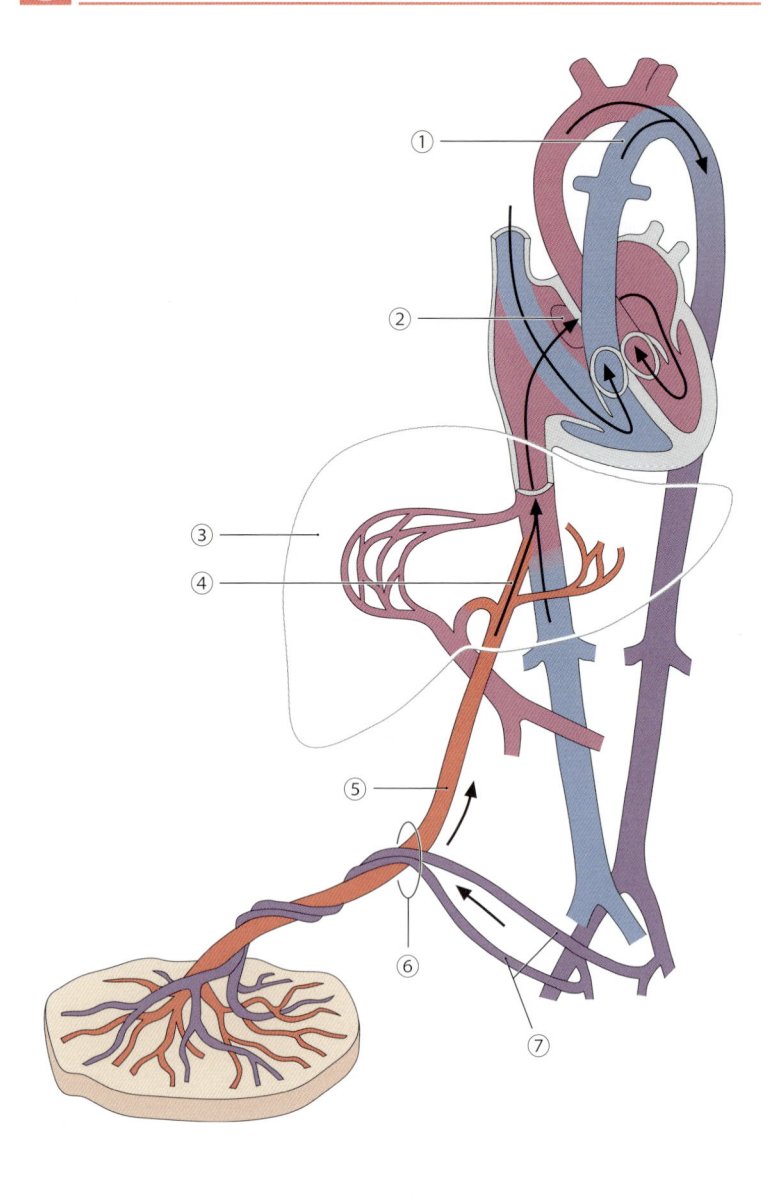

出生前の循環

① □ 動脈管（開いている）　□ Ductus arteriosus（patent）
② □ 卵円孔（開いている）　□ Foramen ovale（patent）
③ □ 肝臓　□ Liver
④ □ 静脈管　□ Ductus venosus
⑤ □ 臍静脈　□ Umbilical vein
⑥ □ 臍　□ Umbilicus
⑦ □ 臍動脈　□ Umbilical arteries

1 図 7.23（Fritsch and Kühnel による）．p.94　2 図 8.23（Fritsch and Kühnel による）．p.102

144 Thorax

Postnatal Circulation

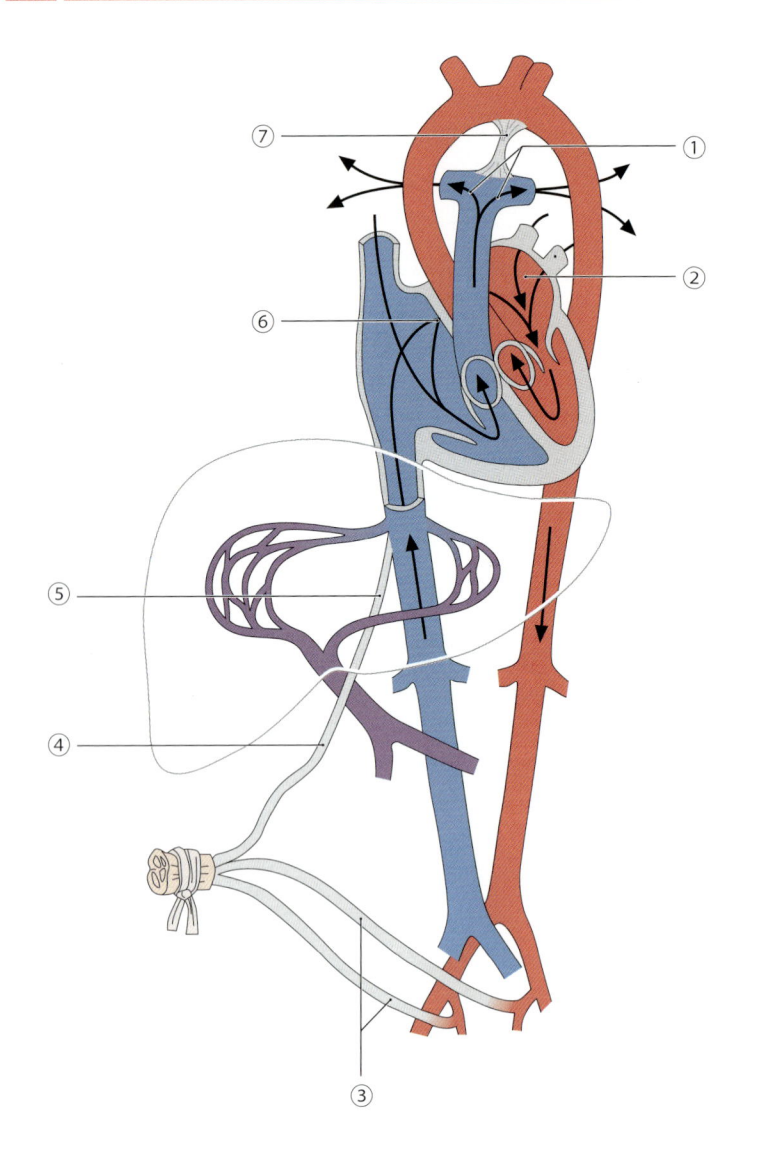

出生後の循環

① ☐ 肺動脈（血流が豊富） ☐ Pulmonary arteries (perfused)

② ☐ 左心房 ☐ Left atrium

③ ☐ 臍動脈の遺残（内側臍索） ☐ Obliterated umbilical arteries (medial umbilical ligaments)

④ ☐ 肝円索（臍静脈の遺残） ☐ Round ligament of liver (obliterated umbilical vein)

⑤ ☐ 静脈管索（静脈管の遺残） ☐ Ligamentum venosum (obliterated ductus venosus)

⑥ ☐ 卵円孔（閉じている） ☐ Foramen ovale (closed)

⑦ ☐ 動脈管索（動脈管の遺残） ☐ Ligamentum arteriosum (obliterated ductus arteriosus)

臨床

先天的な心臓疾患のなかで最も一般的な中隔欠損症では，収縮期に左心の血液が右心へと流入してしまう．心室中隔欠損症（VSD）は最も一般的な型である．心房中隔欠損症（ASD）の最も一般的な型は，卵円孔開存症であり，胎児期のシャントの閉鎖が不完全であったことで生じる．

1 図 7.24（Fritsch and Kühnel による）．p.95　2 図 8.24（Fritsch and Kühnel による）．p.103

Parietal Pleura

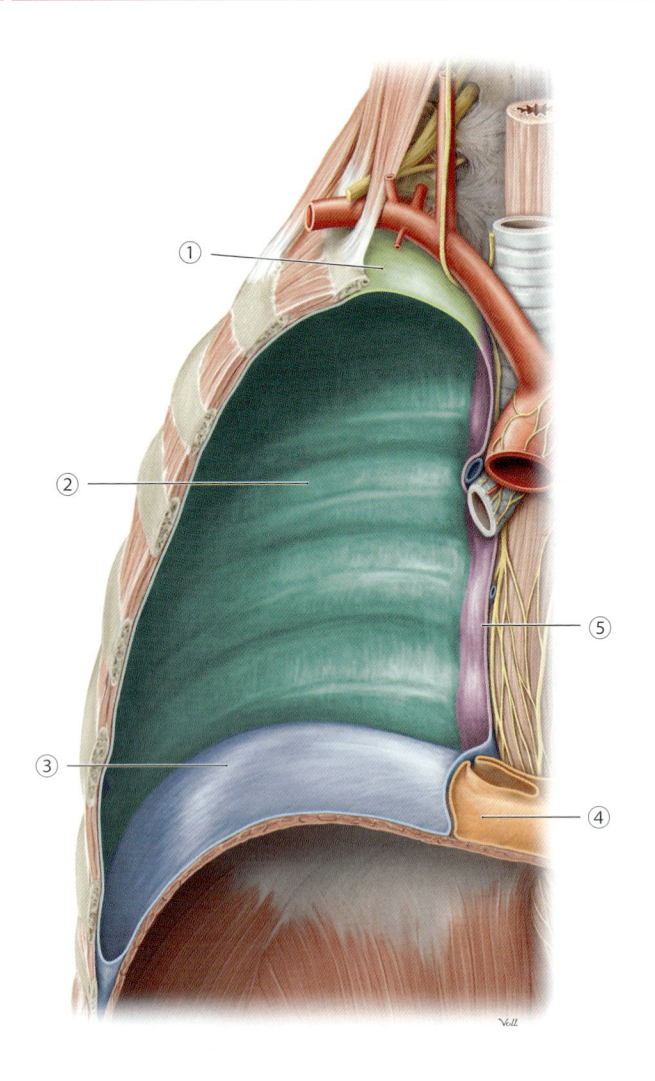

壁側胸膜

右胸膜腔を開く，前面

① □ 胸膜頂　　　　　　　　　　□ Cervical part

② □ 肋骨部（肋骨胸膜）　　　　□ Costal part

③ □ 横隔部（横隔胸膜）　　　　□ Diaphragmatic part

④ □ 線維性心膜　　　　　　　　□ Fibrous pericardium

⑤ □ 縦隔部（縦隔胸膜）　　　　□ Mediastinal part

解説

　胸膜腔は2つの漿膜で囲まれる．臓側胸膜（肺胸膜）は肺を包み，壁側胸膜は胸腔の内面を覆う．壁側胸膜の4つの部分である肋骨胸膜，横隔胸膜，縦隔胸膜，胸膜頂は連続している．

1 図 8.3A. p.103　　2 図 9.2A. p.111

Lungs in Situ

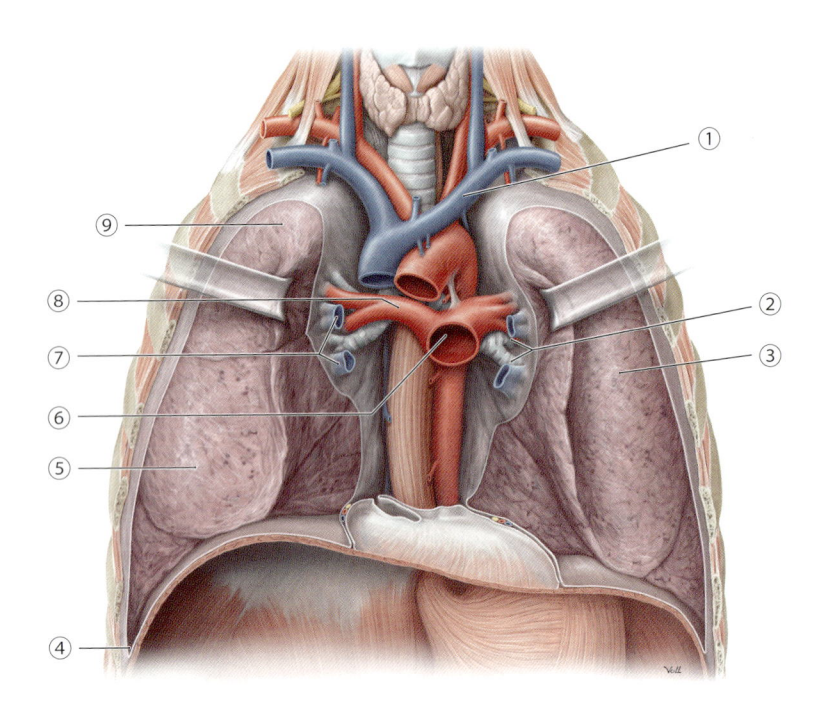

原位置の肺

前面

① □ 左腕頭静脈 — □ Left brachiocephalic vein
② □ 上・下葉気管支 — □ Superior and inferior lobar bronchi
③ □ 左肺（上葉） — □ Left lung (superior lobe)
④ □ 肋骨横隔洞 — □ Costodiaphragmatic recess
⑤ □ 右肺（中葉） — □ Right lung (middle lobe)
⑥ □ 肺動脈幹 — □ Pulmonary trunk
⑦ □ 右肺静脈 — □ Right pulmonary veins
⑧ □ 右肺動脈 — □ Right pulmonary artery
⑨ □ 肺尖 — □ Pulmonary apex

解説

両肺は胸膜腔全体を占めている．心臓の位置のズレのために，左肺は右肺よりもわずかに小さい．

[1] 図 8.4B, p.104　[2] 図 9.6B, p.114

Right Lung

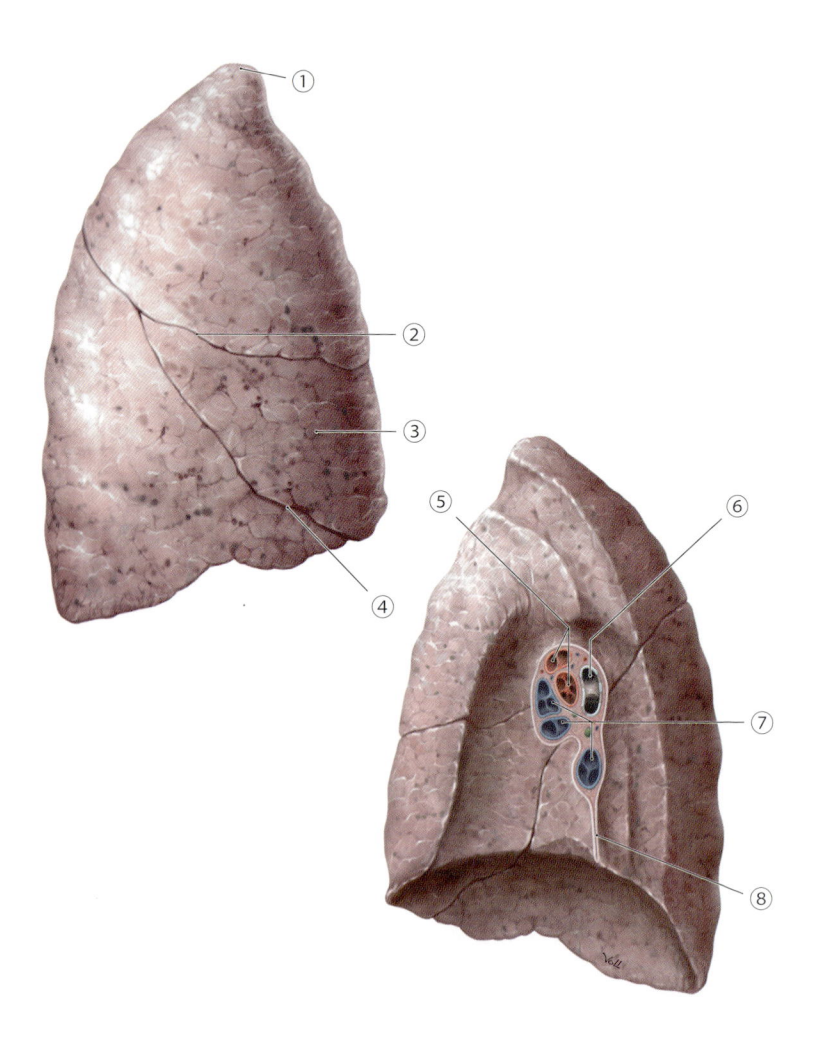

右肺

上:外側面, 下:内側面

① □ 肺尖 □ Apex
② □ 水平裂 □ Horizontal fissure
③ □ 中葉 □ Middle lobe
④ □ 斜裂 □ Oblique fissure
⑤ □ 右肺動脈の枝 □ Branches of right pulmonary artery
⑥ □ 上葉気管支斜裂 □ Superior lobar bronchus
⑦ □ 右肺静脈の枝 □ Branches of right pulmonary veins
⑧ □ 肺間膜 □ Pulmonary ligament

解説

右肺は斜裂と水平裂によって上葉・中葉・下葉の3葉に分けられる.両肺の肺尖は頸の基部に入りこんでいる.

1 図 8.5A,C. p.105   2 図 9.7A,C. p.115

Left Lung

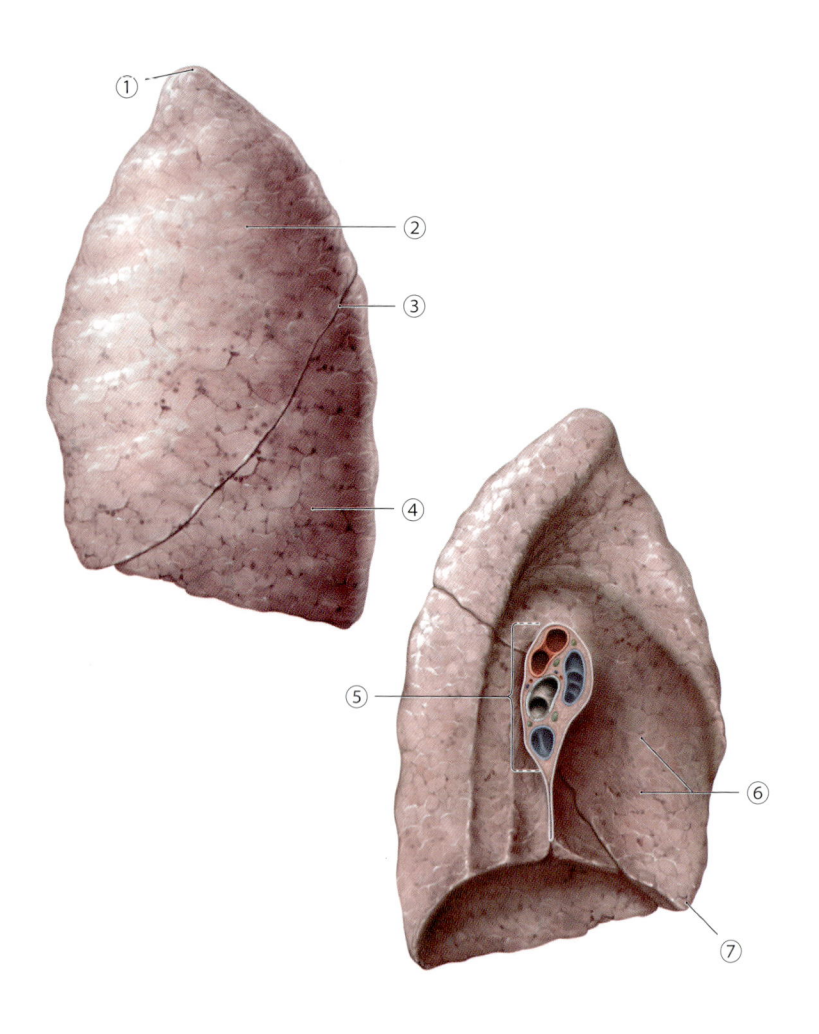

左肺

上:外側面,下:内側面

① □ 肺尖　　　　　　　□ Apex

② □ 上葉　　　　　　　□ Superior lobe

③ □ 斜裂　　　　　　　□ Oblique fissure

④ □ 下葉　　　　　　　□ Inferior lobe

⑤ □ 肺門　　　　　　　□ Hilum

⑥ □ 心圧痕　　　　　　□ Cardiac impression

⑦ □ 小舌　　　　　　　□ Lingula

解説

左肺は斜裂によって上葉と下葉に分けられる．肺門は気管支や神経・脈管が肺に出入りする部位．

1 図 8.5B,D. p.105　2 図 9.7B,D. p.115

Trachea

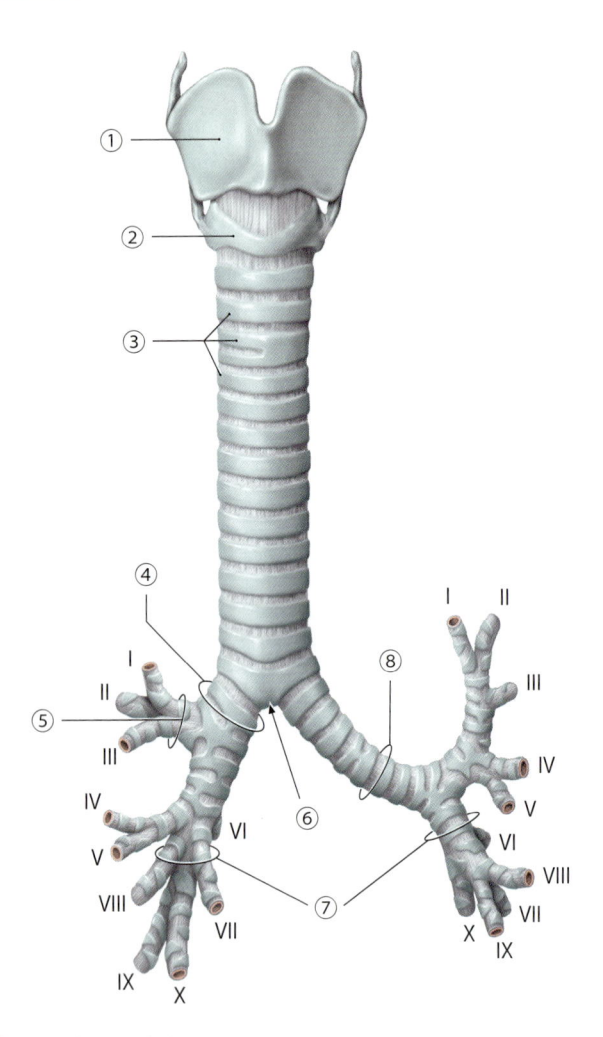

気管竜骨とは何か？

気管

前面

① □ 甲状軟骨 　　　　　　□ Thyroid cartilage
② □ 輪状軟骨 　　　　　　□ Cricoid cartilage
③ □ 気管軟骨 　　　　　　□ Tracheal cartilages
④ □ 右主気管支 　　　　　□ Right main bronchus
⑤ □ 右上葉気管支 　　　　□ Right superior lobar bronchus
⑥ □ 気管分岐部 　　　　　□ Tracheal bifurcation
⑦ □ 右・左下葉気管支 　　□ Right / left inferior lobar bronchi
⑧ □ 左主気管支 　　　　　□ Left main bronchus

A 気管竜骨は気管の最下部にあり，左主気管支と右主気管支を分ける．

[1] 図 8.12B. p.110　[2] 図 9.14B. p.120

Divisions of the Bronchial Tree

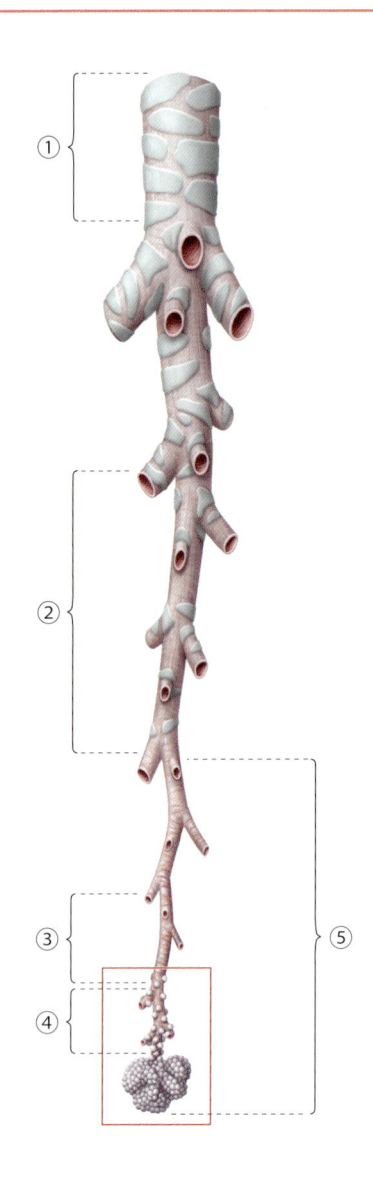

気管支樹の区分

① ☐ 区域気管支 　　　　　　　☐ Segmental bronchus
② ☐ 小さい亜区域気管支 　　　☐ Small subsegmental bronchus
③ ☐ 終末細気管支 　　　　　　☐ Terminal bronchiole
④ ☐ 呼吸細気管支 　　　　　　☐ Respiratory bronchiole
⑤ ☐ 細気管支（軟骨がない） 　 ☐ Bronchiole（cartilage-free wall）

解説

気管支樹の伝導部は気管分岐部から終末細気管支に及び，呼吸部は呼吸細気管支，肺胞管，肺胞嚢，肺胞を含む．

１ 図 8.13A. p.111　 ２ 図 9.15A. p.121

Respiratory Portion of the Bronchial Tree

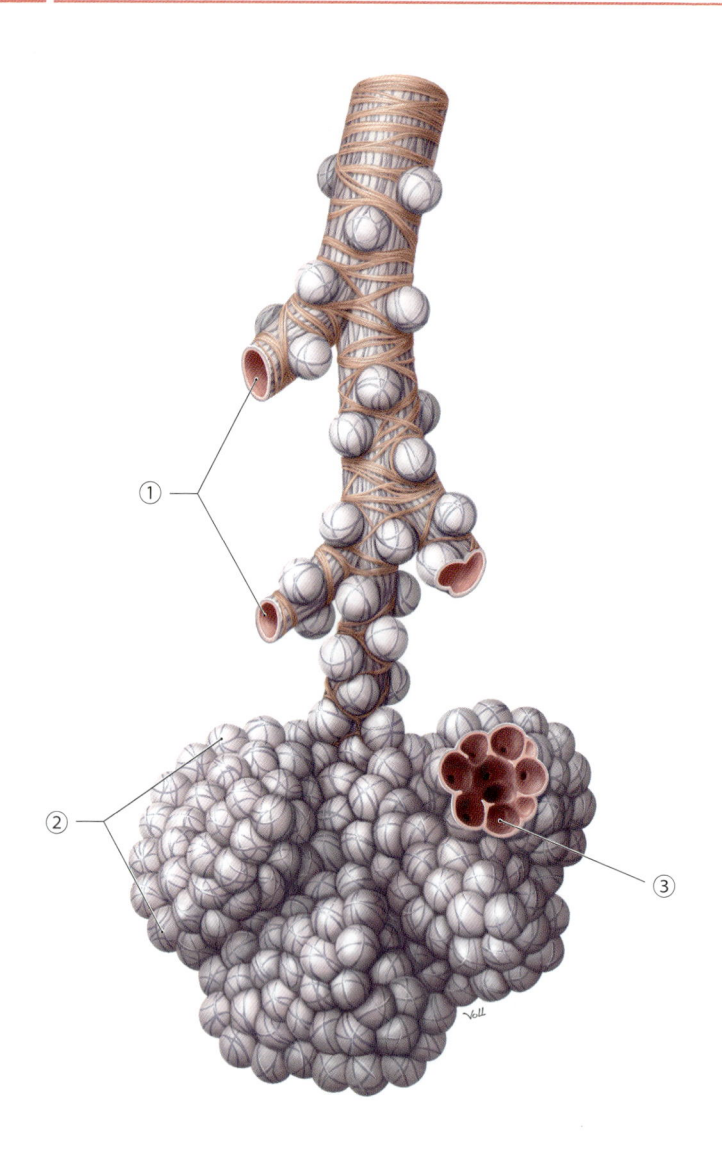

気管支樹の呼吸部

① □ 呼吸細気管支　　　　　　□ Respiratory bronchioles

② □ 肺胞嚢　　　　　　　　　□ Alveolar sac

③ □ 肺胞　　　　　　　　　　□ Alveolus

臨床

気管支レベルでの呼吸器不全の最も一般的な原因は喘息である．肺胞レベルでの呼吸不全は拡散距離の増大，低換気(肺気腫)，液体浸潤(肺炎など)から起こる．

1 図 8.13B. p.111　　2 図 9.15B. p.121

160 Thorax

Pulmonary Arteries & Veins

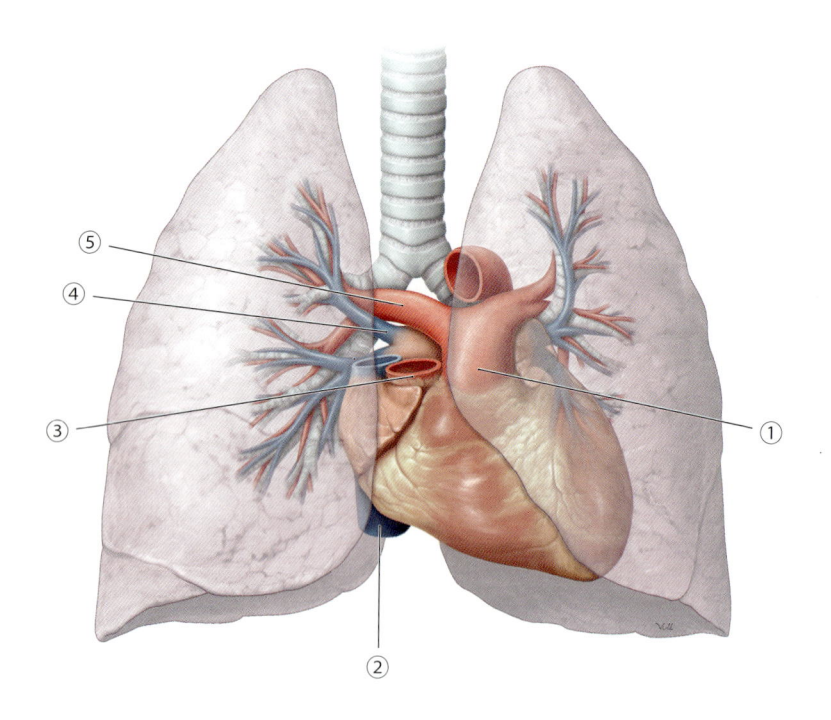

肺動脈と肺静脈

前面

① □ 肺動脈幹　　　　　　□ Pulmonary trunk
② □ 下大静脈　　　　　　□ Inferior vena cava
③ □ 上行大動脈　　　　　□ Ascending aorta
④ □ 右上肺静脈　　　　　□ Superior right pulmonary vein
⑤ □ 右肺動脈　　　　　　□ Right pulmonary artery

解説

　肺動脈は右心室から起こり，両肺への左右の肺動脈に分かれる．肺静脈が左右それぞれ2本ずつ両側から左心房に注ぐ．肺動脈は気管支樹に沿って，追随しながら分岐していくが，肺静脈は肺小葉の辺縁部にあり，気管支樹に随伴しない．

1 図 8.21C. p.114　 2 図 9.23C. p.124

Lymph Nodes of the Pleural Cavity

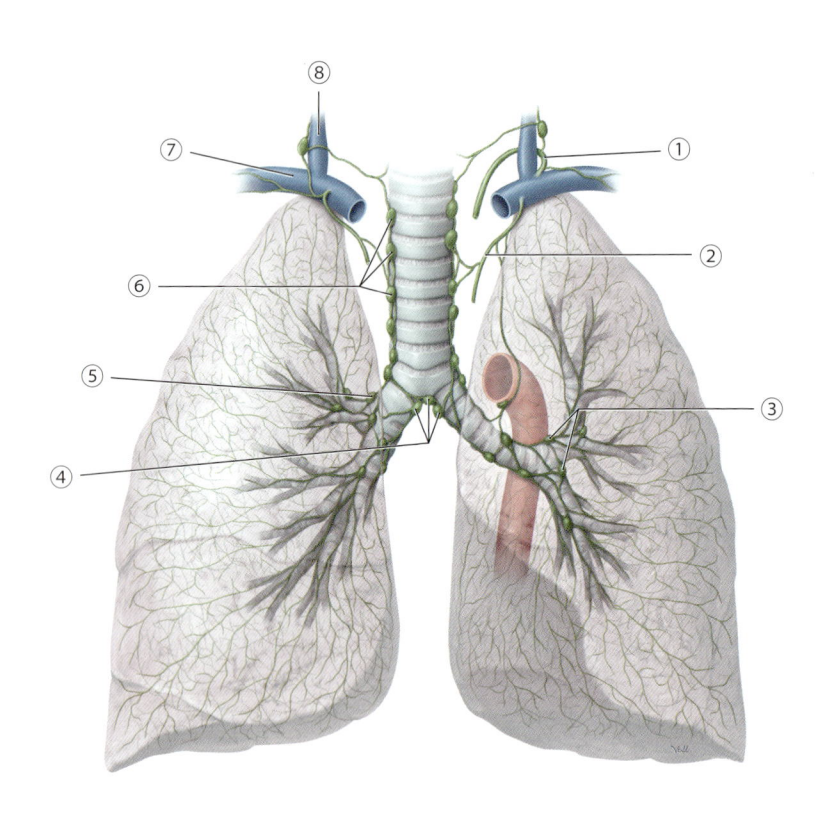

各肺のリンパ流路はどのようなものか？

胸膜腔のリンパ節

前面

① □ 胸管　　　　　　　　　　　□ Thoracic duct
② □ 左気管支縦隔リンパ本幹　　　□ Left broncho-mediastinal trunk
③ □ 気管支肺リンパ節　　　　　　□ Bronchopulmonary lymph node
④ □ 下気管気管支リンパ節　　　　□ Inferior tracheobronchial lymph node
⑤ □ 上気管気管支リンパ節　　　　□ Superior tracheobronchial lymph node
⑥ □ 気管傍リンパ節　　　　　　　□ Paratracheal lymph node
⑦ □ 右鎖骨下静脈　　　　　　　　□ Right subclavian vein
⑧ □ 右内頸静脈　　　　　　　　　□ Right internal jugular vein

A 　右肺と左肺の下半分は右側の気管気管支リンパ節に流入する．左側の気管気管支リンパ節に流入するのは左肺の上葉だけである．

Surface Anatomy

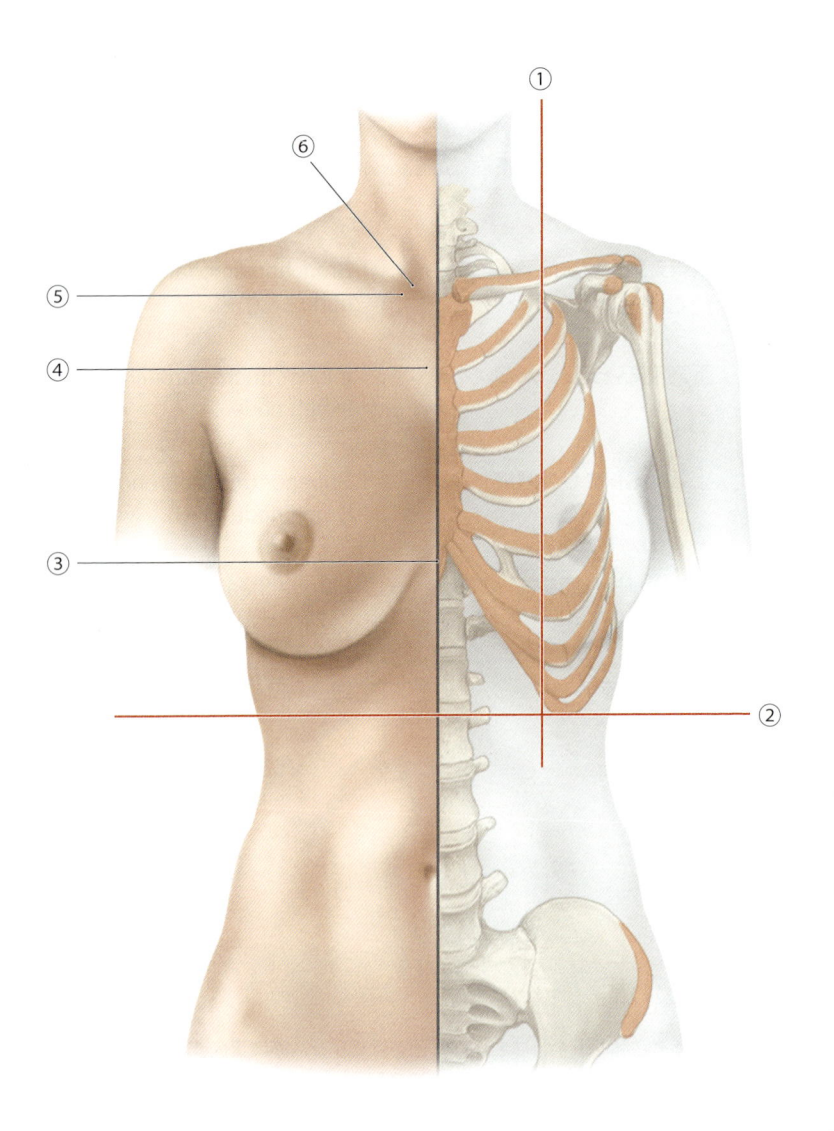

胸部の体表解剖

胸部の触知可能構造，前面

① ☐ 鎖骨中線　　　　　　　　☐ Midclavicular line (MCL)

② ☐ 肋骨下平面　　　　　　　☐ Subcostal plane

③ ☐ 剣状突起　　　　　　　　☐ Xiphoid process

④ ☐ 胸骨角　　　　　　　　　☐ Sternal angle

⑤ ☐ 鎖骨，内側頭　　　　　　☐ Clavicle, medial head

⑥ ☐ 頸切痕　　　　　　　　　☐ Jugular notch

1 図 9.1A. p.120　2 図 5.2A. p.50

腹部・骨盤 Abdomen & Pelvis

寛骨	168
下肢帯	170
骨盤の靱帯1	172
骨盤の靱帯2	174
腹壁の筋1	176
腹壁の筋2	178
腹壁の筋3	180
鼡径部1	182
鼡径部2	184
男性の骨盤底	186
女性の骨盤底1	188
女性の骨盤底2	190
腹腔：骨盤腔	192
腹膜腔	194
網嚢	196
腸間膜と臓器	198
腹膜腔の後壁	200
男性骨盤の内容	202
女性骨盤の内容	204
腹部の水平断面	206
原位置の胃	208
十二指腸	210
大腸	212
原位置の直腸	214
直腸と肛門管	216
肝臓の表面1	218
肝臓の表面2	220
肝外胆管	222
原位置の胆路	224
膵臓	226
原位置の腎臓と尿管	228
女性の膀胱と尿道	230
膀胱三角	232
子宮と卵管1	234
子宮と卵管2	236
女性の外生殖器	238
女性の勃起組織	240
女性会陰の神経・血管	242
陰茎の横断面	244
陰茎	246
精巣と精巣上体	248
精巣の被膜	250
男性の付属生殖腺	252
原位置の前立腺	254
男性会陰の神経・血管	256
腹大動脈	258
腎動脈	260
腹腔動脈1	262
腹腔動脈2	264
上腸間膜動脈	266
下腸間膜動脈	268
下大静脈の支脈	270
腎動脈・静脈	272
門脈の分布	274
原位置の門脈	276
女性骨盤の血管	278
直腸の血管	280
男性生殖器の血管	282
壁側リンパ節	284
自律神経叢	286
女性骨盤の神経支配	288
男性骨盤の神経支配	290
腹部・骨盤の体表解剖	292

Hip Bone

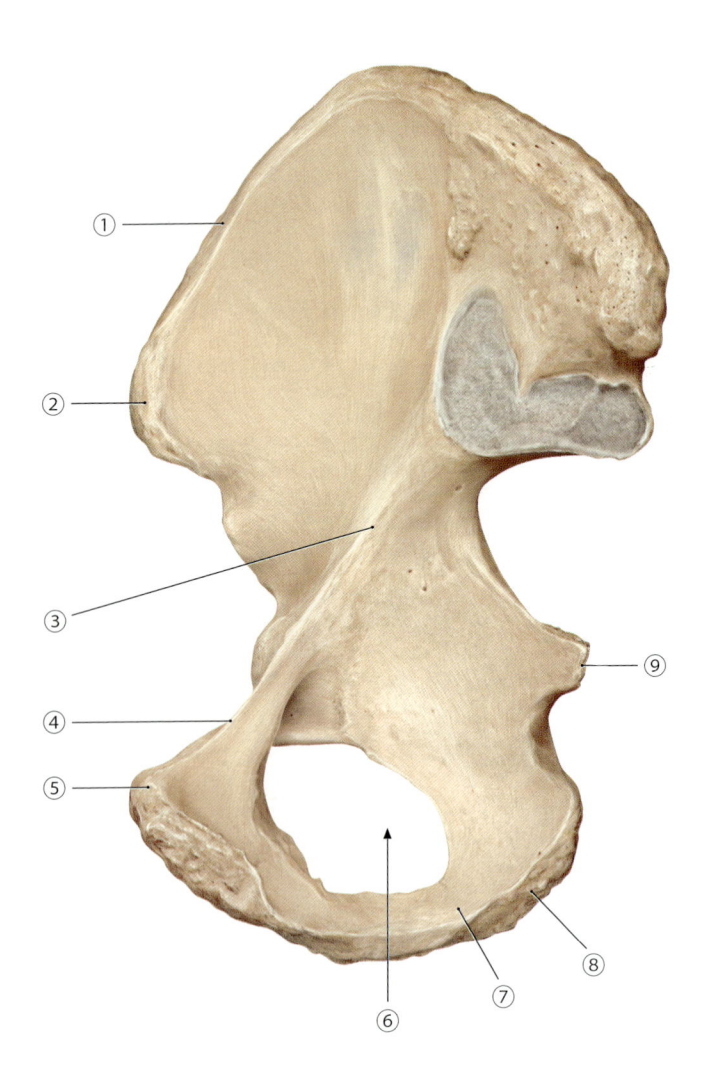

寛骨

内側面

① ☐ 腸骨稜　　　　　　　☐ Iliac crest

② ☐ 上前腸骨棘　　　　　☐ Anterior superior iliac spine

③ ☐ 弓状線　　　　　　　☐ Arcuate line

④ ☐ 恥骨筋線　　　　　　☐ Pectineal line

⑤ ☐ 恥骨結節　　　　　　☐ Pubic tubercle

⑥ ☐ 閉鎖孔　　　　　　　☐ Obturator foramen

⑦ ☐ 坐骨枝　　　　　　　☐ Ischial ramus

⑧ ☐ 坐骨結節　　　　　　☐ Ischial tuberosity

⑨ ☐ 坐骨棘　　　　　　　☐ Ischial spine

1 図 10.2B. p.124　　2 図 16.1B. p.216

Pelvic Girdle

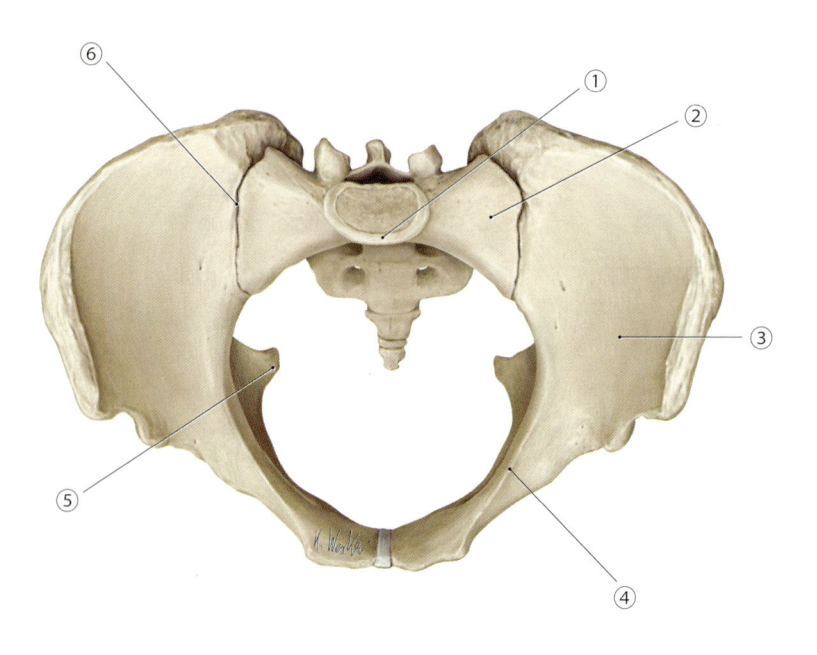

骨盤上口の境界をなすのは何か？

下肢帯

女性骨盤 Female pelvis，上面

① □ 岬角　　　　　　　　□ Promontory

② □ 仙骨翼　　　　　　　□ Ala of sacrum

③ □ 腸骨窩　　　　　　　□ Iliac fossa

④ □ 恥骨櫛　　　　　　　□ Pecten pubis

⑤ □ 坐骨棘　　　　　　　□ Ischial spine

⑥ □ 仙腸関節　　　　　　□ Sacroiliac joint

A 　骨盤上口は恥骨結合の上縁，恥骨稜，恥骨櫛，腸骨の弓状線，仙骨翼の前縁，仙骨の岬角からなる．

[1] 図 10.7B．p.127　[2] 図 16.5C．p.218

Pelvic Ligaments I

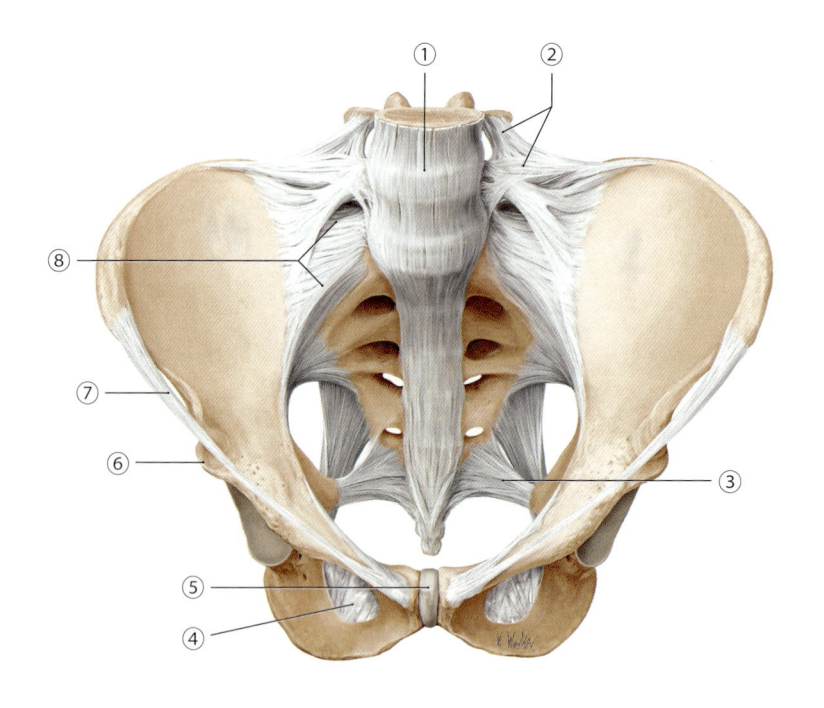

骨盤の靱帯 1

男性骨盤 Male pelvis，前上面

① □ 前縦靱帯　　　　　　　　□ Anterior longitudinal ligament
② □ 腸腰靱帯　　　　　　　　□ Iliolumbar ligament
③ □ 仙棘靱帯　　　　　　　　□ Sacrospinous ligament
④ □ 閉鎖膜　　　　　　　　　□ Obturator membrane
⑤ □ 恥骨結合　　　　　　　　□ Pubic symphysis
⑥ □ 下前腸骨棘　　　　　　　□ Anterior inferior iliac spine
⑦ □ 鼡径靱帯　　　　　　　　□ Inguinal ligament
⑧ □ 前仙腸靱帯　　　　　　　□ Anterior sacroiliac ligaments

1 図 10.9A. p.128　2 図 11.2A. p.134（または図 16.10A. p. 222）

Pelvic Ligaments II

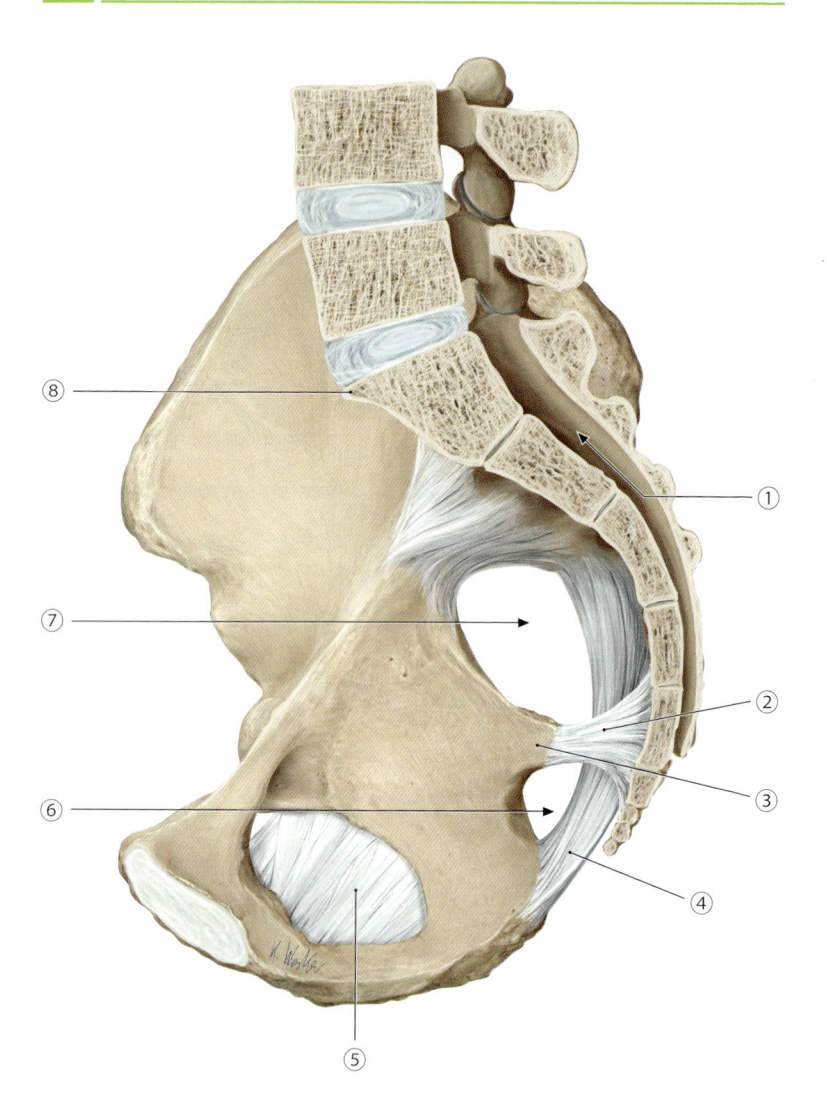

骨盤の靱帯 2

骨盤の右半分，内側面

① □ 仙骨管　　　　　　□ Sacral canal
② □ 仙棘靱帯　　　　　□ Sacrospinous ligament
③ □ 坐骨棘　　　　　　□ Ischial spine
④ □ 仙結節靱帯　　　　□ Sacrotuberous ligament
⑤ □ 閉鎖膜　　　　　　□ Obturator membrane
⑥ □ 小坐骨孔　　　　　□ Lesser sciatic foramen
⑦ □ 大坐骨孔　　　　　□ Greater sciatic foramen
⑧ □ 岬角　　　　　　　□ Promontory

1 図 10.10A. p.129　2 図 16.11A. p.223

Abdominal Wall Muscles I

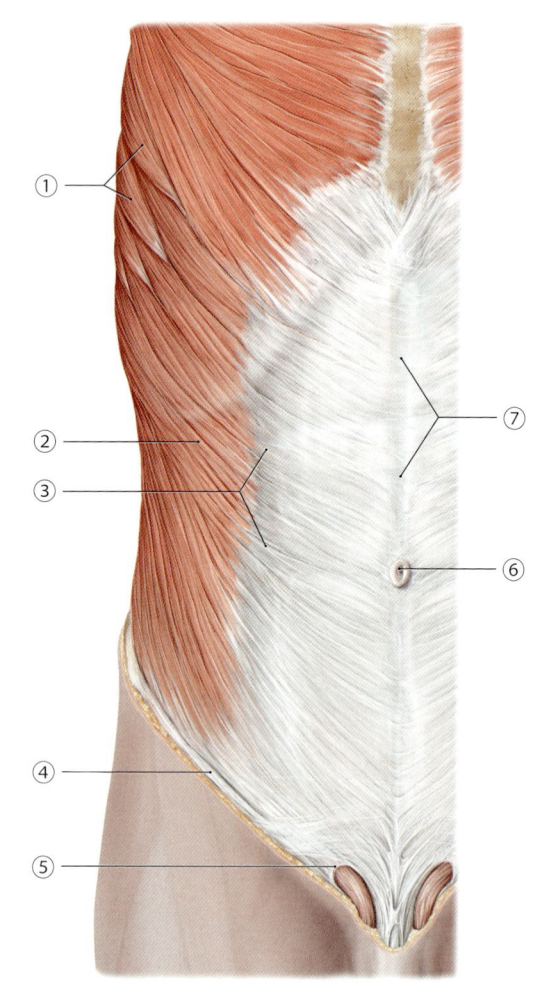

白線とは何か？

腹壁の筋 1

浅層の筋 Superficial muscles，前面

① ☐ 前鋸筋　　　　　　　☐ Serratus anterior
② ☐ 外腹斜筋　　　　　　☐ External oblique
③ ☐ 外腹斜筋の腱膜　　　☐ External oblique aponeurosis
④ ☐ 鼡径靱帯　　　　　　☐ Inguinal ligament
⑤ ☐ 浅鼡径輪　　　　　　☐ Superficial inguinal ring
⑥ ☐ 臍　　　　　　　　　☐ Umbilicus
⑦ ☐ 白線　　　　　　　　☐ Linea alba

A 白線は正中線上を剣状突起から恥骨まで伸びる．白線は左右の前側腹壁にある筋肉の腱膜の線維が重なり合ってできる比較的血管の少ない面であり，しばしば外科手術において切開される．

1 図 11.1A, p.130　2 図 11.4A, p.136

Abdominal Wall Muscles II

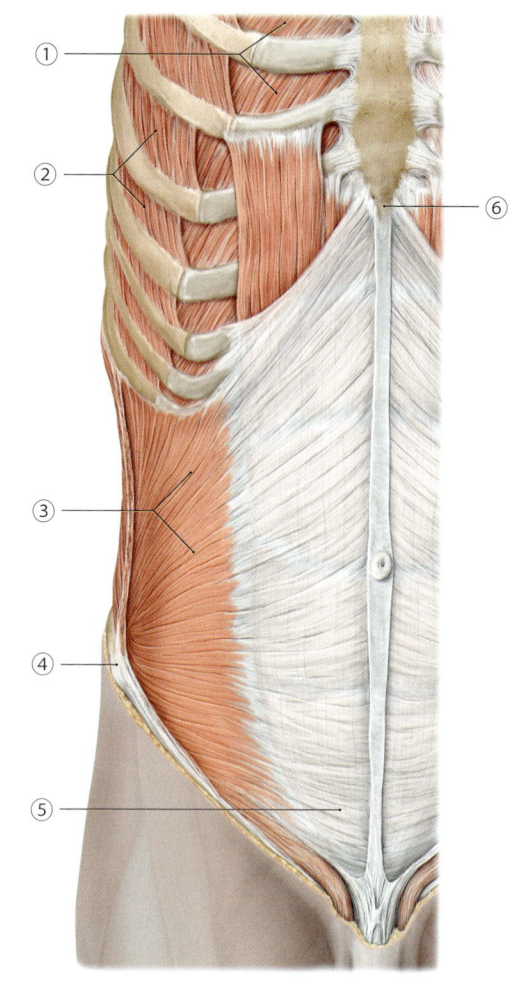

前側腹壁の支配神経は何か？

腹壁の筋 2

中層の筋 Intermediate muscles，**前面**

① □ 内肋間筋　　　　　　　　□ Internal intercostals
② □ 外肋間筋　　　　　　　　□ External intercostals
③ □ 内腹斜筋　　　　　　　　□ Internal oblique
④ □ 上前腸骨棘　　　　　　　□ Anterior superior iliac spine
⑤ □ 腹直筋鞘，前葉　　　　　□ Anterior rectus sheath
⑥ □ 剣状突起　　　　　　　　□ Xiphoid process

A 　前側腹壁の筋肉（外腹斜筋，内腹斜筋，腹横筋）はT7-T12の肋間神経によって支配される．デルマトームの指標として，T10が臍を支配することが用いられる．

1 図 11.1B. p.130　　2 図 11.4B. p.136

Abdominal Wall Muscles III

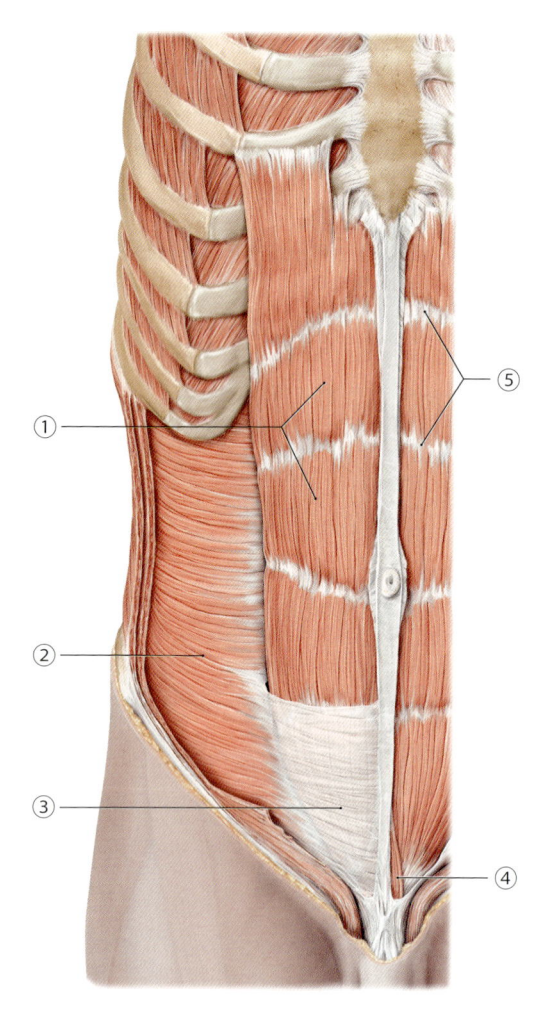

Q 弓状線より下の部分の腹直筋鞘の前葉と後葉を構成するのは何か？

腹壁の筋 3

深層の筋 Deep muscles，前面

① ☐ 腹直筋 ☐ Rectus abdominis
② ☐ 腹横筋 ☐ Transversus abdominis
③ ☐ 腹横筋の腱膜（腹直筋鞘，前葉） ☐ Transversus abdominis aponeurosis（anterior rectus sheath）
④ ☐ 錐体筋 ☐ Pyramidalis
⑤ ☐ 腱画 ☐ Tendinous intersections

A 弓状線より下では，腹壁筋の腱膜は腹直筋の前面に集まり，腹直筋鞘の前葉を構成する．後葉は横筋筋膜と壁側筋膜からのみなる．

1 図 11.1C. p.131 2 図 11.4C. p.137

Inguinal Region I

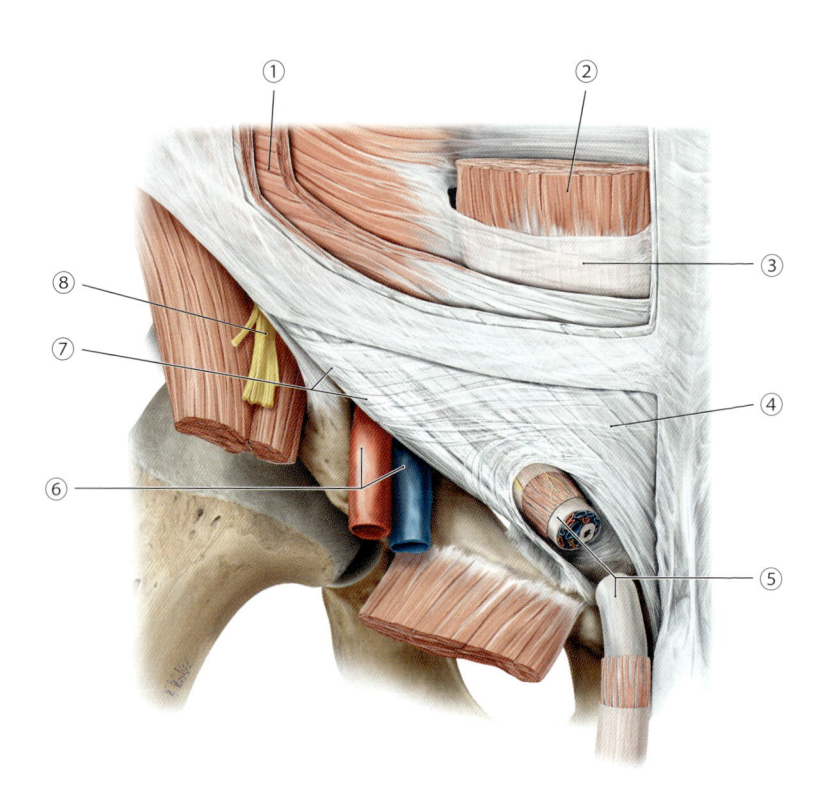

Q 鼠径管の経路を説明せよ．

鼡径部 1

右側，前面

① □ 内腹斜筋 　　　　　　　□ Internal oblique
② □ 腹直筋 　　　　　　　　□ Rectus abdominis
③ □ 腹直筋鞘，前葉 　　　　□ Anterior rectus sheath
④ □ 外腹斜筋の腱膜 　　　　□ External oblique aponeurosis
⑤ □ 精索 　　　　　　　　　□ Spermatic cord
⑥ □ 大腿動脈・静脈 　　　　□ Femoral artery and vein
⑦ □ 鼡径靱帯 　　　　　　　□ Inguinal ligament
⑧ □ 大腿神経 　　　　　　　□ Femoral nerve

A 　鼡径管は前腹壁の下部を斜めに貫通し，最深層外側の深鼡径輪から始まる．深鼡径輪は鼡径靱帯の中点のやや外側にあり，鼡径管の最浅層は内側で終わり，恥骨結節の外側で浅鼡径輪が開口する．

1 図 11.2. p.132　　2 図 11.11A. p.142

Inguinal Region II

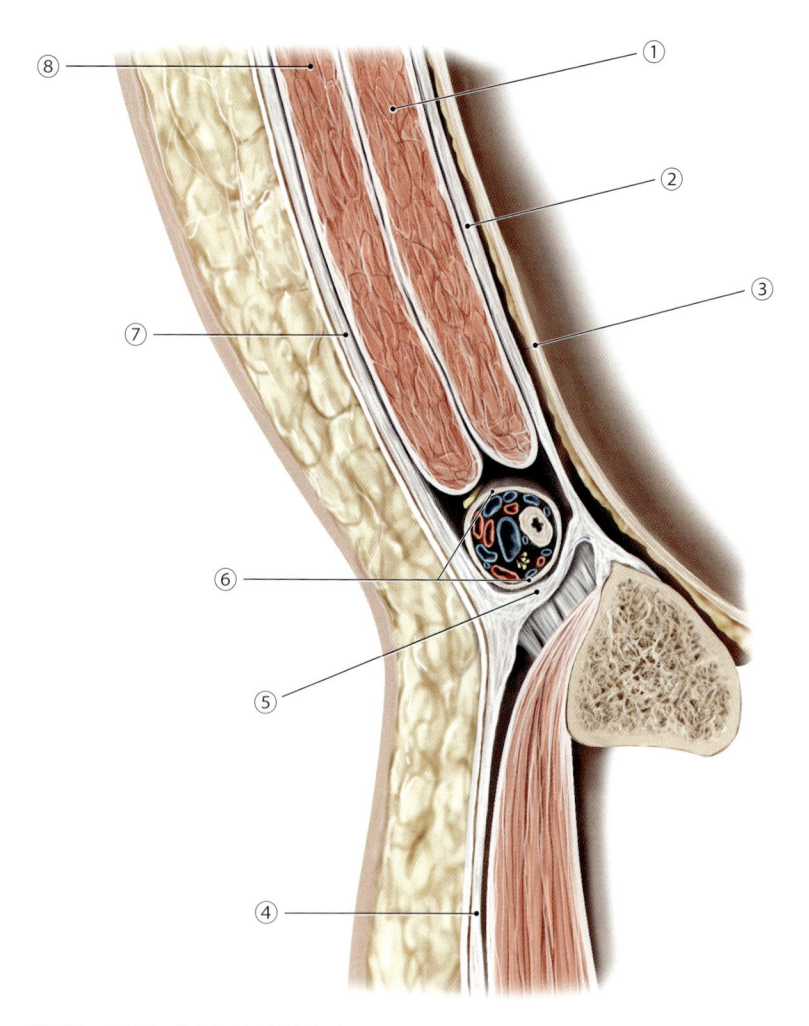

Q 精索に含まれるのは何か？

鼡径部 2

矢状断面

① □ 腹横筋　　　　　　　　　□ Transversus abdominis
② □ 横筋筋膜　　　　　　　　□ Transversalis fascia
③ □ 壁側腹膜　　　　　　　　□ Parietal peritoneum
④ □ 大腿筋膜　　　　　　　　□ Fascia lata
⑤ □ 鼡径靱帯　　　　　　　　□ Inguinal ligament
⑥ □ 精索　　　　　　　　　　□ Spermatic cord
⑦ □ 外腹斜筋の腱膜　　　　　□ External oblique aponeurosis
⑧ □ 内腹斜筋　　　　　　　　□ Internal oblique muscles

A 精索には，精管，精巣動脈，蔓状静脈叢，自律神経，リンパ管，鞘状突起の遺残が含まれる．

[1] 表 11.1. p.133　[2] 表 11.3. p.143

Male Pelvic Floor

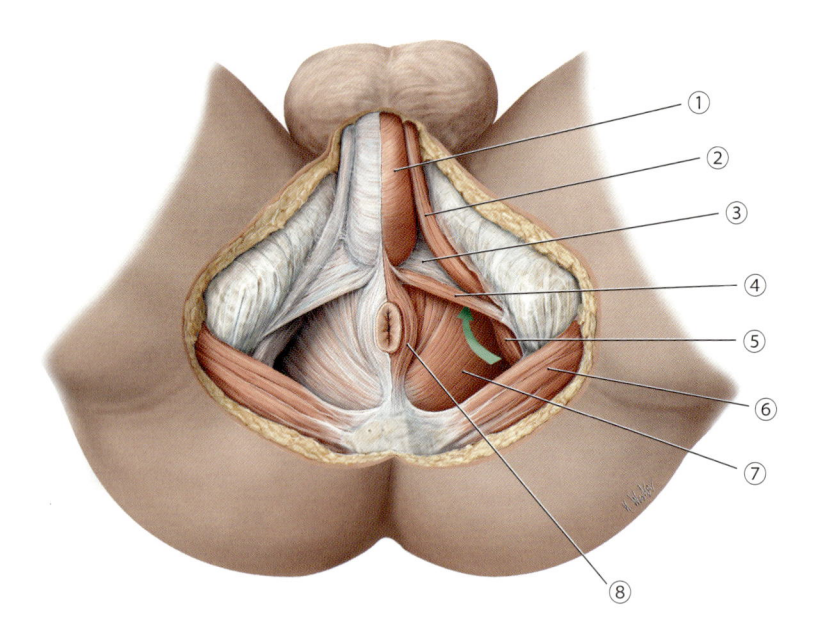

男性の骨盤底

男性の骨盤，切石位，尾側（下面）

① □ 球海綿体筋　　　　　　　　□ Bulbospongiosus

② □ 坐骨海綿体筋　　　　　　　□ Ischiocavernosus

③ □ 下尿生殖隔膜筋膜（会陰膜）　□ Perineal membrane

④ □ 浅会陰横筋　　　　　　　　□ Superficial transverse perineal

⑤ □ 内閉鎖筋　　　　　　　　　□ Obturator internus

⑥ □ 大殿筋　　　　　　　　　　□ Gluteus maximus

⑦ □ 肛門挙筋　　　　　　　　　□ Levator ani

⑧ □ 外肛門括約筋　　　　　　　□ External anal sphincter

解説

男女を問わず会陰の左右の境界をなすのは，恥骨結合，坐骨恥骨枝，坐骨結節，仙結節靱帯，尾骨である．

1 図 11.8B, p.137　　2 図 16.14B, p.225

Female Pelvic Floor I

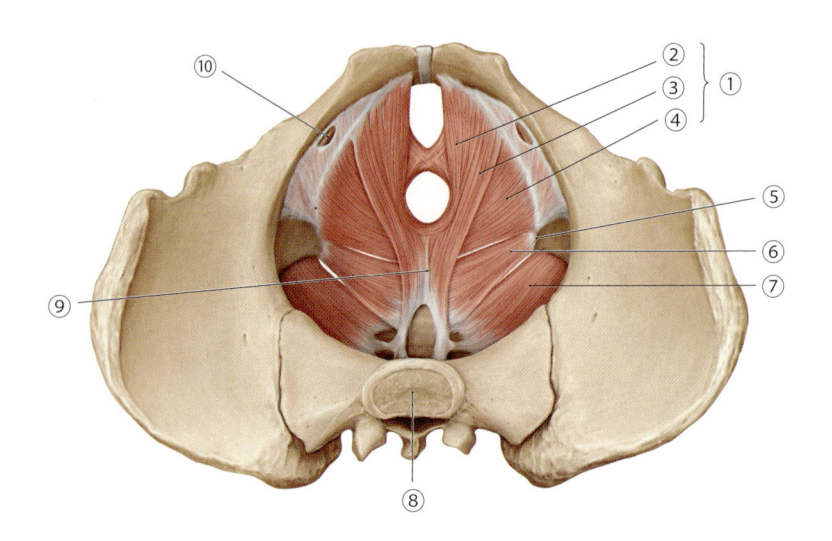

骨盤隔膜をなす筋肉は何か？

女性の骨盤底 1

上面

① □ 肛門挙筋　　　　　　　□ Levator ani
② □ 恥骨直腸筋　　　　　　□ Puborectalis
③ □ 恥骨尾骨筋　　　　　　□ Pubococcygeus
④ □ 腸骨尾骨筋　　　　　　□ Iliococcygeus
⑤ □ 坐骨棘　　　　　　　　□ Ischial spine
⑥ □ 尾骨筋　　　　　　　　□ Coccygeus
⑦ □ 梨状筋　　　　　　　　□ Piriformis
⑧ □ 仙骨　　　　　　　　　□ Sacrum
⑨ □ 肛門尾骨縫線　　　　　□ Anococcygeal raphe
⑩ □ 閉鎖管　　　　　　　　□ Obturator canal

A 　肛門挙筋(恥骨直腸筋, 恥骨尾骨筋, 腸骨尾骨筋)と尾骨筋が骨盤隔膜として知られる骨盤底をなしている.

① 図 11.15A. p.141　② 図 16.13A. p.224

Female Pelvic Floor II

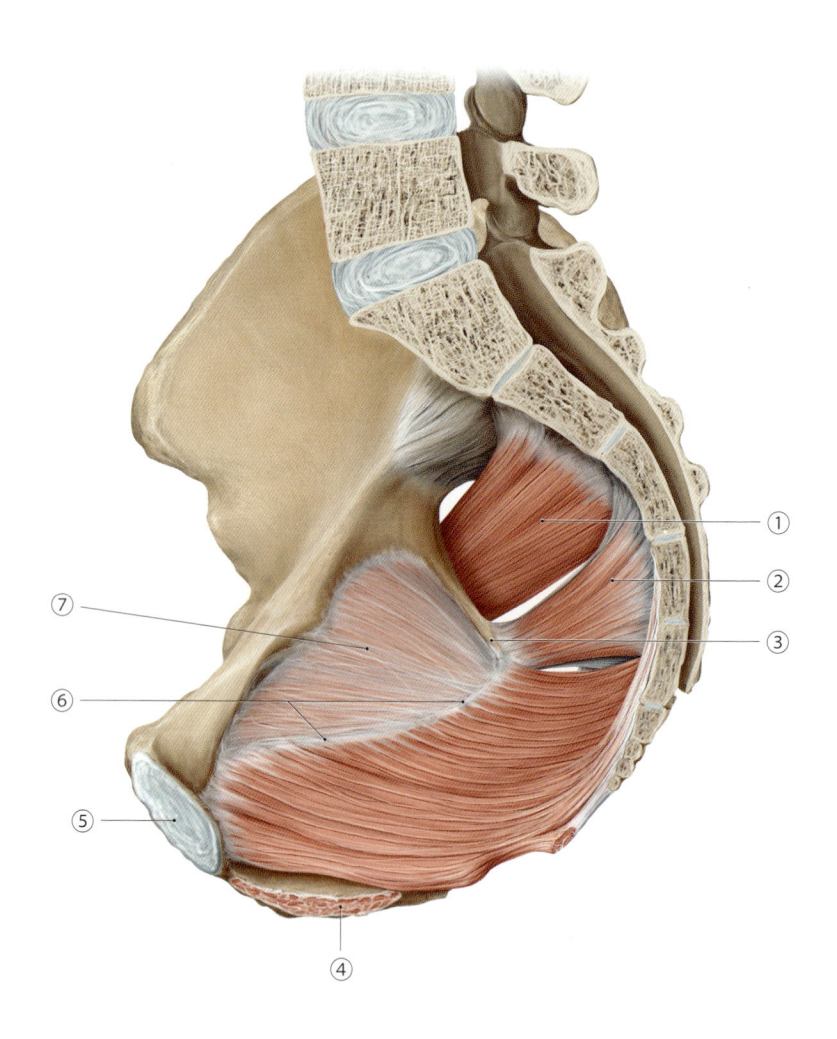

女性の骨盤底 2

骨盤の右半分，内側面

① □ 梨状筋　　　　　　　□ Piriformis
② □ 尾骨筋　　　　　　　□ Coccygeus
③ □ 坐骨棘　　　　　　　□ Ischial spine
④ □ 深会陰横筋　　　　　□ Deep transverse perineal
⑤ □ 恥骨結合　　　　　　□ Pubic symphysis
⑥ □ 肛門挙筋腱弓　　　　□ Tendinous arch of levator ani
⑦ □ 内閉鎖筋筋膜　　　　□ Obturator internus fascia

Abdominopelvic Cavity

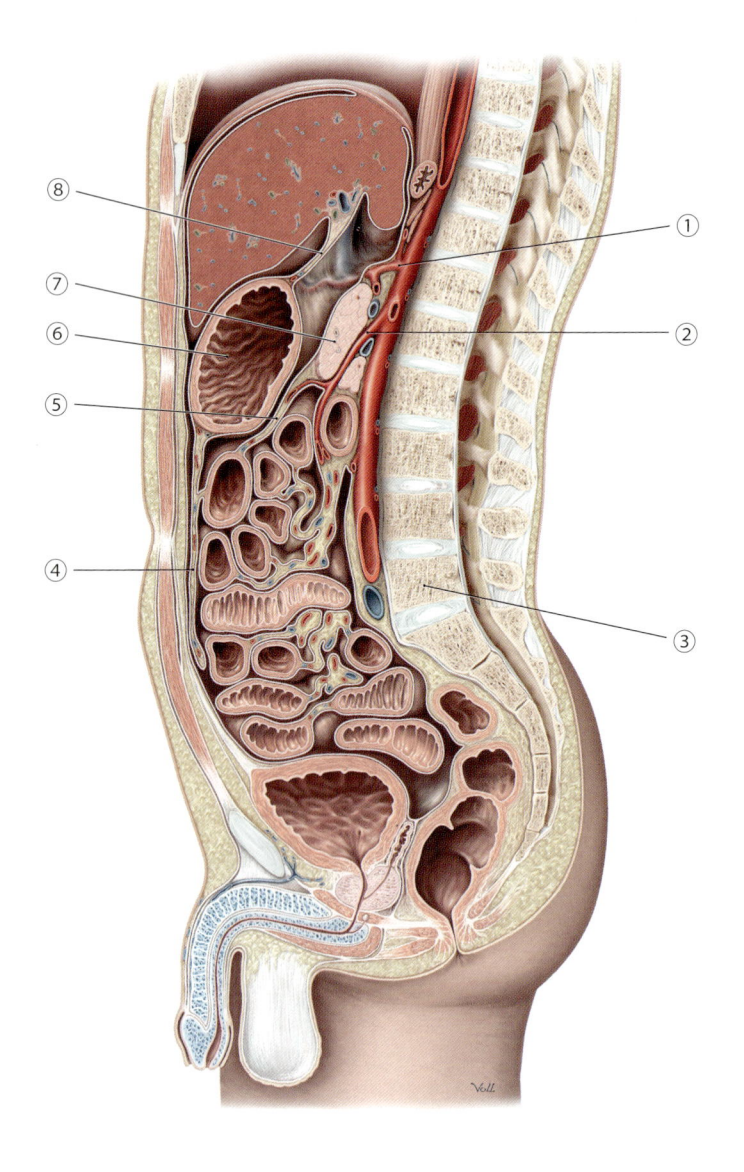

腹腔：骨盤腔

正中矢状断面，左側面

① □ 腹腔動脈　　　　　　　□ Celiac trunk
② □ 上腸間膜動脈　　　　　□ Superior mesenteric artery
③ □ 第5腰椎　　　　　　　 □ L5 vertebra
④ □ 大網　　　　　　　　　□ Greater omentum
⑤ □ 横行結腸間膜　　　　　□ Transverse mesocolon
⑥ □ 胃　　　　　　　　　　□ Stomach
⑦ □ 膵臓　　　　　　　　　□ Pancreas
⑧ □ 肝胃間膜（小網）　　　 □ Hepatogastric ligament

解説

腹膜内器官は臓側腹膜に包まれ，血管と神経を腸間膜を通して受け取る．腹膜後器官は後腹壁に位置し，前面だけが臓側腹膜に覆われる．

① 図 12.3B, p.143　② 図 12.2, p.149

Greater Sac (Peritoneal Cavity)

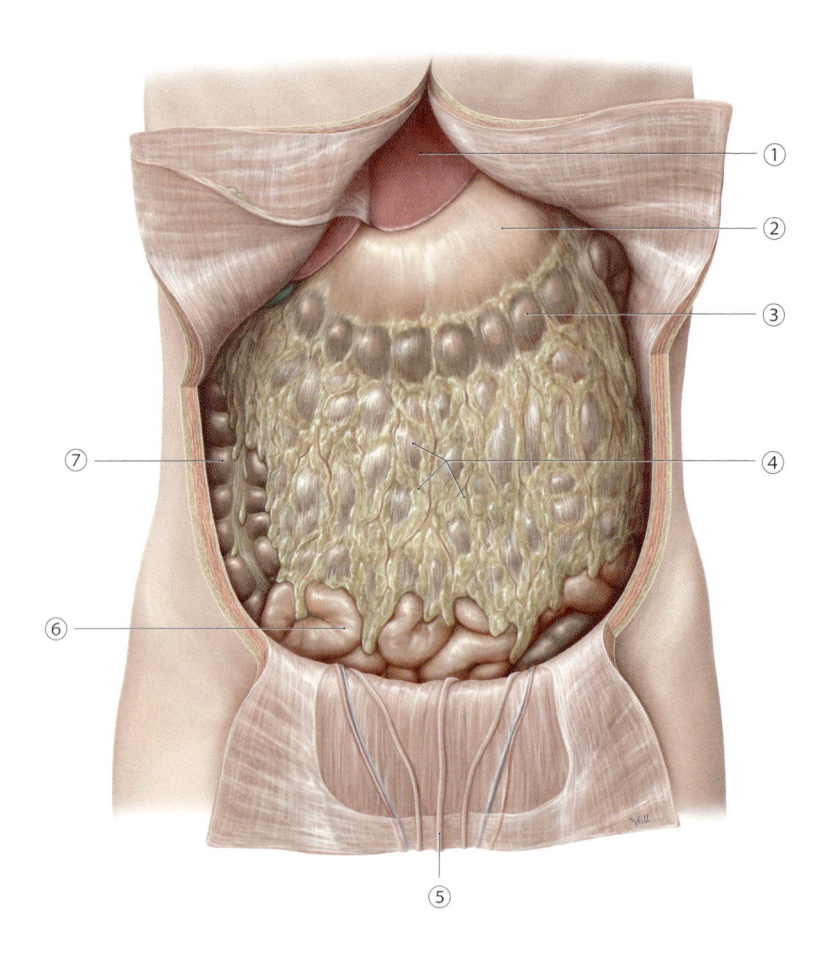

Q 大網とは何か？

腹膜腔

前面

① ☐ 肝臓, 左葉 ☐ Liver, left lobe
② ☐ 胃 ☐ Stomach
③ ☐ 横行結腸 ☐ Transverse colon
④ ☐ 大網 ☐ Greater omentum
⑤ ☐ 正中臍ヒダ(中に閉鎖した尿膜管が走る) ☐ Median umbilical fold (with obliterated urachus)
⑥ ☐ 回腸 ☐ Ileum
⑦ ☐ 上行結腸 ☐ Ascending colon

A 大網は胃の大弯から垂れ下がり, 横行結腸と小腸の前面を覆っているエプロン状の4層の腹膜のヒダである. 横行結腸と小腸の前面で折れ返り, 横行結腸より上では後腹壁に付着する.

1 図 12.4A. p.144 2 図 12.3A. p.150

Omental Bursa

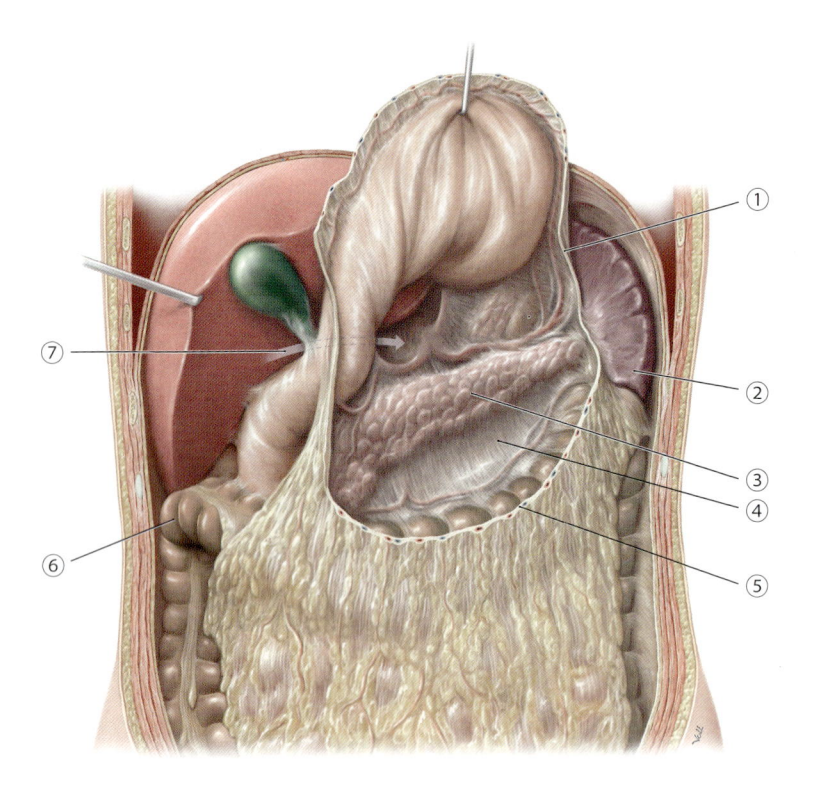

網嚢

前面

① ☐ 胃脾間膜　　　　　　　☐ Gastrosplenic ligament

② ☐ 脾臓　　　　　　　　　☐ Spleen

③ ☐ 膵臓　　　　　　　　　☐ Pancreas

④ ☐ 横行結腸間膜　　　　　☐ Transverse mesocolon

⑤ ☐ 胃結腸間膜　　　　　　☐ Gastrocolic ligament

⑥ ☐ 右結腸曲　　　　　　　☐ Right colic flexure

⑦ ☐ 網嚢孔　　　　　　　　☐ Omental foramen

198 Abdomen & Pelvis

Mesenteries & Organs

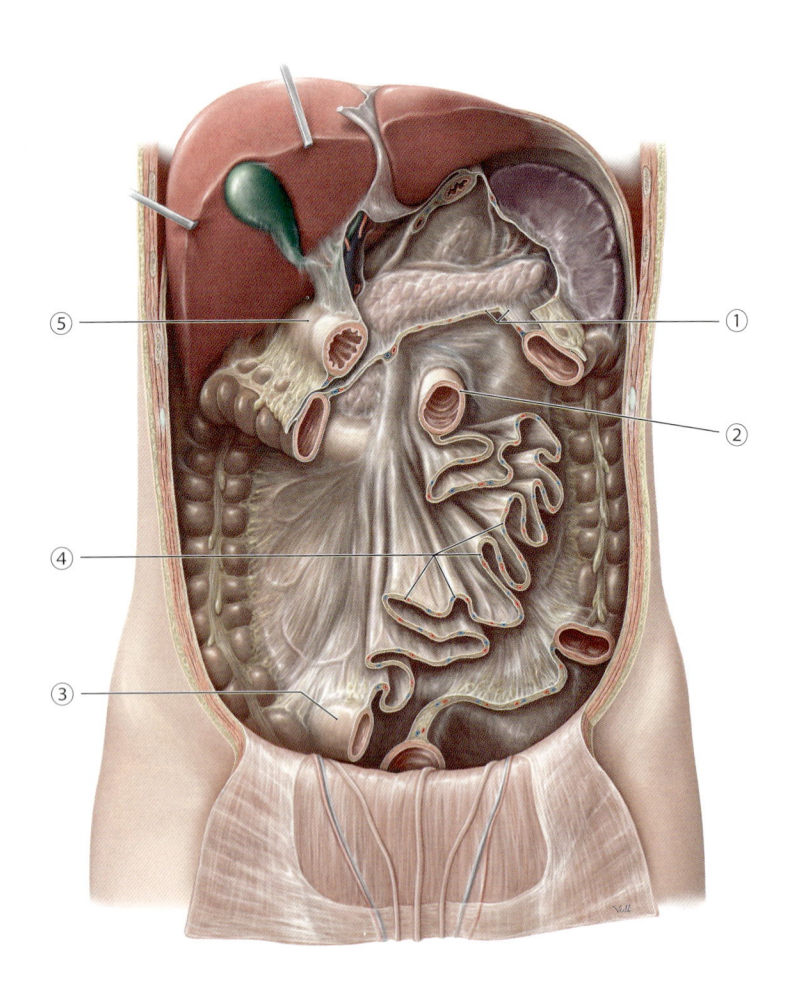

Q 小腸と大腸のうち，腸間膜が付着するのはどの部分か？

腸間膜と臓器

前面

① ☐ 横行結腸間膜，根　　☐ Transverse mesocolon, root

② ☐ 十二指腸空腸曲　　　☐ Duodenojejunal flexure

③ ☐ 回腸　　　　　　　　☐ Ileum

④ ☐ 腸間膜（断端）　　　☐ Mesentery (cut)

⑤ ☐ 十二指腸上部　　　　☐ Duodenum, superior part

A 　小腸の空腸と回腸，大腸の横行結腸とS状結腸は腸間膜によって，吊り下げられている．

1 図 12.8. p.148　2 図 12.7. p.154

Posterior Wall of the Peritoneal Cavity

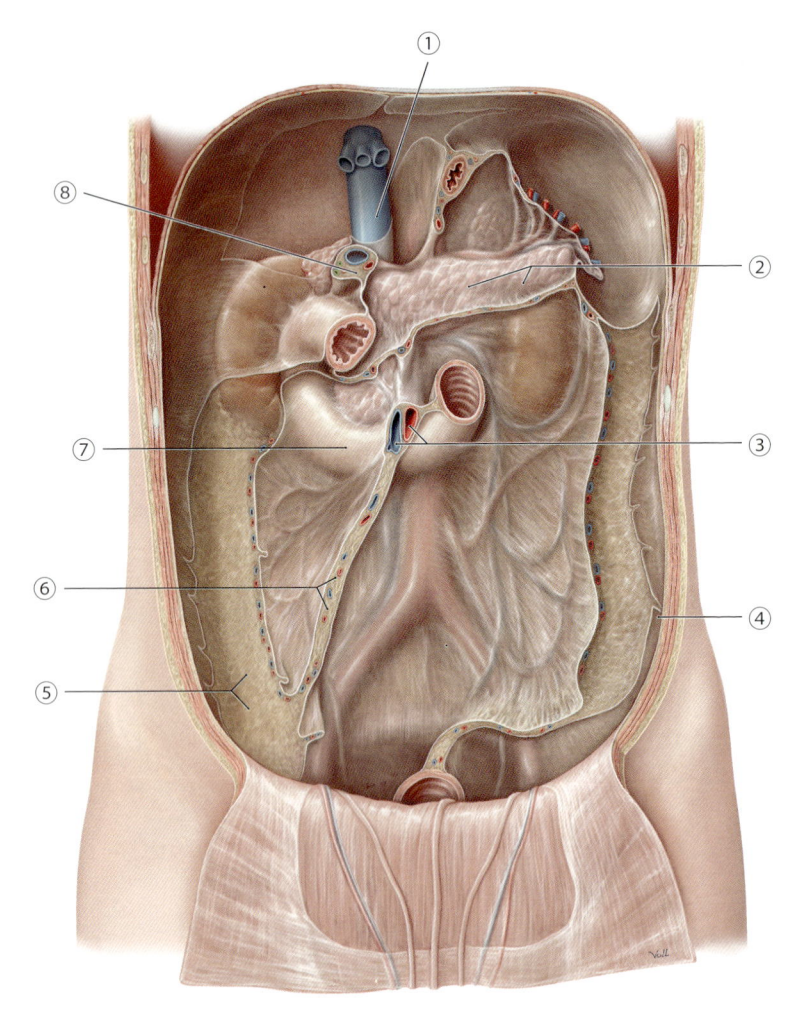

結腸の右下半領域の境界をなすもののうち，排液を制限するのはどれか？

腹膜腔の後壁

前面

① ☐ 下大静脈 — ☐ Inferior vena cava
② ☐ 膵臓（膵体，膵尾） — ☐ Pancreas
③ ☐ 上腸間膜動脈・静脈 — ☐ Superior mesenteric artery and vein
④ ☐ 結腸傍溝 — ☐ Paracolic gutter
⑤ ☐ 上行結腸（付着部） — ☐ Ascending colon (site of attachment)
⑥ ☐ 腸間膜根 — ☐ Mesenteric root
⑦ ☐ 十二指腸水平部 — ☐ Horizontal part of duodenum
⑧ ☐ 肝十二指腸間膜（門脈，固有肝動脈，総胆管が入っている） — ☐ Hepatoduodenal ligament (with portal vein, proper hepatic artery, and common bile duct)

A 結腸の右下半領域は後腹壁上の三角形の部分であり，横行結腸間膜，腸間膜根，上行結腸が境界をなしている．液体の移動はこの境界によって制限されるが，腹膜腔においては結腸傍溝に沿って下へと移動して骨盤に至ることが可能である．

1 図 12.9, p.149　2 図 12.8, p.155

Contents of the Male Pelvis

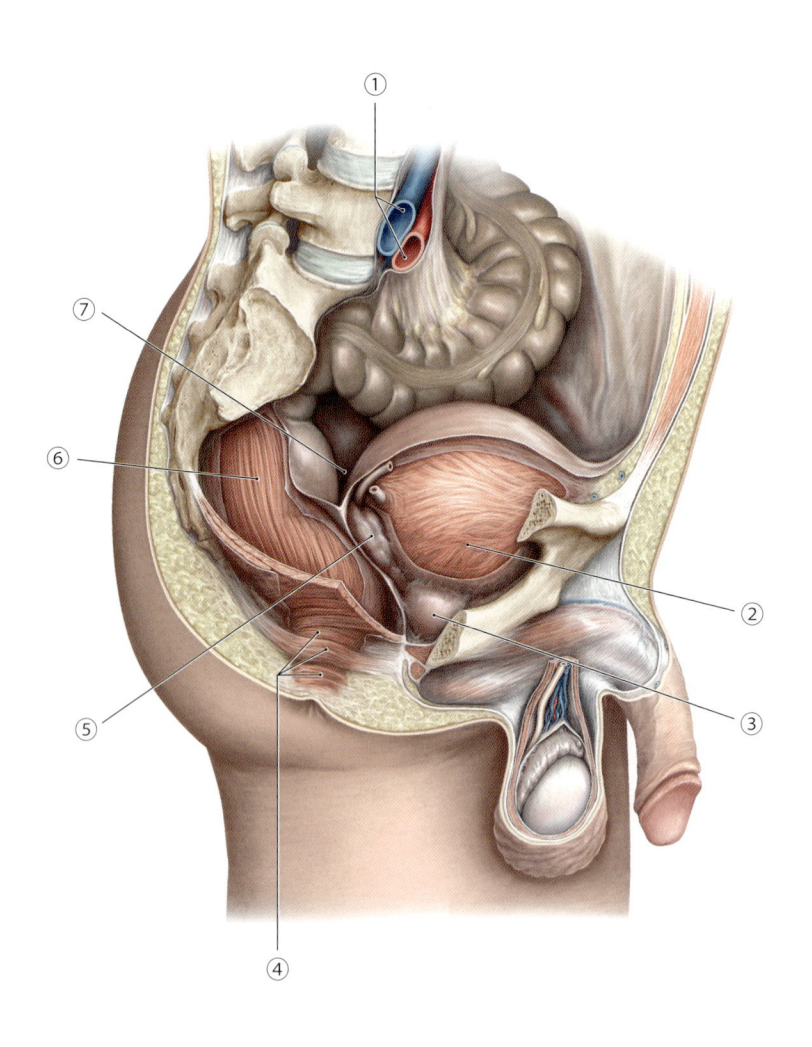

男性骨盤の内容

傍矢状断面，右側面

① ☐ 右総腸骨動脈・静脈　　☐ Right common iliac artery and vein

② ☐ 膀胱　　☐ Urinary bladder

③ ☐ 前立腺　　☐ Prostate

④ ☐ 外肛門括約筋　　☐ External anal sphincter

⑤ ☐ 右の精嚢　　☐ Right seminal vesicle

⑥ ☐ 直腸　　☐ Rectum

⑦ ☐ 直腸膀胱窩　　☐ Rectovesical pouch

1 図 12.10A. p.150　2 図 17.1. p.228

Contents of the Female Pelvis

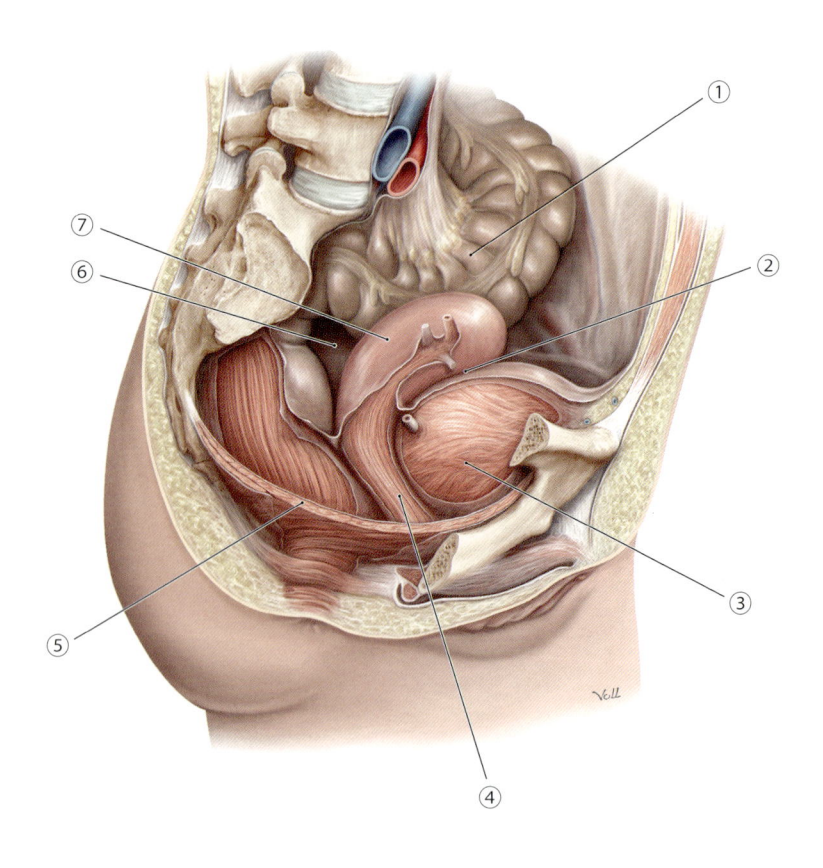

女性骨盤の内容

傍矢状断面，右側面

① □ S状結腸　　　　　　　□ Sigmoid colon
② □ 膀胱子宮窩　　　　　　□ Vesicouterine pouch
③ □ 膀胱　　　　　　　　　□ Urinary bladder
④ □ 腟　　　　　　　　　　□ Vagina
⑤ □ 肛門挙筋　　　　　　　□ Levator ani muscle
⑥ □ 直腸子宮窩　　　　　　□ Rectouterine pouch
⑦ □ 子宮　　　　　　　　　□ Uterus

Transverse Section of the Abdomen

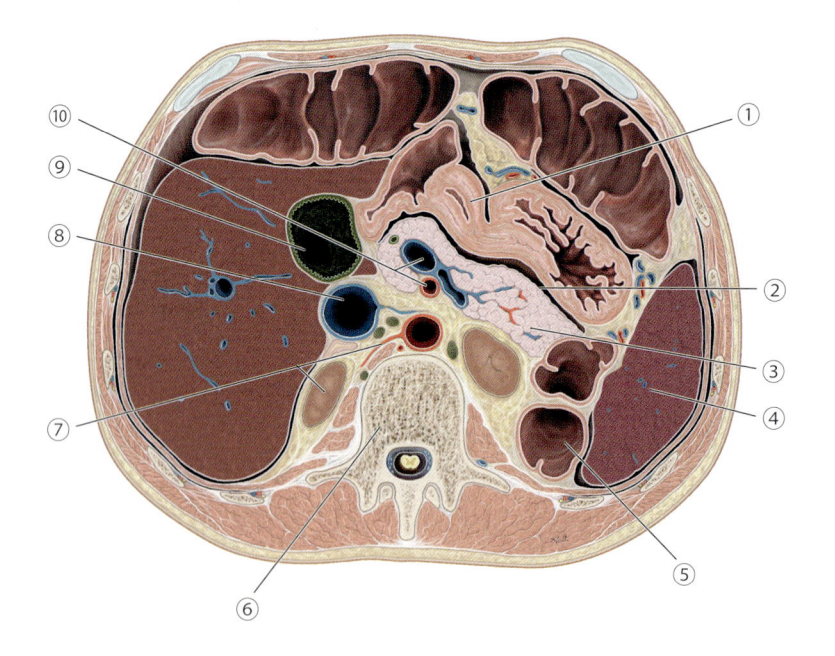

腹部の水平断面

下面

① □ 胃の幽門部　　　　　　　□ Pyloric part of stomach
② □ 網嚢　　　　　　　　　　□ Omental bursa
③ □ 膵臓　　　　　　　　　　□ Pancreas
④ □ 脾臓　　　　　　　　　　□ Spleen
⑤ □ 下行結腸　　　　　　　　□ Descending colon
⑥ □ 第 1 腰椎　　　　　　　　□ L1 vertebra
⑦ □ 腎臓（右腎動脈）　　　　□ Kidney (with right renal artery)
⑧ □ 下大静脈　　　　　　　　□ Inferior vena cava
⑨ □ 胆嚢　　　　　　　　　　□ Gallbladder
⑩ □ 上腸間膜動脈・静脈　　　□ Superior mesenteric artery and vein

Stomach in Situ

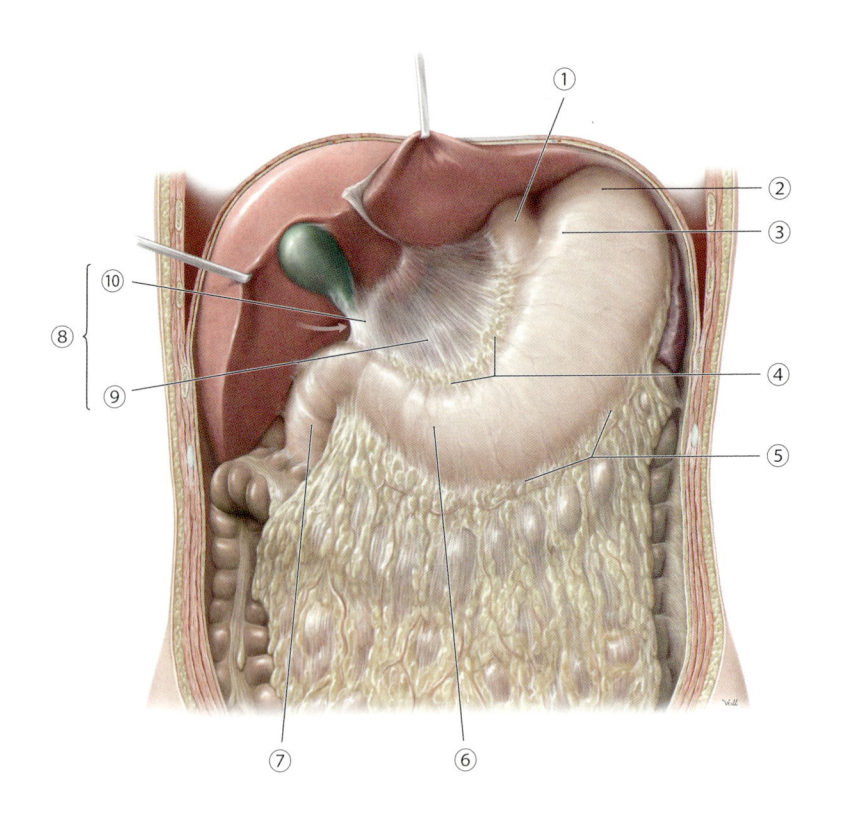

原位置の胃

前面

① □ 食道 　　　　　　　□ Esophagus
② □ 胃底 　　　　　　　□ Fundus
③ □ 噴門 　　　　　　　□ Cardia
④ □ 小弯 　　　　　　　□ Lesser curvature
⑤ □ 大弯 　　　　　　　□ Greater curvature
⑥ □ 幽門洞 　　　　　　□ Pyloric antrum
⑦ □ 十二指腸 　　　　　□ Duodenum
⑧ □ 小網 　　　　　　　□ Lesser omentum
⑨ □ 肝胃間膜 　　　　　□ Hepatogastric ligament
⑩ □ 肝十二指腸間膜 　　□ Hepatoduodenal ligament

臨床

よく知られた胃の疾患である胃炎と胃潰瘍は，胃酸産生過多と関連し，アルコールやアスピリンなどの薬物，細菌のヘリコバクター・ピロリが原因となる．食欲減退，胃痛が症状として現れるが，出血があった場合には，黒色便や吐瀉物中に暗褐色の物質が見られることもある．胃炎は胃壁の内側面に限られるが，胃潰瘍は胃壁に及ぶ．

1 図 13.4. p.159　2 図 13.4. p.157

Duodenum

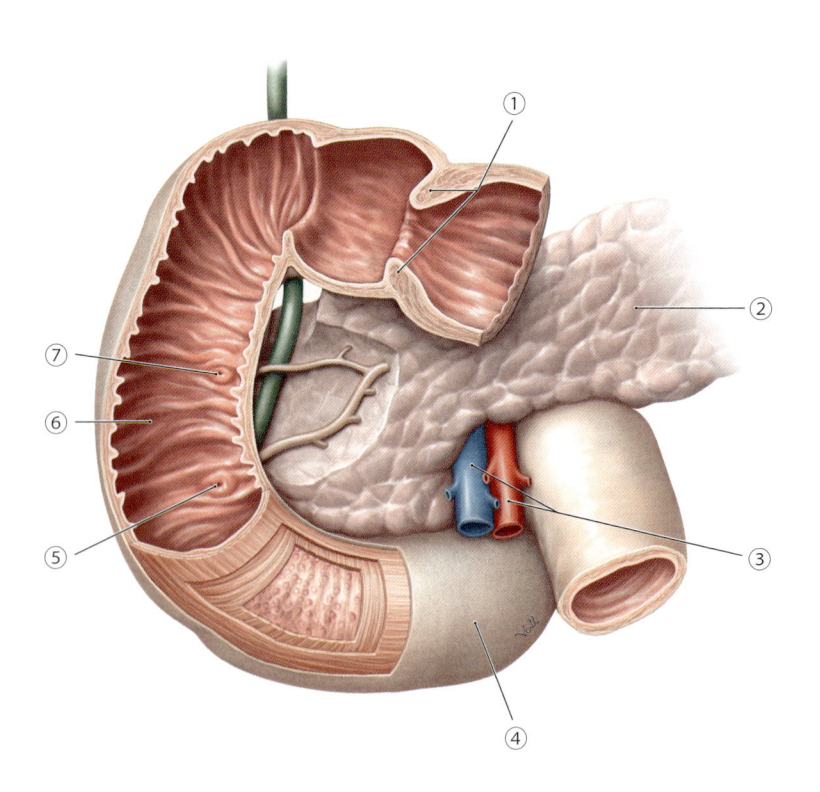

十二指腸を支える靭帯は何か？

十二指腸

前面

① □ 幽門括約筋　　□ Pyloric sphincter
② □ 膵臓　　□ Pancreas
③ □ 上腸間膜動脈・静脈　　□ Superior mesenteric artery and vein
④ □ 十二指腸水平部　　□ Duodenum (horizontal part)
⑤ □ 大十二指腸乳頭　　□ Major duodenal papilla
⑥ □ 十二指腸下行部　　□ Duodenum (descending part)
⑦ □ 小十二指腸乳頭　　□ Minor duodenal papilla

A 　トライツ靱帯は線維筋性のヒモであり，十二指腸空腸曲において十二指腸を横隔膜右脚から吊り下げる．

① 図 13.7. p.160　② 図 13.7. p.158

Large Intestine

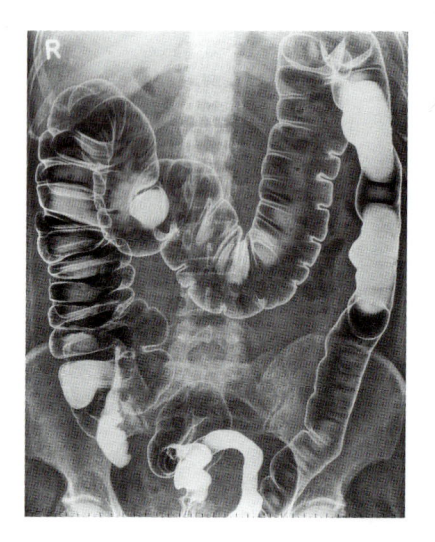

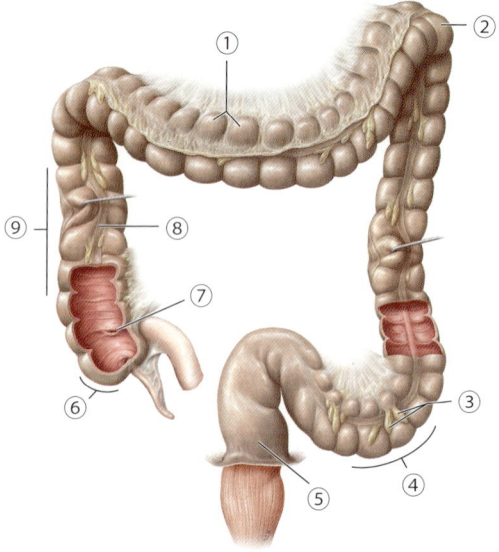

大腸

前面

① □ 膨起　　　　　　　　　□ Haustra

② □ 左結腸曲　　　　　　　□ Left colic flexure

③ □ 腹膜垂　　　　　　　　□ Epiploic appendices

④ □ S状結腸　　　　　　　 □ Sigmoid colon

⑤ □ 直腸（腹膜反転部）　　□ Rectum (with peritoneal reflection)

⑥ □ 盲腸　　　　　　　　　□ Cecum

⑦ □ 回腸口　　　　　　　　□ Ileocecal orifice

⑧ □ 自由ヒモ　　　　　　　□ Taeniae coli

⑨ □ 上行結腸　　　　　　　□ Ascending colon

解説

　発生学的には，大腸は腹膜内器官として発生するが，腸の回転に伴って上行結腸と下行結腸は後腹壁に固定されて間膜を失う．腎臓などの一次性腹膜後器官は後腹壁の壁側腹膜の後方で形成されるので，間膜と結合することはない．

1 図 13.15, 13.16B. p.164, 165　　2 図 13.15, 13.16B. p.162, 163

Rectum in Situ

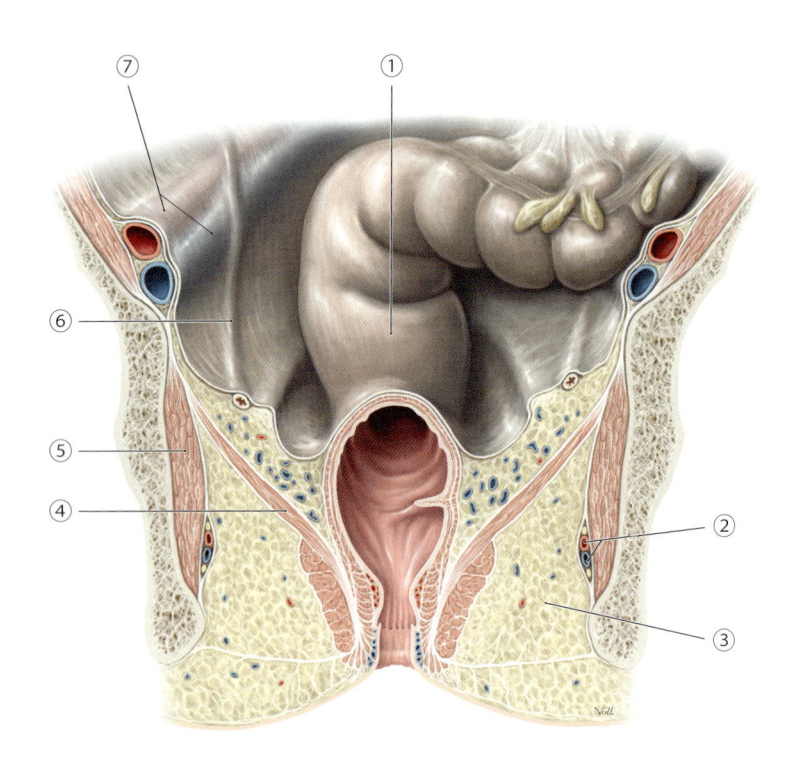

Q S状結腸と直腸の移行部には何があるか？

原位置の直腸

冠状断面，女性骨盤の前面

① □ 直腸　　　　　　　　　□ Rectum
② □ 内陰部動脈・静脈　　　□ Internal pudendal artery and vein
③ □ 坐骨肛門窩（坐骨直腸窩）□ Ischioanal fossa
④ □ 肛門挙筋　　　　　　　□ Levator ani
⑤ □ 内閉鎖筋　　　　　　　□ Obturator internus
⑥ □ 尿管　　　　　　　　　□ Ureter
⑦ □ 外腸骨動脈・静脈　　　□ External iliac artery and vein

A　直腸とS状結腸の移行部はほぼS3の高さであり，S状結腸間膜と結腸ヒモの終端が見られる．

1 図13.19. p.166　2 図18.3. p.234

Rectum & Anal Canal

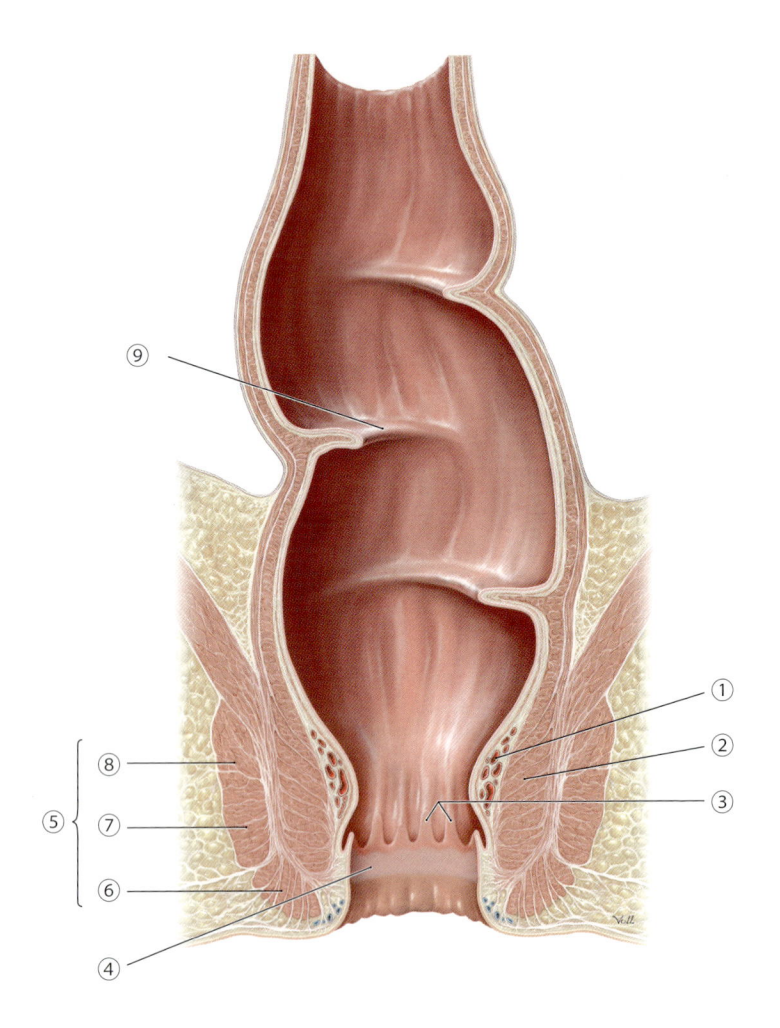

直腸静脈叢と皮下静脈叢のうち，どちらの痔疾がより強い痛みを伴うか？

直腸と肛門管

冠状断面，前面

① □ 直腸静脈叢　　　　　　□ Hemorrhoidal plexus

② □ 内肛門括約筋　　　　　□ Internal anal sphincter

③ □ 肛門柱　　　　　　　　□ Anal columns

④ □ 肛門櫛（白帯）　　　　□ Anal pecten (white zone)

⑤ □ 外肛門括約筋　　　　　□ External anal sphincter

⑥ □ 皮下部　　　　　　　　□ Subcutaneous part

⑦ □ 浅部　　　　　　　　　□ Superficial part

⑧ □ 深部　　　　　　　　　□ Deep part

⑨ □ 中直腸横ヒダ　　　　　□ Middle transverse rectal fold

A　皮下静脈叢は櫛状線より下部に位置し，体性神経からなる下直腸神経が分布する．そのため，この領域は疼痛刺激に対して強く反応する．直腸静脈叢は櫛状線より上部にあり自律神経のみが分布するため，疼痛に対する反応が鈍い．

1 図 13.20. p.167　　2 図 18.4. p.235

Surfaces of the Liver I

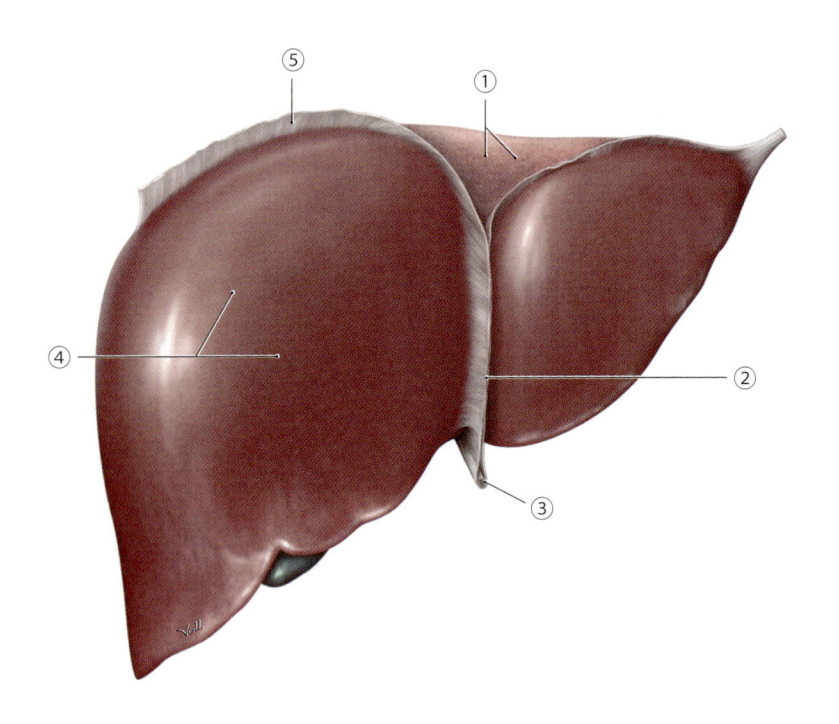

肝臓の無漿膜野はどこか？

肝臓の表面 1

前面

① ☐ 無漿膜野（横隔面） ☐ Bare area (diaphragmatic surface of liver)

② ☐ 肝鎌状間膜 ☐ Falciform ligament

③ ☐ 肝円索（痕跡化した臍静脈を含む） ☐ Ligamentum teres (contains obliterated umbilical vein)

④ ☐ 肝臓の右葉，横隔面 ☐ Right lobe, diaphragmatic surface

⑤ ☐ 肝冠状間膜 ☐ Coronary ligament

A 　肝臓の上面と後面は腹膜に覆われない無漿膜野であり，横隔膜の下面に直接接している．無漿膜野の境界をなすのは，肝冠状間膜と三角間膜の折れ返り部分である．

1 図 13.27A, p.171　2 図 13.23A, p.167

Surfaces of the Liver II

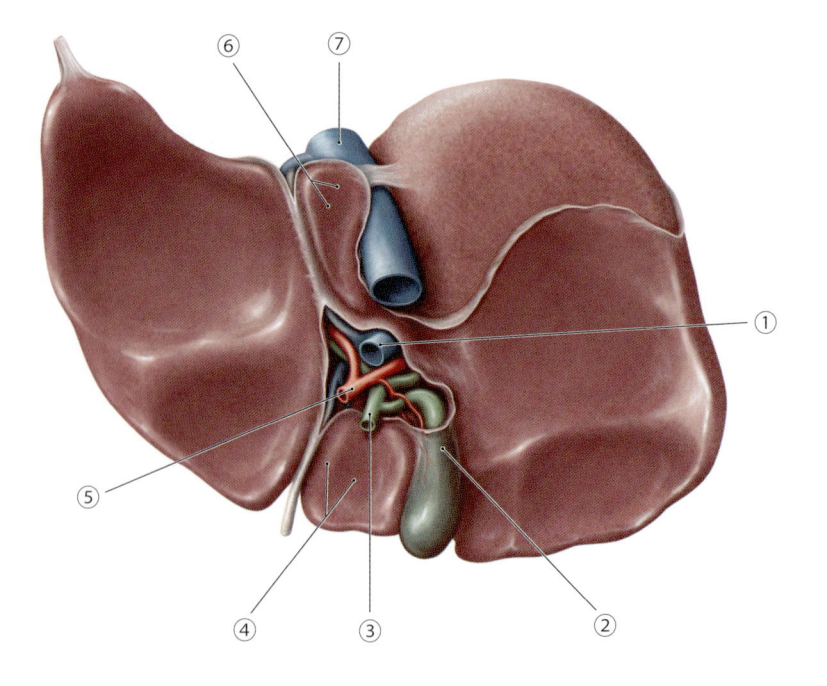

肝臓の表面 2

下面

① ☐ 門脈　　　　　　　☐ Portal vein

② ☐ 胆嚢　　　　　　　☐ Gallbladder

③ ☐ 総胆管　　　　　　☐ Bile duct

④ ☐ 方形葉　　　　　　☐ Quadrate lobe

⑤ ☐ 固有肝動脈　　　　☐ Proper hepatic artery

⑥ ☐ 尾状葉　　　　　　☐ Caudate lobe

⑦ ☐ 下大静脈　　　　　☐ Inferior vena cava

1 図 13.27B. p.171　2 図 13.23B. p.167

Extrahepatic Bile Ducts

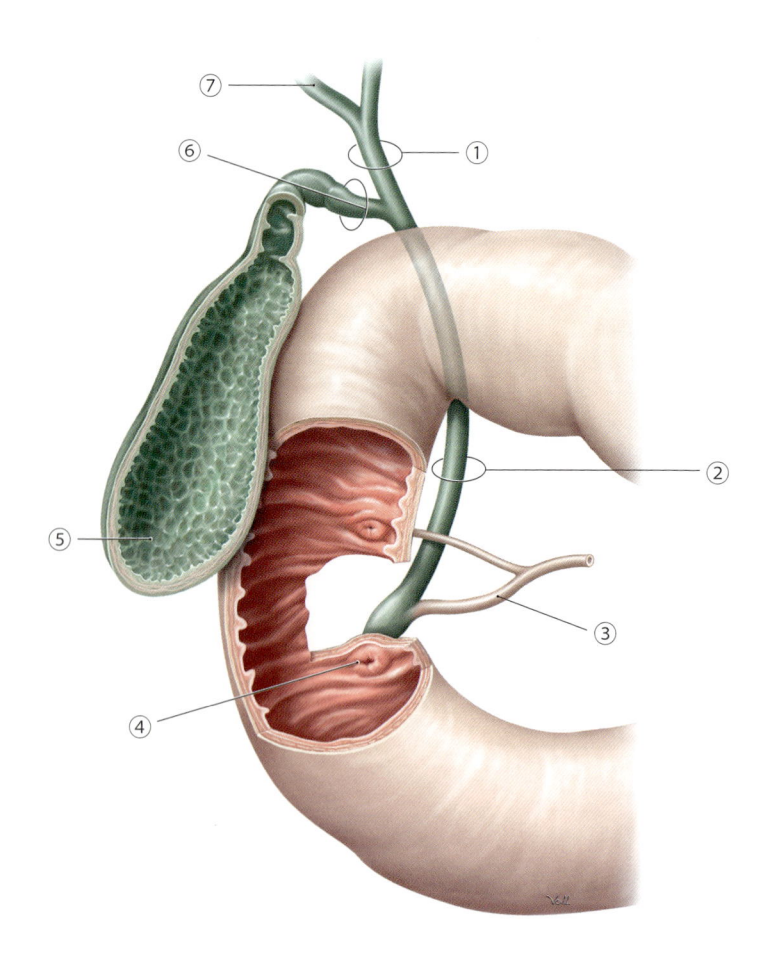

肝外胆管

前面

① □ 総肝管　　　　　　□ Common hepatic duct

② □ 総胆管　　　　　　□ Bile duct

③ □ 膵管　　　　　　　□ Pancreatic duct

④ □ 大十二指腸乳頭　　□ Major duodenal papilla

⑤ □ 胆嚢底　　　　　　□ Fundus

⑥ □ 胆嚢管　　　　　　□ Cystic duct

⑦ □ 右肝管　　　　　　□ Right hepatic duct

臨床

胆汁が胆嚢で貯蔵・濃縮される間に，コレステロールなどの物質は結晶化し胆石となる．胆石が胆管に移動すると激しい痛み（疝痛）を起こす．胆石は十二指腸乳頭で膵管の閉塞を起こすことがあり，死に至らしめるような重度の急性膵炎を起こす．

1 図 13.31. p.172　 2 図 13.27. p.168

Biliary Tract in Situ

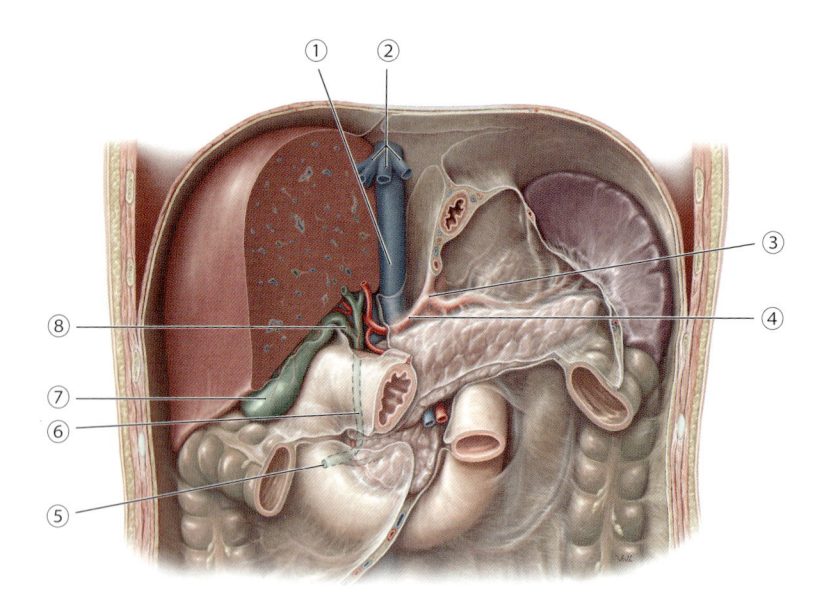

Q 肝十二指腸間膜内にある構造は何か？

原位置の胆路

前面

① ☐ 下大静脈 — ☐ Inferior vena cava
② ☐ 肝静脈 — ☐ Hepatic veins
③ ☐ 腹腔動脈 — ☐ Celiac trunk
④ ☐ 総肝動脈 — ☐ Common hepatic artery
⑤ ☐ 胆膵管（大十二指腸乳頭へ開口）— ☐ Hepatopancreatic duct (opening on major duodenal papilla)
⑥ ☐ 総胆管 — ☐ Bile duct
⑦ ☐ 胆嚢 — ☐ Gallbladder
⑧ ☐ 胆嚢管 — ☐ Cystic duct

A 総胆管，肝動脈，門脈が肝十二指腸間膜内を通る．

Pancreas

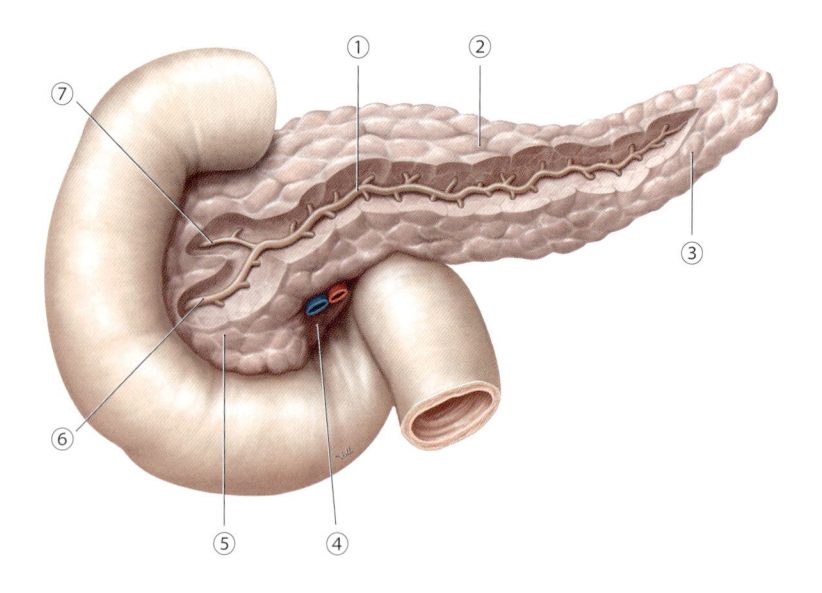

膵臓

前面

① ☐ 膵管 — ☐ Pancreatic duct
② ☐ 膵体 — ☐ Body of pancreas
③ ☐ 膵尾 — ☐ Tail of pancreas
④ ☐ 膵臓（鉤状突起） — ☐ Uncinate process of pancreas
⑤ ☐ 膵頭 — ☐ Head of pancreas
⑥ ☐ 膵管（腹側膵芽から由来） — ☐ Pancreatic duct (from the ventral pancreatic bud)
⑦ ☐ 副膵管（背側膵芽から由来） — ☐ Accessory pancreatic duct (from the dorsal pancreatic bud)

解説

膵管は胎生期の腹側膵と背側膵から生じる．主膵管の近位部は腹側膵に由来し，大十二指腸乳頭で十二指腸に開口する．残りの背側膵から起こった部分は副膵管であり，大十二指腸乳頭の近傍で十二指腸に開口する．膵管の走行には変異が多い．

1 図 13.34. p.174　2 図 13.30. p.170

Kidneys & Ureters in Situ

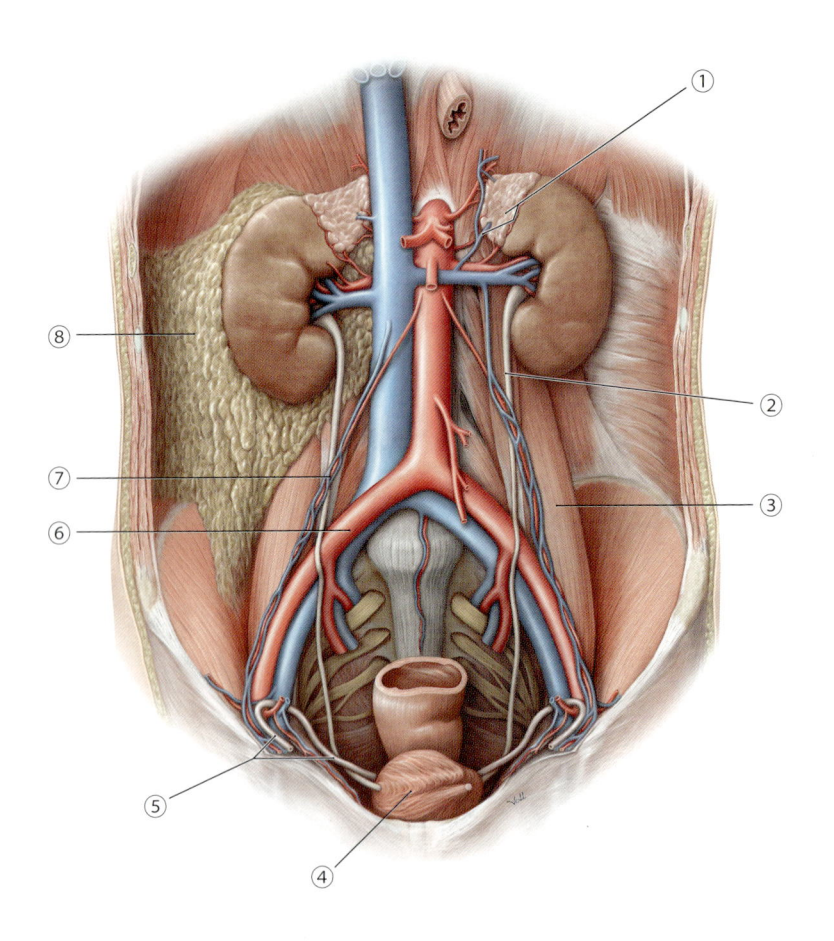

尿管の狭窄が起こりやすい部位はどこか？

原位置の腎臓と尿管

男性腹部，前面

① ☐ 左の副腎，左副腎静脈　　　☐ Left suprarenal gland and vein

② ☐ 尿管（腹部）　　　☐ Ureter（abdominal part）

③ ☐ 大腰筋　　　☐ Psoas major

④ ☐ 膀胱　　　☐ Urinary bladder

⑤ ☐ 右の精管　　　☐ Right ductus deferens

⑥ ☐ 右総腸骨動脈　　　☐ Right common iliac artery

⑦ ☐ 右精巣動脈・静脈　　　☐ Right ovarian / testicular artery and vein

⑧ ☐ 脂肪被膜　　　☐ Perirenal fat capsule

A 　尿管は次の3ヵ所で狭窄を起こしやすい．腎盂が狭くなって尿管になる部位（腎盂尿管移行部），総腸骨動静脈の遠位端で骨盤上口と交差する部位，膀胱を貫通する部位．

① 図 13.47. p.180　② 図 18.5. p.236

Female Urinary Bladder & Urethra

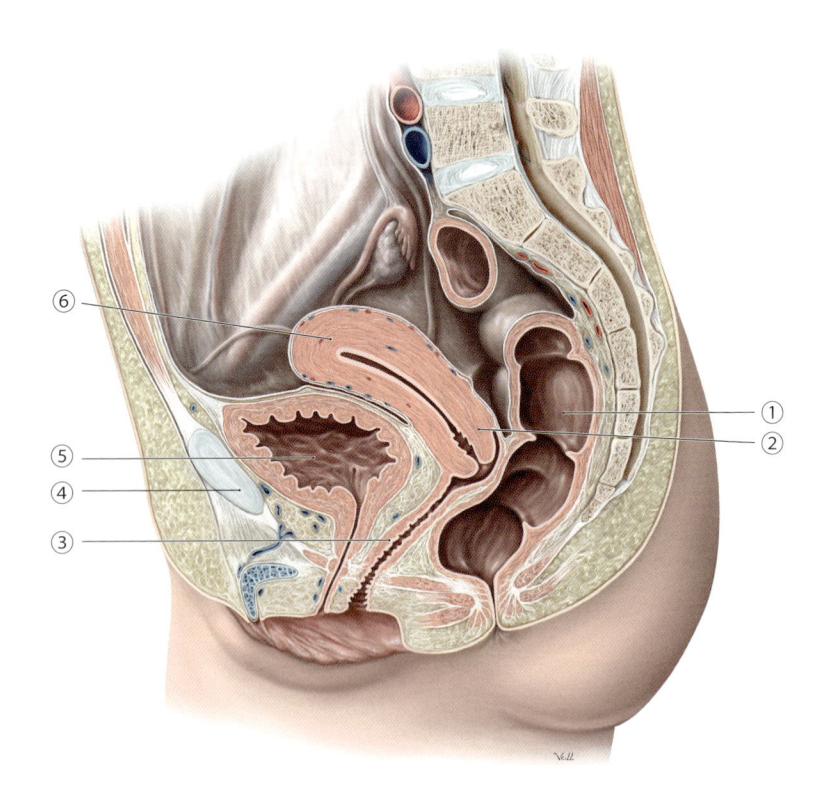

女性の膀胱と尿道

正中矢状断面，左側面

① □ 直腸　　　　　　　　□ Rectum
② □ 子宮頸　　　　　　　□ Uterine cervix
③ □ 腟　　　　　　　　　□ Vagina
④ □ 恥骨結合　　　　　　□ Pubic symphysis
⑤ □ 膀胱　　　　　　　　□ Urinary bladder
⑥ □ 子宮底　　　　　　　□ Uterine fundus

① 図 13.52B. p.184　② 図 18.8A. p.238

Trigone of the Bladder

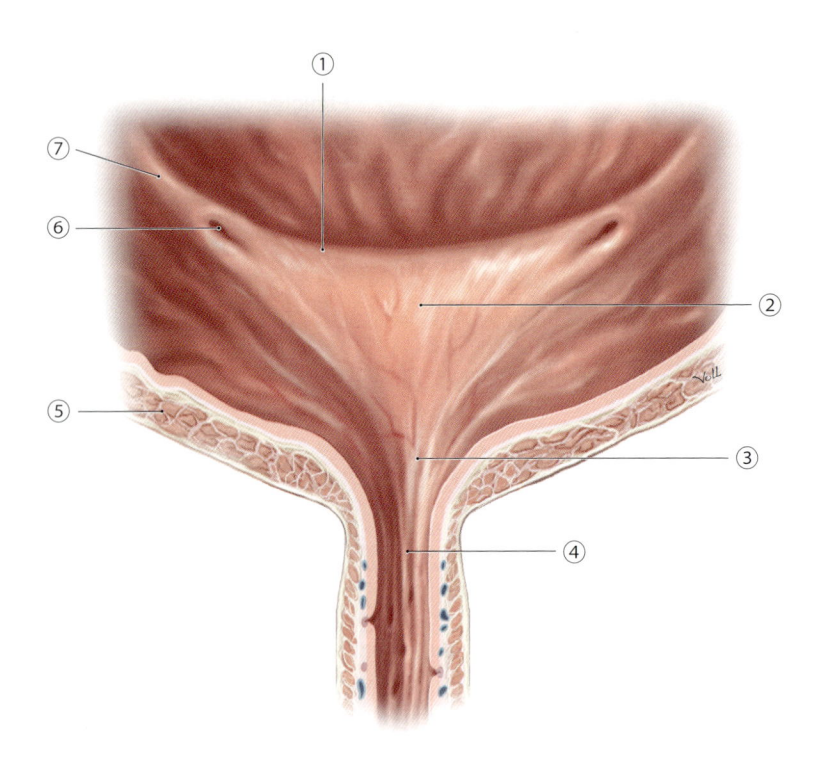

膀胱三角

冠状断面, 前面

① ☐ 尿管間ヒダ　　　　　　　　☐ Interureteral fold
② ☐ 膀胱三角　　　　　　　　　☐ Bladder trigone
③ ☐ 膀胱頸　　　　　　　　　　☐ Neck
④ ☐ 尿道　　　　　　　　　　　☐ Urethra
⑤ ☐ 筋層(＝排尿筋)　　　　　　☐ Muscularis (＝ detrusor vesicae)
⑥ ☐ 尿管口　　　　　　　　　　☐ Ureteral orifice
⑦ ☐ 右の尿管, 壁内部　　　　　☐ Right ureter, intramural part

1 図 13.54. p.185　2 図 18.10. p.239

Uterus & Uterine Tube I

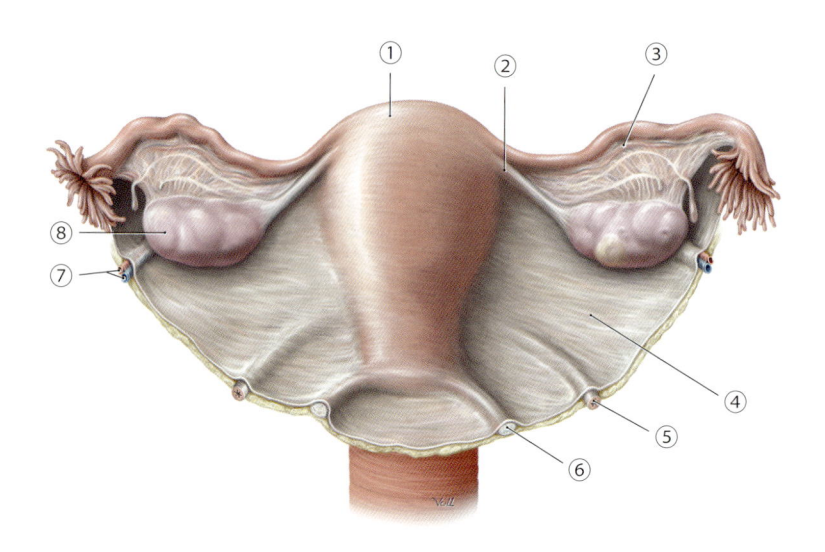

子宮と卵管 1

後上面

① ☐ 子宮底　　　　　　　　　　　☐ Uterine fundus

② ☐ 固有卵巣索　　　　　　　　　☐ Proper ovarian ligament

③ ☐ 卵管間膜（中を子宮動脈・　　☐ Mesosalpinx（with tubal
　　　静脈の卵管枝が走る）　　　　　　branches of uterine artery
　　　　　　　　　　　　　　　　　　　and vein）

④ ☐ 子宮間膜　　　　　　　　　　☐ Mesometrium

⑤ ☐ 右の尿管　　　　　　　　　　☐ Right ureter

⑥ ☐ 直腸子宮靱帯　　　　　　　　☐ Uterosacral ligament
　　　（直腸子宮ヒダの中を走る）　　　（in uterosacral fold）

⑦ ☐ 卵巣動脈・静脈　　　　　　　☐ Ovarian artery and vein
　　　（卵巣提靱帯の中を走る）　　　　（in ovarian suspensory
　　　　　　　　　　　　　　　　　　　ligament）

⑧ ☐ 左の卵巣　　　　　　　　　　☐ Left ovary

臨床

通常，卵子は受精後に子宮腔の壁に着床するが，他の場所（卵管や場合によっては腹膜腔）に着床することもある．最も一般的な異所性妊娠である卵管妊娠では卵管壁が破裂し，腹膜腔内に出血することで生命の危機に陥る可能性がある．卵管妊娠の多くは炎症の後に卵管粘膜に癒着が生じることにより起こる．

[1] 図 14.6A, p.189　[2] 図 18.16A, p.243

Uterus & Uterine Tube II

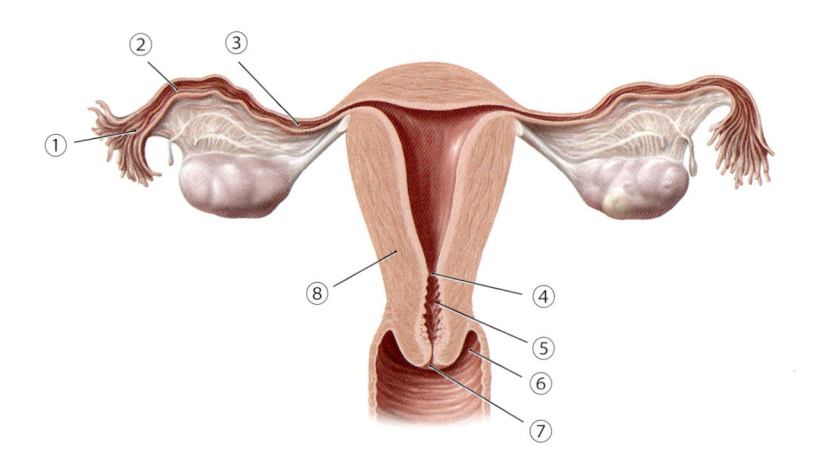

Q 受精が起こるのは通常は女性生殖路のどこか？

子宮と卵管 2

冠状断面，子宮を垂直に示し，後方から見たところ

① □ 卵管漏斗　　　　　　　□ Infundibulum
② □ 卵管膨大部　　　　　　□ Ampulla
③ □ 卵管峡部　　　　　　　□ Isthmus
④ □ 内子宮口（子宮峡部の）　□ Internal os (at uterine isthmus)
⑤ □ 子宮頸管　　　　　　　□ Cervical canal
⑥ □ 腟円蓋，外側部　　　　□ Vaginal fornix, lateral part
⑦ □ 外子宮口　　　　　　　□ External os
⑧ □ 子宮筋層　　　　　　　□ Myometrium

A 卵子と精子の受精は，通常は卵管漏斗か卵管膨大部で起こる．

Female External Genitalia

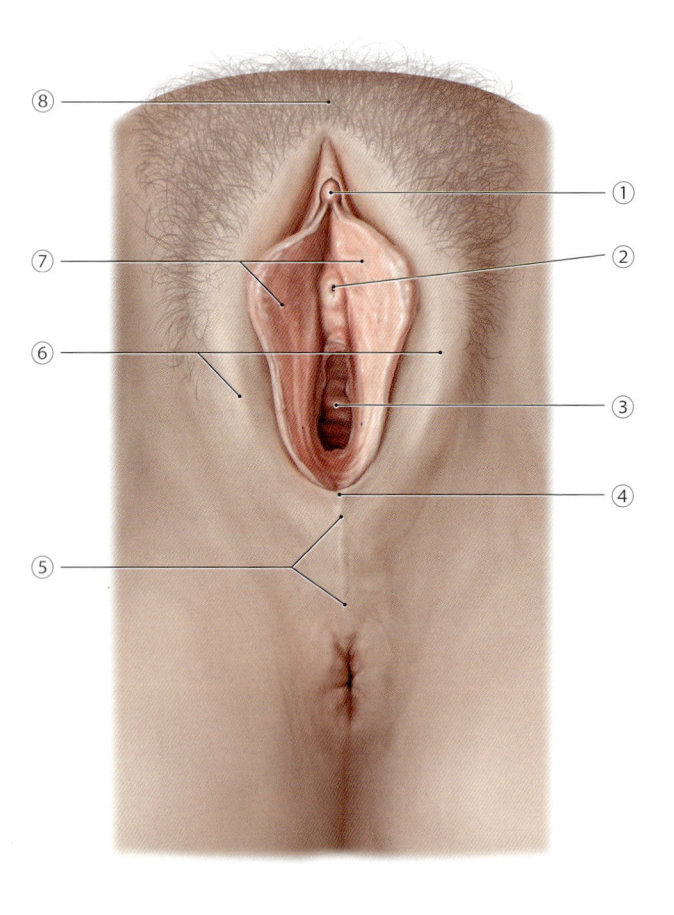

女性の外生殖器

切石位

① ☐ 陰核　　　　　　　　☐ Clitoris

② ☐ 外尿道口　　　　　　☐ External urethral orifice

③ ☐ 腟前庭　　　　　　　☐ Vestibule

④ ☐ 後陰唇交連　　　　　☐ Posterior labial commissure

⑤ ☐ 会陰縫線　　　　　　☐ Perineal raphe

⑥ ☐ 大陰唇　　　　　　　☐ Labia majora

⑦ ☐ 小陰唇　　　　　　　☐ Labia minora

⑧ ☐ 恥丘　　　　　　　　☐ Mons pubis

1 図 14.12. p.192　2 図 18.25. p.248

Female Erectile Muscles & Tissue

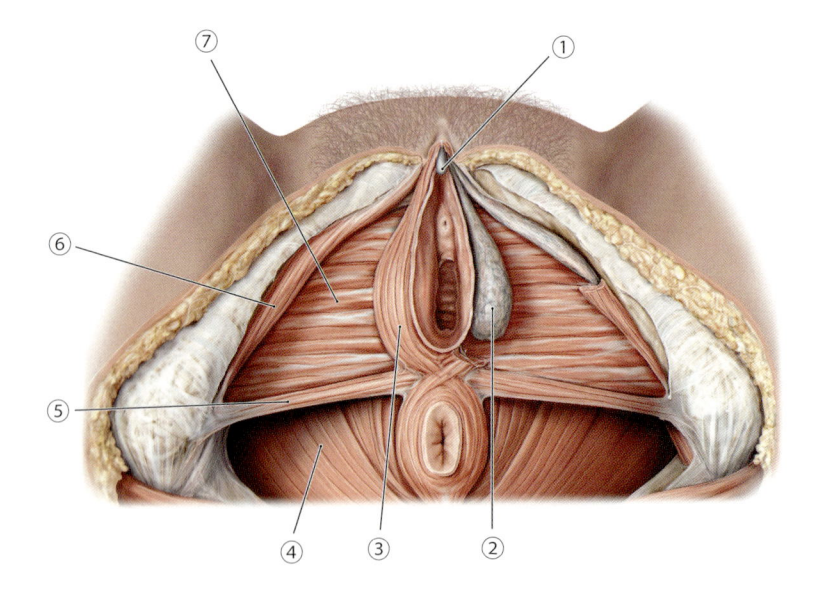

女性の勃起組織

切石位

① □ 陰核亀頭　　　　　　□ Glans of clitoris

② □ 前庭球　　　　　　　□ Vestibular bulb

③ □ 球海綿体筋　　　　　□ Bulbospongiosus

④ □ 肛門挙筋　　　　　　□ Levator ani

⑤ □ 浅会陰横筋　　　　　□ Superficial transverse perineal

⑥ □ 坐骨海綿体筋　　　　□ Ischiocavernosus

⑦ □ 深会陰横筋　　　　　□ Deep transverse perineal

臨床

会陰切開術は分娩の娩出期に産道を拡大する産科的手技である．この手技は一般には，娩出期の低酸素症を防ぎ娩出を早めるために用いられる．そのほか，会陰の皮膚が白色になった場合(血流の低下を表す)は，会陰裂傷の危険が切迫しており，会陰切開術がしばしば行われる．側切開が切開の幅を最も広くとれるが，回復は難しくなる．

1 図 14.14. p.193　2 図 18.27. p.249

Neurovasculature of the Female Perineum

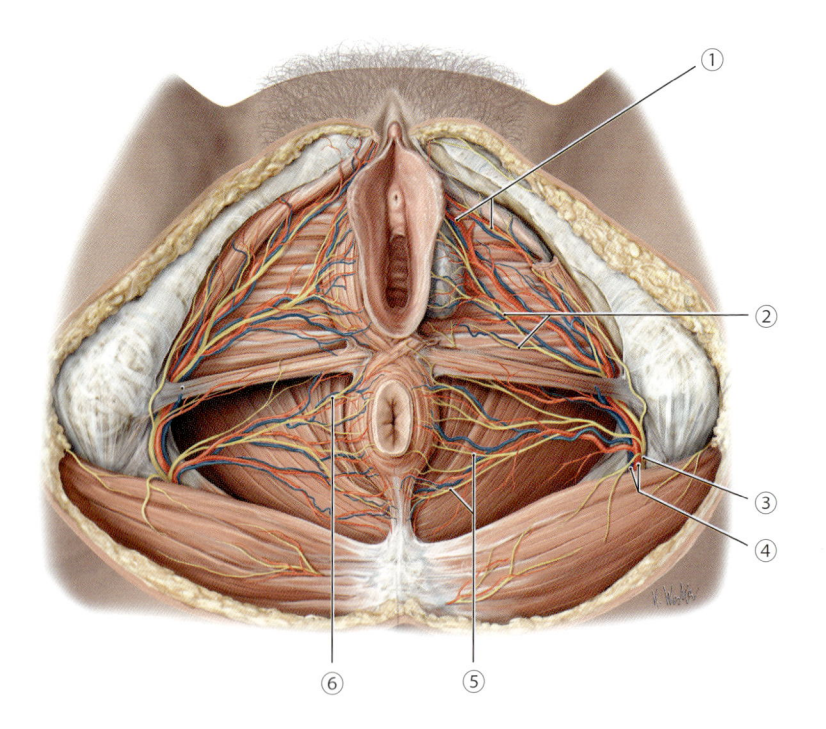

陰部神経の起始と走行は？

女性会陰の神経・血管

切石位

① ☐ 陰核背動脈・神経　　　　　☐ Dorsal clitoral artery and nerve

② ☐ 後陰唇神経(陰部神経の枝)　☐ Posterior labial branches (pudendal nerve)

③ ☐ 陰部神経　　　　　　　　　☐ Pudendal nerve

④ ☐ 内陰部動脈・静脈　　　　　☐ Internal pudendal artery and vein

⑤ ☐ 下直腸神経　　　　　　　　☐ Inferior rectal nerves

⑥ ☐ 会陰神経　　　　　　　　　☐ Perineal nerves

A　陰部神経は S2-S4 の前枝から仙骨神経叢の一枝として起こり，大坐骨孔から骨盤外に出て，仙棘靱帯の後方を通り，小坐骨孔から会陰へ至る．陰部神経の枝は肛門三角と尿生殖三角の各構造に分布する．

[1] 図 14.17. p.195　[2] 図 19.20. p.267

Cross Section of the Penis

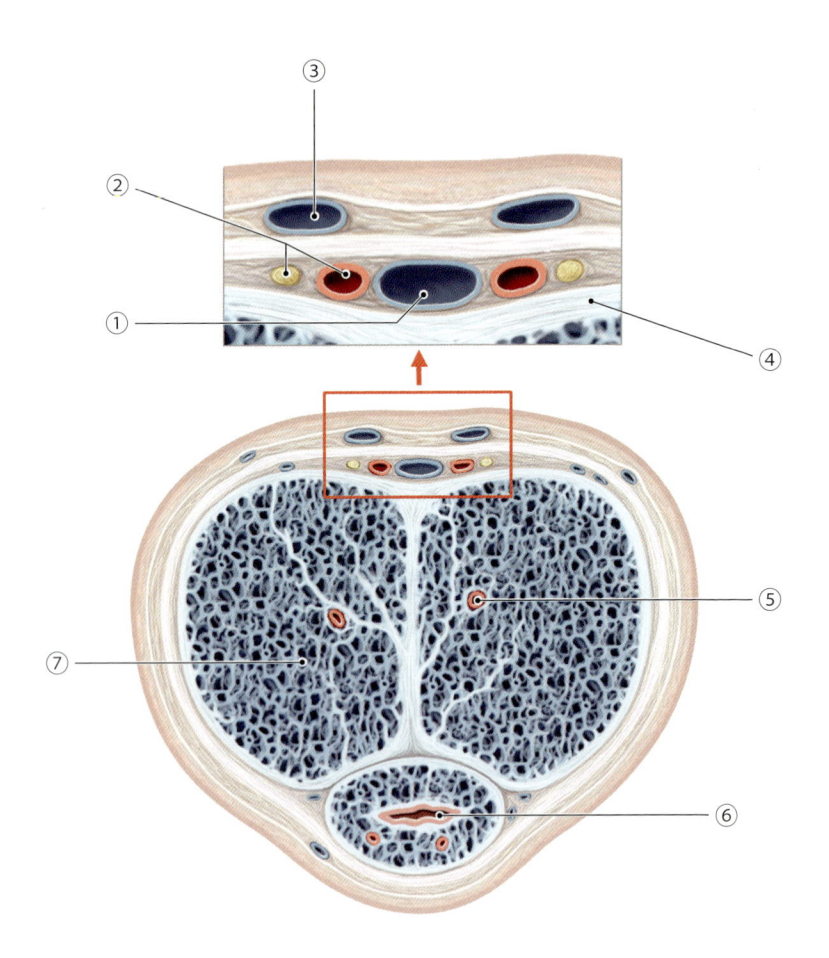

陰茎の横断面

陰茎幹での横断面

① □ 深陰茎背静脈　　　　　　　□ Deep dorsal penile vein
② □ 陰茎背動脈・神経　　　　　□ Dorsal penile artery and nerve
③ □ 浅陰茎背静脈　　　　　　　□ Superficial dorsal penile vein
④ □ 陰茎海綿体白膜　　　　　　□ Tunica albuginea of corpus cavernosum
⑤ □ 陰茎深動脈　　　　　　　　□ Deep penile artery
⑥ □ 尿道（海綿体部）　　　　　□ Urethra (spongy part)
⑦ □ 陰茎海綿体　　　　　　　　□ Corpus cavernosum

1 図 14.20B. p.197　　2 図 18.28D. p.250

Penis

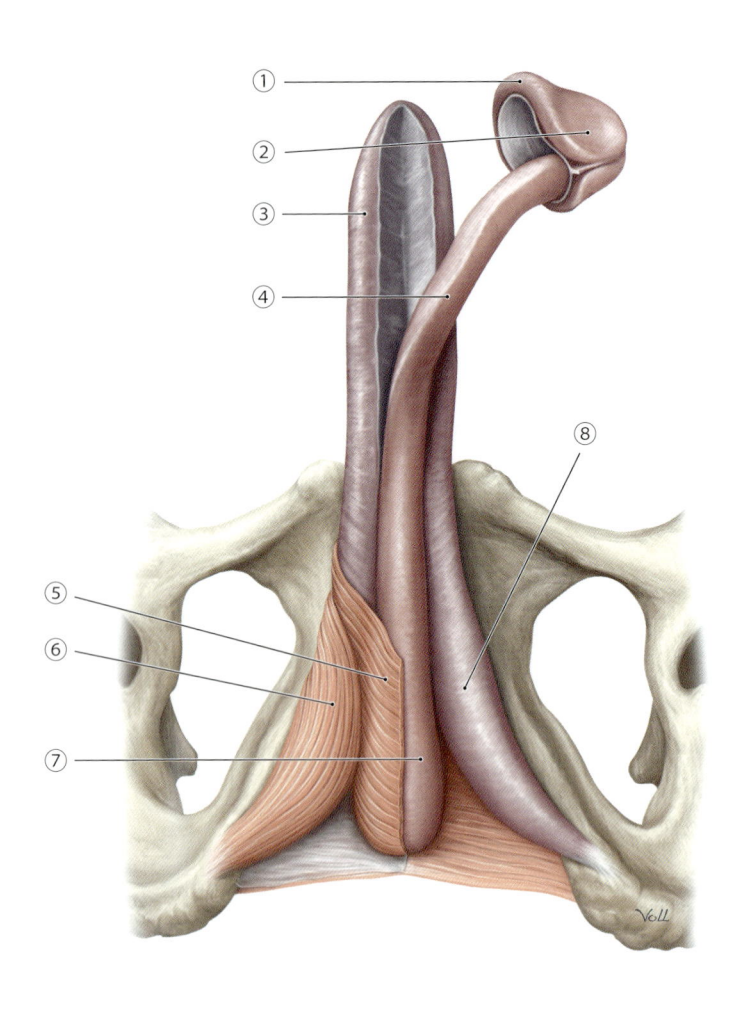

陰茎

下面

① ☐ 亀頭冠 ☐ Corona of glans
② ☐ 陰茎亀頭 ☐ Glans penis
③ ☐ 陰茎海綿体 ☐ Corpus cavernosum
④ ☐ 尿道海綿体 ☐ Corpus spongiosum
⑤ ☐ 球海綿体筋 ☐ Bulbospongiosus
⑥ ☐ 坐骨海綿体筋 ☐ Ischiocavernosus
⑦ ☐ 尿道球 ☐ Bulb of penis
⑧ ☐ 陰茎脚 ☐ Crus of penis

Testis & Epididymis

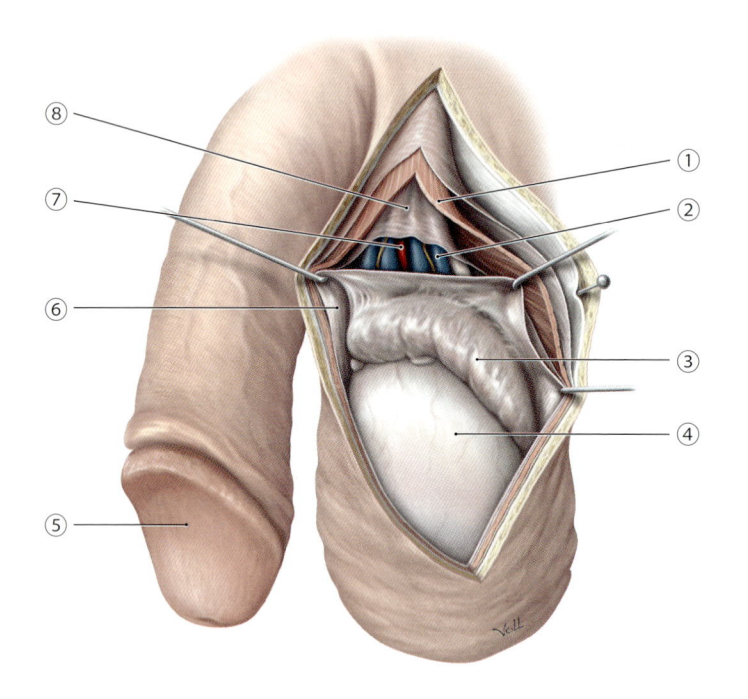

Q 精巣上体とは何か？

精巣と精巣上体

左外側面

① ☐ 精巣挙筋,精巣挙筋膜 ☐ Cremaster muscle and fascia
② ☐ 蔓状静脈叢（精巣静脈） ☐ Pampiniform plexus (testicular veins)
③ ☐ 精巣上体体 ☐ Epididymis, body
④ ☐ 精巣と精巣鞘膜の臓側板 ☐ Testis with tunica vaginalis, visceral layer
⑤ ☐ 陰茎亀頭 ☐ Glans penis
⑥ ☐ 精巣鞘膜の壁側板 ☐ Tunica vaginalis, parietal layer
⑦ ☐ 精巣動脈 ☐ Testicular artery
⑧ ☐ 内精筋膜 ☐ Internal spermatic fascia

A 精巣上体は大きく曲がりくねった管であり，精巣から未成熟な精子を受け取って貯蔵する．尾部は精管につながる．

Coverings of the Testis

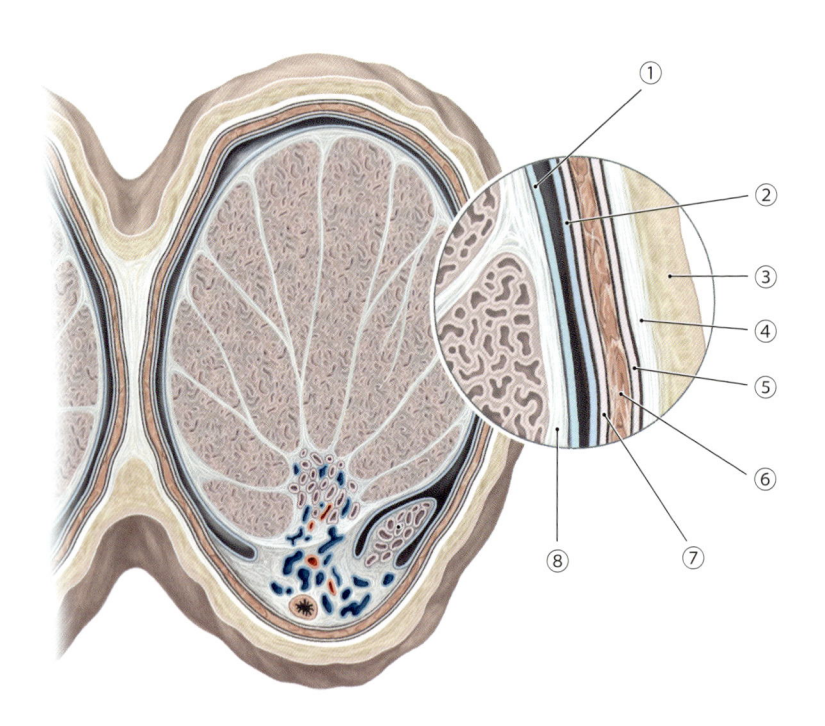

Q 腹壁を構成する層のうち，精索と精巣の被膜に関与しないのはどれか？

精巣の被膜

横断面，上面

① □ 精巣鞘膜の臓側板　　□ Tunica vaginalis, visceral layer

② □ 精巣鞘膜の壁側板　　□ Tunica vaginalis, parietal layer

③ □ 陰嚢の皮膚　　□ Scrotal skin

④ □ 肉様膜　　□ Tunica dartos

⑤ □ 外精筋膜　　□ External spermatic fascia

⑥ □ 精巣挙筋，精巣挙筋膜　　□ Cremaster muscle and fascia

⑦ □ 内精筋膜　　□ Internal spermatic fascia

⑧ □ 白膜　　□ Tunica albuginea

A 腹横筋は精索と精巣の被膜に関与しない．

① 表 14.3. p.199

Male Accessory Sex Glands

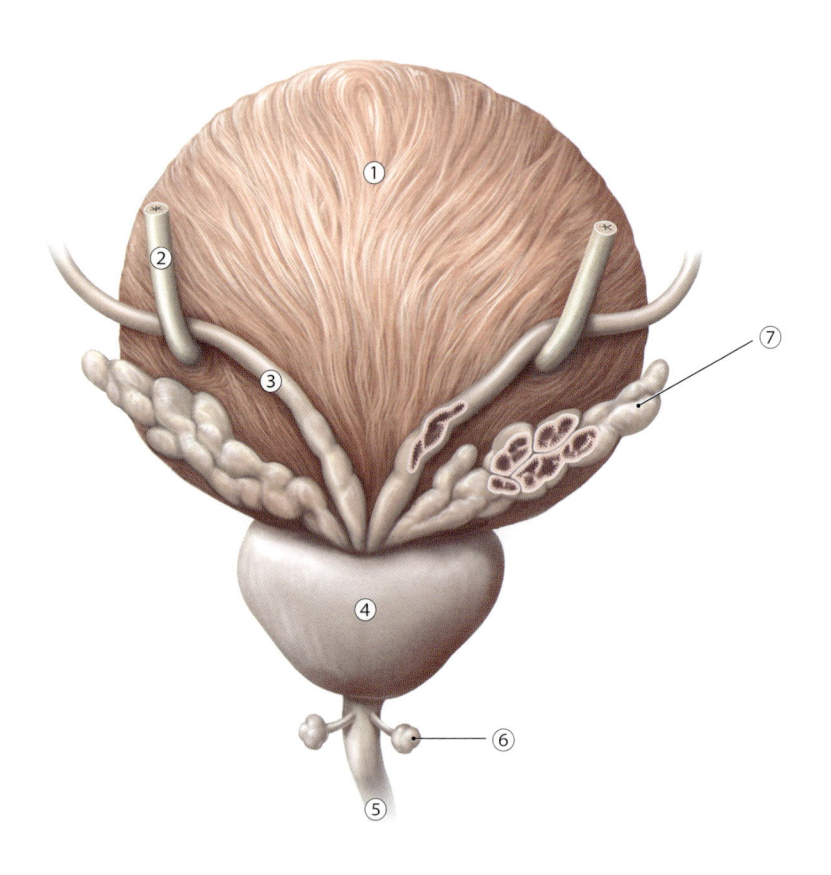

男性の付属生殖腺

後面

① □ 膀胱 □ Urinary bladder
② □ 尿管(海綿体部) □ Ureter (spongy part)
③ □ 精管 □ Ductus deferens
④ □ 前立腺 □ Prostate
⑤ □ 尿道 □ Urethra
⑥ □ 尿道球腺 □ Bulbourethral gland
⑦ □ 精嚢 □ Seminal vesicle

Prostate in Situ

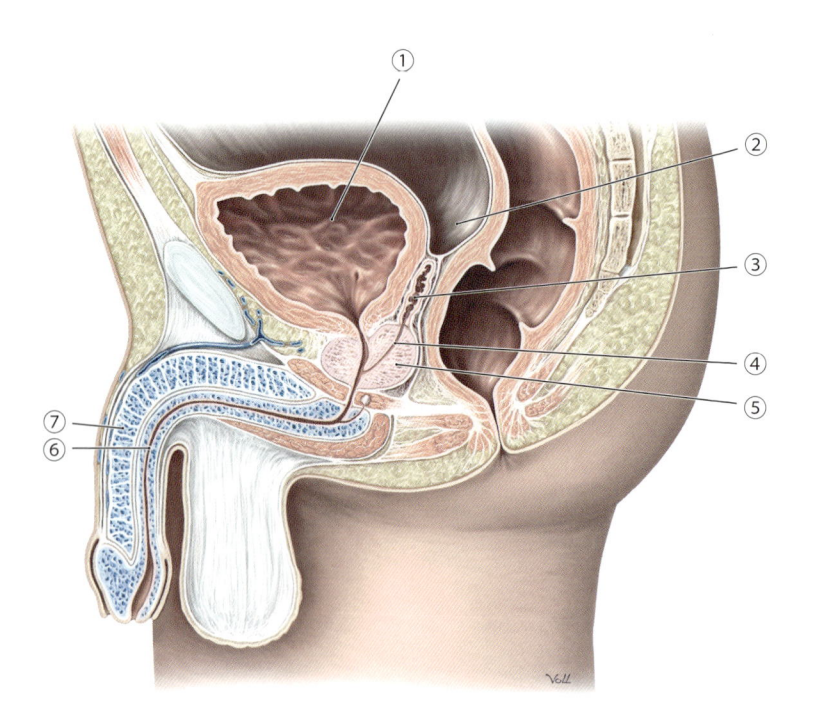

原位置の前立腺

矢状断面，左外側面

① □ 膀胱体 □ Urinary bladder (body)
② □ 直腸膀胱窩 □ Rectovesical pouch
③ □ 精嚢 □ Seminal vesicle
④ □ 射精管 □ Ejaculatory duct
⑤ □ 前立腺 □ Prostate
⑥ □ 尿道の海綿体部 □ Urethra, spongy part
⑦ □ 陰茎海綿体 □ Corpus cavernosum of penis

臨床

　前立腺癌は，高齢の男性において最もよく見られる悪性腫瘍の1つで，前立腺の辺縁領域の被膜下に増殖する．良性の前立腺肥大が中心領域で生じるのとは対照的に，前立腺癌は早期では尿路を閉塞しない．辺縁領域にある腫瘍は，直腸内診によって直腸の前壁を介して硬い塊として触知される．

1 図 14.25, p.201　2 図 18.33, p.253

Neurovasculature of the Male Perineum

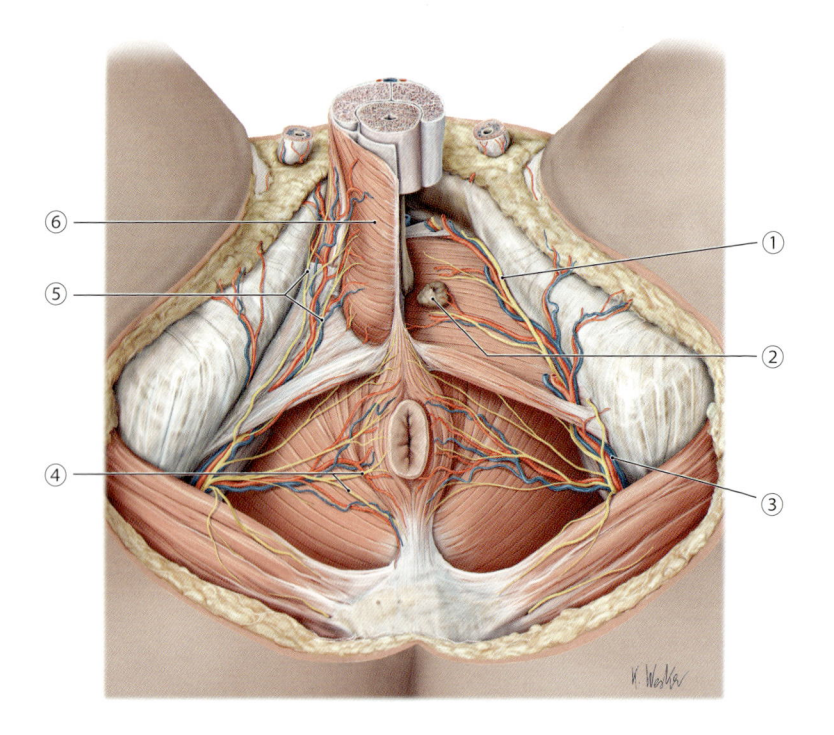

男性会陰の神経・血管

切石位

① □ 陰茎背神経　　　　　　□ Dorsal penile nerve
② □ 尿道球腺　　　　　　　□ Bulbourethral gland
③ □ 内陰部動脈・静脈　　　□ Internal pudendal artery and vein
④ □ 下直腸神経　　　　　　□ Inferior rectal nerves
⑤ □ 後陰嚢神経　　　　　　□ Posterior scrotal nerves
⑥ □ 球海綿体筋　　　　　　□ Bulbospongiosus

Abdominal Aorta

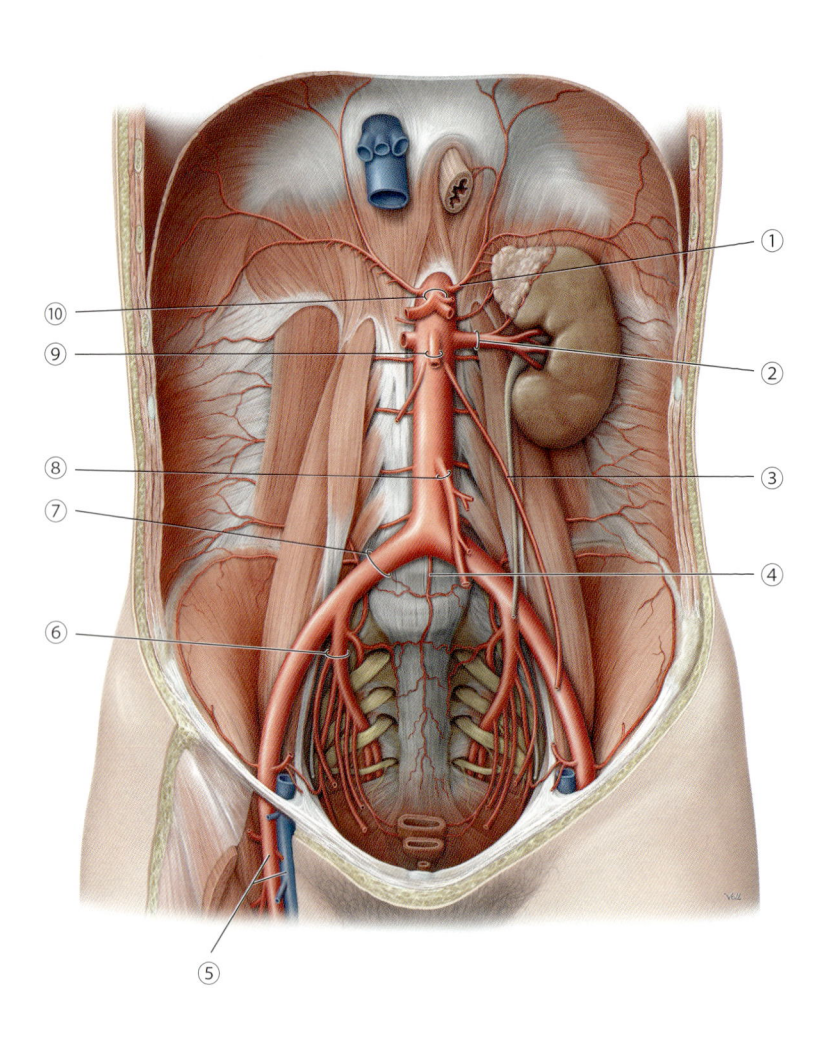

腹大動脈

女性の腹部，前面

① □ 左下横隔動脈　　　　　　　　□ Left inferior phrenic artery

② □ 左腎動脈　　　　　　　　　　□ Left renal artery

③ □ 左卵巣動脈（男性の場合は　　　□ Left ovarian artery (testicular
　　　精巣動脈）　　　　　　　　　　　artery in males)

④ □ 正中仙骨動脈　　　　　　　　□ Median sacral artery

⑤ □ 大腿動脈・静脈　　　　　　　□ Femoral artery and vein

⑥ □ 右内腸骨動脈　　　　　　　　□ Right internal iliac artery

⑦ □ 右総腸骨動脈　　　　　　　　□ Right common iliac artery

⑧ □ 下腸間膜動脈　　　　　　　　□ Inferior mesenteric artery

⑨ □ 上腸間膜動脈　　　　　　　　□ Superior mesenteric artery

⑩ □ 腹腔動脈　　　　　　　　　　□ Celiac trunk

解説

腹大動脈は胸大動脈の延長であり，T12の高さで腹部に入り，L4の高さで二分岐して総腸骨動脈になる．

Renal Arteries

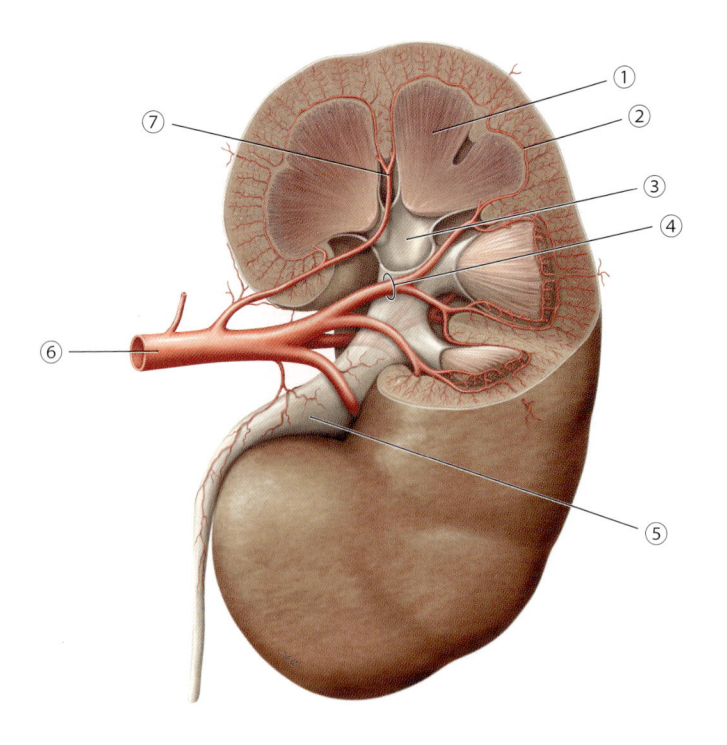

腎動脈

左の腎臓，前面

① ☐ 腎錐体 ☐ Medullary pyramid

② ☐ 弓状動脈（腎錐体の錐体底に） ☐ Arcuate artery (at base of medullary pyramids)

③ ☐ 大腎杯 ☐ Major calix

④ ☐ 上前区動脈 ☐ Anterior superior segmental artery

⑤ ☐ 左の尿管〔腎盂（腎盤）からの起始〕 ☐ Left ureter (origin from renal pelvis)

⑥ ☐ 左腎動脈（本幹） ☐ Left renal artery (main trunk)

⑦ ☐ 葉間動脈（腎錐体の間） ☐ Interlobar artery (between the medullary pyramids)

🏥 臨床

　腎臓は血圧を感知して制御する重要な器官である．腎動脈の狭窄によって腎臓の血流量が減少すると，アンギオテンシノゲンを開裂させてアンギオテンシンIを遊離させるホルモンであるレニンの分泌が促進される．さらに，開裂することで血管収縮を促進して血圧を高めるアンギオテンシンIIが生じる．腎性高血圧症は高血圧症の診断において除外されるか，確定される必要がある．

1 図 15.7. p.209　2 図 14.8. p.179

Celiac Trunk I

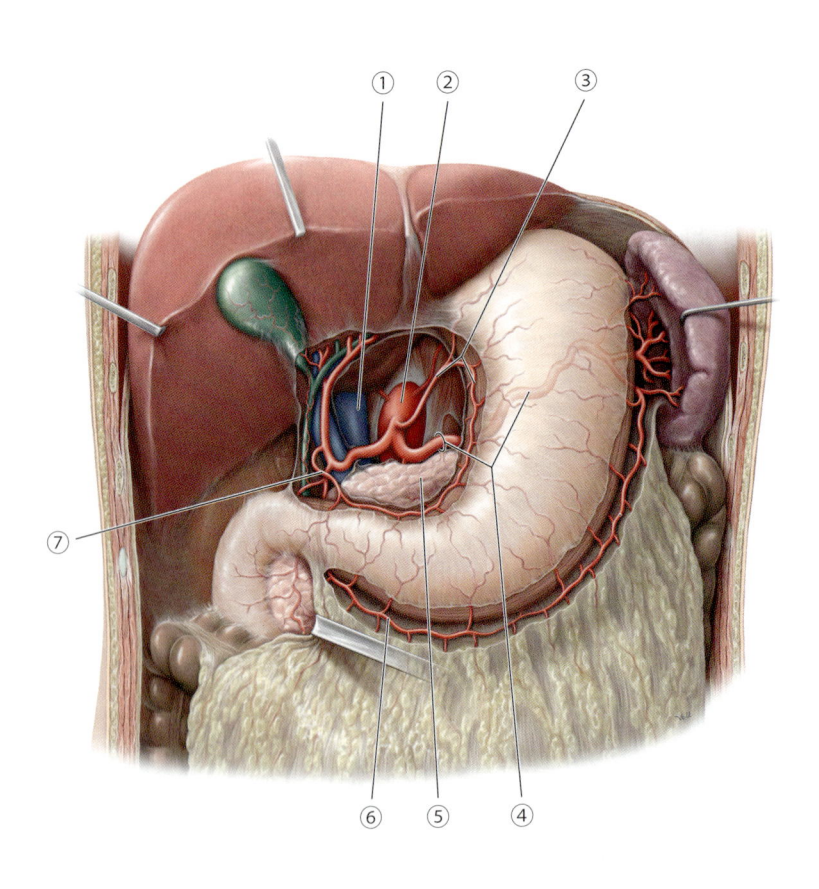

腹腔動脈は前腸に血液を供給する．ここに含まれる構造は何か？

腹腔動脈 1

前面

① ☐ 下大静脈 　　　　　　　　☐ Inferior vena cava
② ☐ 腹大動脈 　　　　　　　　☐ Abdominal aorta
③ ☐ 左胃動脈 　　　　　　　　☐ Left gastric artery
④ ☐ 脾動脈 　　　　　　　　　☐ Splenic artery
⑤ ☐ 膵臓 　　　　　　　　　　☐ Pancreas
⑥ ☐ 右胃大網動脈 　　　　　　☐ Right gastroomental artery
⑦ ☐ 右胃動脈 　　　　　　　　☐ Right gastric artery

A 　腹腔動脈はL1の高さで腹大動脈から起こり，前腸の諸構造に分布する．腹腔動脈から枝を受けるものには，食道の遠位半，胃，十二指腸の近位半，肝臓，胆嚢，脾臓，膵臓の上部がある．

1 図 15.8. p.210　2 図 14.9. p.180

Celiac Trunk II

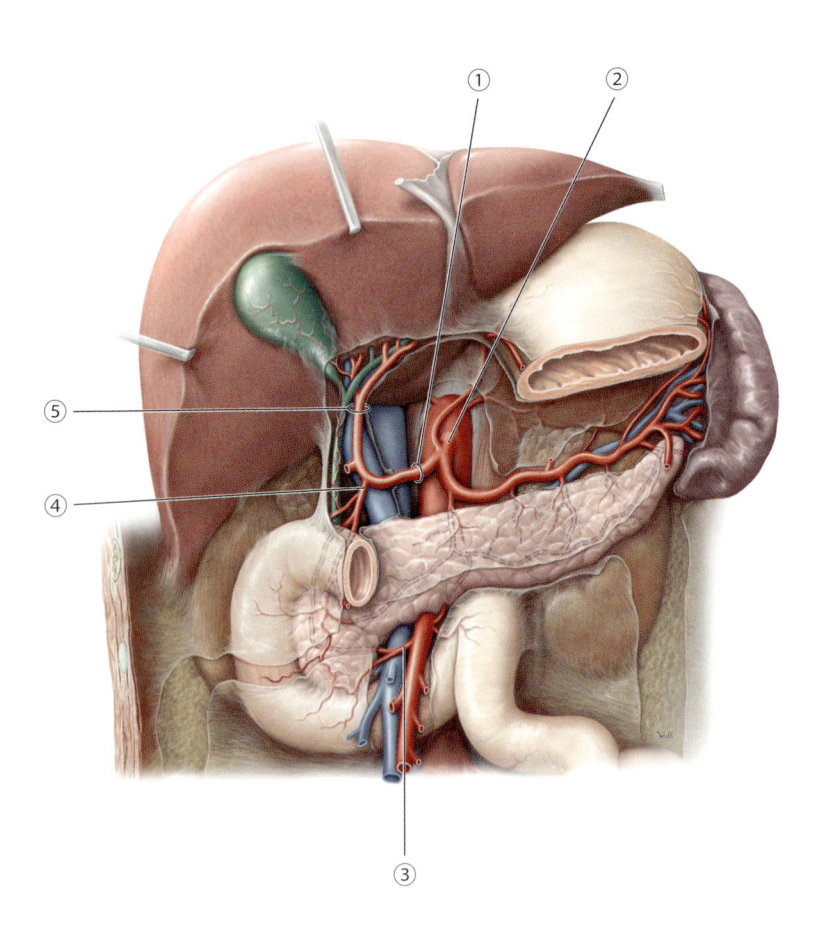

膵十二指腸動脈弧はどの動脈から生じるか？

腹腔動脈 2

前面

① □ 総肝動脈　　　　　　□ Common hepatic artery
② □ 腹腔動脈　　　　　　□ Celiac trunk
③ □ 下膵十二指腸動脈　　□ Inferior pancreaticoduodenal artery
④ □ 胃十二指腸動脈　　　□ Gastroduodenal artery
⑤ □ 固有肝動脈　　　　　□ Proper hepatic artery

A 　膵十二指腸動脈弓は腹腔動脈と上腸間膜動脈の重要な吻合である．上膵十二指腸動脈は胃十二指腸動脈から起こり，下膵十二指腸動脈は上腸間膜動脈から起こる．上・下膵十二指腸動脈はともに前後に分かれ，膵頭内で吻合する．

1 図 15.9. p.211　2 図 14.10. p.181

Superior Mesenteric Artery

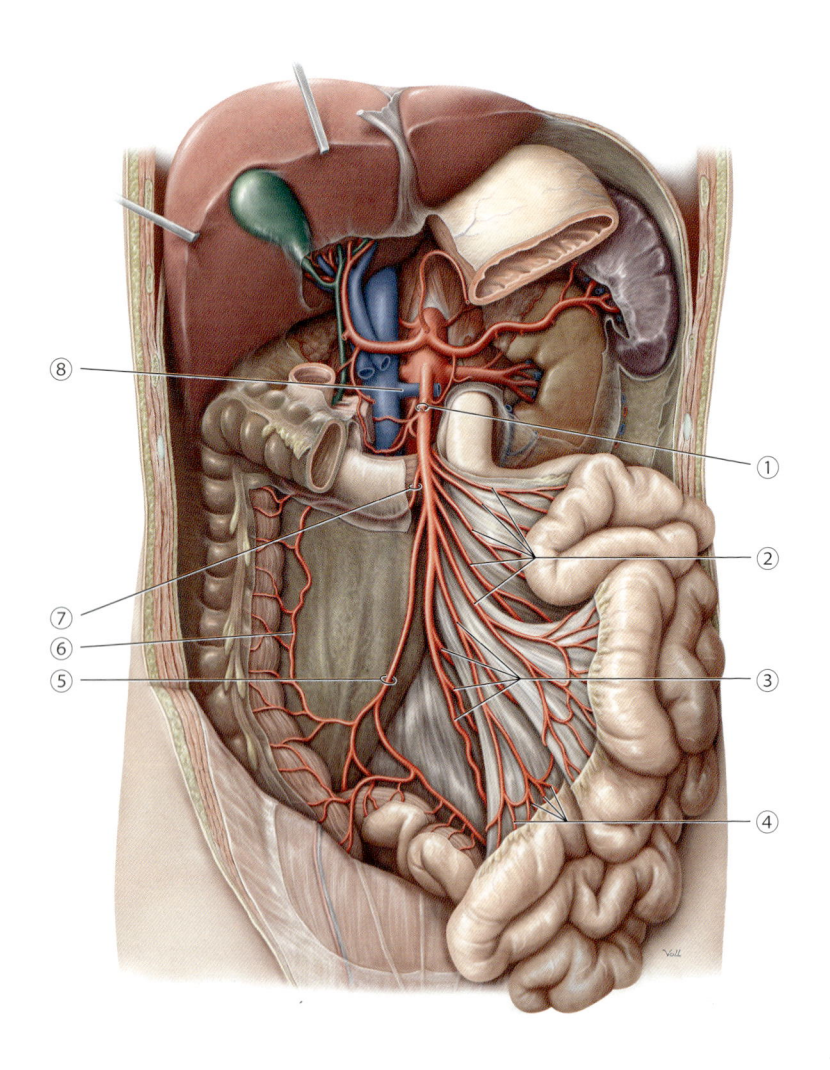

上腸間膜動脈

前面

① ☐ 中結腸動脈　　　　　☐ Middle colic artery
② ☐ 空腸動脈　　　　　　☐ Jejunal arteries
③ ☐ 回腸動脈　　　　　　☐ Ileal arteries
④ ☐ 直細動脈　　　　　　☐ Vasa recta
⑤ ☐ 回結腸動脈　　　　　☐ Ileocolic artery
⑥ ☐ 結腸辺縁動脈　　　　☐ Marginal artery
⑦ ☐ 右結腸動脈　　　　　☐ Right colic artery
⑧ ☐ 左腎静脈　　　　　　☐ Left renal vein

解説

　上腸間膜動脈は中腸に分布し，そこには十二指腸の遠位部(膵臓の一部も含む)，空腸，回腸，左結腸曲までの結腸が含まれる．結腸辺縁動脈は上腸間膜動脈の結腸枝を結び，下腸間膜動脈の枝と吻合する．

① 図 15.10. p.212　② 図 14.11. p.182

Inferior Mesenteric Artery

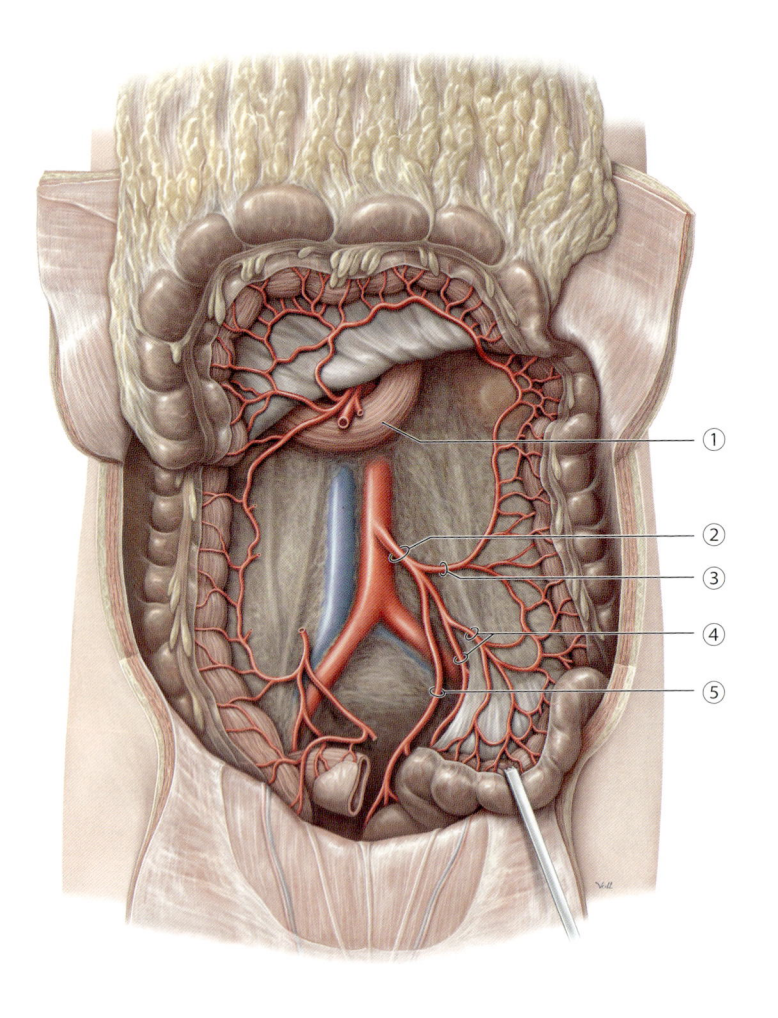

下腸間膜動脈

前面

① □ 十二指腸　　　　　　　　　□ Duodenum
② □ 下腸間膜動脈　　　　　　　□ Inferior mesenteric artery
③ □ 左結腸動脈　　　　　　　　□ Left colic artery
④ □ S状結腸動脈　　　　　　　 □ Sigmoid arteries
⑤ □ 上直腸動脈　　　　　　　　□ Superior rectal artery

解説

　下腸間膜動脈は左結腸曲，下行結腸，S状結腸，および直腸の大部分に分布する．下腸間膜動脈は上腸間膜動脈とは結腸辺縁動脈において吻合し，骨盤内では直腸の動脈と上直腸動脈によって吻合する．

1 図 15.11. p.213　　2 図 14.12. p.183

Tributaries of the Inferior Vena Cava

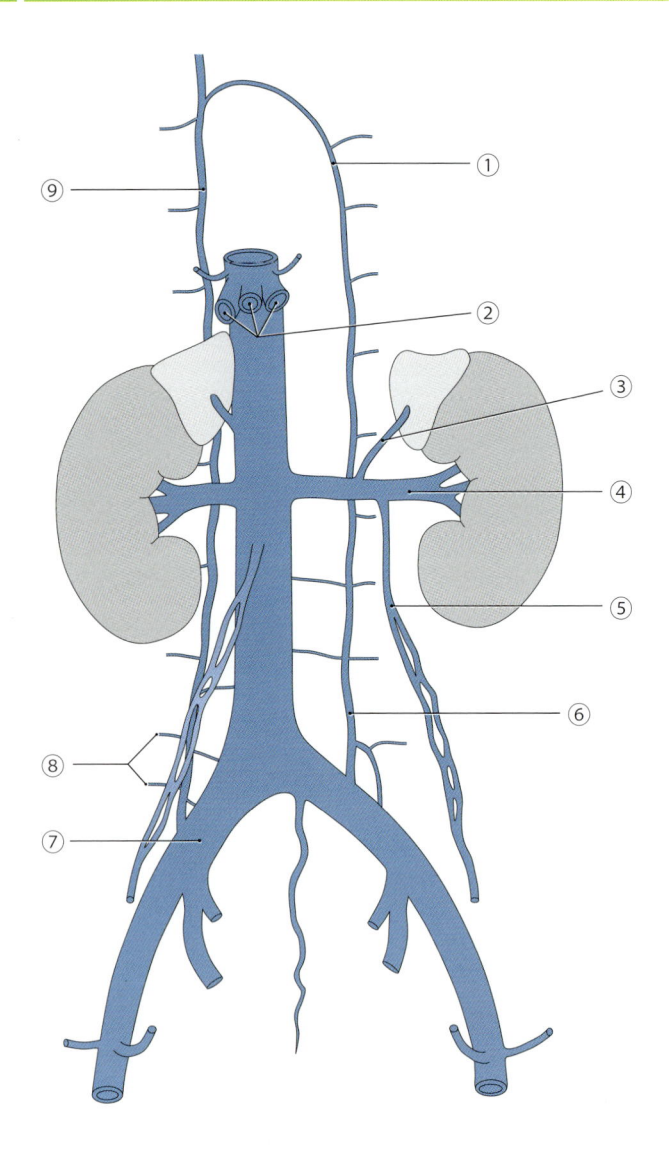

下大静脈の支脈

① □ 半奇静脈　　　　　□ Hemiazygos vein
② □ 肝静脈　　　　　　□ Hepatic veins
③ □ 上副腎静脈　　　　□ Suprarenal vein
④ □ 腎静脈　　　　　　□ Renal vein
⑤ □ 精巣 / 卵巣静脈　　□ Testicular / ovarian vein
⑥ □ 上行腰静脈　　　　□ Ascending lumbar vein
⑦ □ 総腸骨静脈　　　　□ Common iliac vein
⑧ □ 腰静脈　　　　　　□ Lumbar veins
⑨ □ 奇静脈　　　　　　□ Azygos vein

1 表 15.2. p.214　2 表 14.2. p.184

Renal Arteries & Veins

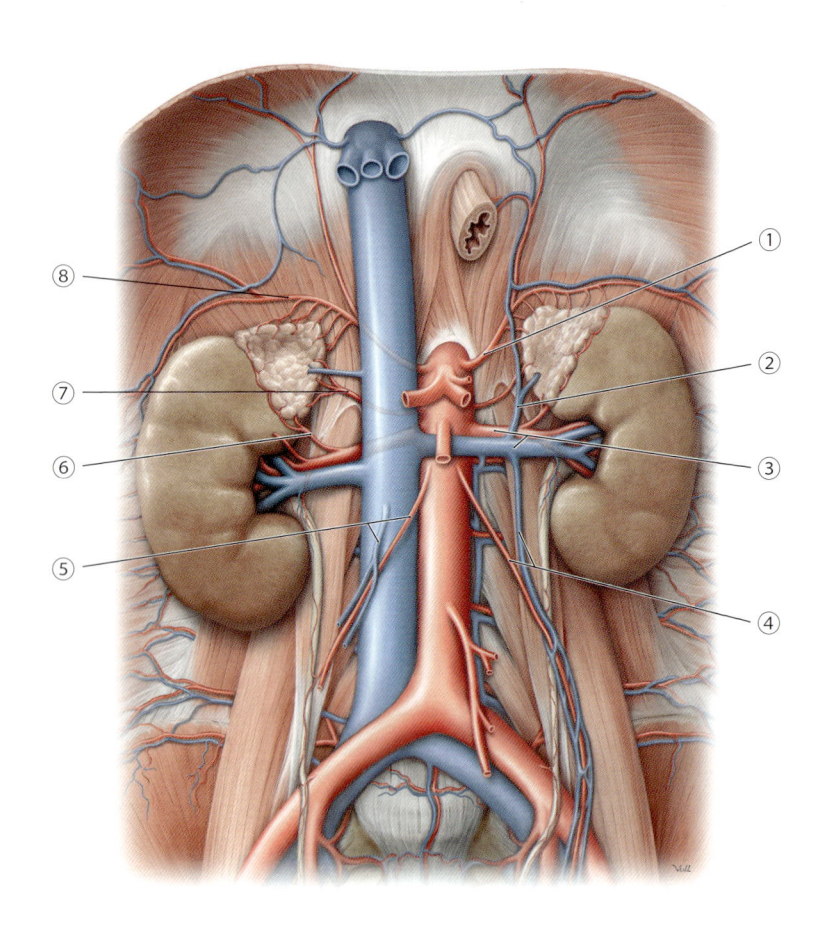

右腎静脈と左腎静脈の走行と枝を比較せよ．

腎動脈・静脈

前面

① ☐ 左下横隔動脈　　　　　　　☐ Left inferior phrenic artery

② ☐ 左副腎静脈（一般的に　　　☐ Left suprarenal vein (typically
　　　左腎静脈に開口）　　　　　　　opens into left renal vein)

③ ☐ 左腎動脈・静脈　　　　　　☐ Left renal artery and vein

④ ☐ 左精巣 / 卵巣動脈・静脈　　☐ Left testicular / ovarian artery and vein

⑤ ☐ 右精巣 / 卵巣動脈・静脈　　☐ Right testicular / ovarian artery and vein

⑥ ☐ 右下副腎動脈　　　　　　　☐ Right inferior suprarenal artery

⑦ ☐ 右中副腎動脈　　　　　　　☐ Right middle suprarenal artery

⑧ ☐ 右上副腎動脈　　　　　　　☐ Right superior suprarenal artery

A 左腎静脈には左副腎静脈と左精巣・卵巣静脈が注ぐが，右副腎静脈と右精巣・卵巣静脈は直接下大静脈に注ぐ．尿管から細い静脈が左右の腎静脈に注ぐ．

[1] 図 15.16, p.217　[2] 図 14.17, p.187

Portal Vein Distribution

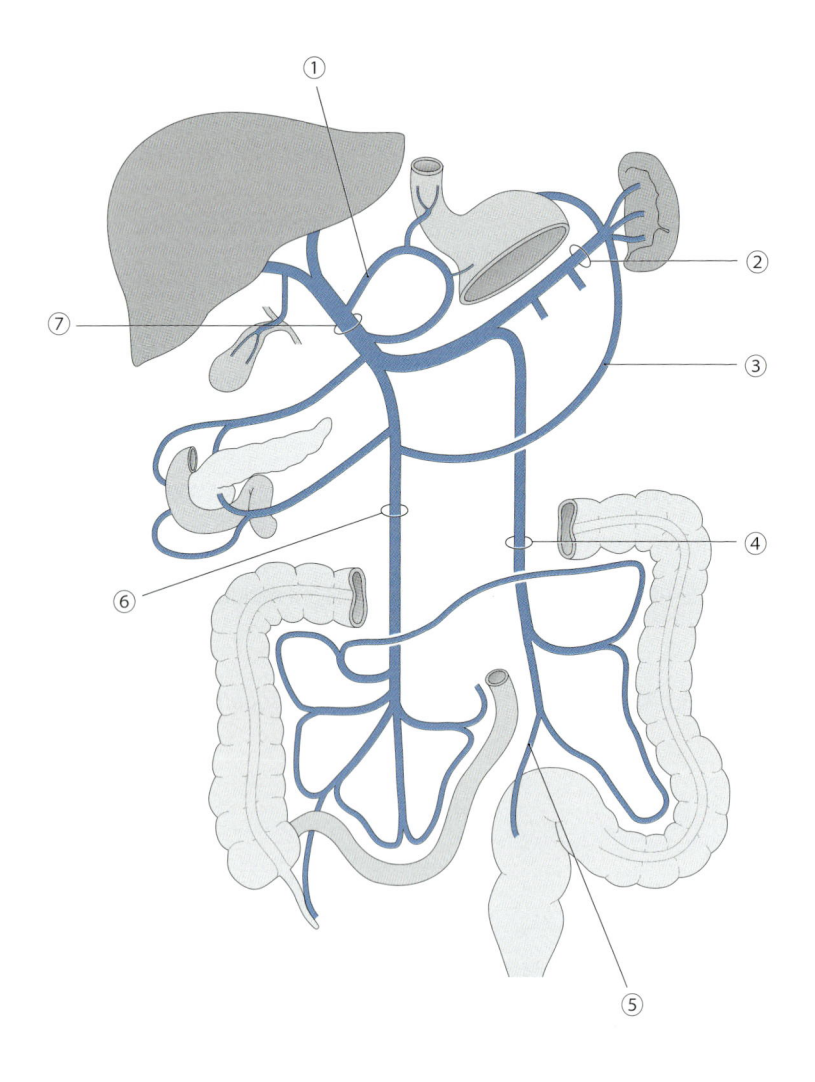

門脈の分布

① □ 左胃静脈と食道静脈　　□ Left gastric vein (with esophageal veins)

② □ 脾静脈　　□ Splenic vein

③ □ 左胃大網静脈　　□ Left gastro-omental vein

④ □ 下腸間膜静脈　　□ Inferior mesenteric vein

⑤ □ 上直腸静脈　　□ Superior rectal vein

⑥ □ 上腸間膜静脈　　□ Superior mesenteric vein

⑦ □ 門脈　　□ Portal vein

臨床

上直腸静脈が分布する部位の腫瘍は，門脈系を介して肝臓の毛細血管床に広がる（肝臓転移）．中直腸静脈と下直腸静脈が分布する部位の腫瘍は，下大静脈と右心を介して肺の毛細血管床に転移する（肺転移）．

1 図 15.14B. p.215　2 図 14.15B. p.185

Portal Vein in Situ

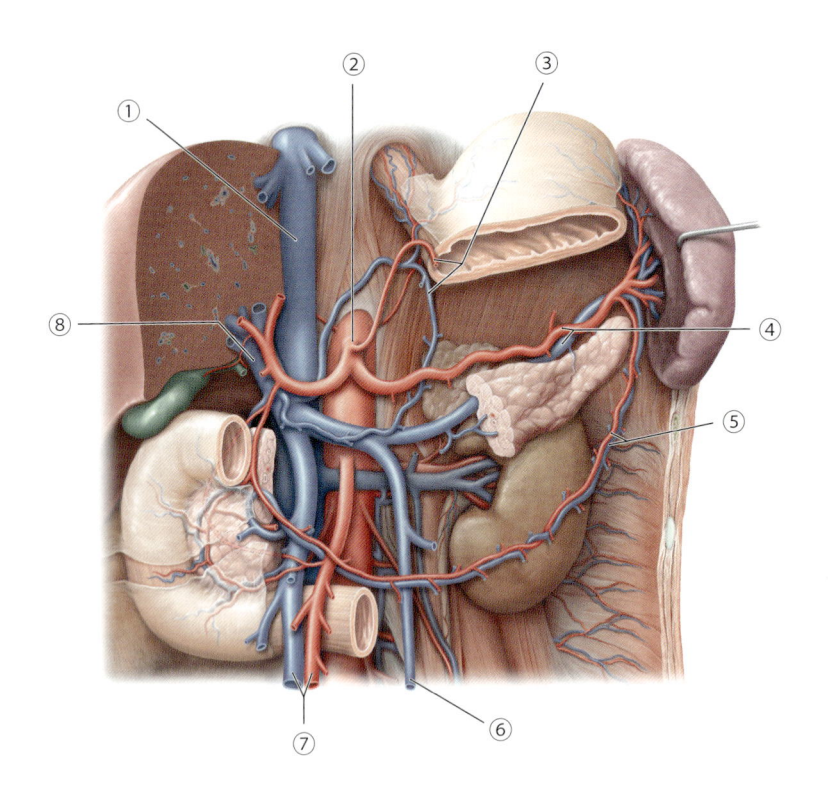

門脈系が分布する腹部内臓は何か？

原位置の門脈

前面

① ☐ 下大静脈 — ☐ Inferior vena cava
② ☐ 腹腔動脈 — ☐ Celiac trunk
③ ☐ 左胃動脈・静脈 — ☐ Left gastric artery and vein
④ ☐ 脾動脈・静脈 — ☐ Splenic artery and vein
⑤ ☐ 左胃大網動脈・静脈 — ☐ Left gastro-omental artery and vein
⑥ ☐ 下腸間膜静脈 — ☐ Inferior mesenteric vein
⑦ ☐ 上腸間膜動脈・静脈 — ☐ Superior mesenteric artery and vein
⑧ ☐ 門脈 — ☐ Portal vein

A 門脈系は食道下部から直腸上部までの胃腸管，また肝臓，胆嚢，膵臓，脾臓に分布する．

Blood Vessels of the Female Pelvis

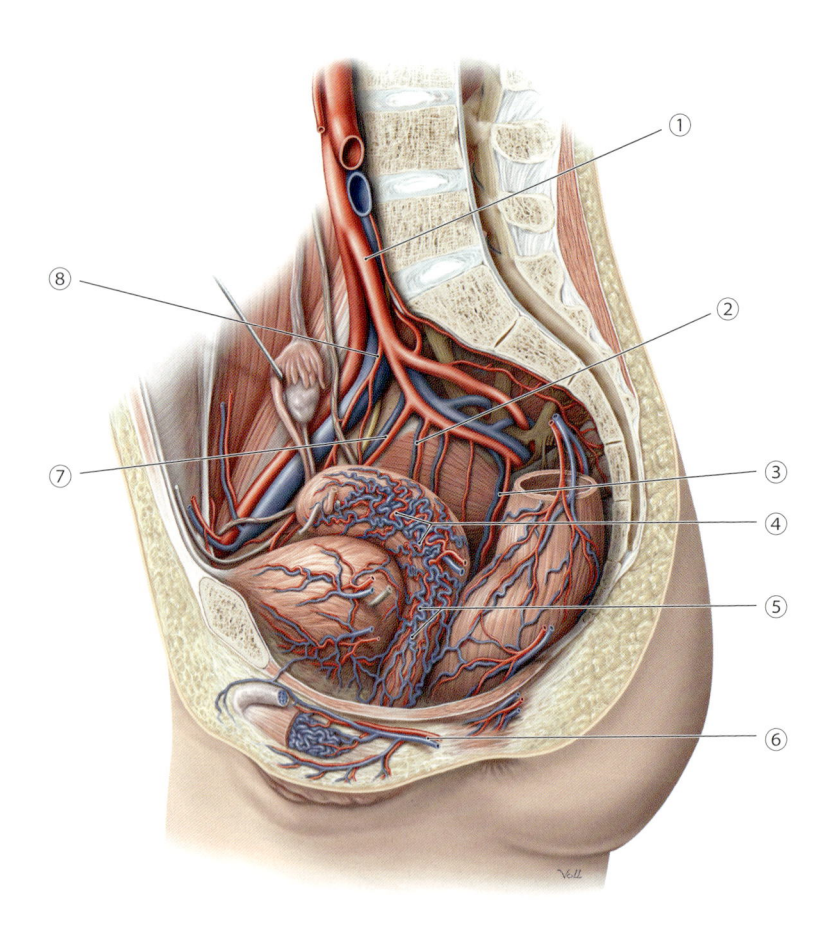

外科手術において，脈管遮断の危険を恐れることなく内腸骨動脈を切断できるのはなぜか？

女性骨盤の血管

骨盤の右半分，左外側面

① □ 右内腸骨動脈　　　　　　□ Right internal iliac artery
② □ 右子宮動脈・静脈　　　　□ Right uterine artery and vein
③ □ 右中直腸動脈・静脈　　　□ Right middle rectal artery and vein
④ □ 子宮静脈叢　　　　　　　□ Uterine venous plexus
⑤ □ 腟静脈叢　　　　　　　　□ Vaginal venous plexus
⑥ □ 左内陰部動脈・静脈　　　□ Left internal pudendal artery and vein
⑦ □ 右閉鎖動脈・静脈　　　　□ Right obturator artery and vein
⑧ □ 右臍動脈　　　　　　　　□ Right umbilical artery

A 　内腸骨動脈は同側および対側の枝との間に多くの吻合がある．また，内腸骨動脈は外腸骨動脈，大腿動脈，下腸間膜動脈，卵巣動脈との間に側副路がある．

1 図 15.21B. p.223　2 図 19.1B. p.255

Blood Vessels of the Rectum

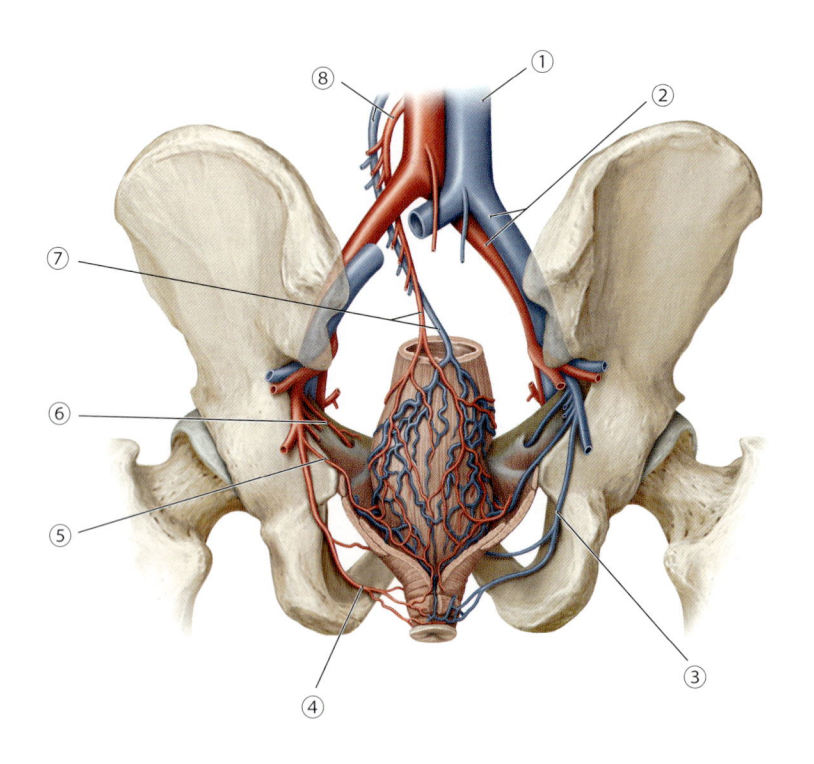

直腸の血管

後面

① □ 下大静脈　　□ Inferior vena cava

② □ 右総腸骨動脈・静脈　　□ Right common iliac artery and vein

③ □ 右内陰部静脈　　□ Right internal pudendal vein

④ □ 左下直腸動脈　　□ Left inferior rectal artery

⑤ □ 左中直腸動脈　　□ Left middle rectal artery

⑥ □ 左閉鎖動脈　　□ Left obturator artery

⑦ □ 上直腸動脈・静脈　　□ Superior rectal artery and vein

⑧ □ 下腸間膜動脈・静脈　　□ Inferior mesenteric artery and vein

解説

主に直腸に分布するのは上直腸動脈である．中直腸動脈は上直腸動脈と下直腸動脈との間の吻合路となっている．

1 図 15.22. p.224　　2 図 19.2. p.256

Blood Vessels of the Male Genitalia

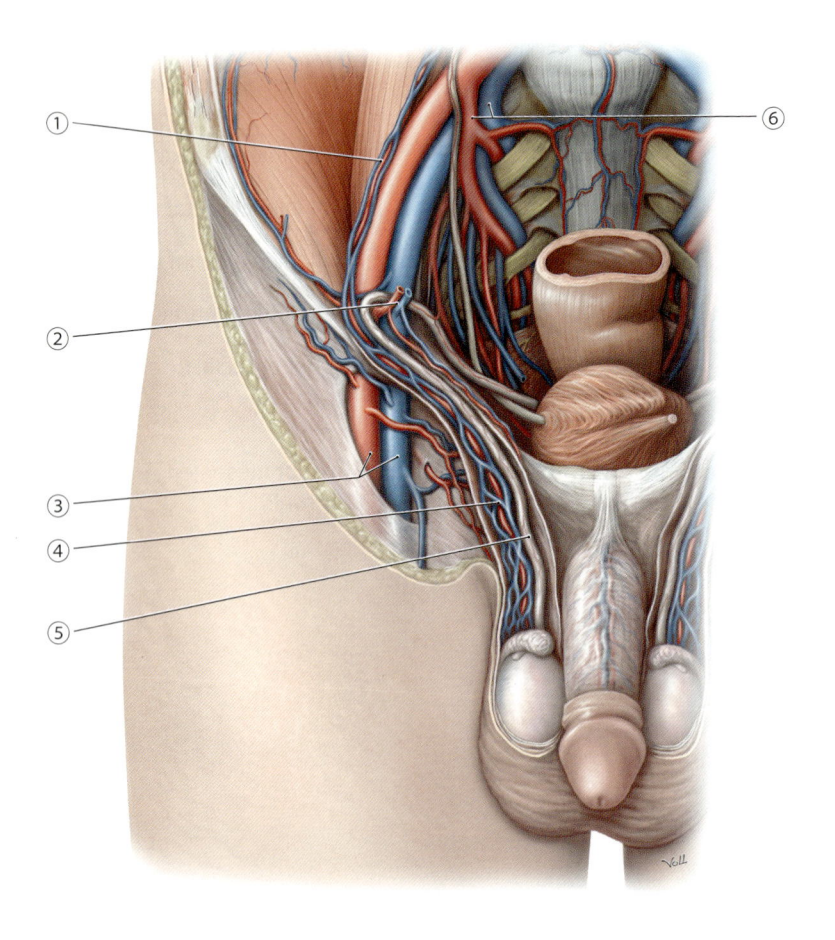

男性生殖器の血管

前面

① □ 精巣動脈・静脈　　　　　　　□ Testicular artery and vein
② □ 下腹壁動脈・静脈　　　　　　□ Inferior epigastric artery and vein
③ □ 大腿動脈・静脈　　　　　　　□ Femoral artery and vein
④ □ 蔓状静脈叢（精巣静脈）　　　□ Pampiniform plexus (testicular veins)
⑤ □ 右の精管　　　　　　　　　　□ Right ductus deferens
⑥ □ 内腸骨動脈・静脈　　　　　　□ Internal iliac artery and vein

Parietal Lymph Nodes

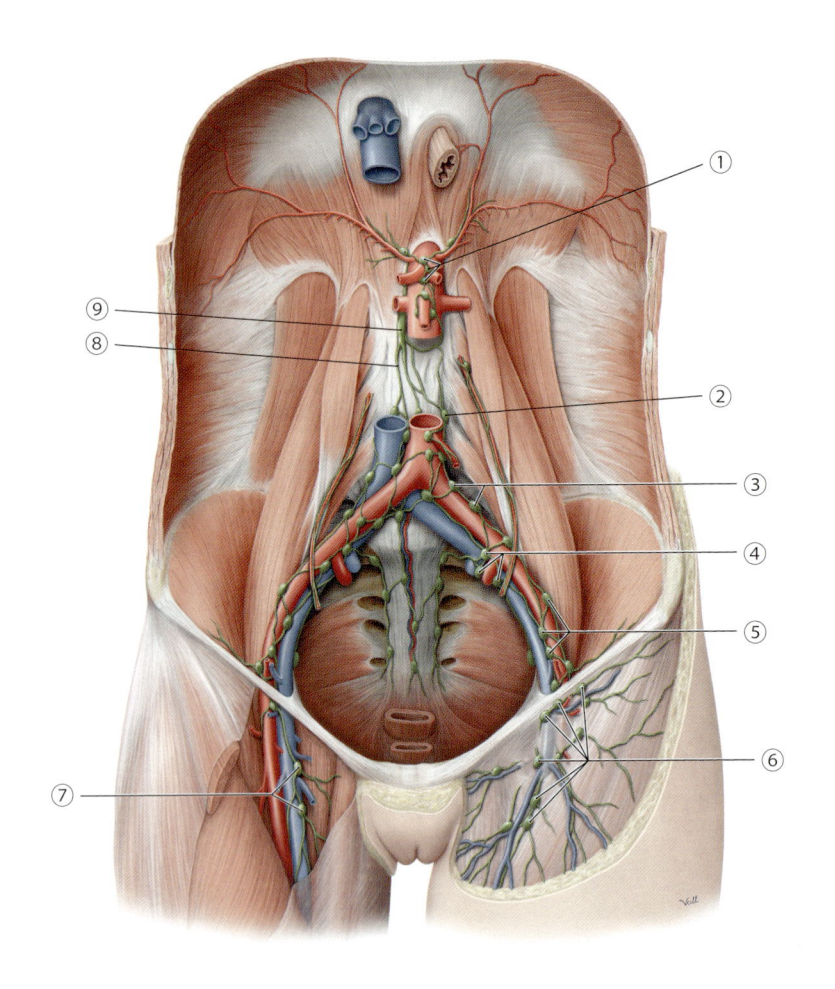

腸のリンパ流路について簡単に説明せよ．

壁側リンパ節

前面

① □ 腹腔リンパ節 □ Celiac lymph node
② □ 左外側大動脈リンパ節 □ Left lateral aortic lymph node
③ □ 総腸骨リンパ節 □ Common iliac lymph node
④ □ 内腸骨リンパ節 □ Internal iliac lymph node
⑤ □ 外腸骨リンパ節 □ External iliac lymph node
⑥ □ 浅鼠径リンパ節(水平群と垂直群) □ Superficial inguinal lymph node (horizontal and vertical groups)
⑦ □ 深鼠径リンパ節 □ Deep inguinal lymph node
⑧ □ 右腰リンパ本幹 □ Right lumbar trunk
⑨ □ 乳ビ槽 □ Cisterna chyli

> 腸のリンパ系は動脈の走行に従い,腹腔動脈・上腸間膜動脈・下腸間膜動脈周辺の大動脈前リンパ節を通過することになる.最終的には乳ビ槽に至り,そこから胸管へ入っていく.

1 図 16.6. p.228 2 図 14.24. p.194

Autonomic Plexuses

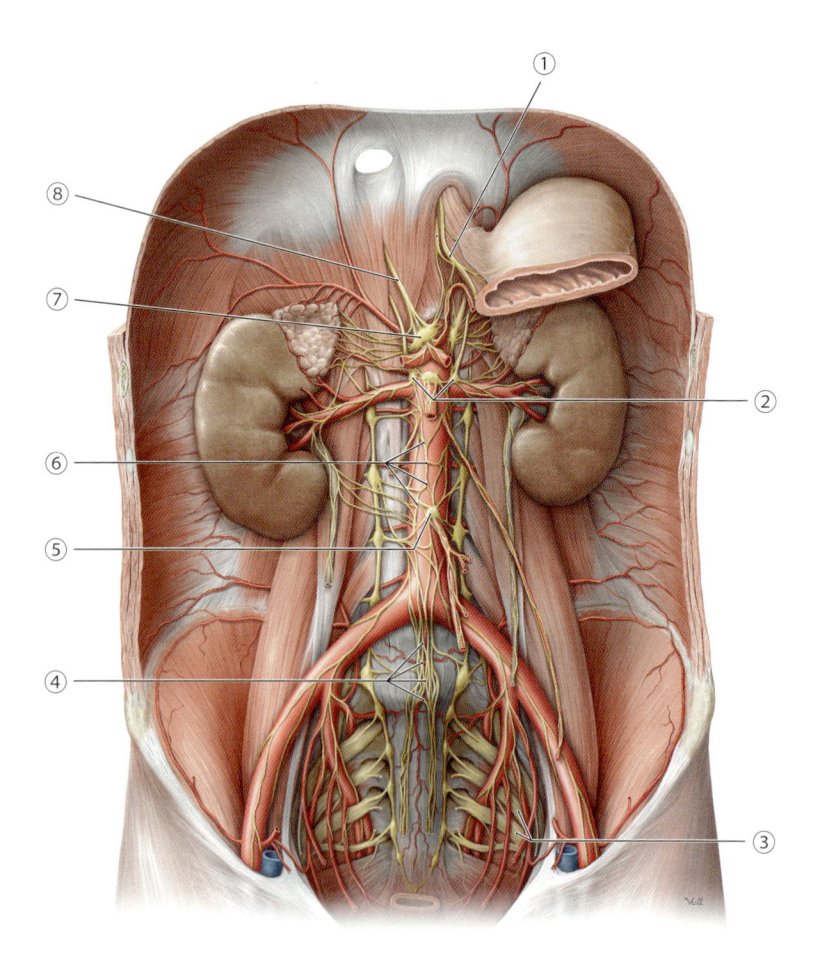

自律神経叢

男性腹部，前面

① □ 前迷走神経幹 □ Anterior vagal trunk
② □ 大動脈腎動脈神経節 □ Aorticorenal ganglia
③ □ 仙骨神経叢 □ Sacral plexus
④ □ 上下腹神経叢 □ Superior hypogastric plexus
⑤ □ 下腸間膜動脈神経節 □ Inferior mesenteric ganglion
⑥ □ 腸間膜動脈間神経叢 □ Intermesenteric plexus
⑦ □ 腹腔神経節 □ Celiac ganglion
⑧ □ 右大内臓神経 □ Right greater splanchnic nerve

Innervation of the Female Pelvis

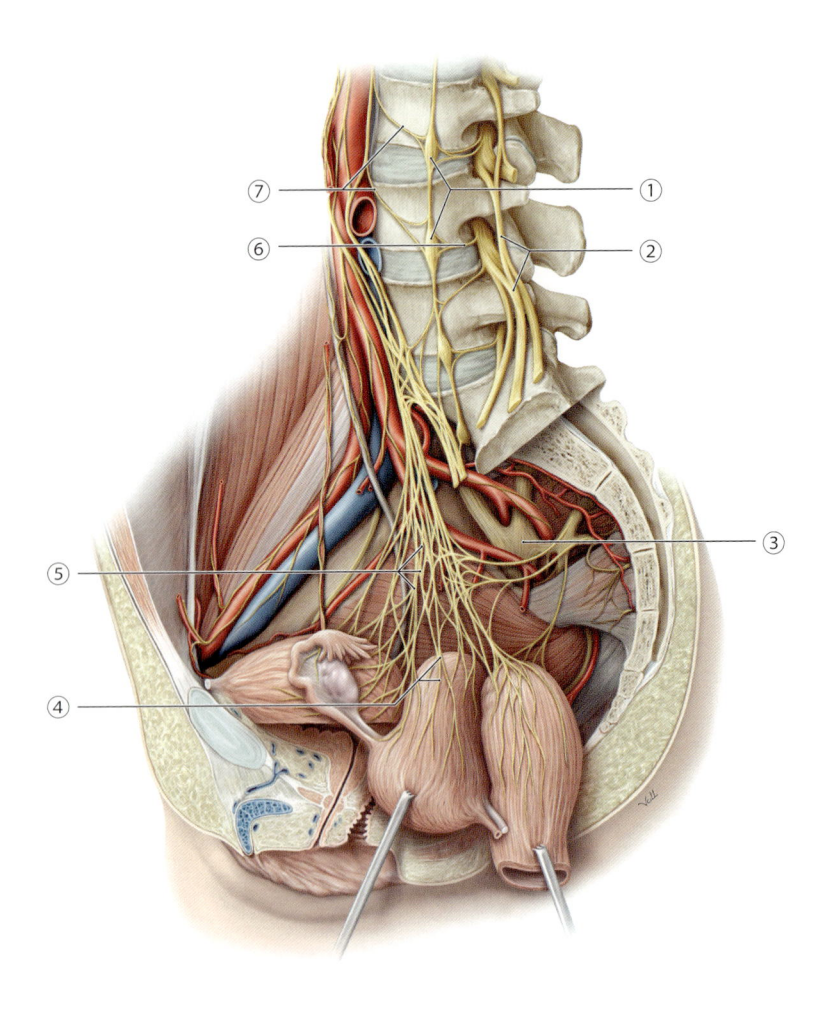

女性骨盤の神経支配

右骨盤，左外側面

① ☐ 交感神経幹，腰神経節 　　　☐ Sympathetic trunk, lumbar ganglia

② ☐ 腰神経，前枝 　　　☐ Lumbar nerves, anterior rami

③ ☐ 仙骨神経叢 　　　☐ Sacral plexus

④ ☐ 右子宮腟神経叢 　　　☐ Right uterovaginal plexus

⑤ ☐ 右下下腹神経叢 　　　☐ Right inferior hypogastric plexus

⑥ ☐ 灰白交通枝 　　　☐ Gray ramus communicans

⑦ ☐ 腰内臓神経 　　　☐ Lumbar splanchnic nerve

Innervation of the Male Pelvis

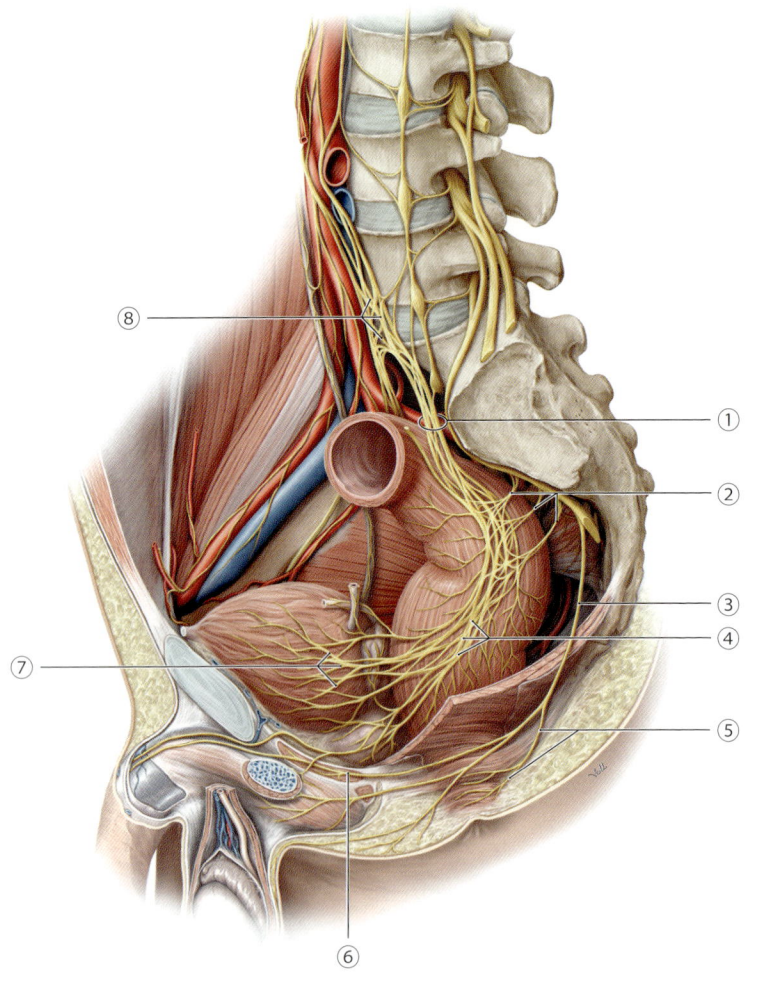

Q 骨盤内臓の副交感神経系の起始はどこか？

男性骨盤の神経支配

右骨盤，左外側面

① ☐ 左下腹神経　　　　　　☐ Left hypogastric nerve
② ☐ 骨盤内臓神経　　　　　☐ Pelvic splanchnic nerves
③ ☐ 陰部神経　　　　　　　☐ Pudendal nerve
④ ☐ 下直腸動脈神経叢　　　☐ Inferior rectal plexus
⑤ ☐ 下直腸神経　　　　　　☐ Inferior rectal nerves
⑥ ☐ 陰茎背神経　　　　　　☐ Dorsal nerve of the penis
⑦ ☐ 膀胱神経叢　　　　　　☐ Vesical plexus
⑧ ☐ 上下腹神経叢　　　　　☐ Superior hypogastric plexus

A 骨盤内臓神経は仙髄から起こり，仙骨神経を通って左右の下腹神経叢に至り，そこで骨盤神経叢を作る．

1 図 17.7. p.243　　2 図 19.15. p.263

Surface Anatomy

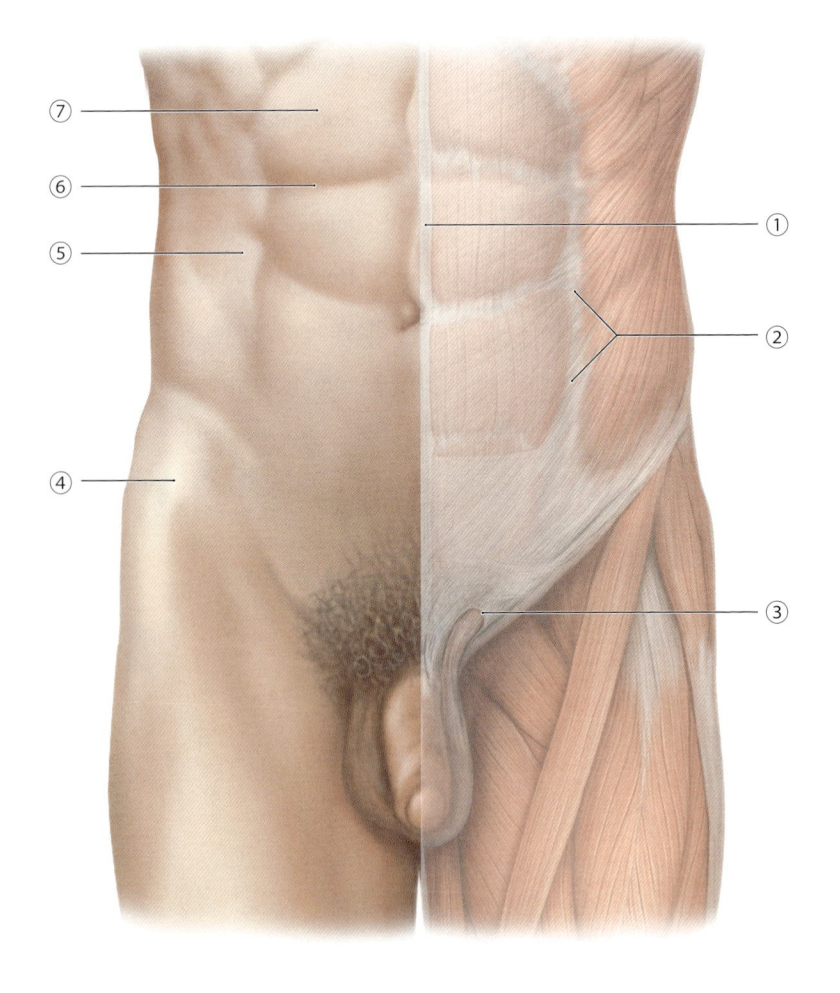

腹部・骨盤の体表解剖

前面

① ☐ 白線　　　　　☐ Linea alba
② ☐ 半月線　　　　☐ Semilunar line
③ ☐ 浅鼠径輪　　　☐ Superficial inguinal ring
④ ☐ 上前腸骨棘　　☐ Anterior superior iliac spine (ASIS)
⑤ ☐ 外腹斜筋　　　☐ External oblique
⑥ ☐ 腱の付着　　　☐ Tendinous insertion
⑦ ☐ 腹直筋　　　　☐ Rectus abdominis

上肢 Upper Limb

上肢の骨格	296
鎖骨	298
肩甲骨 1	300
肩甲骨 2	302
上腕骨 1	304
上腕骨 2	306
上肢帯の関節	308
胸鎖関節	310
肩関節(肩甲上腕関節) 1	312
肩関節(肩甲上腕関節) 2	314
肩の前額断面	316
肩と上腕の筋(前面) 1	318
肩と上腕の筋(前面) 2	320
肩と上腕の筋(前面) 3	322
肩と上腕の筋(前面) 4	324
肩と上腕の筋(後面) 1	326
肩と上腕の筋(後面) 2	328
肩と上腕の筋(後面) 3	330
橈骨と尺骨	332
肘関節 1	334
肘関節 2	336
前腕の筋(前面) 1	338
前腕の筋(前面) 2	340
前腕の筋(前面) 3	342
前腕の筋(後面) 1	344
前腕の筋(後面) 2	346
手首と手の骨格 1	348
手首と手の骨格 2	350
手首と手の関節	352
手の筋 1	354
手の筋 2	356
手の筋 3	358
手の筋 4	360
手背	362
上肢の動脈	364
上肢の皮静脈	366
腕神経叢の構造	368
腕神経叢の走行	370
腕神経叢からの神経 1(腋窩神経)	372
腕神経叢からの神経 2(橈骨神経)	374
腕神経叢からの神経 3(筋皮神経)	376
腕神経叢からの神経 4(正中神経)	378
腕神経叢からの神経 5(尺骨神経)	380
肩の後部における神経・血管 1	382
肩の後部における神経・血管 2	384
腋窩の神経・血管 1	386
腋窩の神経・血管 2	388
腋窩の神経・血管 3	390
上腕の神経・血管	392
前腕の神経・血管	394
手根管	396
浅掌動脈弓	398
深掌動脈弓	400
解剖学的嗅ぎタバコ入れ	402
手における感覚神経の分布 1	404
手における感覚神経の分布 2	406
上腕の横断面	408
前腕の横断面	410
手の体表解剖	412

Bones of the Upper Limb

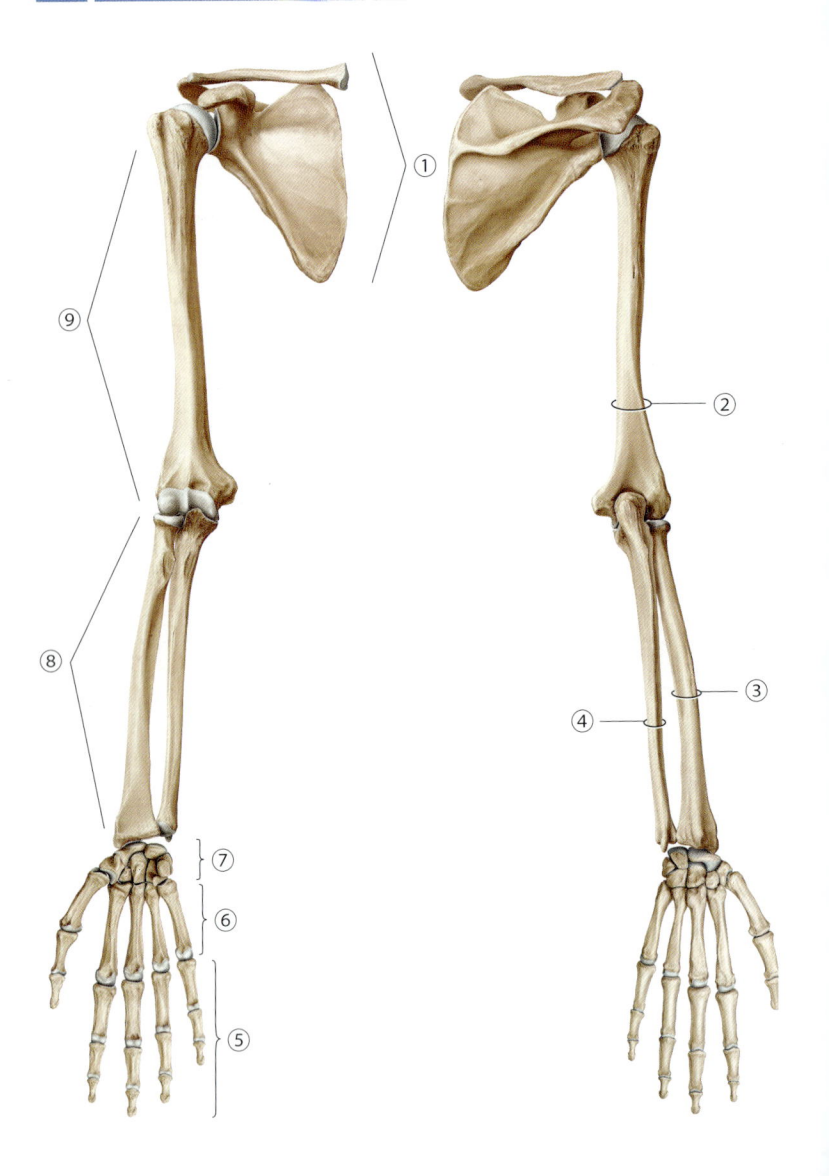

上肢の骨格

右上肢，左：前面，右：後面

① □ 上肢帯　　　　　　　□ Shoulder girdle
② □ 上腕骨　　　　　　　□ Humerus
③ □ 橈骨　　　　　　　　□ Radius
④ □ 尺骨　　　　　　　　□ Ulna
⑤ □ 指骨（指節骨）　　　□ Phalanges
⑥ □ 中手骨　　　　　　　□ Metacarpals
⑦ □ 手根骨　　　　　　　□ Carpal bones
⑧ □ 前腕　　　　　　　　□ Forearm
⑨ □ 上腕　　　　　　　　□ Arm

1 図 19.1A, B. p.252　2 図 21.1A, B. p.276

Clavicle

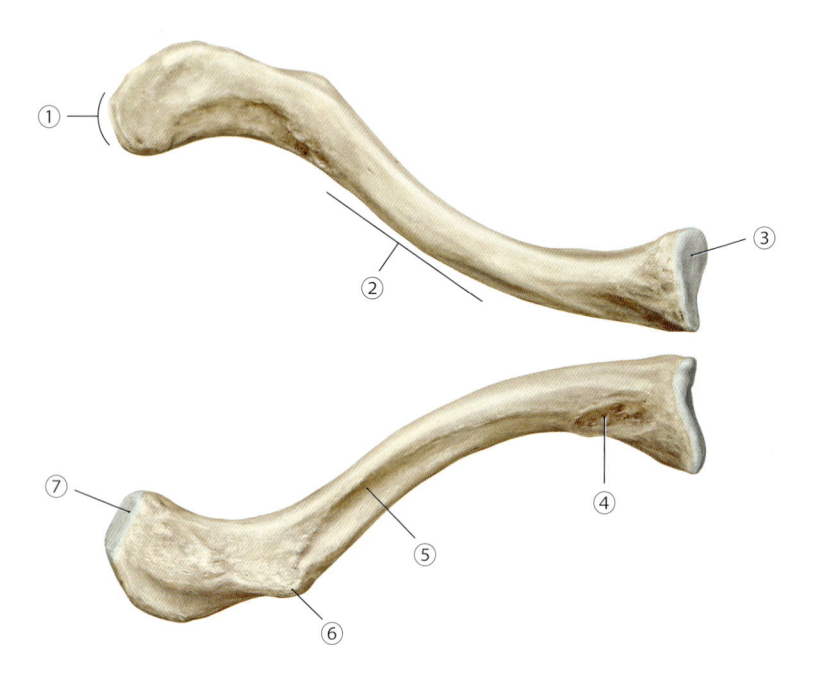

鎖骨

右鎖骨，上：上面，下：下面

① □ 肩峰端　　　　　　　　□ Acromial end
② □ 鎖骨体　　　　　　　　□ Shaft of clavicle
③ □ 胸骨関節面　　　　　　□ Sternal articular surface
④ □ 肋鎖靱帯圧痕　　　　　□ Impression for costoclavicular ligament
⑤ □ 鎖骨下筋溝　　　　　　□ Groove for subclavius muscle
⑥ □ 円錐靱帯結節　　　　　□ Conoid tubercle
⑦ □ 肩峰関節面　　　　　　□ Acromial articular surface

解説

　鎖骨はＳ字のような形をしており，全長（12〜15 cm）を体表から触知できる．鎖骨の内側端（胸骨端）は胸骨との間で胸鎖関節をなす．一方，外側端（肩峰端）は肩甲骨（肩峰）との間に肩鎖関節をなす．

1 図 19.3A, B. p.254　2 図 21.3A, B. p.278

Scapula I

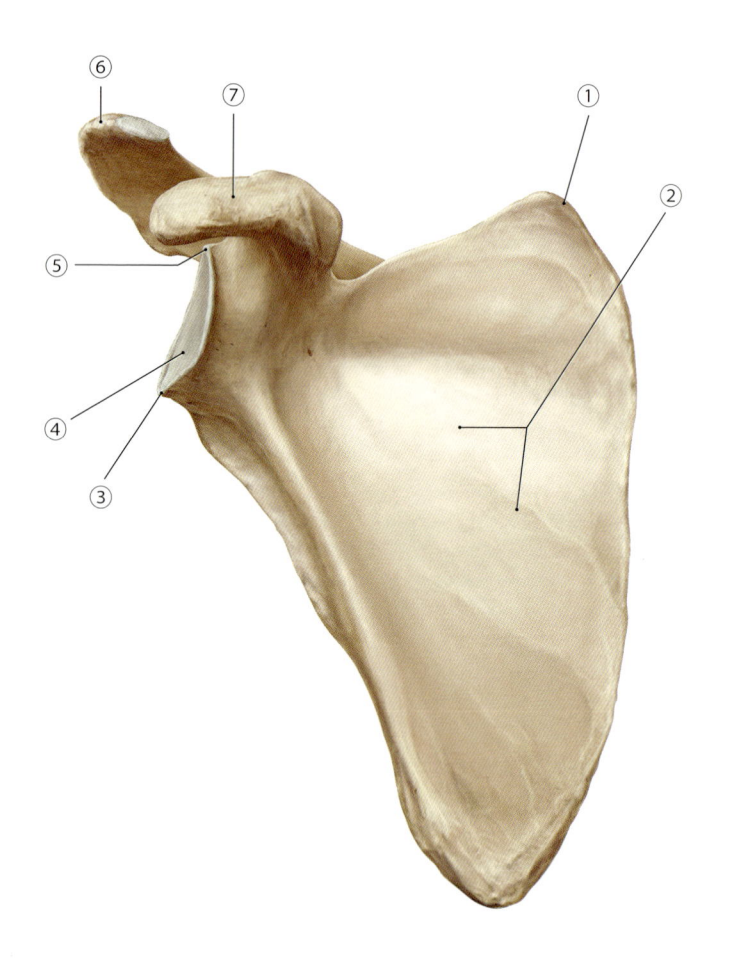

肩甲骨 1

右肩甲骨,前面

① □ 上角　　　　　　　　　□ Superior angle

② □ 肩甲下窩　　　　　　　□ Subscapular fossa

③ □ 関節下結節　　　　　　□ Infraglenoid tubercle

④ □ 関節窩　　　　　　　　□ Glenoid cavity

⑤ □ 関節上結節　　　　　　□ Supraglenoid tubercle

⑥ □ 肩峰　　　　　　　　　□ Acromion

⑦ □ 烏口突起　　　　　　　□ Coracoid process

解説

解剖学的正位では,肩甲骨は第2肋骨から第7肋骨の間に位置する.

1 図 19.4A. p.255　　2 図 21.4A. p.279

Scapula II

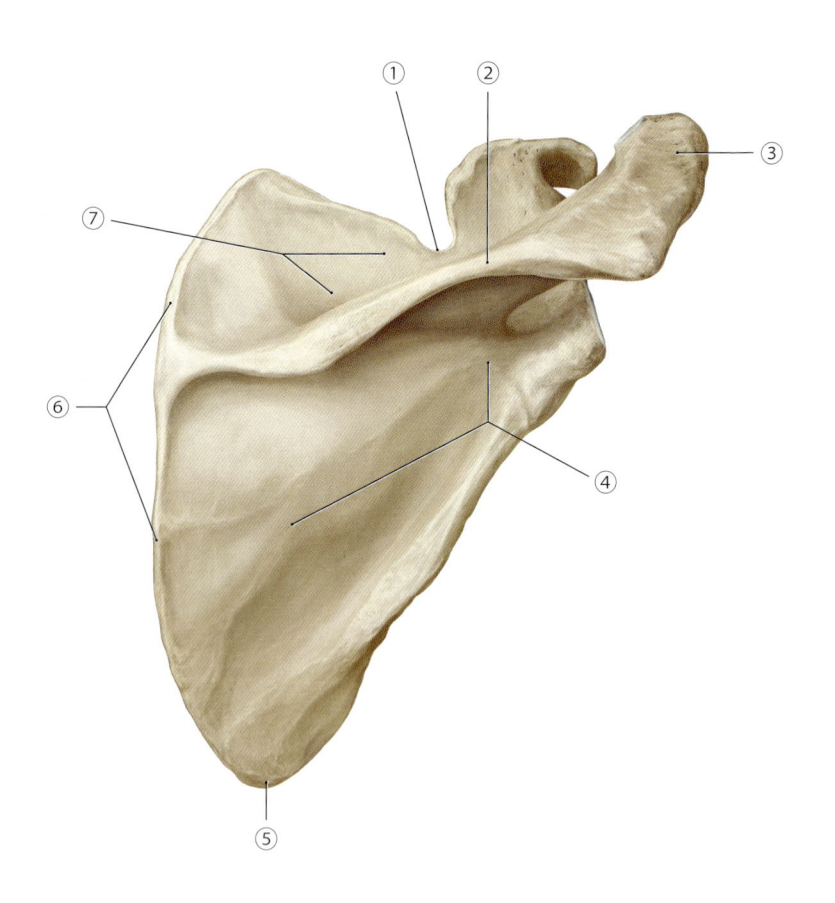

肩甲骨 2

右肩甲骨，後面

① □ 肩甲切痕　　　　　　□ Scapular notch
② □ 肩甲棘　　　　　　　□ Scapular spine
③ □ 肩峰　　　　　　　　□ Acromion
④ □ 棘下窩　　　　　　　□ Infraspinous fossa
⑤ □ 下角　　　　　　　　□ Inferior angle
⑥ □ 内側縁　　　　　　　□ Medial border
⑦ □ 棘上窩　　　　　　　□ Supraspinous fossa

臨床

上肩甲横靱帯の骨化により，肩甲切痕が骨性の孔（肩甲孔）となる場合がある．肩甲上神経は肩甲切痕を通過するので，上肩甲横靱帯の骨化に伴い，この神経が圧迫される場合がある．

[1] 図 19.4C. p.255　[2] 図 21.4C. p.279

Humerus I

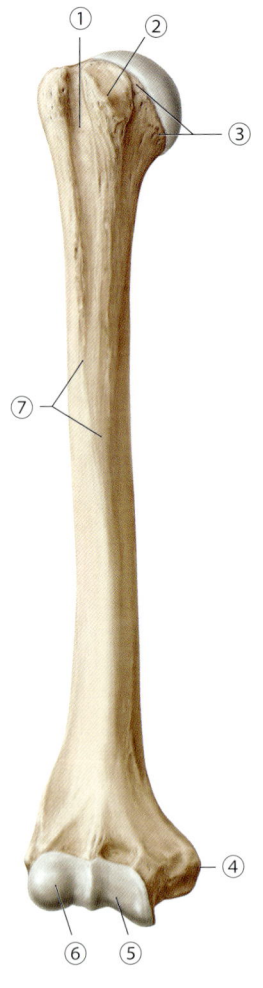

上腕骨外科頸の骨折で損傷される場合がある神経・血管は何か？

上腕骨 1

右上腕骨，前面

① □ 結節間溝　　　　　□ Intertubercular groove

② □ 小結節　　　　　　□ Lesser tuberosity

③ □ 解剖頸　　　　　　□ Anatomical neck

④ □ 内側上顆　　　　　□ Medial epicondyle

⑤ □ 上腕骨滑車　　　　□ Trochlea

⑥ □ 上腕骨小頭　　　　□ Capitellum

⑦ □ 三角筋粗面　　　　□ Deltoid tuberosity

A 　腋窩神経と前・後上腕回旋動脈が上腕骨外科頸の骨折で損傷される場合がある．

1 図 19.5A. p.256　　2 図 21.5A. p.280

Humerus II

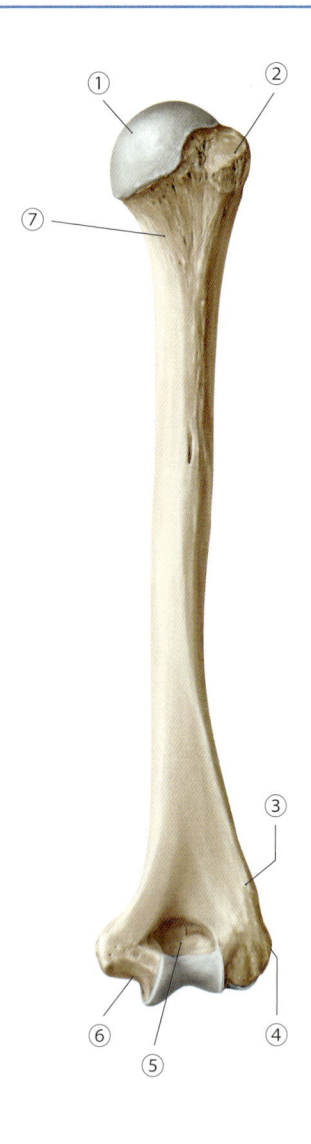

上腕骨 2

右上腕骨, 後面

① □ 上腕骨頭　　　　　□ Head of humerus
② □ 大結節　　　　　　□ Greater tuberosity
③ □ 外側顆上稜　　　　□ Lateral supracondylar ridge
④ □ 外側上顆　　　　　□ Lateral epicondyle
⑤ □ 肘頭窩　　　　　　□ Olecranon fossa
⑥ □ 尺骨神経溝　　　　□ Ulnar groove (for ulnar nerve)
⑦ □ 外科頸　　　　　　□ Surgical neck

1 図 19.5C. p.256　 2 図 21.5C. p.280

Joints of the Shoulder Girdle

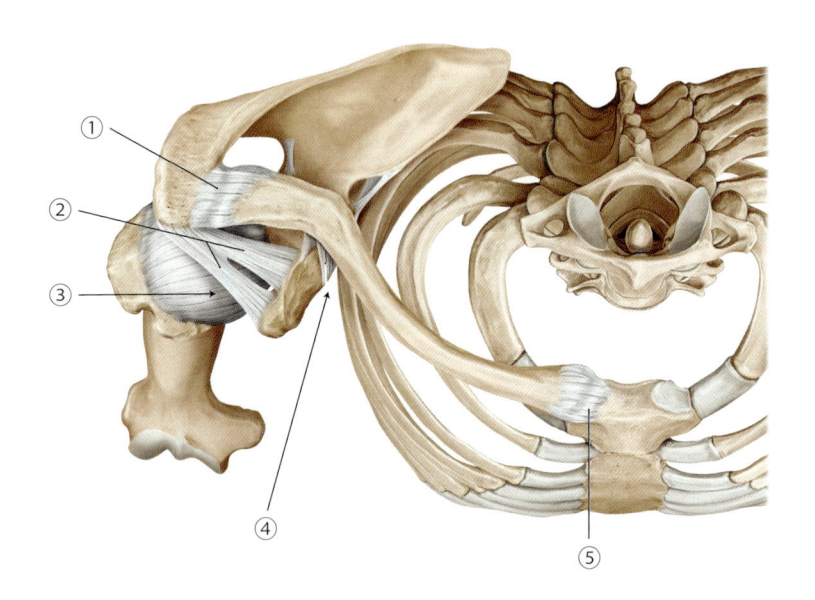

①
②
③
④
⑤

Q 上肢帯を体幹に連結する関節はどれか？

上肢帯の関節

右肩，上面

① ☐ 肩鎖関節（肩鎖靱帯）　　　☐ Acromioclavicular joint (with acromioclavicular ligament)

② ☐ 烏口肩峰靱帯　　　☐ Coracoacromial ligament

③ ☐ 肩関節（肩甲上腕関節）　　　☐ Glenohumeral joint

④ ☐ 肩甲胸郭関節　　　☐ Scapulothoracic joint

⑤ ☐ 胸鎖関節（前胸鎖靱帯）　　　☐ Sternoclavicular joint (with anterior sternoclavicular ligament)

A 　上肢帯の骨格は胸鎖関節のみによって体幹と連結する．肩甲骨は体幹の骨とは直接連結しない．上肢帯のすべての運動において，肩甲骨は胸郭の表面に存在する粗性結合組織（前鋸筋と肩甲下筋の間に形成される）の上を滑走する．肩甲骨とこの滑走面でできる連結を肩甲胸郭関節と呼ぶ場合がある．

1 図 19.7. p.258　2 図 21.7. p.282

Sternoclavicular Joint

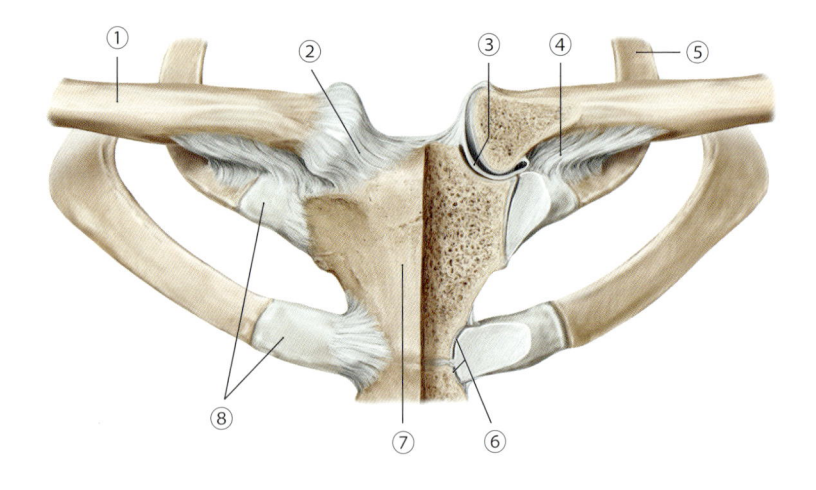

胸鎖関節

前面,左胸鎖関節の前額断面が見えている

① ☐ 鎖骨　　　　　　　　　☐ Clavicle
② ☐ 前胸鎖靱帯　　　　　　☐ Anterior sternoclavicular ligament
③ ☐ 関節円板　　　　　　　☐ Articular disk
④ ☐ 肋鎖靱帯　　　　　　　☐ Costoclavicular ligament
⑤ ☐ 第1肋骨　　　　　　　☐ 1st rib
⑥ ☐ 胸肋関節　　　　　　　☐ Sternocostal joint
⑦ ☐ 胸骨柄　　　　　　　　☐ Manubrium sterni
⑧ ☐ 肋軟骨　　　　　　　　☐ Costal cartilage

解説

　線維軟骨でできた関節円板を介して,鎖骨の胸骨端と胸骨柄の関節面が密着する.

1 図19.9. p.259　2 図21.9. p.283

Shoulder Joint (Glenohumeral Joint) I

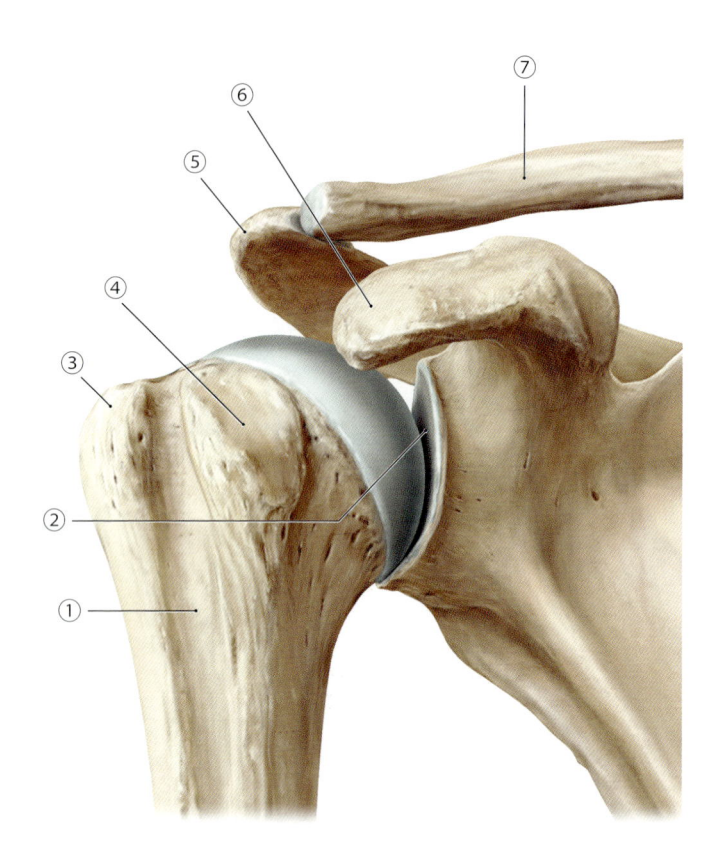

肩関節（肩甲上腕関節） 1

右肩，前面

① ☐ 結節間溝　　　　　☐ Intertubercular groove

② ☐ 関節窩　　　　　　☐ Glenoid cavity

③ ☐ 大結節　　　　　　☐ Greater tuberosity

④ ☐ 小結節　　　　　　☐ Lesser tuberosity

⑤ ☐ 肩峰　　　　　　　☐ Acromion

⑥ ☐ 烏口突起　　　　　☐ Coracoid process

⑦ ☐ 鎖骨　　　　　　　☐ Clavicle

1 図 19.11A. p.260　　2 図 21.11A. p.284

Shoulder Joint (Glenohumeral Joint) II

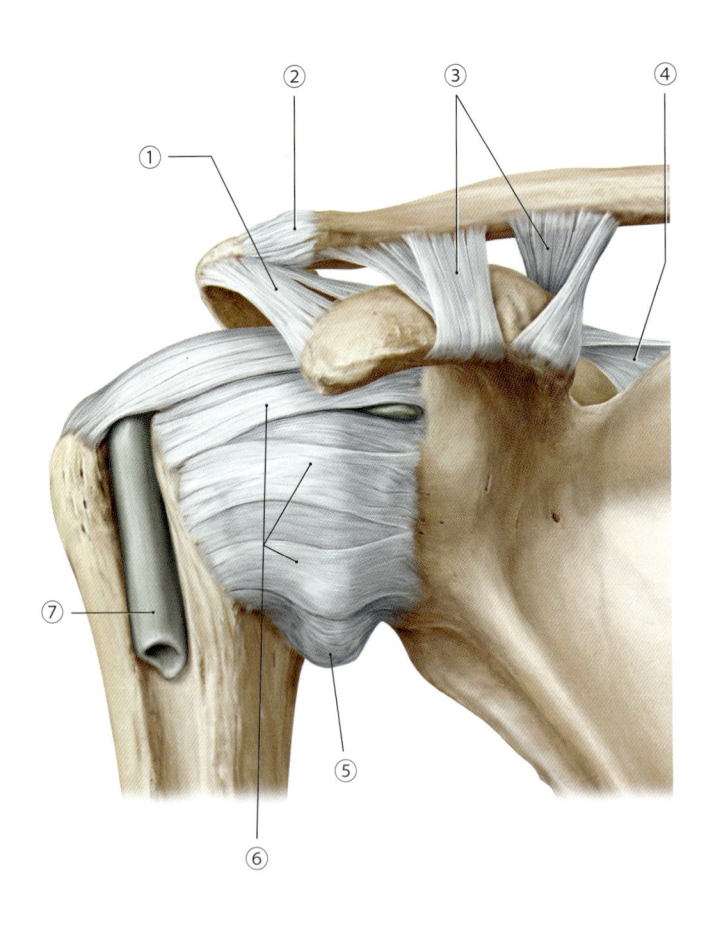

肩関節（肩甲上腕関節） 2

右肩，前面

① ☐ 烏口肩峰靱帯　　　　　☐ Coracoacromial ligament

② ☐ 肩鎖靱帯　　　　　　　☐ Acromioclavicular ligament

③ ☐ 烏口鎖骨靱帯　　　　　☐ Coracoclavicular ligament

④ ☐ 上肩甲横靱帯　　　　　☐ Superior transverse scapular ligament

⑤ ☐ 腋窩陥凹　　　　　　　☐ Axillary recess

⑥ ☐ 関節包，関節上腕靱帯　☐ Joint capsule, glenohumeral ligaments

⑦ ☐ 結節間滑液鞘　　　　　☐ Intertubercular synovial sheath

1 図 19.13A. p.261　2 図 21.13A. p.285

Coronal Section of the Shoulder

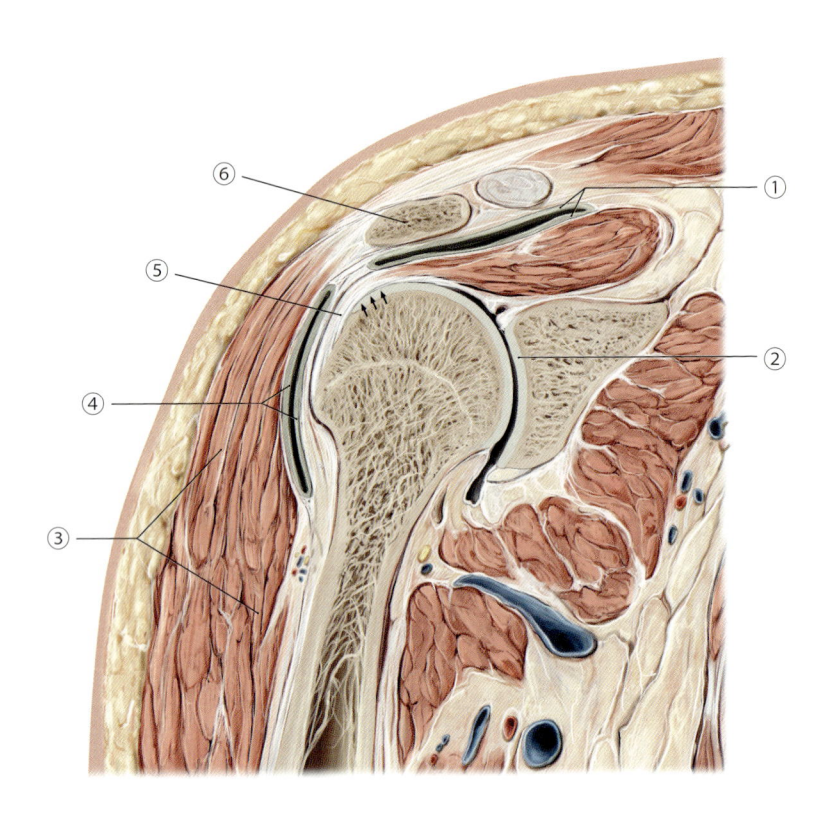

棘上筋腱が断裂した場合，肩関節の運動にどのような影響が及ぶか？

肩の前額断面

右肩，前面

① □ 肩峰下包　　　　　　　□ Subacromial bursa

② □ 肩甲骨，関節窩　　　　□ Scapula, glenoid cavity

③ □ 三角筋　　　　　　　　□ Deltoid

④ □ 三角筋下包　　　　　　□ Subdeltoid bursa

⑤ □ 棘上筋（腱）　　　　　□ Supraspinatus tendon

⑥ □ 肩峰　　　　　　　　　□ Acromion

A 　棘上筋は主として肩関節における外転運動の開始（最初の 10 度）に関与する．したがって，棘上筋腱の断裂（肩回旋腱板の断裂のうち一般的なもの）により，棘上筋による外転開始機能が損なわれる．棘上筋腱は肩峰の下にできる狭い空間を通過するので，この腱に石灰化や退行性変性が生じ，腱の厚みが増すと，肩峰の直下で腱が損傷を受ける．

1 図 19.18B. p.263　　2 図 21.18B. p.287

Anterior Muscles of the Shoulder & Arm I

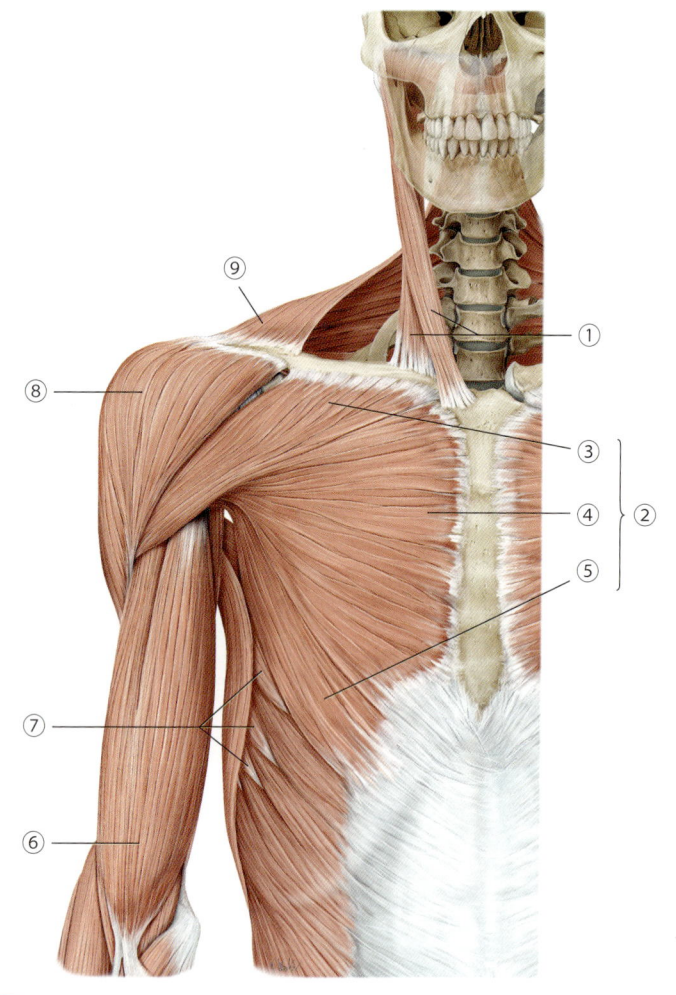

Q 大胸筋の作用は何か？

肩と上腕の筋（前面）1

右側，前面

① □ 胸鎖乳突筋　　　　　□ Sternocleidomastoid

② □ 大胸筋　　　　　　　□ Pectoralis major

③ □ 鎖骨部　　　　　　　□ Clavicular part

④ □ 胸肋部　　　　　　　□ Sternocostal part

⑤ □ 腹部　　　　　　　　□ Abdominal part

⑥ □ 上腕二頭筋　　　　　□ Biceps brachii

⑦ □ 前鋸筋　　　　　　　□ Serratus anterior

⑧ □ 三角筋　　　　　　　□ Deltoid

⑨ □ 僧帽筋　　　　　　　□ Trapezius

A 　大胸筋は上腕の内転と内旋に関与する強力な筋である．また，大胸筋の鎖骨部は肩関節を屈曲させ，胸肋部は屈曲位からの伸展に関与する．

1 図 19.19A. p.264　　2 図 21.19A. p.288

Anterior Muscles of the Shoulder & Arm II

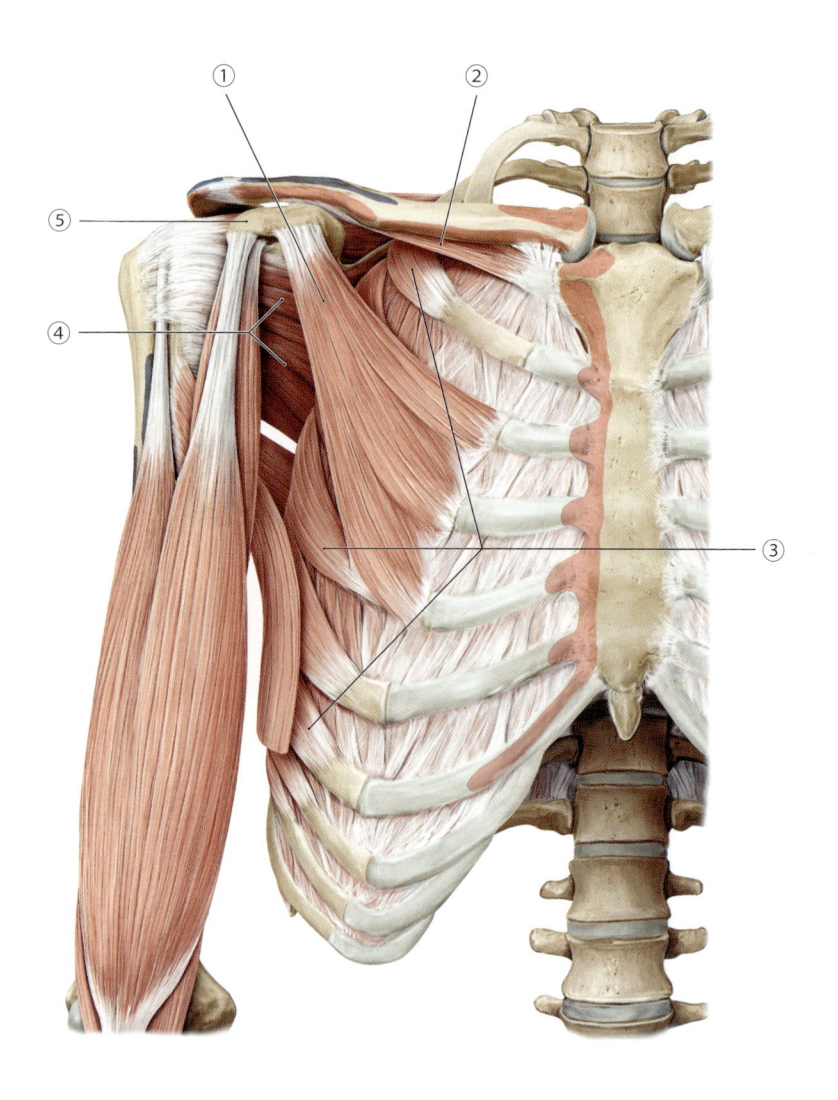

肩と上腕の筋（前面）2

右側，前面

① □ 小胸筋　　　　　□ Pectoralis minor
② □ 鎖骨下筋　　　　□ Subclavius
③ □ 前鋸筋　　　　　□ Serratus anterior
④ □ 肩甲下筋　　　　□ Subscapularis
⑤ □ 烏口突起　　　　□ Coracoid process

Anterior Muscles of the Shoulder & Arm III

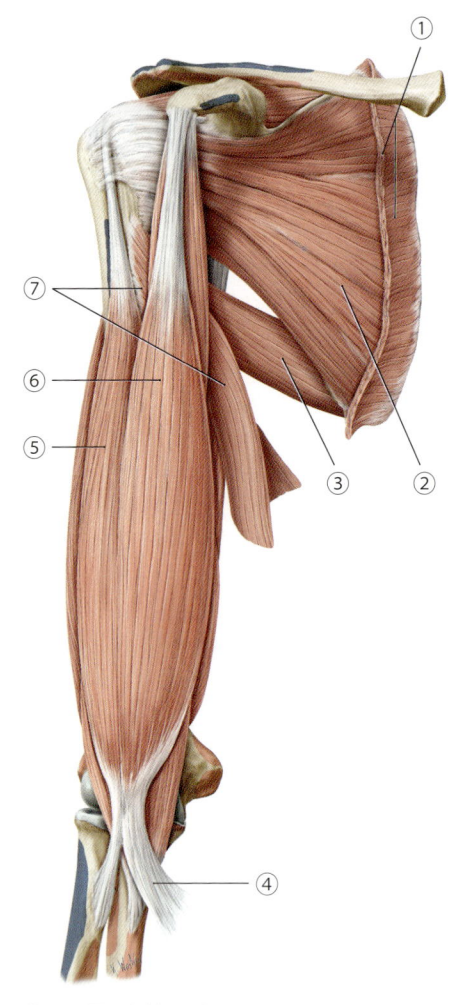

Q 上腕二頭筋の長頭の起始はどこか？

肩と上腕の筋（前面）3

右上肢，前面

① □ 前鋸筋　　　　　　　□ Serratus anterior

② □ 肩甲下筋　　　　　　□ Subscapularis

③ □ 大円筋　　　　　　　□ Teres major

④ □ 上腕二頭筋腱膜　　　□ Bicipital aponeurosis

⑤ □ 上腕二頭筋，長頭　　□ Biceps brachii, long head

⑥ □ 上腕二頭筋，短頭　　□ Biceps brachii, short head

⑦ □ 広背筋　　　　　　　□ Latissimus dorsi

A 　上腕二頭筋の長頭は肩甲骨の関節上結節から起始する．長頭の腱は滑膜に包まれた状態で肩関節腔を通過し，上腕骨の転子間溝に現れる．一方，上腕二頭筋の短頭は，小胸筋や烏口腕筋とともに，肩甲骨の烏口突起から起始する．

1 図 19.20A．p.266　2 図 21.20A．p.290

Anterior Muscles of the Shoulder & Arm IV

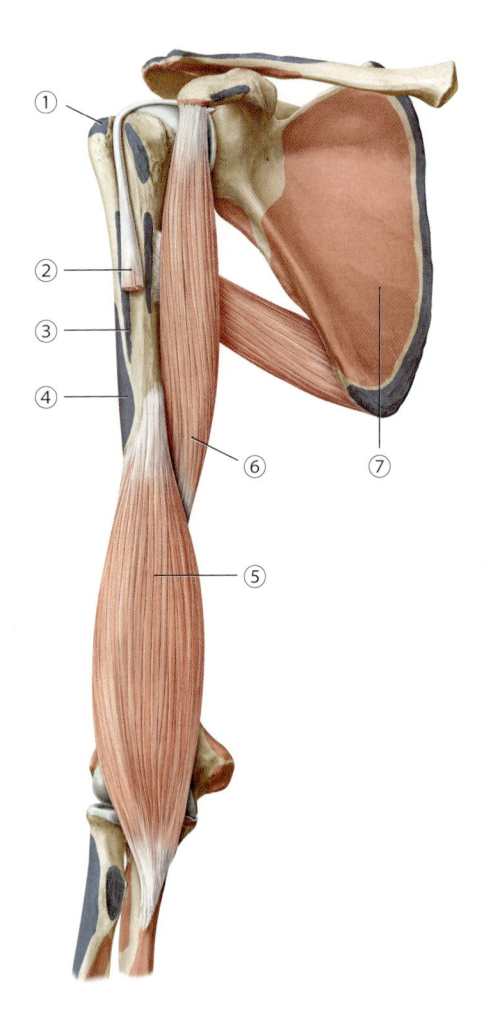

Q 上腕筋の作用は何か？

肩と上腕の筋（前面） 4

右上肢，前面

① ☐ 棘上筋（筋の停止）　　☐ Supraspinatus（insertion）

② ☐ 上腕二頭筋，長頭　　　☐ Biceps brachii, long head

③ ☐ 大胸筋（筋の停止）　　☐ Pectoralis major（insertion）

④ ☐ 三角筋（筋の停止）　　☐ Deltoid（insertion）

⑤ ☐ 上腕筋　　　　　　　　☐ Brachialis

⑥ ☐ 烏口腕筋　　　　　　　☐ Coracobrachialis

⑦ ☐ 肩甲下筋（筋の起始）　☐ Subscapularis（origin）

A 　上腕筋は肘関節の屈曲に関与する．上腕二頭筋も肘関節を屈曲するが，上腕二頭筋は橈骨に停止するので，前腕の回外にも関与する．上腕筋は尺骨に停止するため，上腕二頭筋のような回外作用を持たない．

1 図 19.20C. p.267　2 図 21.20C. p.291

Posterior Muscles of the Shoulder & Arm I

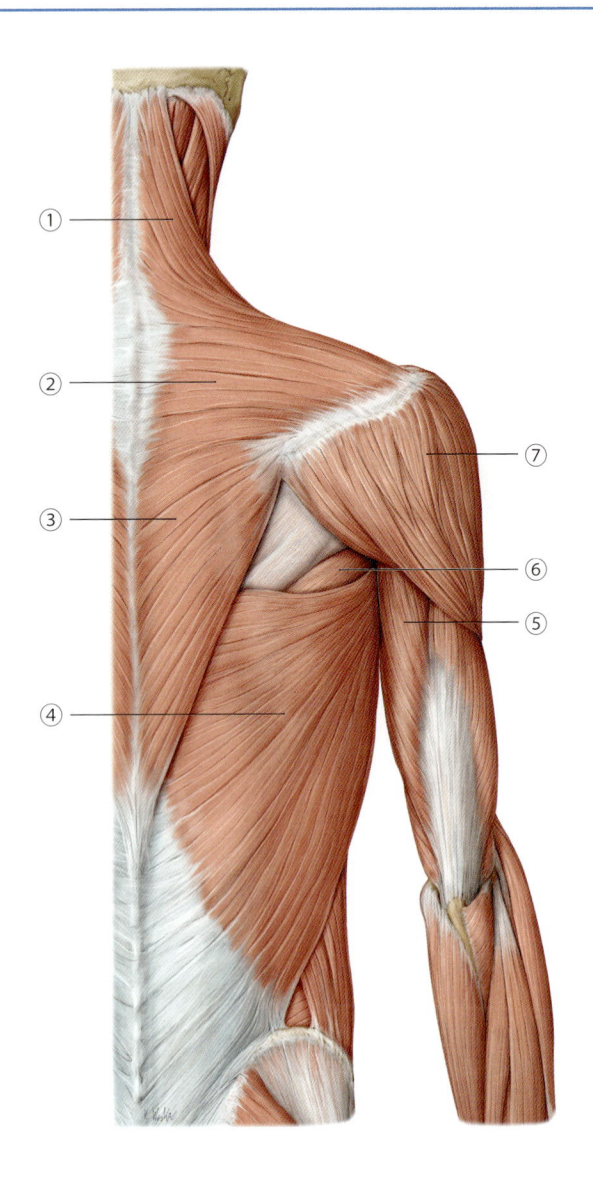

肩と上腕の筋（後面）1

右側，後面

① ☐ 僧帽筋，下行部　　　　　☐ Descending part of trapezius

② ☐ 僧帽筋，横行部（水平部）　☐ Transverse part of trapezius

③ ☐ 僧帽筋，上行部　　　　　☐ Ascending part of trapezius

④ ☐ 広背筋　　　　　　　　　☐ Latissimus dorsi

⑤ ☐ 上腕三頭筋，長頭　　　　☐ Long head of triceps brachii

⑥ ☐ 大円筋　　　　　　　　　☐ Teres major

⑦ ☐ 三角筋　　　　　　　　　☐ Deltoid

Posterior Muscles of the Shoulder & Arm II

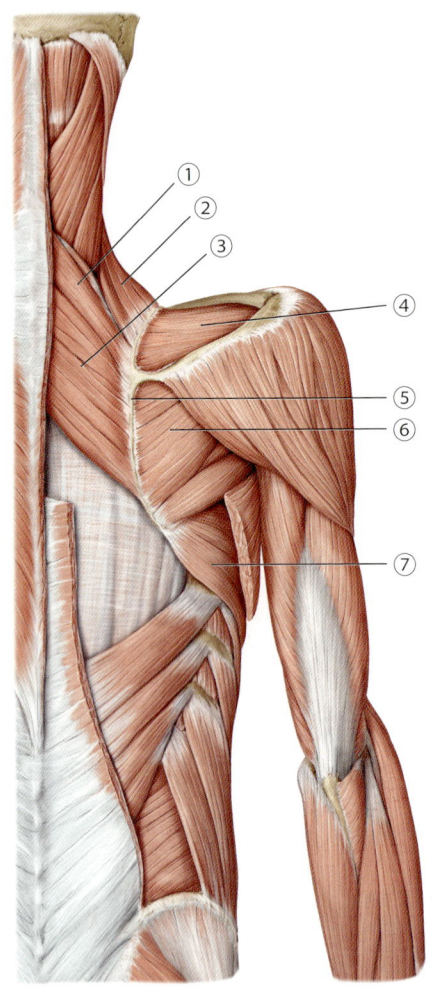

Q 翼状肩甲(肩甲骨の内側縁が後方に突出した状態)が見られる場合，どの筋の障害が示唆されるか？

肩と上腕の筋(後面) 2

右側,後面

① □ 小菱形筋　　　　　□ Rhomboid minor

② □ 肩甲挙筋　　　　　□ Levator scapulae

③ □ 大菱形筋　　　　　□ Rhomboid major

④ □ 棘上筋　　　　　　□ Supraspinatus

⑤ □ 肩甲骨,内側縁　　□ Scapula, medial border

⑥ □ 棘下筋　　　　　　□ Infraspinatus

⑦ □ 前鋸筋　　　　　　□ Serratus anterior

A 前鋸筋が麻痺すると,肩甲骨の内側縁が胸郭から遊離して,後方に突出し,翼のような外観(翼状肩甲)を呈する.

1 図 19.21B. p.269　2 図 21.21B. p.293

Posterior Muscles of the Shoulder & Arm III

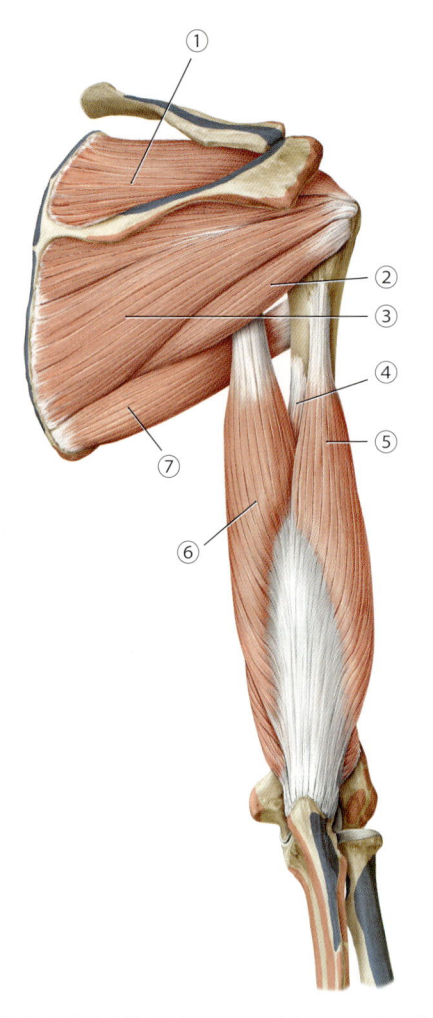

Q 回旋筋腱板を形成する筋はどれか？ また，これらの筋の支配神経は何か？

肩と上腕の筋（後面） 3

右上肢，後面

① □ 棘上筋　　　　　　　　□ Supraspinatus
② □ 小円筋　　　　　　　　□ Teres minor
③ □ 棘下筋　　　　　　　　□ Infraspinatus
④ □ 上腕三頭筋，内側頭　　　□ Triceps brachii, medial head
⑤ □ 上腕三頭筋，外側頭　　　□ Triceps brachii, lateral head
⑥ □ 上腕三頭筋，長頭　　　　□ Triceps brachii, long head
⑦ □ 大円筋　　　　　　　　□ Teres major

A 　回旋筋腱板を構成する筋（4種類）とその支配神経は以下のとおりである．これらの支配神経は，いずれも腕神経叢の後神経幹に由来する．

　棘上筋・棘下筋 ── 肩甲上神経
　小円筋 ──────── 腋窩神経
　肩甲下筋 ─────── 肩甲下神経

1 図 19.22B, p.270　 2 図 21.22B, p.294

Radius & Ulna

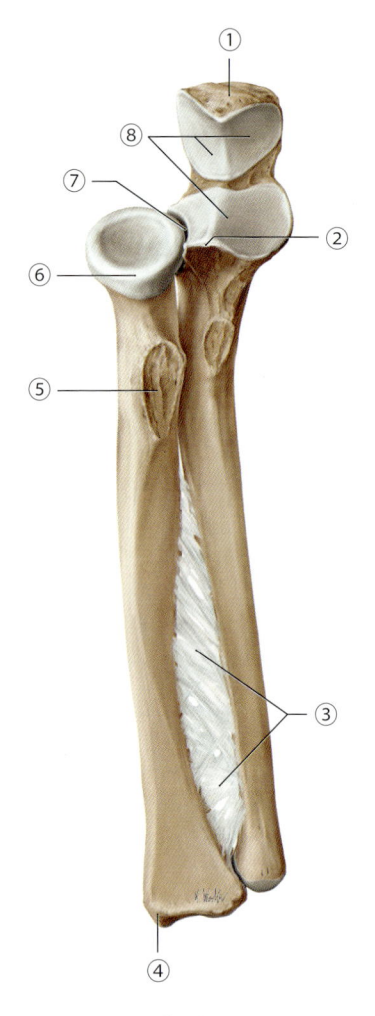

上・下橈尺関節で行われる運動は何か？

橈骨と尺骨

右前腕，前上方面

① □ 肘頭　　　　　　　□ Olecranon
② □ 鈎状突起　　　　　□ Coronoid process
③ □ 前腕骨間膜　　　　□ Interosseous membrane
④ □ 橈骨の茎状突起　　□ Styloid process of radius
⑤ □ 橈骨粗面　　　　　□ Radial tuberosity
⑥ □ 橈骨頭　　　　　　□ Head of radius
⑦ □ 上橈尺関節　　　　□ Proximal radioulnar joint
⑧ □ 滑車切痕　　　　　□ Trochlear notch

A 回内と回外が上・下橈尺関節で行われる．

1 図 20.1C. p.281　2 図 22.1C. p.305

Intact Joint Capsule of the Elbow

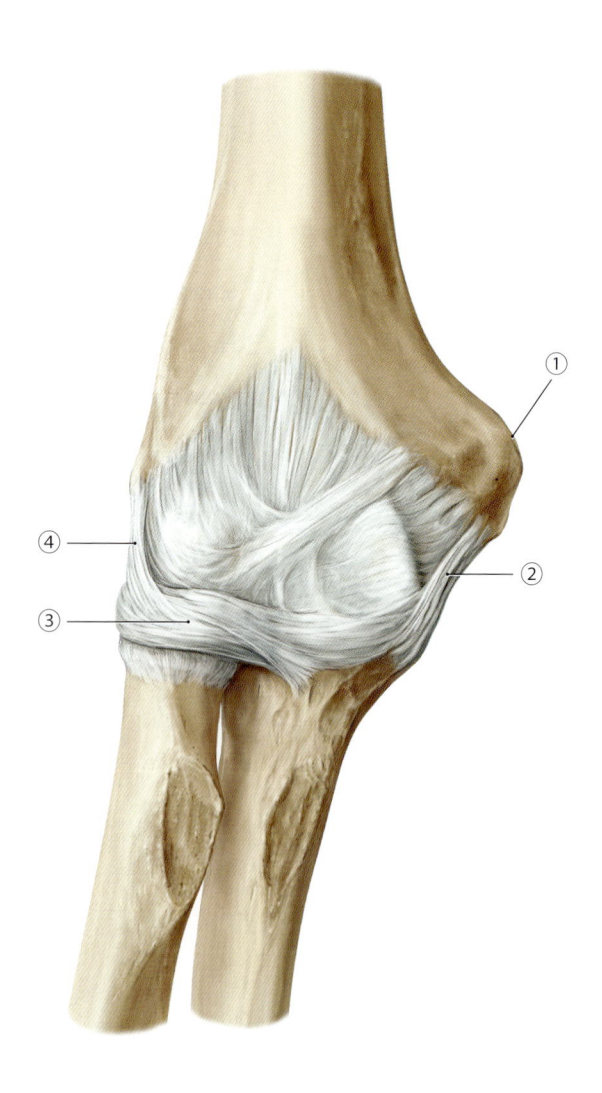

肘関節 1

右肘，伸展位，前面

① ☐ 内側上顆　　　　　　　　　☐ Medial epicondyle
② ☐ 内側側副靱帯　　　　　　　☐ Ulnar collateral ligament
③ ☐ 橈骨輪状靱帯　　　　　　　☐ Annular ligament of radius
④ ☐ 外側側副靱帯　　　　　　　☐ Radial collateral ligament

1 図 20.6A. p.285　　2 図 22.6A. p.309

Windowed Joint Capsule of the Elbow

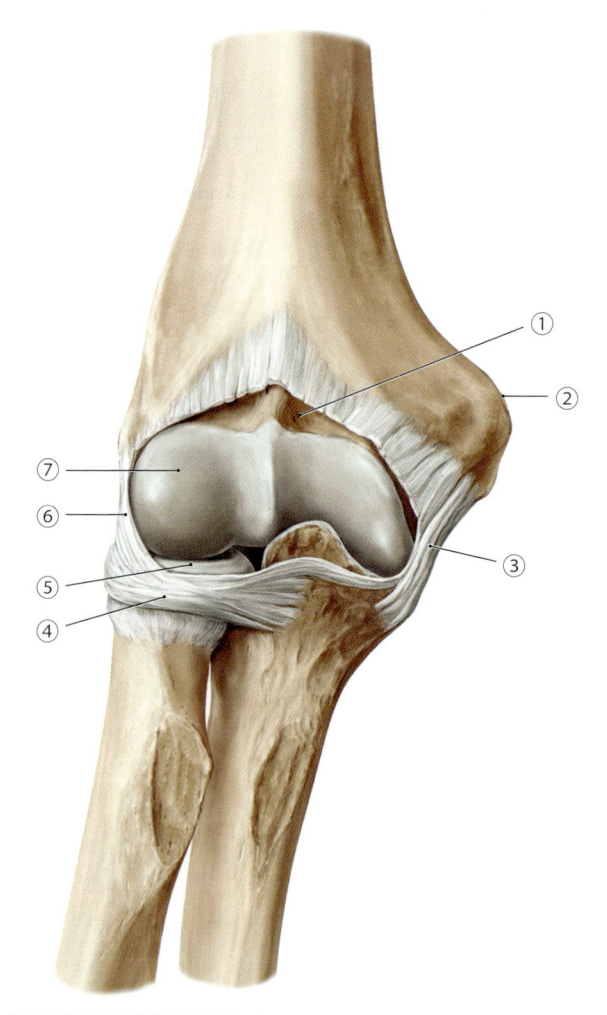

肘内障（子守り肘）とは何か？

肘関節 2

右肘, 伸展位, 前面

① ☐ 鈎突窩　　　　　　　☐ Coronoid fossa
② ☐ 内側上顆　　　　　　☐ Medial epicondyle
③ ☐ 内側側副靱帯　　　　☐ Ulnar collateral ligament
④ ☐ 橈骨輪状靱帯　　　　☐ Annular ligament of radius
⑤ ☐ 橈骨頭　　　　　　　☐ Head of radius
⑥ ☐ 外側側副靱帯　　　　☐ Radial collateral ligament
⑦ ☐ 上腕骨小頭　　　　　☐ Capitellum

A 　肘内障は小児によく見られ, 手や手首を引っ張られた際に生じやすい. 未成熟な橈骨頭が橈骨輪状靱帯よりも下方に偏位し, 回外運動が強く制限される. 上肢は一見麻痺したようになるが, 簡単に整復することができる.

[1] 図 20.6B. p.285　[2] 図 22.6B. p.309

Muscles of the Anterior Forearm I

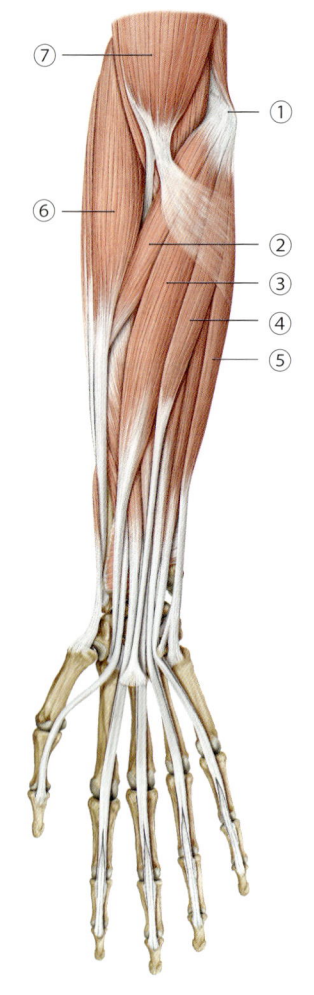

Q 腕橈骨筋の支配神経は何か？

前腕の筋（前面） 1

右前腕，前面

① ☐ 内側上顆（前腕屈筋の共通頭）　☐ Medial epicondyle (common head of flexors)

② ☐ 円回内筋　☐ Pronator teres

③ ☐ 橈側手根屈筋　☐ Flexor carpi radialis

④ ☐ 長掌筋　☐ Palmaris longus

⑤ ☐ 尺側手根屈筋　☐ Flexor carpi ulnaris

⑥ ☐ 腕橈骨筋　☐ Brachioradialis

⑦ ☐ 上腕二頭筋　☐ Biceps brachii

A 腕橈骨筋は前腕の後区画の筋であり，橈骨神経に支配される．しかし，他の後区画の筋と異なり，前腕の前面に位置し，肘関節の屈筋として働く．

1 図 20.11A. p.288　2 図 22.11A. p.312

Muscles of the Anterior Forearm II

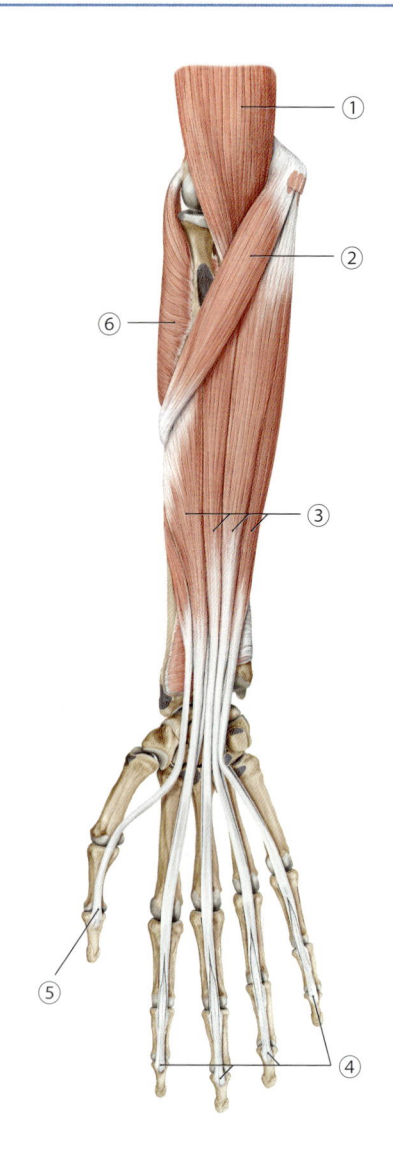

前腕の筋（前面） 2

右前腕，前面

① ☐ 上腕筋　　　　　　　☐ Brachialis

② ☐ 円回内筋　　　　　　☐ Pronator teres

③ ☐ 浅指屈筋　　　　　　☐ Flexor digitorum superficialis

④ ☐ 深指屈筋（腱）　　　☐ Flexor digitorum profundus tendons

⑤ ☐ 長母指屈筋（腱）　　☐ Flexor pollicis longus tendon

⑥ ☐ 回外筋　　　　　　　☐ Supinator

1 図 20.11B. p.288　2 図 22.11B. p.312

Muscles of the Anterior Forearm III

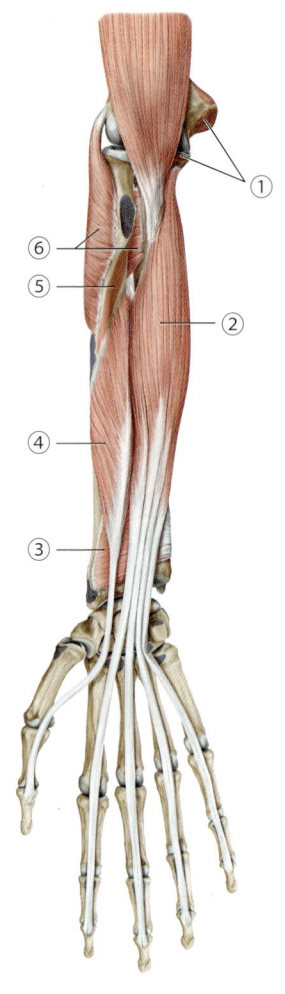

Q 回外に関与する筋は何か？（図示されていないものも含む）

前腕の筋（前面）3

右前腕，前面

① □ 浅指屈筋，上腕尺骨頭（筋の起始） □ Flexor digitorum superficialis, humero-ulnar head (origin)

② □ 深指屈筋 □ Flexor digitorum profundus

③ □ 方形回内筋 □ Pronator quadratus

④ □ 長母指屈筋 □ Flexor pollicis longus

⑤ □ 浅指屈筋，橈骨頭（筋の起始） □ Flexor digitorum superficialis, radial head (origin)

⑥ □ 回外筋 □ Supinator

A 回外筋と上腕二頭筋が回外に関与する．

Muscles of the Posterior Forearm I

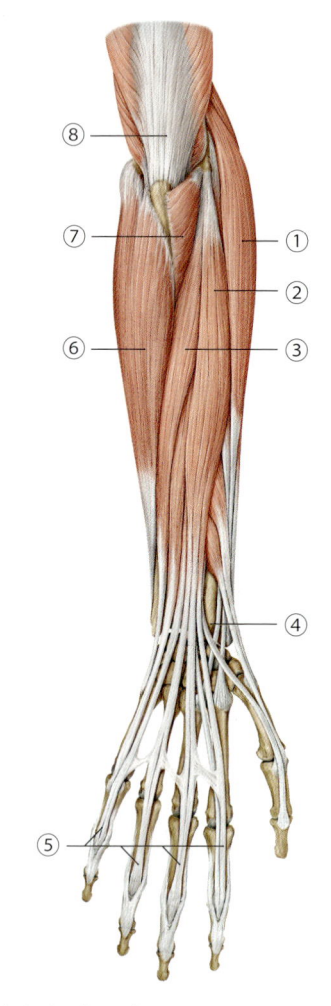

複数の伸筋腱を有する指はどれか？

前腕の筋（後面）1

右前腕，後面

① ☐ 長橈側手根伸筋　　　　　　☐ Extensor carpi radialis longus

② ☐ ［総］指伸筋　　　　　　　☐ Extensor digitorum

③ ☐ 尺側手根伸筋　　　　　　　☐ Extensor carpi ulnaris

④ ☐ （橈骨の）背側結節　　　　　☐ Dorsal tubercle

⑤ ☐ ［総］指伸筋（腱），指背腱膜　☐ Extensor digitorum tendons, dorsal digital expansion

⑥ ☐ 尺側手根屈筋　　　　　　　☐ Flexor carpi ulnaris

⑦ ☐ 肘筋　　　　　　　　　　　☐ Anconeus

⑧ ☐ 上腕三頭筋　　　　　　　　☐ Triceps brachii

A 　第1指〔母指（親指）〕，第2指〔示指（人差し指）〕，第5指（小指）には2本の伸筋腱が停止する．

Muscles of the Posterior Forearm II

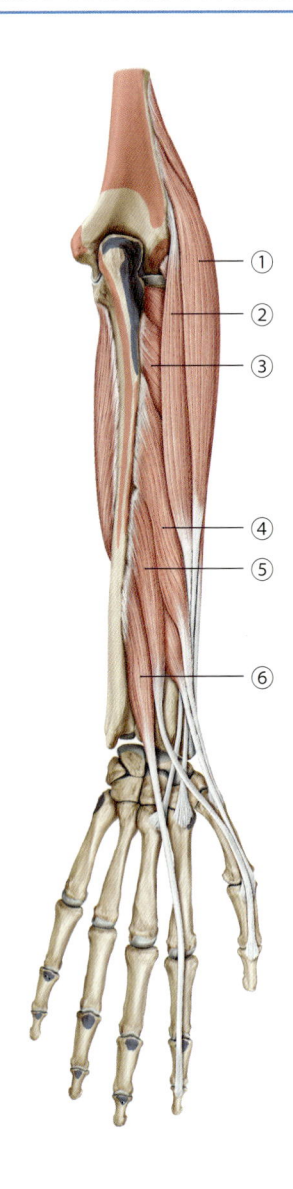

1.
2.
3.
4.
5.
6.

前腕の筋（後面） 2

右前腕，後面

① ☐ 長橈側手根伸筋　　☐ Extensor carpi radialis longus

② ☐ 短橈側手根伸筋　　☐ Extensor carpi radialis brevis

③ ☐ 回外筋　　☐ Supinator

④ ☐ 長母指外転筋　　☐ Abductor pollicis longus

⑤ ☐ 長母指伸筋　　☐ Extensor pollicis longus

⑥ ☐ 示指伸筋　　☐ Extensor indicis

1 図 20.12B. p.290　2 図 22.12B. p.314

Bones of the Wrist & Hand I

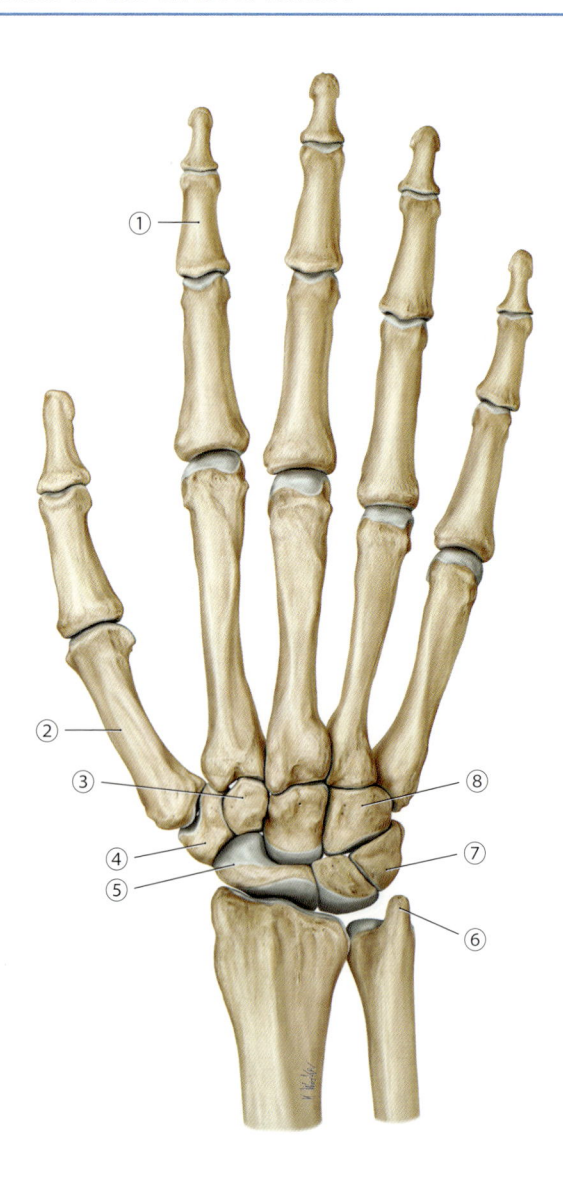

手首と手の骨格 1

右手，後面（背側面）

① □ 第2中節骨　　　　　　　□ 2nd middle phalanx

② □ 第1中手骨　　　　　　　□ 1st metacarpal

③ □ 小菱形骨　　　　　　　　□ Trapezoid

④ □ 大菱形骨　　　　　　　　□ Trapezium

⑤ □ 舟状骨　　　　　　　　　□ Scaphoid

⑥ □ 尺骨の茎状突起　　　　　□ Styloid process of ulna

⑦ □ 三角骨　　　　　　　　　□ Triquetrum

⑧ □ 有鈎骨　　　　　　　　　□ Hamate

臨床

舟状骨骨折は，手根骨骨折の中で最もよく見られ，近位端と遠位端の間にあるくびれた部分で折れる場合が多い．舟状骨を栄養する動脈は遠位端から入るので，舟状骨骨折の際には近位端へ血流が途絶し，骨折が治癒せず，しばしば近位端の無血管性壊死をきたす．

1 図21.1. p.298　　2 図23.1. p.322

Bones of the Wrist & Hand II

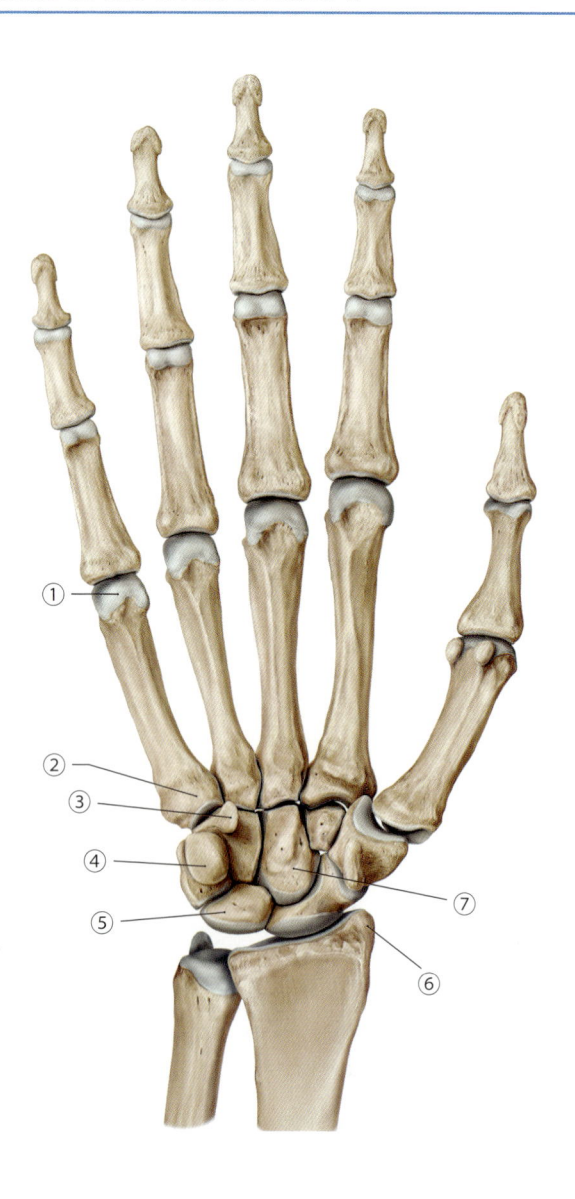

手首と手の骨格 2

右手,前面(掌側面)

① □ 中手骨の頭　　□ Head of metacarpal
② □ 中手骨の底　　□ Base of metacarpal
③ □ 有鈎骨鈎　　　□ Hook of hamate
④ □ 豆状骨　　　　□ Pisiform
⑤ □ 月状骨　　　　□ Lunate
⑥ □ 橈骨の茎状突起　□ Styloid process of radius
⑦ □ 有頭骨　　　　□ Capitate

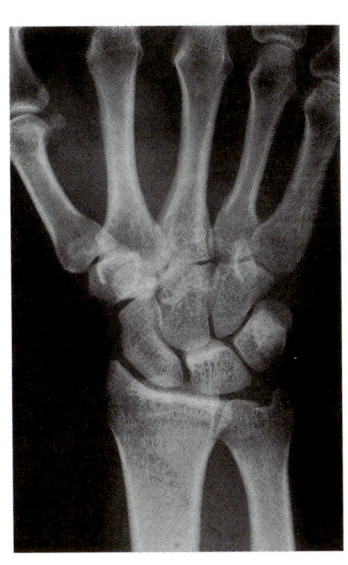

右手(後面)のX線像

1 図21.2, 図21.3. p.299　2 図23.2, 図23.3. p.323

Joints of the Wrist & Hand

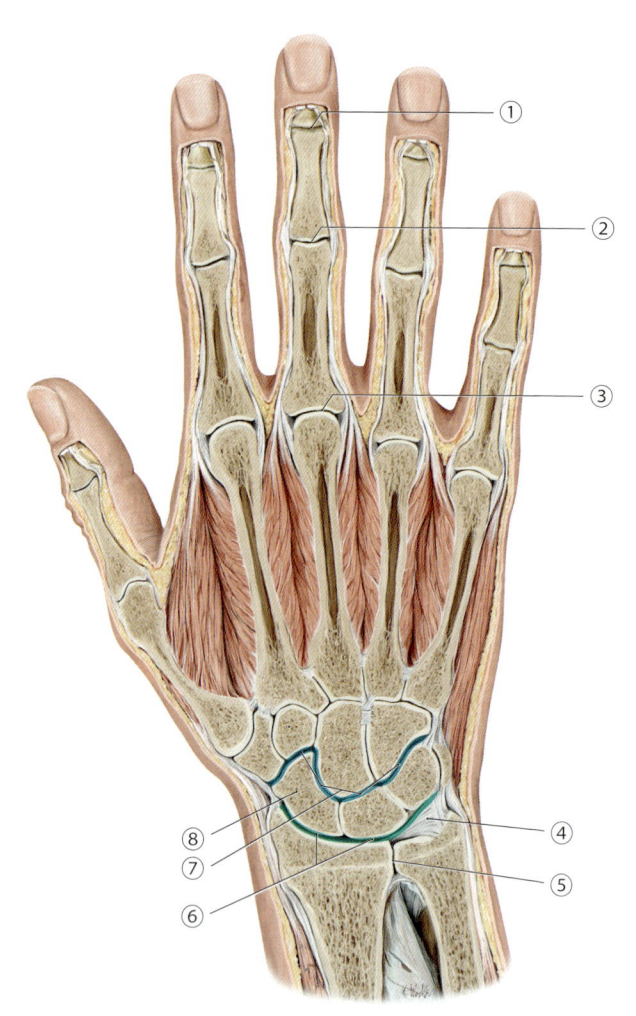

手根骨のうち，第1指（母指）の中手骨と関節をなすのはどれか？

手首と手の関節

右手, 後面(背側面)

① ☐ 遠位指節間(DIP)関節　☐ Distal interphalangeal joint
② ☐ 近位指節間(PIP)関節　☐ Proximal interphalangeal joint
③ ☐ 中手指節(MCP)関節　☐ Metacarpophalangeal joint
④ ☐ 関節円板　☐ Ulnocarpal disk
⑤ ☐ 下橈尺関節　☐ Distal radioulnar joint
⑥ ☐ 橈骨手根関節　☐ Radiocarpal joint
⑦ ☐ 手根中央関節　☐ Midcarpal joint
⑧ ☐ 舟状骨　☐ Scaphoid

A 大菱形骨が第1指(母指)の中手骨と関節をなす.

1 図 21.5A. p.301　2 図 23.6A. p.327

Muscles of the Hand I

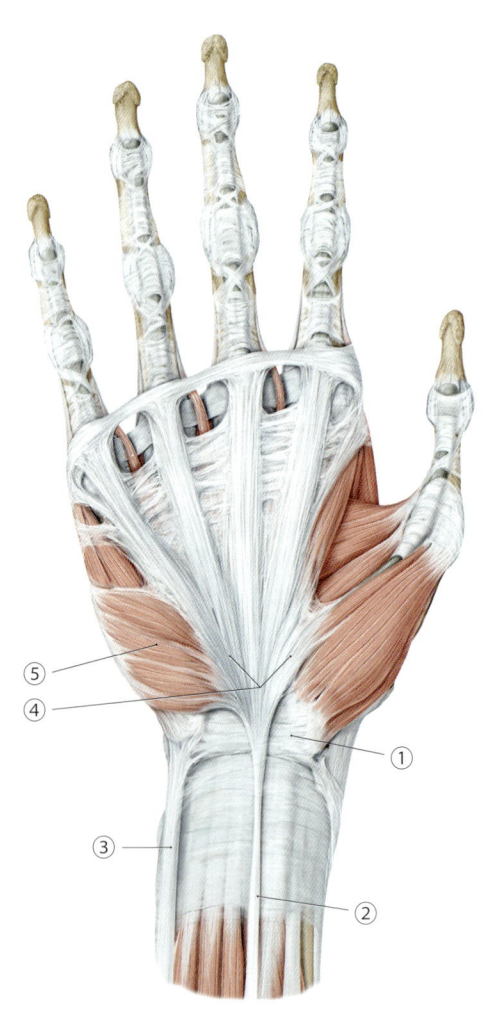

Q デュプイトラン拘縮とは何か？

手の筋 1

右手,前面(掌側面)

① □ 屈筋支帯 □ Flexor retinaculum
② □ 長掌筋(腱) □ Palmaris longus tendon
③ □ 尺側手根屈筋 □ Flexor carpi ulnaris
④ □ 手掌腱膜 □ Palmar aponeurosis
⑤ □ 短掌筋 □ Palmaris brevis

A デュプイトラン拘縮は手掌腱膜が徐々に萎縮することで生じる.手掌腱膜の短縮が進行すると,主に第4・5指〔環指(薬指)・小指〕が屈曲位の状態で拘縮し,手の把握機能が著しく損なわれる.

1 図 21.13A. p.306 2 図 23.15A. p.334

Muscles of the Hand II

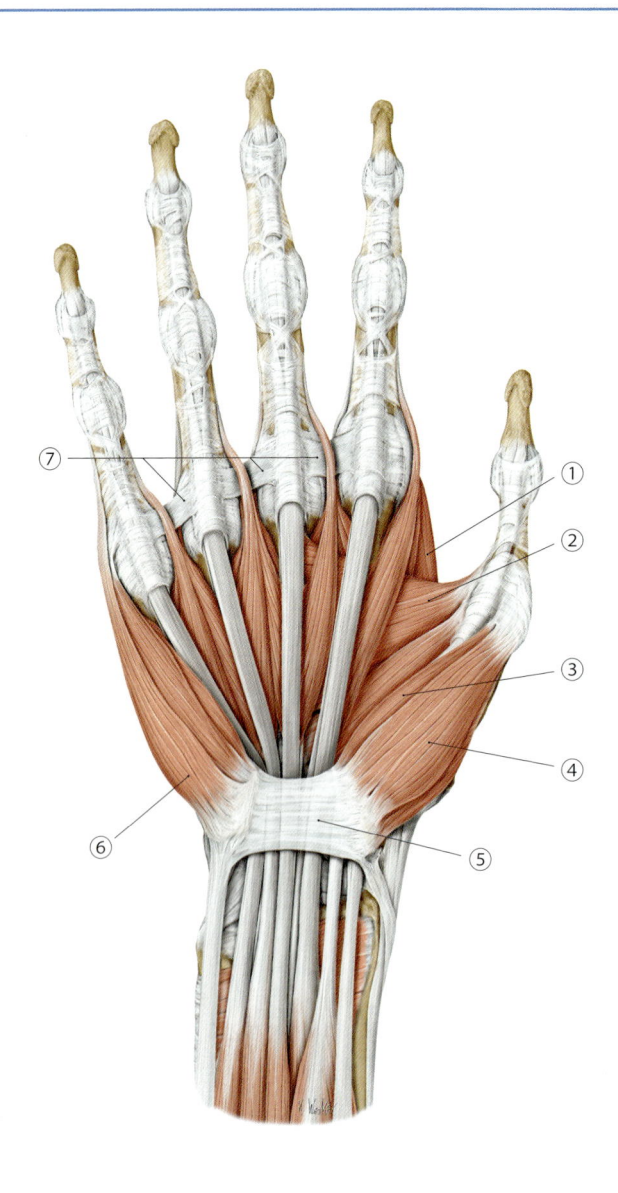

手の筋 2

右手，前面（掌側面）

① ☐ 第1背側骨間筋 ☐ 1st dorsal interosseus

② ☐ 母指内転筋，横頭 ☐ Adductor pollicis, transverse head

③ ☐ 短母指屈筋，浅頭 ☐ Flexor pollicis brevis, superficial head

④ ☐ 短母指外転筋 ☐ Abductor pollicis brevis

⑤ ☐ 屈筋支帯 ☐ Flexor retinaculum

⑥ ☐ 小指外転筋 ☐ Abductor digiti minimi

⑦ ☐ 深横中手靱帯 ☐ Deep transverse metacarpal ligament

臨床

第1指（母指）の腱鞘は，長母指屈筋の腱鞘を介して，指屈筋の総腱鞘と連絡している．母指以外の指でも指の腱鞘と総腱鞘が連絡している場合がある．刺創によって指の腱鞘に感染が生じると，連絡部を介して感染が総腱鞘に広がることがある．

1 図 21.13C. p.307　2 図 23.15C. p.335

358 Upper Limb

Muscles of the Hand III

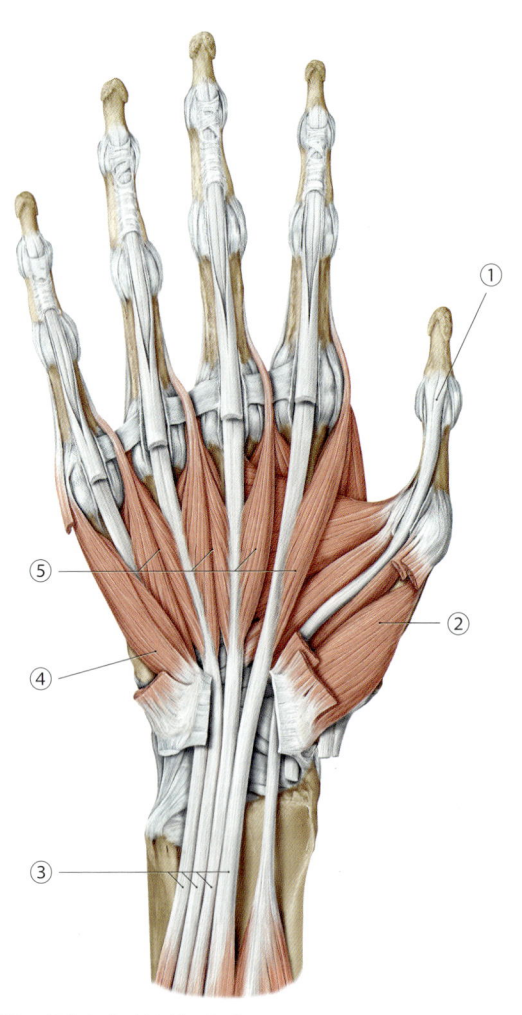

Q 虫様筋の起始と停止はどこか？

手の筋 3

右手, 前面(掌側面)

① □ 長母指屈筋(腱) □ Flexor pollicis longus tendon
② □ 母指対立筋 □ Opponens pollicis
③ □ 深指屈筋 □ Flexor digitorum profundus
④ □ 短小指屈筋 □ Flexor digiti minimi
⑤ □ 虫様筋 □ Lumbricals

A 虫様筋は手掌において深指屈筋腱から起始し, 指の背側面において指背腱膜に停止する.

1 図 21.13D. p.307 2 図 23.15D. p.335

Muscles of the Hand IV

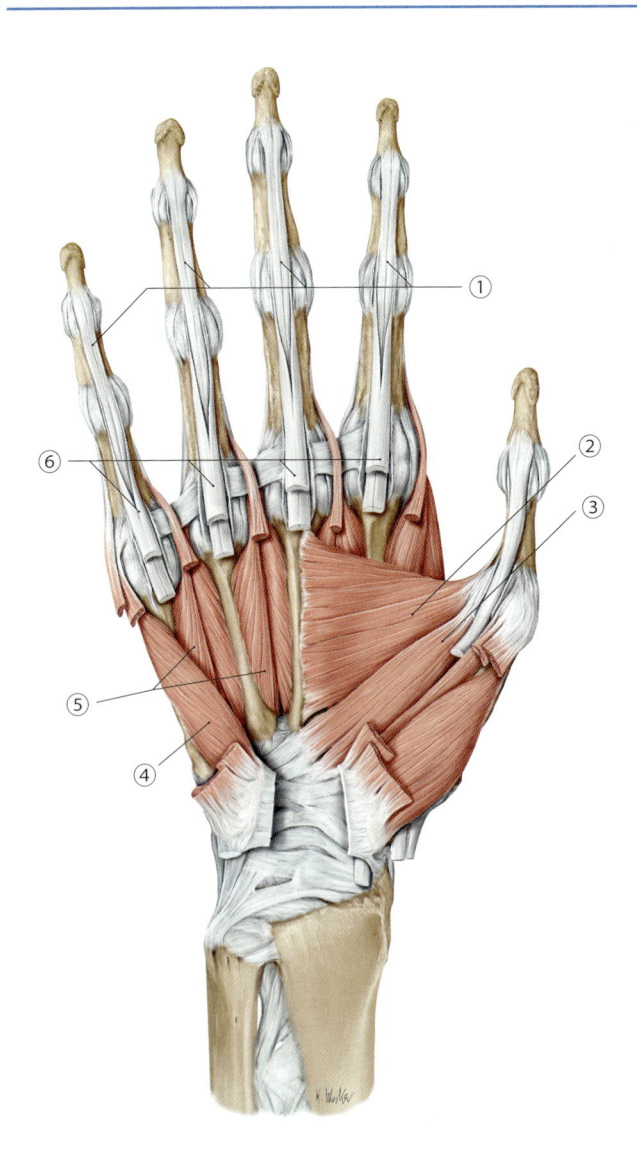

手の筋 4

右手，前面（掌側面）

① ☐ 深指屈筋（腱） ☐ Flexor digitorum profundus tendons

② ☐ 母指内転筋，横頭 ☐ Adductor pollicis, transverse head

③ ☐ 母指内転筋，斜頭 ☐ Adductor pollicis, oblique head

④ ☐ 小指対立筋 ☐ Opponens digiti minimi

⑤ ☐ 第2・3掌側骨間筋 ☐ 2nd and 3rd palmar interossei

⑥ ☐ 浅指屈筋（腱） ☐ Flexor digitorum superficialis tendons

1 図 21.14A. p.308　2 図 23.16A. p.336

Dorsum of the Hand

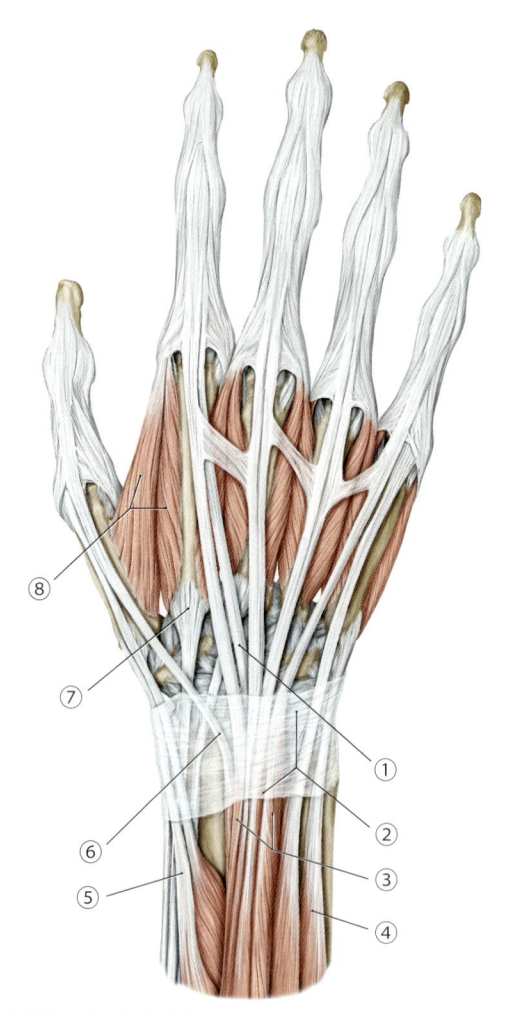

背側骨間筋の支配神経は何か？

手背

右手，後面（背側面）

① □ 示指伸筋（腱）　　□ Extensor indicis tendon
② □ 伸筋支帯　　□ Extensor retinaculum
③ □ ［総］指伸筋　　□ Extensor digitorum
④ □ 尺側手根伸筋　　□ Extensor carpi ulnaris
⑤ □ 長母指外転筋　　□ Abductor pollicis longus
⑥ □ 長母指伸筋（腱）　　□ Extensor pollicis longus tendon
⑦ □ 長橈側手根伸筋（腱）　　□ Extensor carpi radialis longus tendon
⑧ □ 第1背側骨間筋　　□ 1st dorsal interosseus

A 　背側骨間筋，掌側骨間筋はともに尺骨神経によって支配される．橈骨神経は上腕と前腕の後面にある筋を支配するが，手の筋（手内筋）には分布しない．

1 図 21.17A. p.310　　2 図 23.19A. p.338

Arteries of the Upper Limb

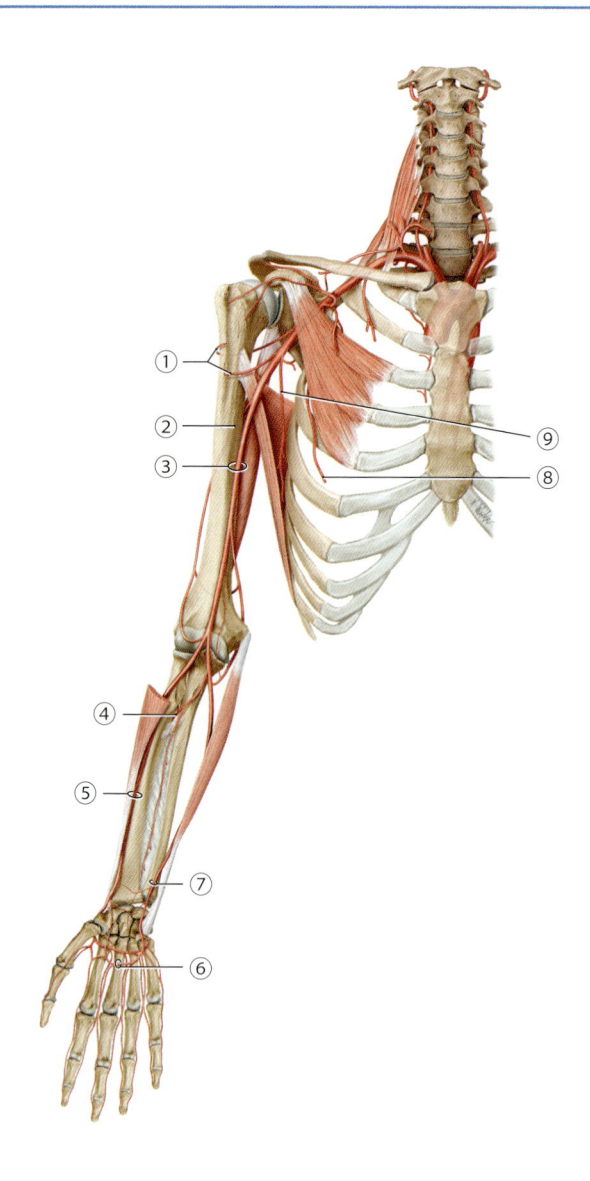

上肢の動脈

右上肢，前面

① □ 前・後上腕回旋動脈　　　□ Anterior and posterior circumflex humeral arteries

② □ 上腕深動脈　　　　　　　□ Profunda brachii artery

③ □ 上腕動脈　　　　　　　　□ Brachial artery

④ □ 後骨間動脈　　　　　　　□ Posterior interosseous artery

⑤ □ 橈骨動脈　　　　　　　　□ Radial artery

⑥ □ 浅掌動脈弓　　　　　　　□ Superficial palmar arch

⑦ □ 尺骨動脈　　　　　　　　□ Ulnar artery

⑧ □ 外側胸動脈　　　　　　　□ Lateral thoracic artery

⑨ □ 胸背動脈　　　　　　　　□ Thoracodorsal artery

解説

上肢に分布する動脈は鎖骨下動脈およびその枝である．鎖骨下動脈は第1肋骨の外側縁を越えたところで，腋窩動脈となる．また，腋窩動脈は大円筋の下縁を過ぎると上腕動脈となる．上腕動脈は肘窩で橈骨動脈と尺骨動脈に分かれる．この2つの動脈は手掌において，2つの動脈弓（浅・深掌動脈弓）を形成する．

1 図 22.1B. p.316　　2 図 24.1B. p.344

Superficial Veins of the Upper Limb

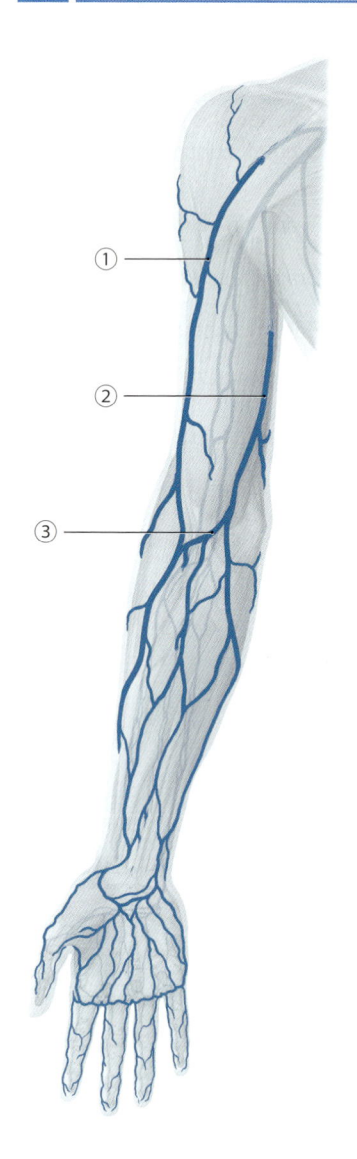

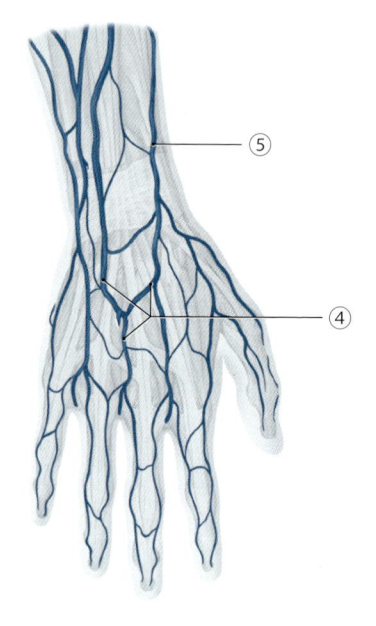

上肢の皮静脈

右上肢，左：前面，右：後面

① □ 橈側皮静脈　　　　□ Cephalic vein

② □ 尺側皮静脈　　　　□ Basilic vein

③ □ 肘正中皮静脈　　　□ Median cubital vein

④ □ 手背静脈網　　　　□ Dorsal venous network

⑤ □ 橈側皮静脈　　　　□ Cephalic vein

臨床

　肘窩の静脈は採血の際に頻繁に利用される．採血の準備として上腕に駆血帯を巻く．この操作では皮静脈は容易に圧迫されるが，動脈は比較的圧迫を受けない．したがって，皮静脈はうっ滞した血液により怒張し，静脈の視認や触知が容易になる．

1 図 22.5A，図 22.6. p.318　2 図 24.5A，図 24.6. p.346

Structure of the Brachial Plexus

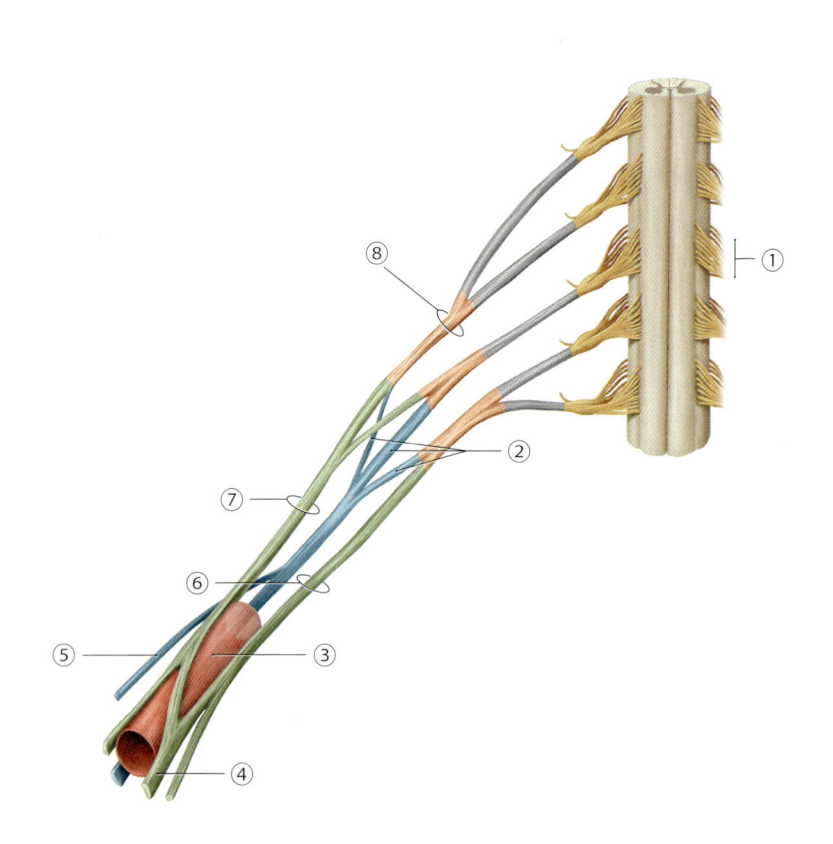

後神経束に含まれる神経はどの根に由来するか？

腕神経叢の構造

右側，前面

① ☐ 第7頸神経 　　　　　　　☐ C7
② ☐ 腕神経叢の後部 　　　　　☐ Posterior divisions of brachial plexus
③ ☐ 腋窩動脈 　　　　　　　　☐ Axillary artery
④ ☐ 正中神経 　　　　　　　　☐ Median nerve
⑤ ☐ 腋窩神経 　　　　　　　　☐ Axillary nerve
⑥ ☐ 内側神経束 　　　　　　　☐ Medial cord
⑦ ☐ 外側神経束 　　　　　　　☐ Lateral cord
⑧ ☐ 上神経幹（第5・6頸神経） ☐ Upper trunk (C5-C6)

A 腕神経叢を構成する根（C5-T1）のすべてが後神経側の形成に関与する．

① 図 22.11A. p.321　② 図 24.11A. p.349

Course of the Brachial Plexus

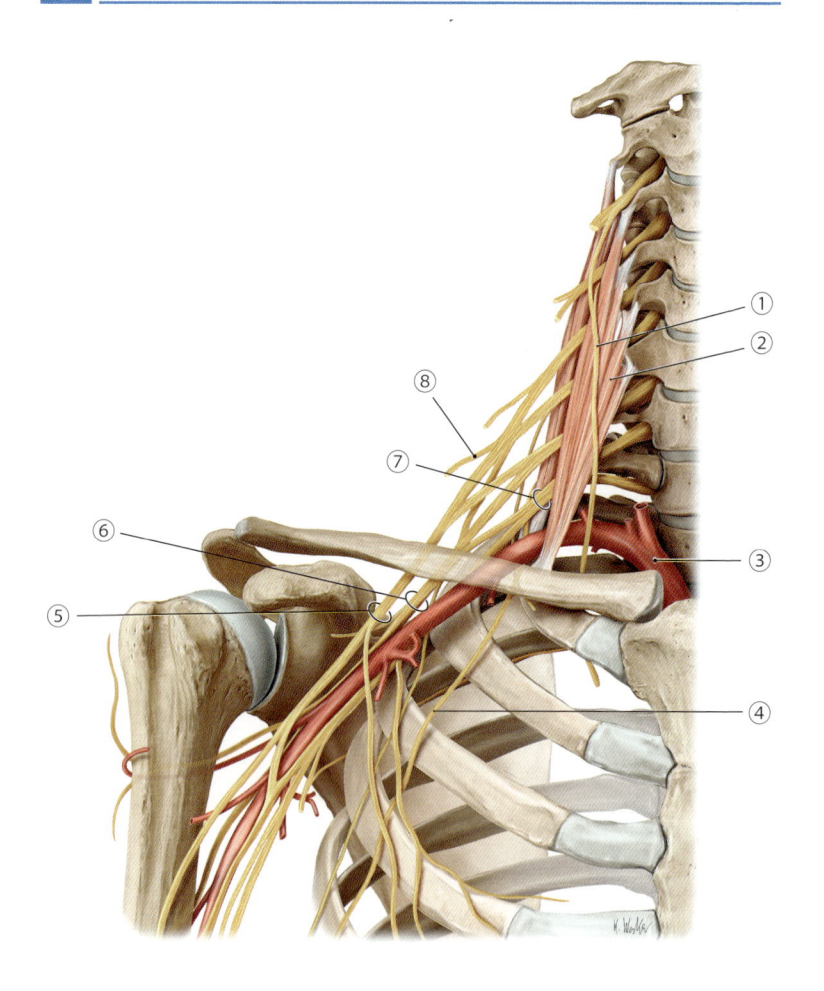

①
②
③
④
⑤
⑥
⑦
⑧

Q 腕神経叢のうち，鎖骨のすぐ後ろの部分を何と呼ぶか？

腕神経叢の走行

右側，前面

① ☐ 横隔神経　　　　　☐ Phrenic nerve
② ☐ 前斜角筋　　　　　☐ Anterior scalene
③ ☐ 鎖骨下動脈　　　　☐ Subclavian artery
④ ☐ 長胸神経　　　　　☐ Long thoracic nerve
⑤ ☐ 外側神経束　　　　☐ Lateral cord
⑥ ☐ 後神経束　　　　　☐ Posterior cord
⑦ ☐ 下神経幹　　　　　☐ Lower trunk
⑧ ☐ 肩甲上神経　　　　☐ Suprascapular nerve

A 鎖骨の後ろには，腕神経叢の神経束が存在する．腕神経叢の根，神経幹，前部，後部は鎖骨上部，神経束とその枝は鎖骨下部と呼ばれる．

1 図 22.11C, p.321　2 図 24.11C, p.349

Nerves of the Brachial Plexus I

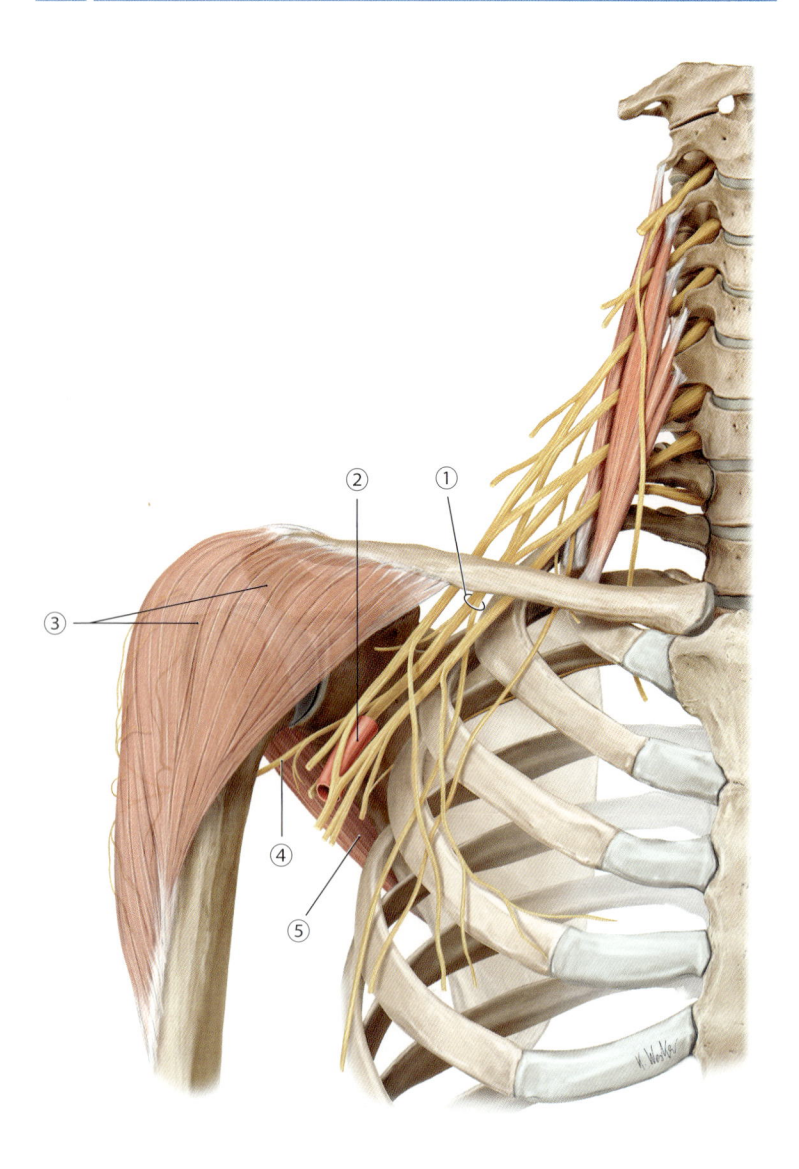

腕神経叢からの神経 1（腋窩神経）

右側，前面

① □ 後神経束　　　　　□ Posterior cord

② □ 腋窩動脈　　　　　□ Axillary artery

③ □ 三角筋　　　　　　□ Deltoid

④ □ 腋窩神経　　　　　□ Axillary nerve

⑤ □ 小円筋　　　　　　□ Teres minor

臨床

腋窩神経は上腕骨近位部の骨折に伴って損傷される場合がある．腋窩神経の損傷では，上肢の外転が制限され，三角筋による肩の盛り上がりが失われることもある．

1 図 22.15. p.324　 2 図 24.15. p.352

Nerves of the Brachial Plexus II

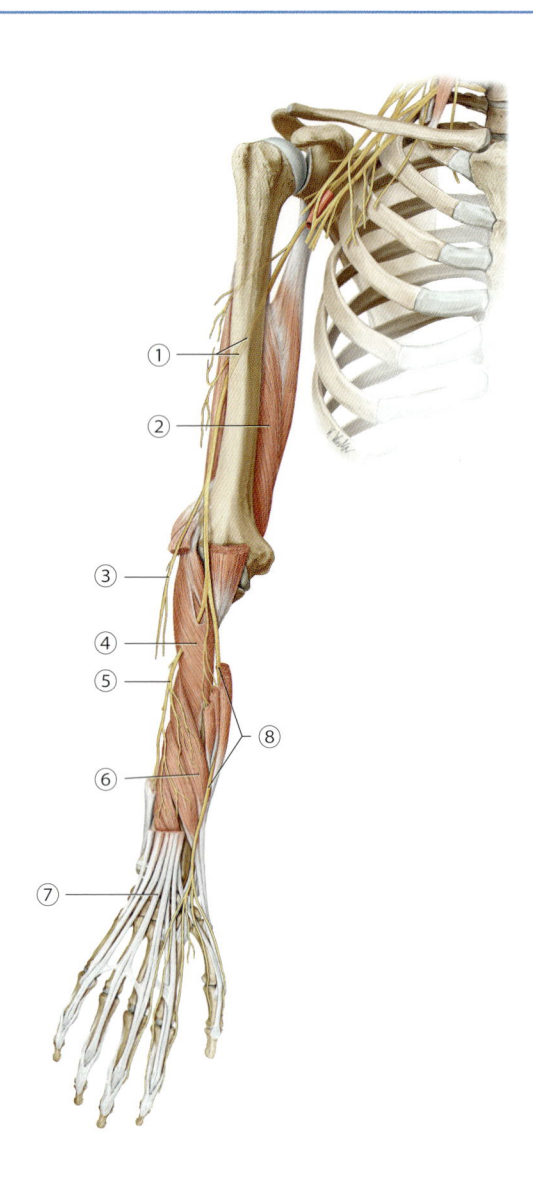

腕神経叢からの神経 2（橈骨神経）

右上肢，回内位，前面

① ☐ 橈骨神経（橈骨神経溝を通る） ☐ Radial nerve (in radial groove)

② ☐ 上腕三頭筋 ☐ Triceps brachii

③ ☐ 後前腕皮神経 ☐ Posterior antebrachial cutaneous nerve

④ ☐ 回外筋 ☐ Supinator

⑤ ☐ 後［前腕］骨間神経 ☐ Posterior interosseous nerve

⑥ ☐ 長母指外転筋 ☐ Abductor pollicis longus

⑦ ☐ ［総］指伸筋（腱） ☐ Extensor digitorum tendon

⑧ ☐ 橈骨神経，浅枝 ☐ Radial nerve, superficial branch

臨床

腋窩において橈骨神経が慢性的な圧迫を受けると（例えば，松葉杖の不適切な使用），上腕，前腕，手の感覚および運動機能が損なわれる場合がある．橈骨神経がより遠位で障害された場合，影響を受ける筋の数は少なくなり，上腕三頭筋の機能は正常だが，下垂手が見られるといった状態となる．

1 図 22.17, p.325　2 図 24.17, p.353

Nerves of the Brachial Plexus III

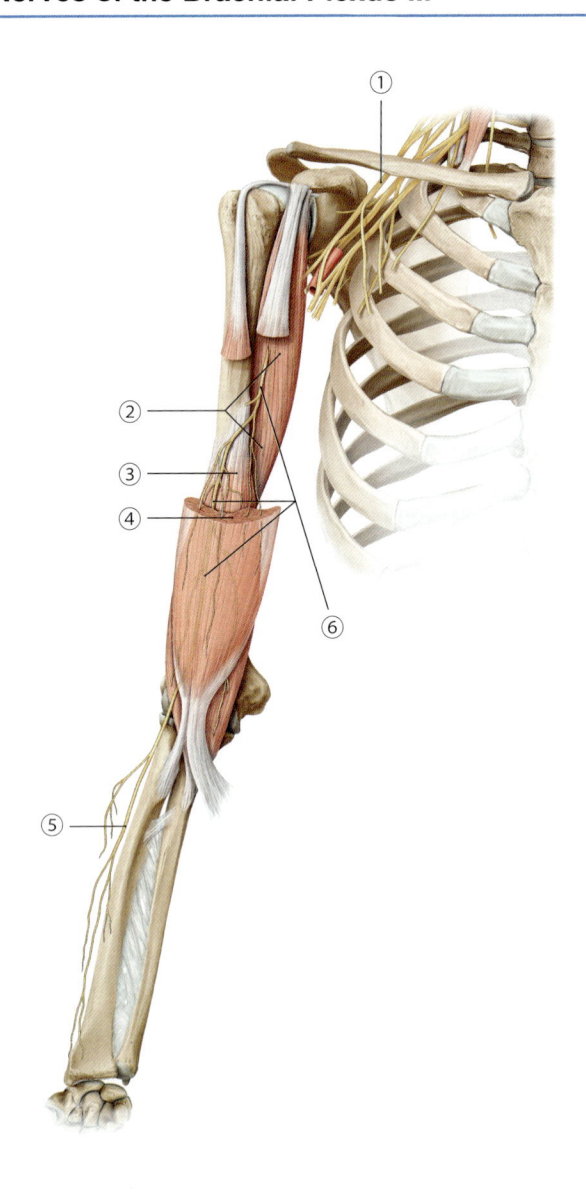

腕神経叢からの神経 3（筋皮神経）

右上肢，前面

① □ 外側神経束　　　　　□ Lateral cord

② □ 烏口腕筋　　　　　　□ Coracobrachialis

③ □ 上腕筋　　　　　　　□ Brachialis

④ □ 上腕二頭筋　　　　　□ Biceps brachii

⑤ □ 外側前腕皮神経　　　□ Lateral antebrachial cutaneous nerve

⑥ □ 筋皮神経　　　　　　□ Musculocutaneous nerve

Nerves of the Brachial Plexus IV

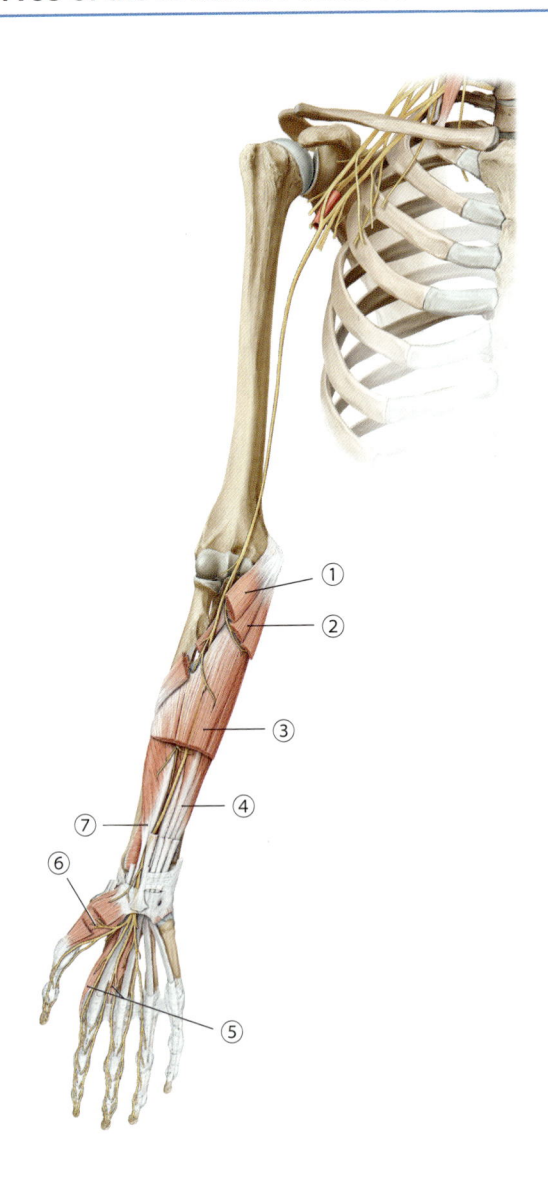

腕神経叢からの神経 4（正中神経）

右上肢，前面

① ☐ 円回内筋，上腕頭　　☐ Pronator teres, humeral head

② ☐ 橈側手根屈筋　　☐ Flexor carpi radialis

③ ☐ 浅指屈筋　　☐ Flexor digitorum superficialis

④ ☐ 深指屈筋　　☐ Flexor digitorum profundus

⑤ ☐ 第1・2虫様筋　　☐ 1st and 2nd lumbricals

⑥ ☐ 母指球筋への筋枝　　☐ Thenar muscular branch

⑦ ☐ 長母指屈筋　　☐ Flexor pollicis longus

臨床

正中神経は腕神経叢から出る主要な神経であり，内側神経束と外側神経束の両方の成分からなる．肘関節の骨折や脱臼によって正中神経が損傷されると，手の把握機能と指先の感覚が損なわれる．

[1] 図22.22. p.328　[2] 図24.22. p.356

Nerves of the Brachial Plexus V

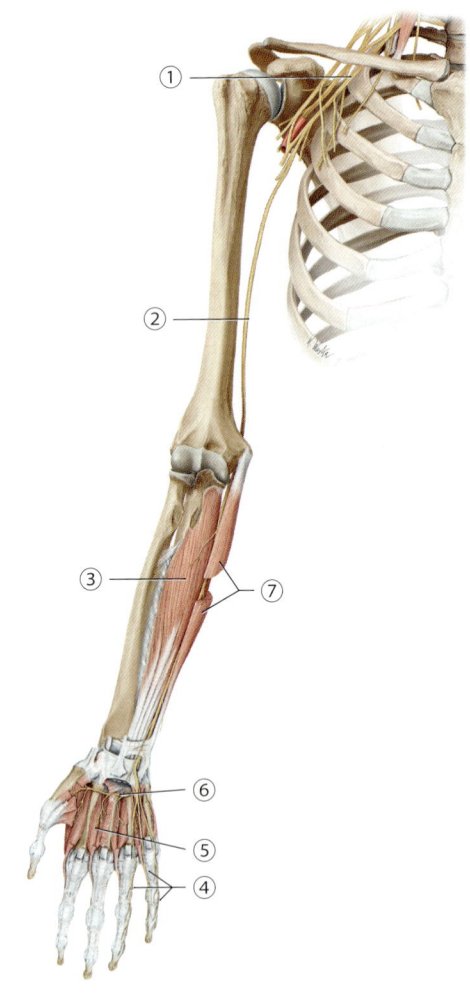

Q 尺骨神経損傷の主要な特徴は何か？

腕神経叢からの神経 5（尺骨神経）

右上肢，前面

① □ 内側神経束　　　　□ Medial cord
② □ 尺骨神経　　　　　□ Ulnar nerve
③ □ 深指屈筋　　　　　□ Flexor digitorum profundus
④ □ 固有掌側指神経　　□ Proper palmar digital nerves
⑤ □ 骨間筋　　　　　　□ Interossei
⑥ □ 深枝　　　　　　　□ Deep branch
⑦ □ 尺側手根屈筋　　　□ Flexor carpi ulnaris

A 尺骨神経の損傷では，いわゆる「鷲手」が見られる．鷲手は，骨間筋（尺骨神経支配）の萎縮により，指が中手指節関節で過伸展位，近位および遠位指節間関節で軽い屈曲位をとるようになった状態を指す．

1 図 22.25, p.329　 2 図 24.25, p.357

Neurovasculature of the Posterior Shoulder I

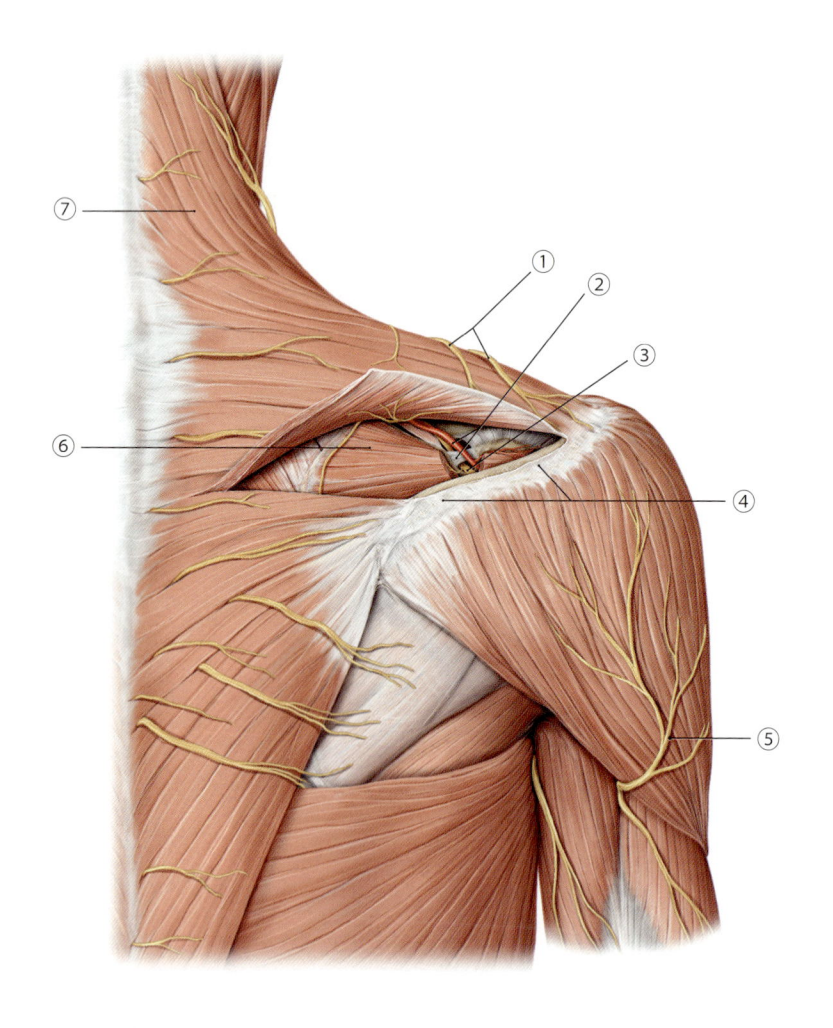

肩の後部における神経・血管 1

右肩，後面

① ☐ 鎖骨上神経 　　　　　　　　　☐ Supraclavicular nerves

② ☐ 肩甲上動脈（上肩甲横靱帯の上を通る） 　☐ Suprascapular artery (with superior transverse scapular ligament)

③ ☐ 肩甲上神経（肩甲切痕を通る） 　☐ Suprascapular nerve (in scapular notch)

④ ☐ 肩甲棘 　　　　　　　　　　　☐ Scapular spine

⑤ ☐ 上外側上腕皮神経（腋窩神経の枝） 　☐ Superior lateral brachial cutaneous nerve (axillary nerve)

⑥ ☐ 棘上筋 　　　　　　　　　　　☐ Supraspinatus

⑦ ☐ 僧帽筋，下行部 　　　　　　　☐ Trapezius, descending part

1 図 22.29. p.332　 2 図 24.29. p.360

Neurovasculature of the Posterior Shoulder II

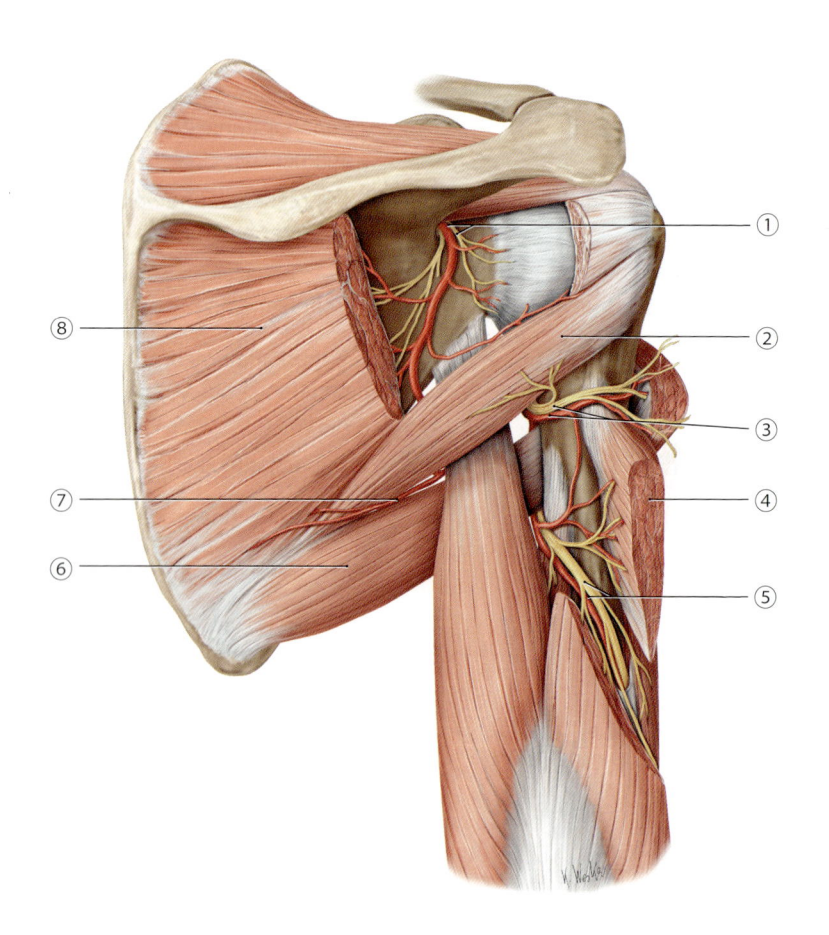

Q 肩甲骨動脈網に加わる主要な動脈は何か？

肩の後部における神経・血管 2

右肩，後面

① □ 肩甲上動脈・神経　　□ Suprascapular artery and nerve

② □ 小円筋　　□ Teres minor

③ □ 腋窩神経と後上腕回旋動脈　　□ Axillary nerve and posterior circumflex humeral artery

④ □ 上腕三頭筋，外側頭　　□ Triceps brachii, lateral head

⑤ □ 上腕深動脈と橈骨神経（橈骨神経溝を通る）　　□ Profunda brachii artery and radial nerve (in radial groove)

⑥ □ 大円筋　　□ Teres major

⑦ □ 肩甲回旋動脈　　□ Circumflex scapular artery

⑧ □ 棘下筋　　□ Infraspinatus

A 　肩甲骨動脈網を形成する主要な動脈は，甲状頸動脈から出る肩甲上動脈と頸横動脈（枝である肩甲背動脈を介して），腋窩動脈から出る肩甲下動脈の3種である．

①図22.30. p.333　②図24.30B. p.361

Neurovasculature of the Axilla I

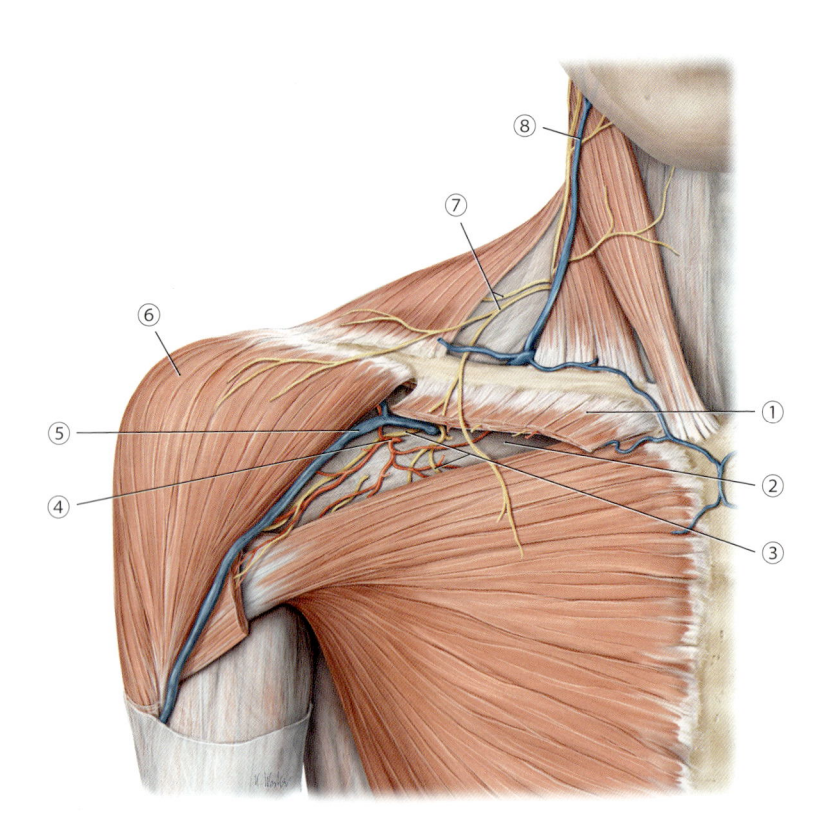

腋窩の神経・血管 1

右肩，前面

① □ 大胸筋，鎖骨部　　　　　□ Pectoralis major, clavicular part

② □ 鎖骨胸筋筋膜　　　　　　□ Clavipectoral fascia

③ □ 内側・外側胸筋神経　　　□ Medial and lateral pectoral nerves

④ □ 胸肩峰動脈　　　　　　　□ Thoracoacromial artery

⑤ □ 橈側皮静脈（三角筋胸筋溝を通る）　□ Cephalic vein (in deltopectoral groove)

⑥ □ 三角筋　　　　　　　　　□ Deltoid

⑦ □ 鎖骨上神経　　　　　　　□ Supraclavicular nerves

⑧ □ 外頸静脈　　　　　　　　□ External jugular vein

1 図 22.31B. p.334　　2 図 24.31B. p.362

Neurovasculature of the Axilla II

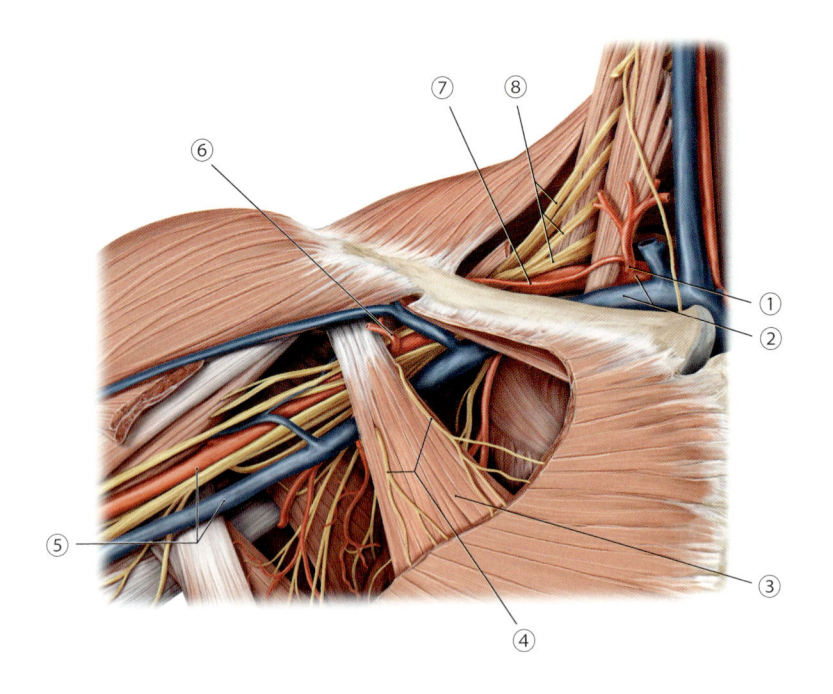

腋窩の神経・血管 2

右肩，前面

① □ 甲状頸動脈　　　　　□ Thyrocervical trunk
② □ 鎖骨下動脈・静脈　　□ Subclavian artery and vein
③ □ 小胸筋　　　　　　　□ Pectoralis minor
④ □ 内側・外側胸筋神経　□ Medial and lateral pectoral nerves
⑤ □ 腋窩動脈・静脈　　　□ Axillary artery and vein
⑥ □ 胸肩峰動脈　　　　　□ Thoracoacromial artery
⑦ □ 肩甲上動脈　　　　　□ Suprascapular artery
⑧ □ 腕神経叢（斜角筋隙から出る）　□ Brachial plexus (emerging from interscalene space)

[1] 図 22.33. p.335　[2] 図 24.33. p.363

Neurovasculature of the Axilla III

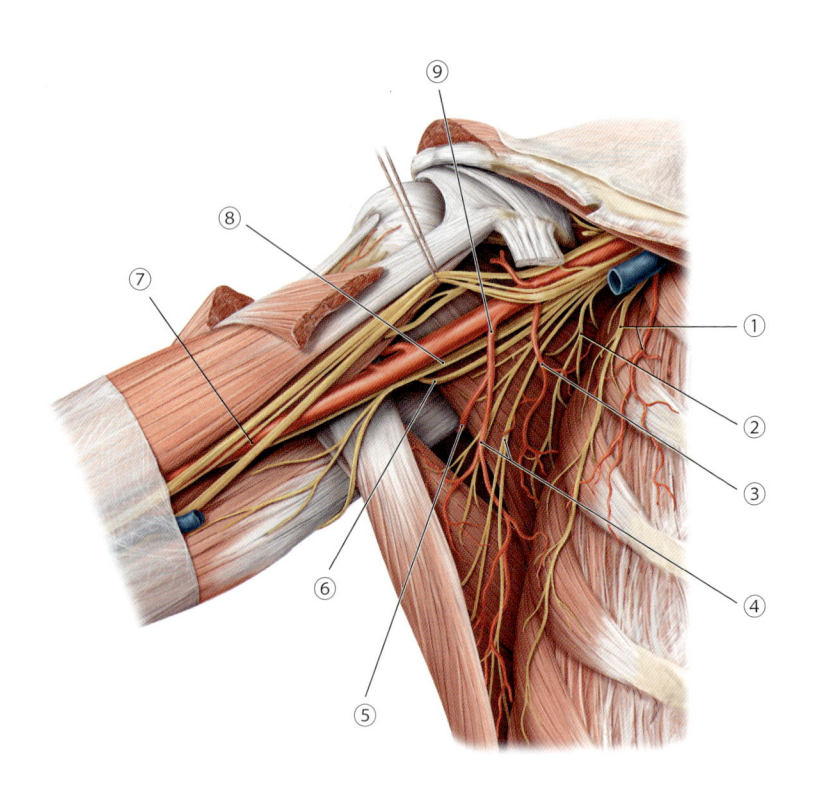

Q 長胸神経の起始はどこか？

腋窩の神経・血管 3

右肩, 前面

① □ 長胸神経, 最上胸動脈　　□ Long thoracic nerve, superior thoracic artery

② □ 上肩甲下神経　　□ Upper subscapular nerve

③ □ 外側胸動脈　　□ Lateral thoracic artery

④ □ 胸背動脈・神経　　□ Thoracodorsal artery and nerve

⑤ □ 肩甲回旋動脈　　□ Circumflex scapular artery

⑥ □ 腋窩神経　　□ Axillary nerve

⑦ □ 上腕動脈　　□ Brachial artery

⑧ □ 橈骨神経　　□ Radial nerve

⑨ □ 肩甲下動脈　　□ Subscapular artery

A 長胸神経は腕神経叢の根(C5-C7)から起始する.

1 図 22.34B. p.337　2 図 24.34B. p.365

Neurovasculature of the Brachial Region

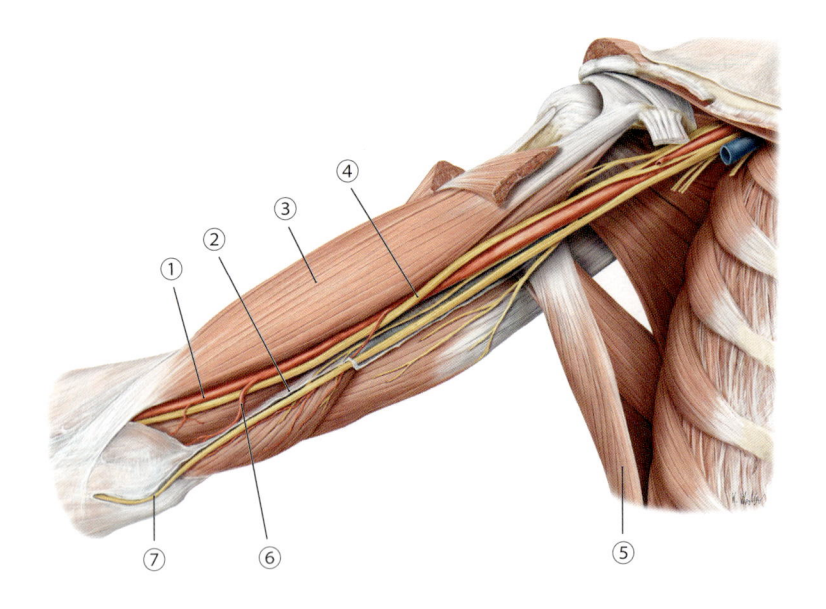

上腕の神経・血管

右上腕，前面

① □ 上腕動脈 □ Brachial artery
② □ 内側上腕筋間中隔 □ Medial intermuscular septum
③ □ 上腕二頭筋 □ Biceps brachii
④ □ 正中神経 □ Median nerve
⑤ □ 広背筋 □ Latissimus dorsi
⑥ □ 下尺側側副動脈 □ Inferior ulnar collateral artery
⑦ □ 尺骨神経（尺骨神経溝を通る） □ Ulnar nerve (in ulnar groove)

1 図 22.35. p.338　2 図 24.35. p.366

394 Upper Limb

Neurovasculature of the Forearm

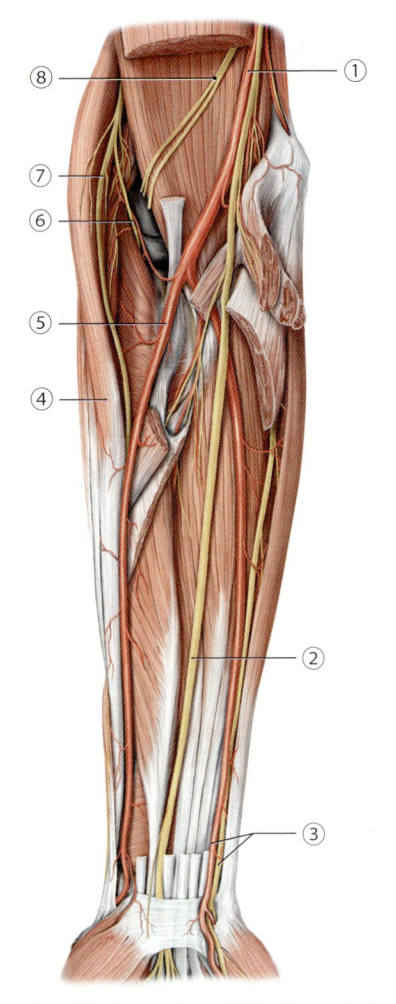

Q 前腕の筋のうち，尺骨神経に支配されるのはどれか？

前腕の神経・血管

右前腕，前面

① □ 上腕動脈　　　　　　　□ Brachial artery

② □ 正中神経　　　　　　　□ Median nerve

③ □ 尺骨動脈・神経　　　　□ Ulnar artery and nerve

④ □ 腕橈骨筋　　　　　　　□ Brachioradialis

⑤ □ 橈骨動脈　　　　　　　□ Radial artery

⑥ □ 橈骨神経，深枝　　　　□ Deep branch of radial nerve

⑦ □ 橈骨神経，浅枝　　　　□ Superficial branch of radial nerve

⑧ □ 筋皮神経
　　　（外側前腕皮神経）　　□ Musculocutaneous nerve (lateral antebrachial cutaneous nerve)

A　尺骨神経は，前腕では尺側手根屈筋と深指屈筋の尺側半分〔第4・5指（環指・小指）に腱を送る〕を支配する．前腕の前区画に位置する残りの筋は正中神経によって支配される．

1 図 22.37C. p.341　　2 図 24.37C. p.369

The Carpal Tunnel

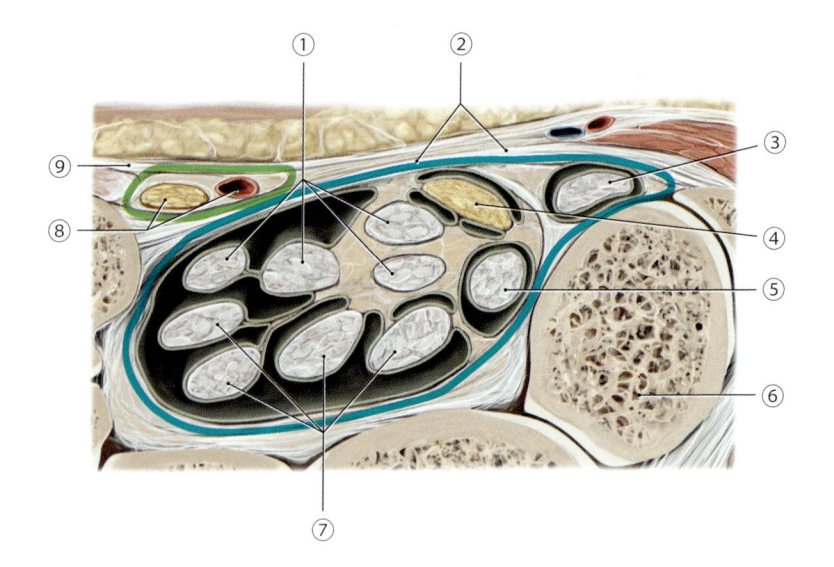

手根管

右手首の横断面，近位面（上面）

① ☐ 浅指屈筋（腱） ☐ Flexor digitorum superficialis tendons
② ☐ 屈筋支帯 ☐ Flexor retinaculum
③ ☐ 橈側手根屈筋（腱） ☐ Flexor carpi radialis tendon
④ ☐ 正中神経 ☐ Median nerve
⑤ ☐ 長母指屈筋（腱） ☐ Flexor pollicis longus tendon
⑥ ☐ 舟状骨 ☐ Scaphoid
⑦ ☐ 深指屈筋（腱） ☐ Flexor digitorum profundus tendons
⑧ ☐ 尺骨動脈・神経 ☐ Ulnar artery and nerve
⑨ ☐ 掌側手根靱帯 ☐ Palmar carpal ligament

解説

手根管は屈筋支帯と手根骨によって囲まれた空間である．正中神経や屈筋腱は手根管を通って手掌に達する．尺骨管は屈筋支帯と掌側手根靱帯によって囲まれた空間であり，ここを尺骨神経と尺骨動脈が通る．

1 図 22.41B. p.343　2 図 24.41B. p.371

Superficial Palmar Arch

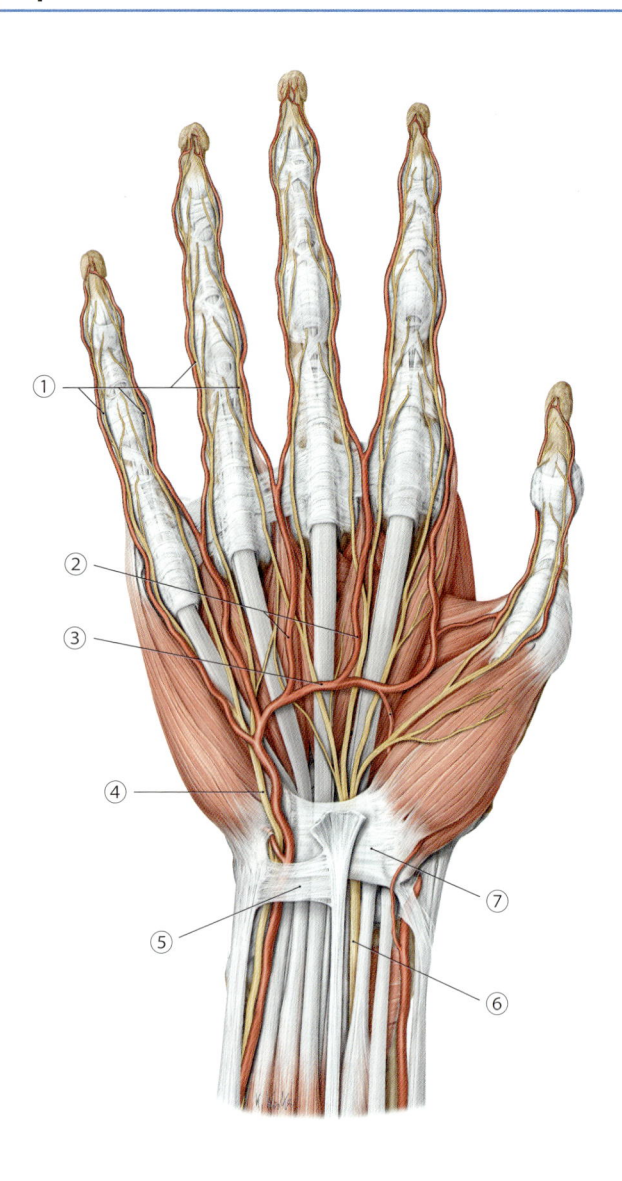

浅掌動脈弓

右手，前面（掌側面）

① ☐ 固有掌側指動脈・神経　☐ Proper palmar digital arteries and nerves

② ☐ 総掌側指動脈　☐ Common palmar digital arteries

③ ☐ 浅掌動脈弓　☐ Superficial palmar arch

④ ☐ 尺骨神経，浅枝　☐ Ulnar nerve, superficial branch

⑤ ☐ 掌側手根靱帯　☐ Palmar carpal ligament

⑥ ☐ 正中神経　☐ Median nerve

⑦ ☐ 屈筋支帯　☐ Flexor retinaculum

臨床

　手根管症候群では，感覚障害は指に現れるが，手掌の感覚は保たれる．これは，指に分布する正中神経の枝（総掌側指神経）が手根管よりも遠位で分かれるためである．なお，正中神経の掌枝は手根管よりも近位で分かれ，手根管の前方を通って手に達する．

1 図 22.44A. p.345　2 図 22.44A. p.373

Deep Palmar Arch

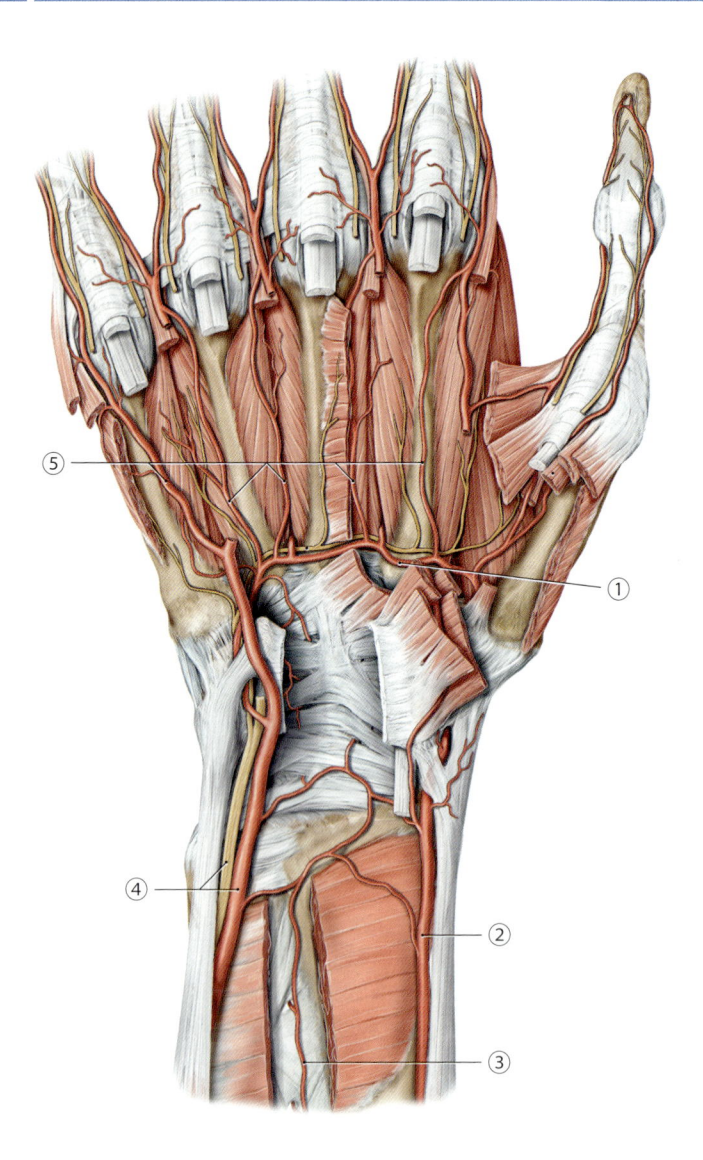

深掌動脈弓

右手,前面(掌側面)

① □ 深掌動脈弓　　　　　□ Deep palmar arch
② □ 橈骨動脈　　　　　　□ Radial artery
③ □ 前骨間動脈　　　　　□ Anterior interosseous artery
④ □ 尺骨動脈・神経　　　□ Ulnar artery and nerve
⑤ □ 掌側中手動脈　　　　□ Palmar metacarpal arteries

1 図 22.44B. p.345　2 図 24.44B. p.373

Anatomic Snuffbox

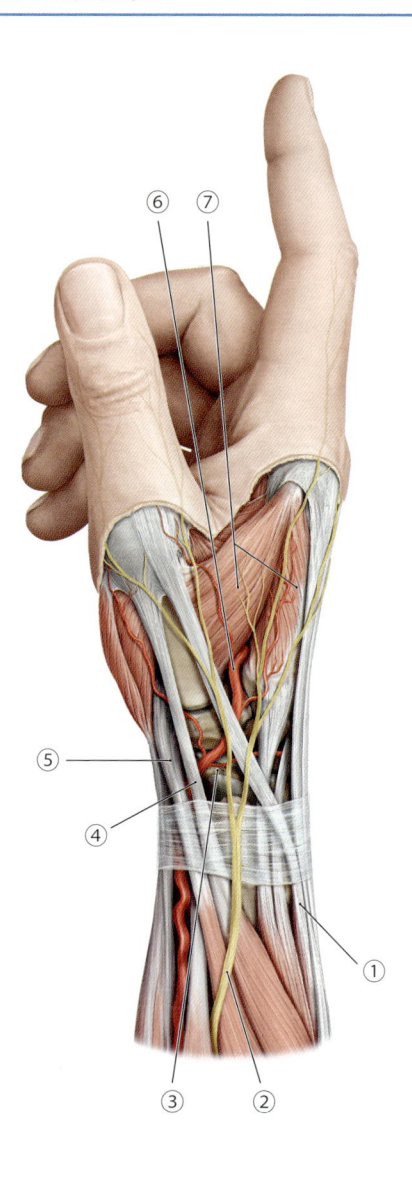

解剖学的嗅ぎタバコ入れ

右手，橈側面（内側面）

① ☐ 長母指伸筋（腱） ☐ Extensor pollicis longus tendon

② ☐ 橈骨神経，浅枝 ☐ Radial nerve, superficial branch

③ ☐ 舟状骨 ☐ Scaphoid

④ ☐ 短母指伸筋（腱） ☐ Extensor pollicis brevis tendon

⑤ ☐ 長母指外転筋（腱） ☐ Abductor pollicis longus tendon

⑥ ☐ 橈骨動脈 ☐ Radial artery

⑦ ☐ 第1背側骨間筋 ☐ 1st dorsal interosseous

臨床

解剖学的嗅ぎタバコ入れは，手首の橈側面（内側面）に位置した小区画であり，境界は長母指伸筋腱，短母指伸筋腱，長母指外転筋腱によって形成される．嗅ぎタバコ入れの床の大部分は舟状骨からなるので，舟状骨骨折では嗅ぎタバコ入れに自発痛や圧痛が見られる．

1 図 22.47. p.346　2 図 24.47. p.374

Sensory Innervation of the Hand I

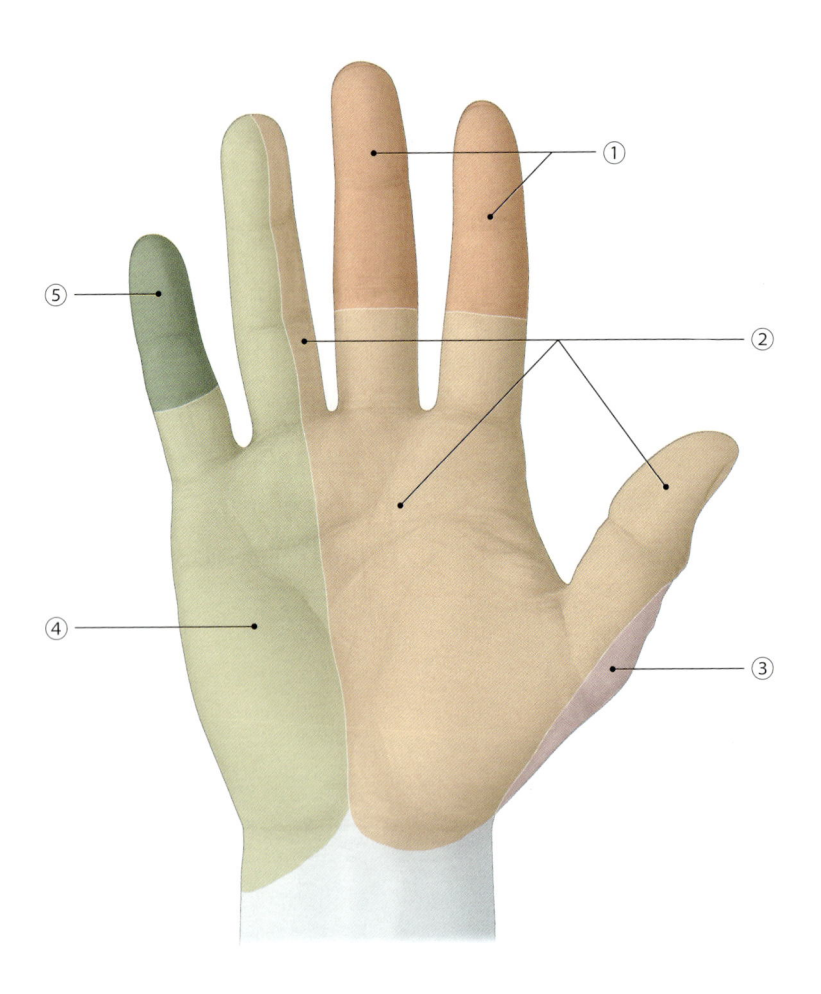

手における感覚神経の分布 1

右手，前面（掌側面）

① ☐ 掌側指神経（正中神経の固有領域） ☐ Palmar digital nerves (exclusive area of median nerve)

② ☐ 正中神経，掌枝 ☐ Median nerve, palmar branch

③ ☐ 橈骨神経，背側指神経 ☐ Radial nerve, dorsal digital nerve

④ ☐ 尺骨神経，掌枝 ☐ Ulnar nerve, palmar branch

⑤ ☐ 掌側指神経（尺骨神経の固有領域） ☐ Palmar digital nerve (exclusive area of ulnar nerve)

Sensory Innervation of the Hand II

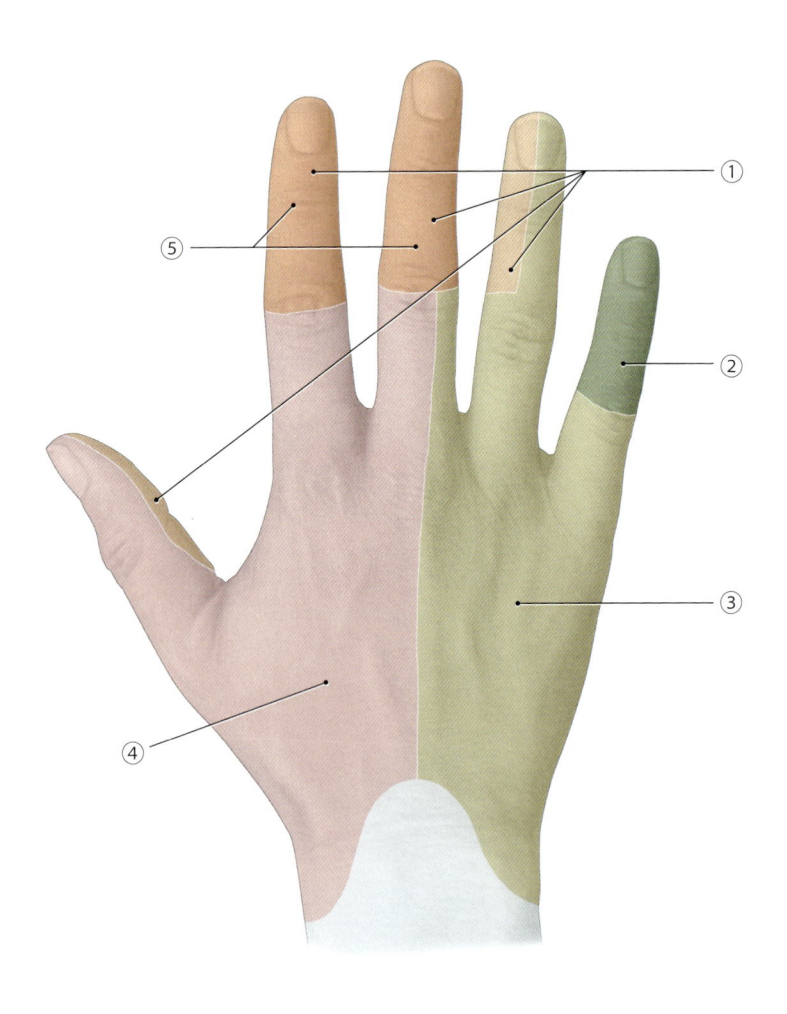

手における感覚神経の分布 2

右手，後面（背側面）

① □ 正中神経，掌側指神経の背側枝 □ Median nerve, dorsal branches of palmar digital nerves

② □ 背側指神経（尺骨神経の固有領域） □ Dorsal digital nerve (exclusive area of ulnar nerve)

③ □ 尺骨神経，背側枝 □ Ulnar nerve, dorsal branch

④ □ 橈骨神経，浅枝と背側指神経 □ Radial nerve, superficial branch and dorsal digital nerves

⑤ □ 正中神経の固有領域 □ Exclusive area of median nerve

Transverse Section of the Arm

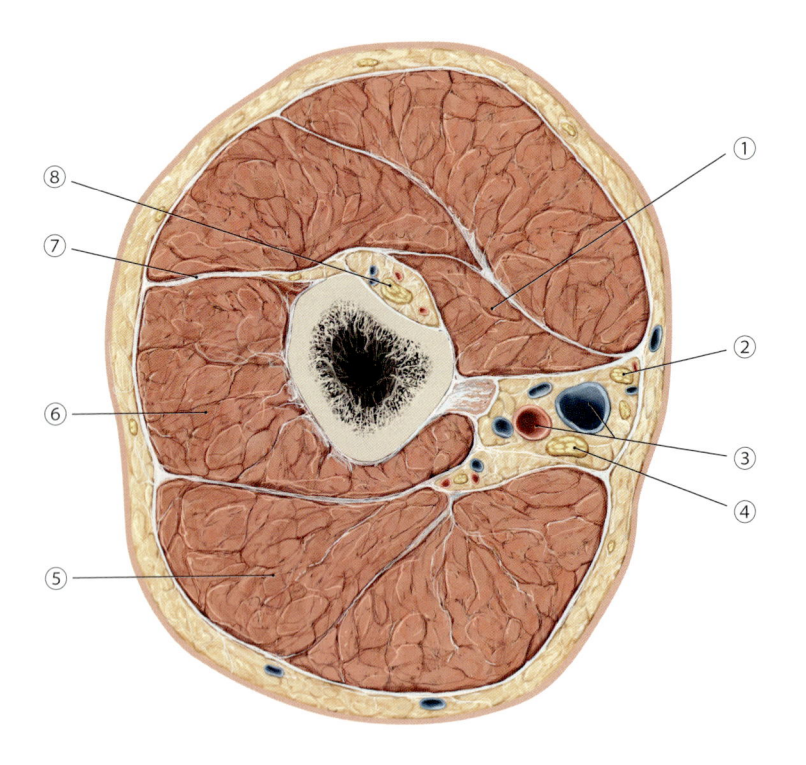

上腕の横断面

右上腕，近位方向（上方）から見たところ

① ☐ 上腕三頭筋，内側頭　　☐ Triceps brachii, medial head
② ☐ 尺骨神経　　☐ Ulnar nerve
③ ☐ 上腕動脈・静脈　　☐ Brachial artery and vein
④ ☐ 正中神経　　☐ Median nerve
⑤ ☐ 上腕二頭筋，長頭　　☐ Biceps brachii, long head
⑥ ☐ 上腕筋　　☐ Brachialis
⑦ ☐ 外側上腕筋間中隔　　☐ Lateral intermuscular septum
⑧ ☐ 橈骨神経　　☐ Radial nerve

解説

　上・下肢の筋は筋間中隔によって，区画化されている．各区画に入る筋どうしは同様の機能を有し，多くの場合，同じ神経と血管が分布する．

1 図 22.50A. p.349　2 図 24.50A. p.377

Transverse Section of the Forearm

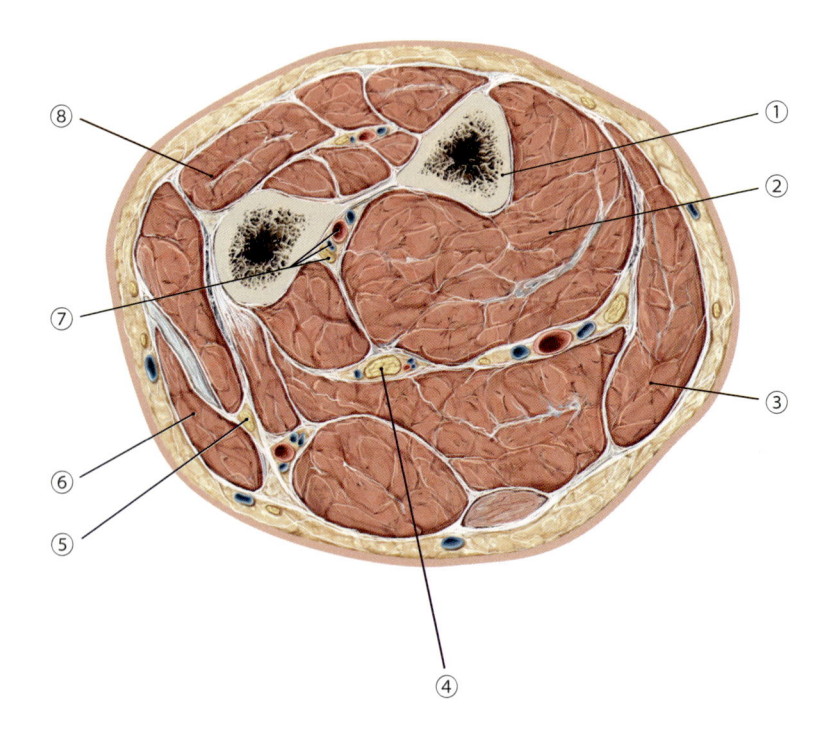

前腕の横断面

右前腕，近位方向（上方）から見たところ

① □ 尺骨　　　　　　　　　□ Ulna
② □ 深指屈筋　　　　　　　□ Flexor digitorum profundus
③ □ 尺側手根屈筋　　　　　□ Flexor carpi ulnaris
④ □ 正中神経　　　　　　　□ Median nerve
⑤ □ 橈骨神経，浅枝　　　　□ Radial nerve, superficial branch
⑥ □ 腕橈骨筋　　　　　　　□ Brachioradialis
⑦ □ 前骨間動脈・静脈，前［前腕］骨間神経　□ Anterior interosseous artery, vein, and nerve
⑧ □ ［総］指伸筋　　　　　□ Extensor digitorum

1 図 22.50B. p.349　2 図 24.50B. p.377

Surface Anatomy

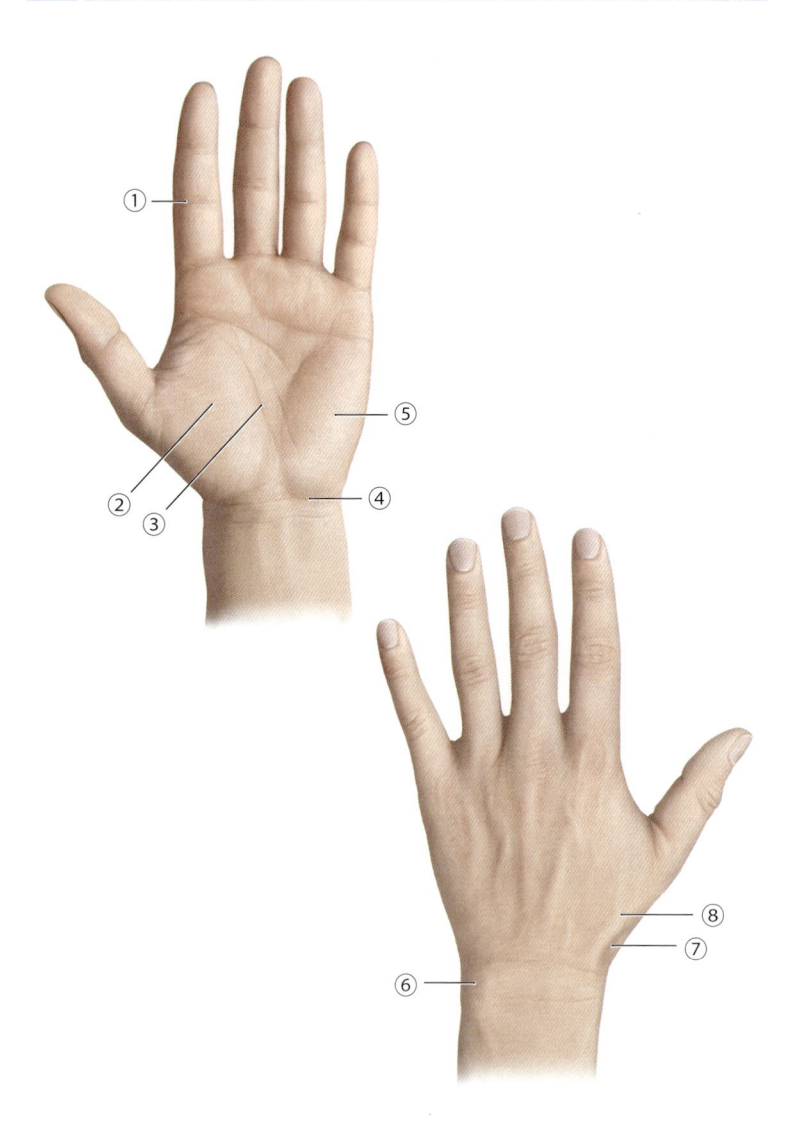

手の体表解剖

左手，上：前面（掌側面），下：後面（背側面）

①	☐ 近位指節間関節線	☐ Proximal interphalangeal (PIP) joint crease
②	☐ 母指球	☐ Thenar eminence
③	☐ 母指球線（"生命線"）	☐ Thenar crease ("life line")
④	☐ 遠位手根線	☐ Distal wrist crease
⑤	☐ 小指球	☐ Hypothenar eminence
⑥	☐ 尺骨の茎状突起	☐ Styloid process of ulna
⑦	☐ 解剖学的嗅ぎタバコ入れ	☐ Anatomic snuffbox
⑧	☐ 長母指伸筋（腱）	☐ Extensor pollicis longus tendon

図 23.7A, 図 23.8A. p.353

下肢 Lower Limb

下肢の骨格 ………………………………… *416*
寛骨の構成 ………………………………… *418*
大腿骨 ……………………………………… *420*
股関節 1 …………………………………… *422*
股関節 2 …………………………………… *424*
股関節の靱帯 1 …………………………… *426*
股関節の靱帯 2 …………………………… *428*
骨盤と大腿の筋(前面) 1 ………………… *430*
骨盤と大腿の筋(前面) 2 ………………… *432*
骨盤と大腿の筋(前面) 3 ………………… *434*
骨盤と大腿の筋(内側面) ………………… *436*
骨盤と大腿の筋(後面) 1 ………………… *438*
骨盤と大腿の筋(後面) 2 ………………… *440*
骨盤と大腿の筋(後面) 3 ………………… *442*
骨盤と大腿の筋(外側面) ………………… *444*
脛骨と腓骨 ………………………………… *446*
膝関節 1 …………………………………… *448*
膝関節 2 …………………………………… *450*
膝関節の靱帯 1 …………………………… *452*
膝関節の靱帯 2 …………………………… *454*
膝関節の靱帯 3 …………………………… *456*
下腿の筋(前面) ………………………… *458*
下腿の筋(外側面) ……………………… *460*
下腿の筋(後面) 1 ……………………… *462*
下腿の筋(後面) 2 ……………………… *464*
下腿の筋(後面) 3 ……………………… *466*
足の骨格 1 ………………………………… *468*
足の骨格 2 ………………………………… *470*
足首と足の関節 1 ………………………… *472*
足首と足の関節 2 ………………………… *474*
足首と足の関節 3 ………………………… *476*
足首と足の靱帯 1 ………………………… *478*
足首と足の靱帯 2 ………………………… *480*
足首と足の靱帯 3 ………………………… *482*
足底の筋 1 ………………………………… *484*
足底の筋 2 ………………………………… *486*
足底の筋 3 ………………………………… *488*
足底の筋 4 ………………………………… *490*
足首と足 …………………………………… *492*
下肢の動脈 1 ……………………………… *494*
下肢の動脈 2 ……………………………… *496*
腰仙骨神経叢 1 …………………………… *498*
腰仙骨神経叢 2 …………………………… *500*
腰神経叢からの神経 1 …………………… *502*
腰神経叢からの神経 2 …………………… *504*
仙骨神経叢からの神経 1 ………………… *506*
仙骨神経叢からの神経 2 ………………… *508*
皮静脈と皮神経 …………………………… *510*
鼡径部 ……………………………………… *512*
坐骨孔 ……………………………………… *514*
大腿前面の神経・血管 …………………… *516*
大腿後面の神経・血管 …………………… *518*
下腿後面の神経・血管 …………………… *520*
足根管 ……………………………………… *522*
下腿外側の神経・血管 …………………… *524*
下腿前面の神経・血管 …………………… *526*
足背の神経・血管 ………………………… *528*
足底の神経・血管 ………………………… *530*
大腿の横断面 ……………………………… *532*
下腿の横断面 ……………………………… *534*
下肢の体表解剖 …………………………… *536*

Bones of the Lower Limb

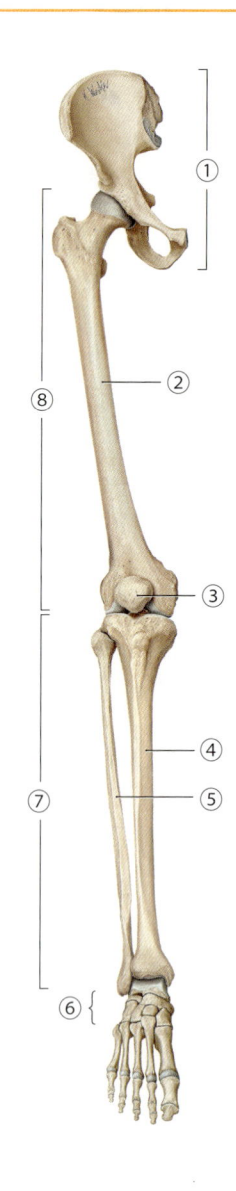

下肢の骨格

右下肢，前面

① □ 下肢帯　　　　　□ Pelvic girdle

② □ 大腿骨　　　　　□ Femur

③ □ 膝蓋骨　　　　　□ Patella

④ □ 脛骨　　　　　　□ Tibia

⑤ □ 腓骨　　　　　　□ Fibula

⑥ □ 足根骨　　　　　□ Tarsal bones

⑦ □ 下腿　　　　　　□ Lower leg

⑧ □ 大腿　　　　　　□ Thigh

Components of the Hip Bone

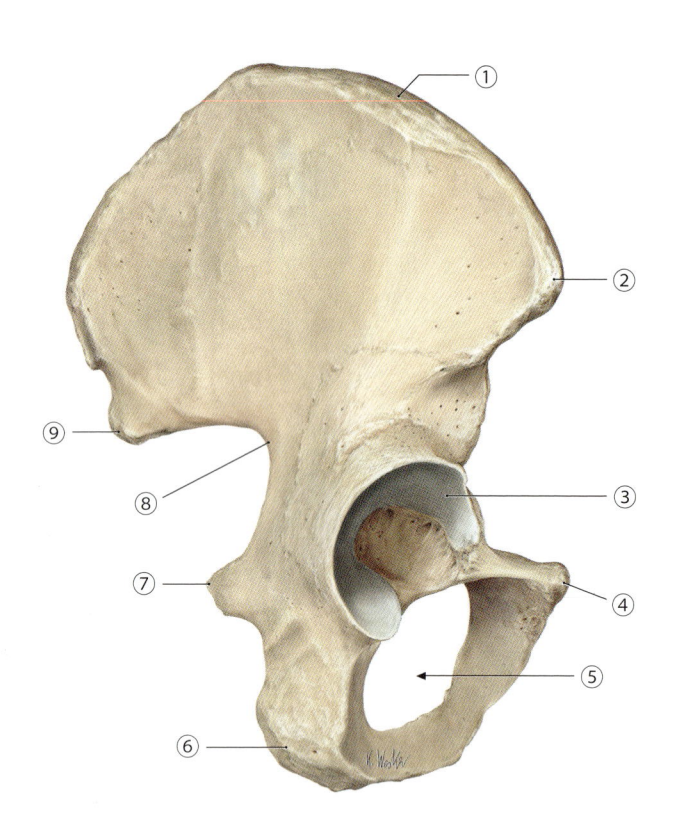

Q 寛骨は3つの骨が寛骨臼で融合してできる．この3つの骨とは何か？

寛骨の構成

右寛骨，外側面

① □ 腸骨稜　　　　　　　□ Iliac crest
② □ 上前腸骨棘　　　　　□ Anterior superior iliac spine
③ □ 寛骨臼　　　　　　　□ Acetabulum
④ □ 恥骨結節　　　　　　□ Pubic tubercle
⑤ □ 閉鎖孔　　　　　　　□ Obturator foramen
⑥ □ 坐骨結節　　　　　　□ Ischial tuberosity
⑦ □ 坐骨棘　　　　　　　□ Ischial spine
⑧ □ 大坐骨切痕　　　　　□ Greater sciatic notch
⑨ □ 下後腸骨棘　　　　　□ Posterior inferior iliac spine

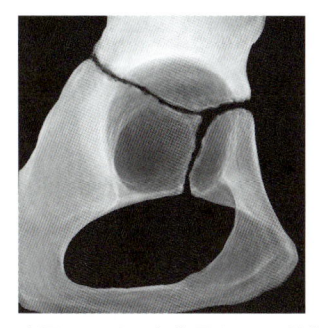

小児における右寛骨臼のX線像

A 寛骨は腸骨，坐骨，恥骨が融合してできる．融合は14〜16歳の間に起こる．

[1] 図24.6B, C. p.359　　[2] 図16.4, 図16.3B. p.217

420 Lower Limb

Femur

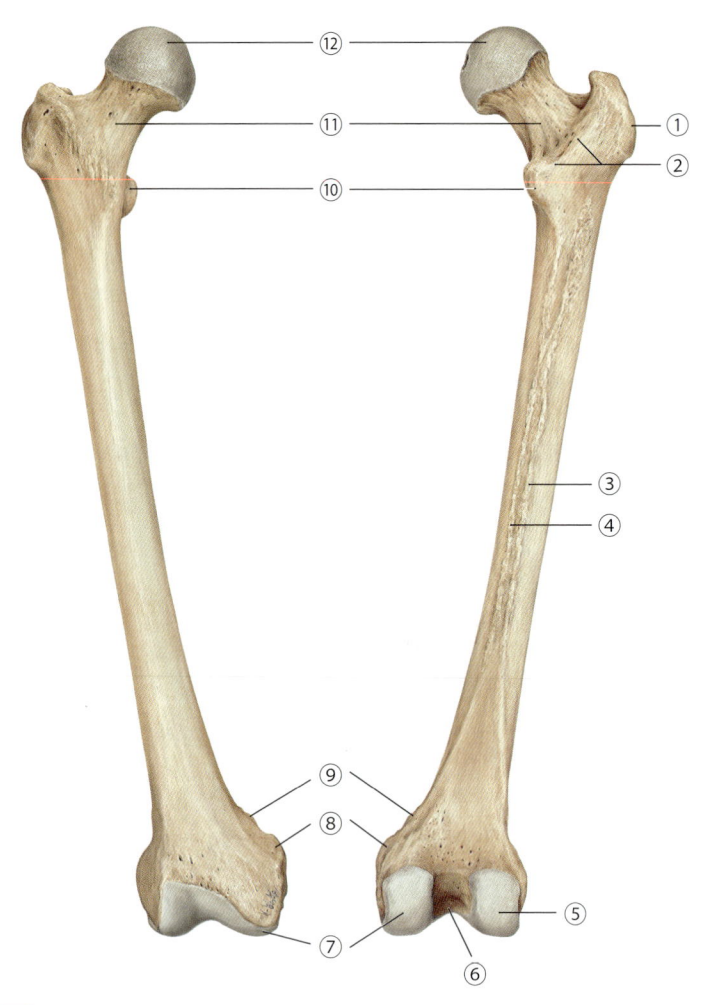

骨粗鬆症患者の大腿骨骨折はどの部位に起こりやすいか？

大腿骨

右大腿骨，左：前面，右：後面

① ☐ 大転子 　　　　　　　　☐ Greater trochanter
② ☐ 転子間稜 　　　　　　　☐ Intertrochanteric crest
③ ☐ 粗線の外側唇 　　　　　☐ Lateral lip of the linea aspera
④ ☐ 粗線の内側唇 　　　　　☐ Medial lip of the linea aspera
⑤ ☐ 外側顆 　　　　　　　　☐ Lateral condyle
⑥ ☐ 顆間窩 　　　　　　　　☐ Intercondylar notch
⑦ ☐ 内側顆 　　　　　　　　☐ Medial condyle
⑧ ☐ 内側上顆 　　　　　　　☐ Medial epicondyle
⑨ ☐ 内転筋結節 　　　　　　☐ Adductor tubercle
⑩ ☐ 小転子 　　　　　　　　☐ Lesser trochanter
⑪ ☐ 大腿骨頸 　　　　　　　☐ Neck
⑫ ☐ 大腿骨頭 　　　　　　　☐ Head

A 骨粗鬆症患者の大腿骨骨折は大腿骨頸に起こりやすい．

[1] 図 24.7A, B. p.360　[2] 図 26.4A, B. p.384

Hip Joint I

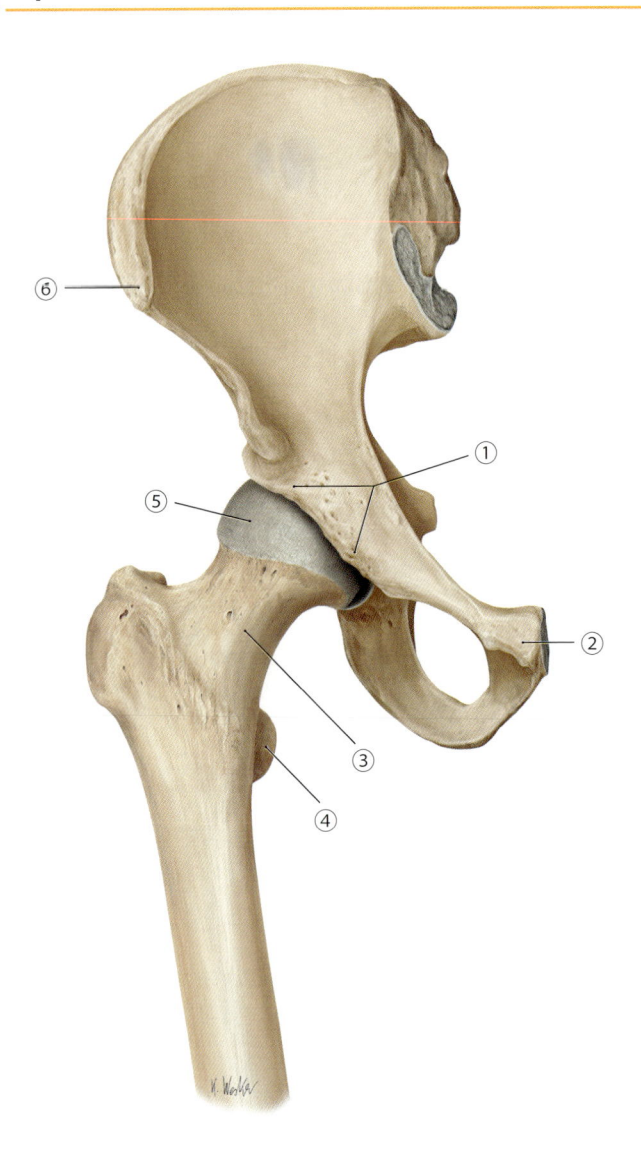

股関節 1

右股関節，前面

① □ 寛骨臼縁　　　　　　□ Bony acetabular rim
② □ 恥骨結節　　　　　　□ Pubic tubercle
③ □ 大腿骨頸　　　　　　□ Neck of femur
④ □ 小転子　　　　　　　□ Lesser trochanter
⑤ □ 大腿骨頭　　　　　　□ Head of femur
⑥ □ 上前腸骨棘　　　　　□ Anterior superior iliac spine

解説

大腿骨頭は寛骨の寛骨臼との間で，球関節の一種である股関節を形成する（球関節とは，ボールとソケットを組み合わせたような様式の関節を指す）．大腿骨頭はほぼ球状であり（平均曲率半径は約 2.5 cm），その大部分が寛骨臼内にはまり込む．

1 図 24.9A. p.362　2 図 26.6A. p.386

Hip Joint II

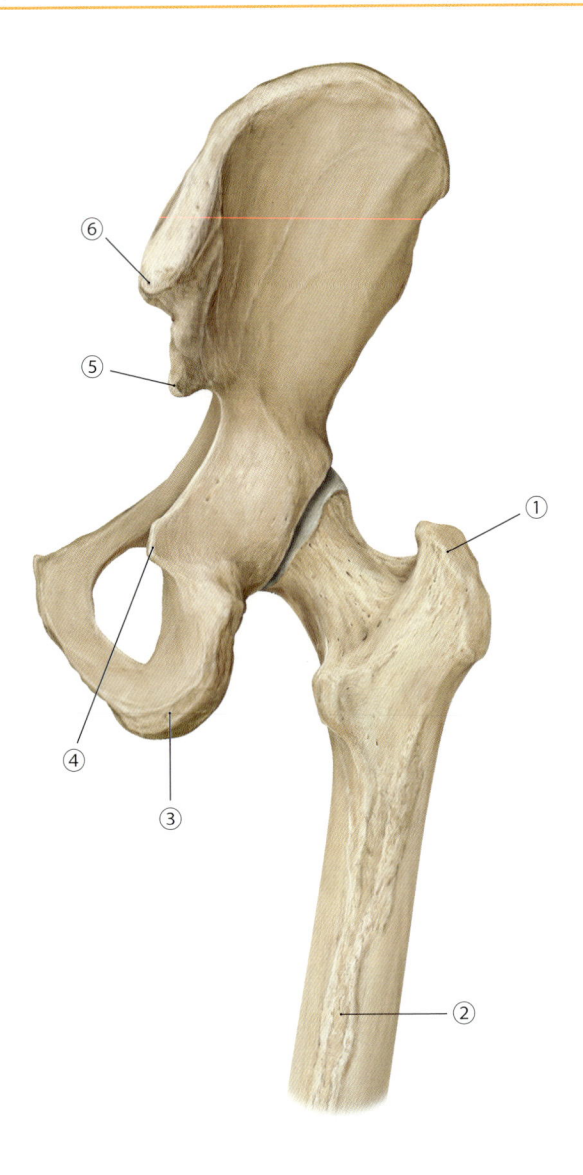

股関節 2

右股関節，後面

① ☐ 大転子 ☐ Greater trochanter
② ☐ 粗線 ☐ Linea aspera
③ ☐ 坐骨結節 ☐ Ischial tuberosity
④ ☐ 坐骨棘 ☐ Ischial spine
⑤ ☐ 下後腸骨棘 ☐ Posterior inferior iliac spine
⑥ ☐ 上後腸骨棘 ☐ Posterior superior iliac spine

臨床

乳幼児における股関節のスクリーニング検査において，超音波検査は最も重要なものである．この検査では，股関節の低形成や脱臼といった形態的な異常を見つけ出すことができる．股関節脱臼の患者では，股関節の不安定性や外転制限，殿溝の非対称を伴った下肢の短縮が見られる．

1 図 24.9B. p.362　 2 図 26.6B. p.386

Ligaments of the Hip Joint I

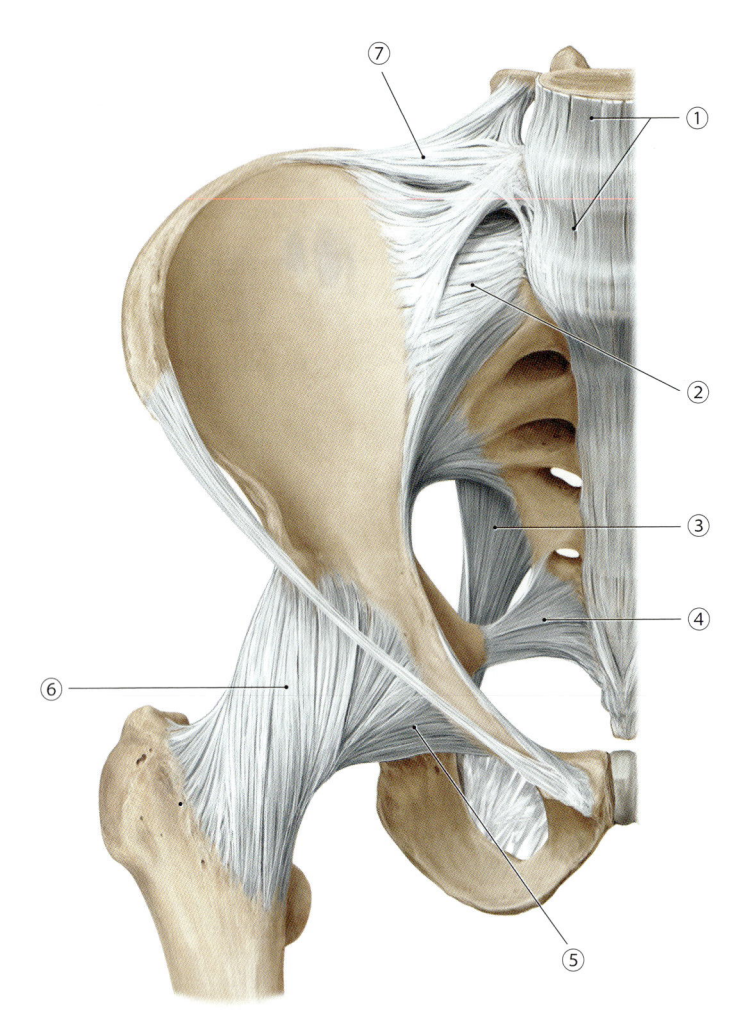

股関節はどの肢位において最も不安定となるか（最も脱臼しやすいか）？

股関節の靱帯 1

右股関節，前面

① ☐ 前縦靱帯　　　　　　　　☐ Anterior longitudinal ligament
② ☐ 前仙腸靱帯　　　　　　　☐ Anterior sacroiliac ligaments
③ ☐ 仙結節靱帯　　　　　　　☐ Sacrotuberous ligament
④ ☐ 仙棘靱帯　　　　　　　　☐ Sacrospinous ligament
⑤ ☐ 恥骨大腿靱帯　　　　　　☐ Pubofemoral ligament
⑥ ☐ 腸骨大腿靱帯　　　　　　☐ Iliofemoral ligament
⑦ ☐ 腸腰靱帯　　　　　　　　☐ Iliolumbar ligament

A　股関節の関節包は，大腿骨頸をラセン状に取り巻く3つの靱帯（腸骨大腿靱帯，恥骨大腿靱帯，坐骨大腿靱帯）で補強されている．これらの靱帯は外転屈曲位において弛緩し，このとき股関節が最も不安定となる．

1 図 24.12B, p.365　　2 図 26.9B, p.389

Ligaments of the Hip Joint II

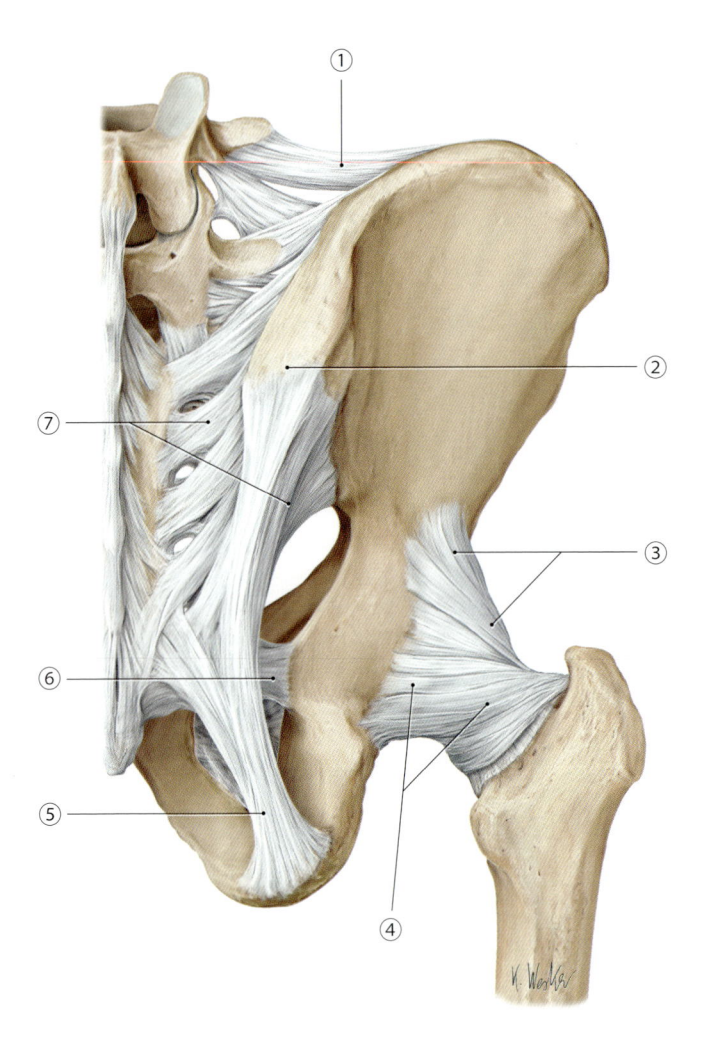

股関節の靱帯 2

右股関節，後面

① □ 腸腰靱帯　　　　　　□ Iliolumbar ligament
② □ 上後腸骨棘　　　　　□ Posterior superior iliac spine
③ □ 腸骨大腿靱帯　　　　□ Iliofemoral ligament
④ □ 坐骨大腿靱帯　　　　□ Ischiofemoral ligament
⑤ □ 仙結節靱帯　　　　　□ Sacrotuberous ligament
⑥ □ 仙棘靱帯　　　　　　□ Sacrospinous ligament
⑦ □ 後仙腸靱帯　　　　　□ Posterior sacroiliac ligaments

Anterior Muscles of the Hip & Thigh I

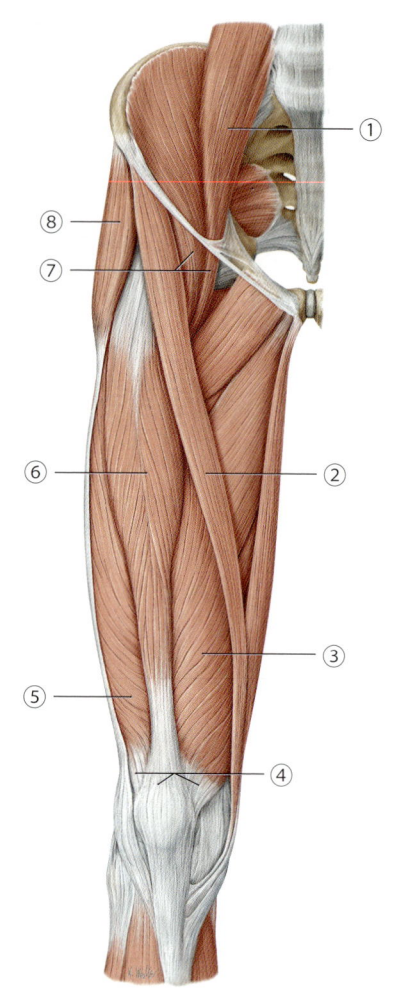

①
⑧
⑦
⑥
②
③
⑤
④

Q 大腿三角とはどこか？

骨盤と大腿の筋(前面) 1

右下肢，前面

① □ 大腰筋　　　　　　　□ Psoas major
② □ 縫工筋　　　　　　　□ Sartorius
③ □ 内側広筋　　　　　　□ Vastus medialis
④ □ 大腿四頭筋(腱)　　　□ Quadriceps femoris tendon
⑤ □ 外側広筋　　　　　　□ Vastus lateralis
⑥ □ 大腿直筋　　　　　　□ Rectus femoris
⑦ □ 腸腰筋　　　　　　　□ Iliopsoas
⑧ □ 大腿筋膜張筋　　　　□ Tensor fasciae latae

A 　大腿三角は鼡径靱帯，縫工筋，長内転筋によって囲まれた大腿前面の領域であり，大腿動脈，大腿静脈，大腿神経がここを通過する．腸腰筋と恥骨筋は大腿三角の後壁(床)を形成する．

1 図 24.14A. p.366　2 図 26.11A. p.390

Anterior Muscles of the Hip & Thigh II

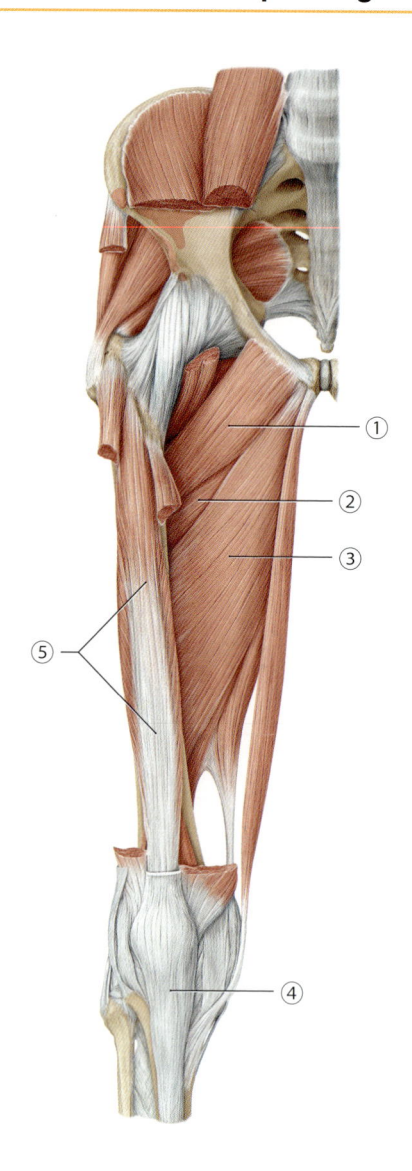

骨盤と大腿の筋（前面）2

右下肢，前面

① □ 恥骨筋　　　　　　　　□ Pectineus

② □ 短内転筋　　　　　　　□ Adductor brevis

③ □ 長内転筋　　　　　　　□ Adductor longus

④ □ 膝蓋靱帯　　　　　　　□ Patellar ligament

⑤ □ 中間広筋　　　　　　　□ Vastus intermedius

1 図 24.14C. p.367　2 図 26.11C. p.391

Anterior Muscles of the Hip & Thigh III

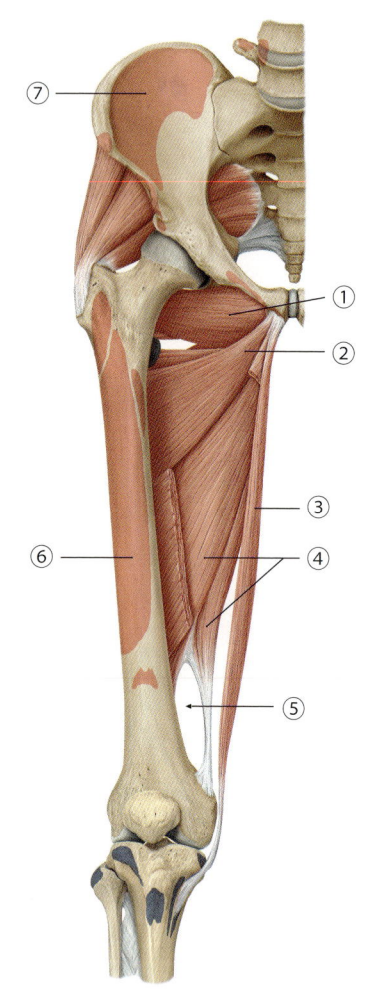

内転筋腱裂孔を通過する血管は何か？

骨盤と大腿の筋（前面） 3

右下肢．前面

① □ 外閉鎖筋　　　　　　□ Obturator externus
② □ 短内転筋　　　　　　□ Adductor brevis
③ □ 薄筋　　　　　　　　□ Gracilis
④ □ 大内転筋　　　　　　□ Adductor magnus
⑤ □ ［内転筋］腱裂孔　　□ Adductor hiatus
⑥ □ 中間広筋（筋の起始）□ Vastus intermedius（origin）
⑦ □ 腸骨筋（筋の起始）　□ Iliacus（origin）

A　大腿動脈と大腿静脈が内転筋腱裂孔を通過し，大腿前面から膝窩に達する．

1 図 24.14D. p.367　2 図 26.11D. p.391

Medial View of Thigh Muscles

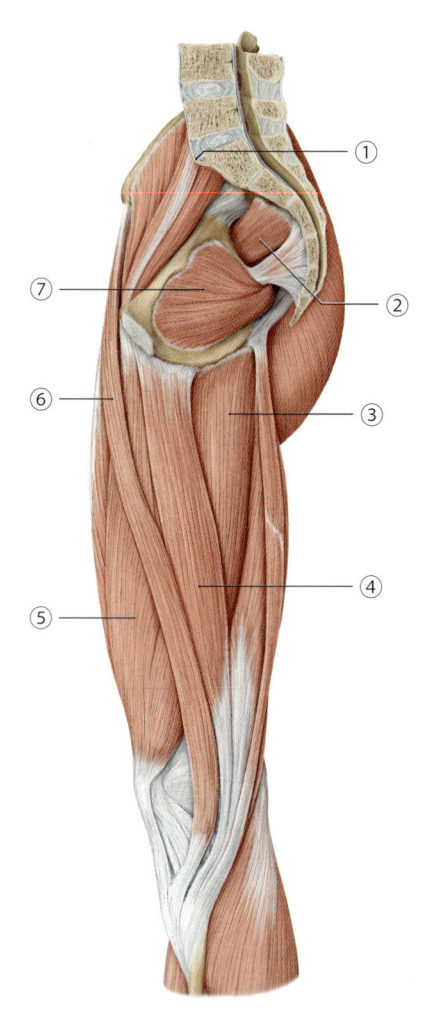

Q 縫工筋，薄筋，半腱様筋の共通停止腱は何と呼ばれるか？

骨盤と大腿の筋（内側面）

右下肢，内側面

① ☐ 岬角　　　　　　　　☐ Promontory
② ☐ 梨状筋　　　　　　　☐ Piriformis
③ ☐ 大内転筋　　　　　　☐ Adductor magnus
④ ☐ 薄筋　　　　　　　　☐ Gracilis
⑤ ☐ 内側広筋　　　　　　☐ Vastus medialis
⑥ ☐ 縫工筋　　　　　　　☐ Sartorius
⑦ ☐ 内閉鎖筋　　　　　　☐ Obturator internus

A　縫工筋，薄筋，半腱様筋は，鵞足と呼ばれる共通停止腱を形成する．鵞足の直下には鵞足包（滑液包の一種）が存在する．

1 図 24.16. p.369　　2 図 26.13. p.393

Posterior Muscles of the Hip & Thigh I

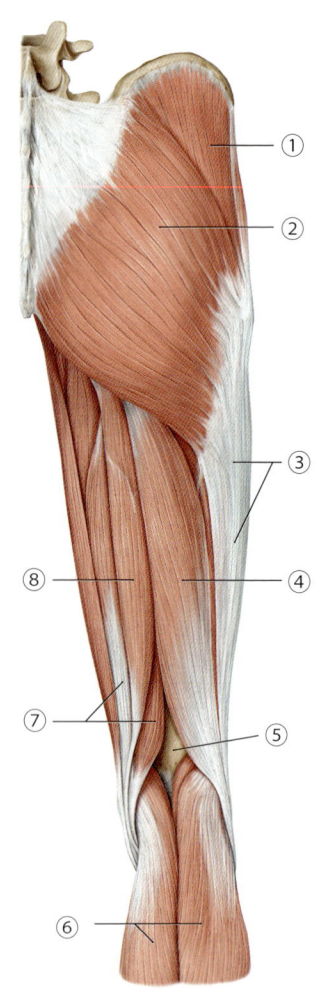

Q 大殿筋の機能は何か？

骨盤と大腿の筋（後面） 1

右下肢，後面

① ☐ 中殿筋　　　　　　　　　　☐ Gluteus medius
② ☐ 大殿筋　　　　　　　　　　☐ Gluteus maximus
③ ☐ 腸脛靱帯　　　　　　　　　☐ Iliotibial tract
④ ☐ 大腿二頭筋，長頭　　　　　☐ Biceps femoris, long head
⑤ ☐ 膝窩　　　　　　　　　　　☐ Popliteal fossa
⑥ ☐ 腓腹筋，内側頭と外側頭　　☐ Gastrocnemius, medial and lateral heads
⑦ ☐ 半膜様筋　　　　　　　　　☐ Semimembranosus
⑧ ☐ 半腱様筋　　　　　　　　　☐ Semitendinosus

A 　大殿筋は股関節を伸展・外旋する強力な筋である．また，大殿筋の上部は股関節の外転作用，下部は股関節の内転作用を有する．

1 図 24.17A, p.370　　2 図 26.14A, p.394

Posterior Muscles of the Hip & Thigh II

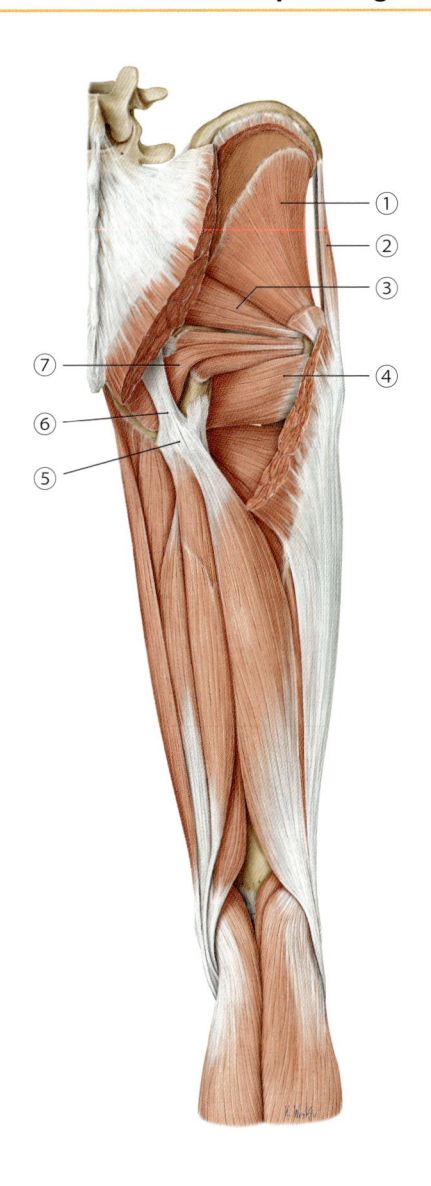

骨盤と大腿の筋（後面）2

右下肢，後面

① □ 小殿筋　　　　　　　□ Gluteus minimus
② □ 大腿筋膜張筋　　　　□ Tensor fasciae latae
③ □ 梨状筋　　　　　　　□ Piriformis
④ □ 大腿方形筋　　　　　□ Quadratus femoris
⑤ □ 坐骨結節　　　　　　□ Ischial tuberosity
⑥ □ 仙結節靱帯　　　　　□ Sacrotuberous ligament
⑦ □ 内閉鎖筋　　　　　　□ Obturator internus

解説

　ハムストリングス（半腱様筋，半膜様筋，大腿二頭筋の長頭）はすべてが坐骨結節から起始し，坐骨神経の脛骨神経部によって支配される．これらの筋は，股関節の伸筋ならびに膝関節の屈筋として働く．

1 図24.17B. p.370　2 図26.14B. p.394

Posterior Muscles of the Hip & Thigh III

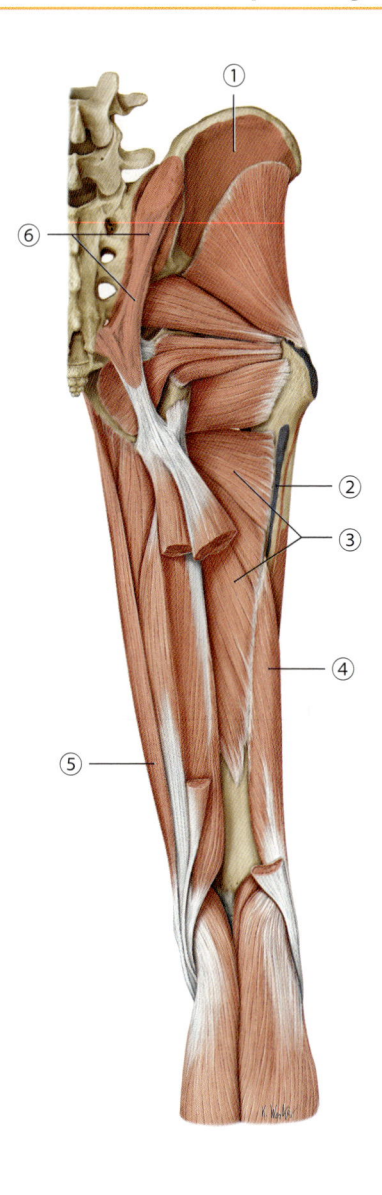

骨盤と大腿の筋(後面) 3

右下肢，後面

① □ 中殿筋(筋の起始)　　□ Gluteus medius (origin)

② □ 大殿筋(筋の停止)　　□ Gluteus maximus (insertion)

③ □ 大内転筋　　□ Adductor magnus

④ □ 大腿二頭筋，短頭　　□ Biceps femoris, short head

⑤ □ 薄筋　　□ Gracilis

⑥ □ 大殿筋(筋の起始)　　□ Gluteus maximus (origin)

1 図 24.17C. p.371　2 図 26.14C. p.395

444 Lower Limb

Lateral View of Hip & Thigh Muscles

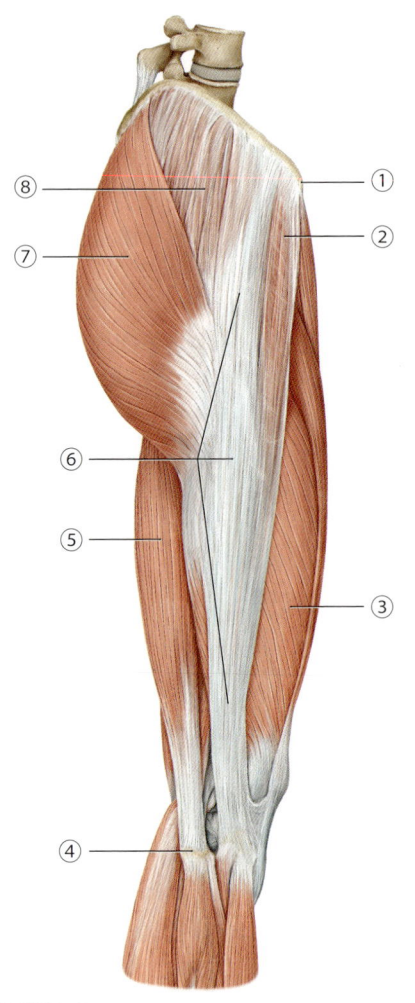

Q 腸脛靭帯とは何か？

骨盤と大腿の筋（外側面）

右下肢．外側面

① □ 上前腸骨棘　　　　　　　　　　□ Anterior superior iliac spine
② □ 大腿筋膜張筋　　　　　　　　　□ Tensor fasciae latae
③ □ 外側広筋　　　　　　　　　　　□ Vastus lateralis
④ □ 腓骨頭　　　　　　　　　　　　□ Head of fibula
⑤ □ 大腿二頭筋，長頭　　　　　　　□ Long head of biceps femoris
⑥ □ 腸脛靱帯　　　　　　　　　　　□ Iliotibial tract
⑦ □ 大殿筋　　　　　　　　　　　　□ Gluteus maximus
⑧ □ 中殿筋　　　　　　　　　　　　□ Gluteus medius

A　腸脛靱帯は大腿筋膜の外側部が肥厚したものであり，長軸方向に発達した線維によって補強されている．腸脛靱帯は幅の広い帯のようであり，腸骨稜と脛骨の前外側面の間に張っている．腸脛靱帯の上部は，大腿筋膜張筋を包み込むとともに，大殿筋腱膜の停止にもなっている．

① 図 24.19. p.373　② 図 26.16. p.397

Tibia & Fibula

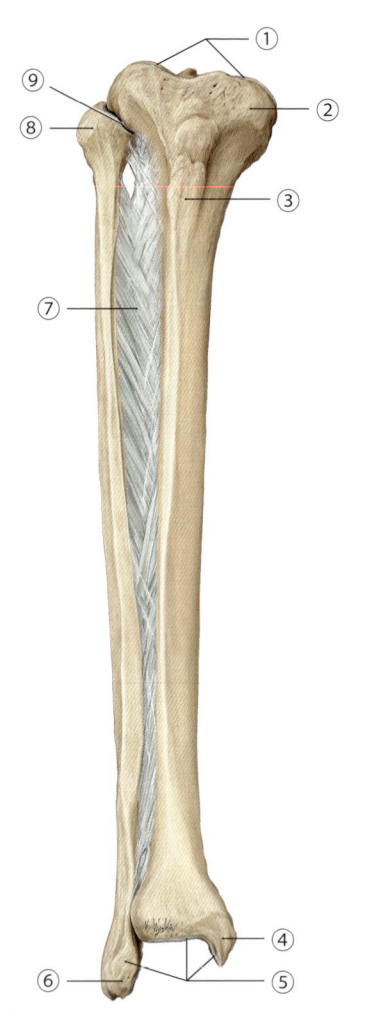

Q 腓骨の役割は何か？

脛骨と腓骨

右下腿，前面

① □ 上関節面　　　　　□ Tibial plateau
② □ 内側顆　　　　　　□ Medial condyle
③ □ 脛骨粗面　　　　　□ Tibial tuberosity
④ □ 内果　　　　　　　□ Medial malleolus
⑤ □ 足関節窩　　　　　□ Ankle mortise
⑥ □ 外果　　　　　　　□ Lateral malleolus
⑦ □ 下腿骨間膜　　　　□ Interosseous membrane
⑧ □ 腓骨頭　　　　　　□ Head of fibula
⑨ □ 脛腓関節　　　　　□ Tibiofibular joint

A 腓骨には体重を支える役割はないが，距腿関節の関節面の一部を形成し，関節の安定性を保つうえで重要な役割をはたす．また，腓骨には下肢のいくつかの筋が起始もしくは停止する．

1 図 25.1A. p.380　2 図 27.1A. p.404

Knee Joint I

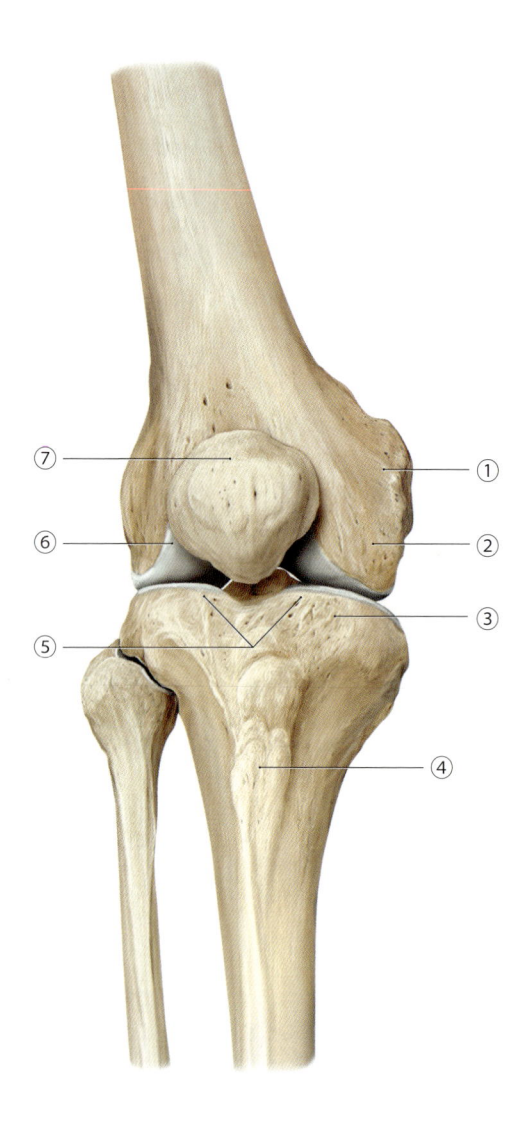

膝関節 1

右膝,前面

① □ 内側上顆　　　　　　　□ Medial epicondyle

② □ 大腿骨の内側顆　　　　□ Medial femoral condyle

③ □ 脛骨の内側顆　　　　　□ Medial tibial condyle

④ □ 脛骨粗面　　　　　　　□ Tibial tuberosity

⑤ □ 上関節面　　　　　　　□ Tibial plateau

⑥ □ 大腿骨の外側顆　　　　□ Lateral femoral condyle

⑦ □ 膝蓋骨　　　　　　　　□ Patella

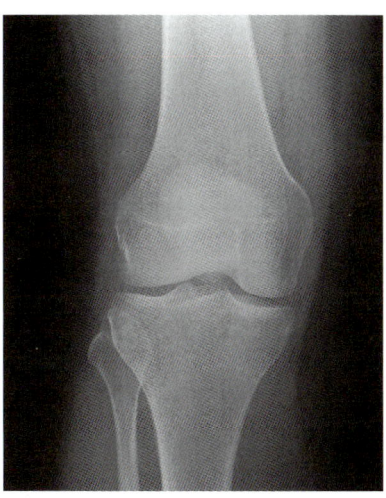

右膝のX線像

1 図25.2A, 図25.3A. p.382-383　　2 図27.2A, 図27.3A. p.406-407

Knee Joint II

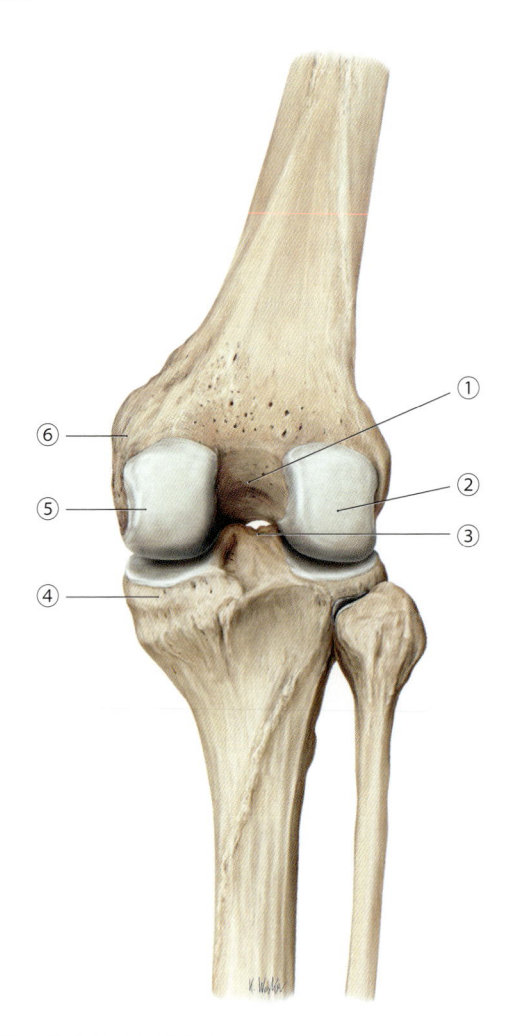

Q 膝関節を構成する骨は何か？

膝関節 2

右膝，後面

① ☐ 顆間窩　　　　　　　☐ Intercondylar notch

② ☐ 大腿骨の外側顆　　　☐ Lateral femoral condyle

③ ☐ 顆間隆起　　　　　　☐ Intercondylar eminence

④ ☐ 脛骨の内側顆　　　　☐ Medial tibial condyle

⑤ ☐ 大腿骨の内側顆　　　☐ Medial femoral condyle

⑥ ☐ 内側上顆　　　　　　☐ Medial epicondyle

A 　膝関節は3つの骨（大腿骨，脛骨，膝蓋骨）からなる．腓骨は膝関節には関与しないが，脛骨との間に脛腓関節と脛腓靱帯結合を形成する．

1 図 25.2B. p.382　2 図 27.2B. p.406

Ligaments of the Knee Joint I

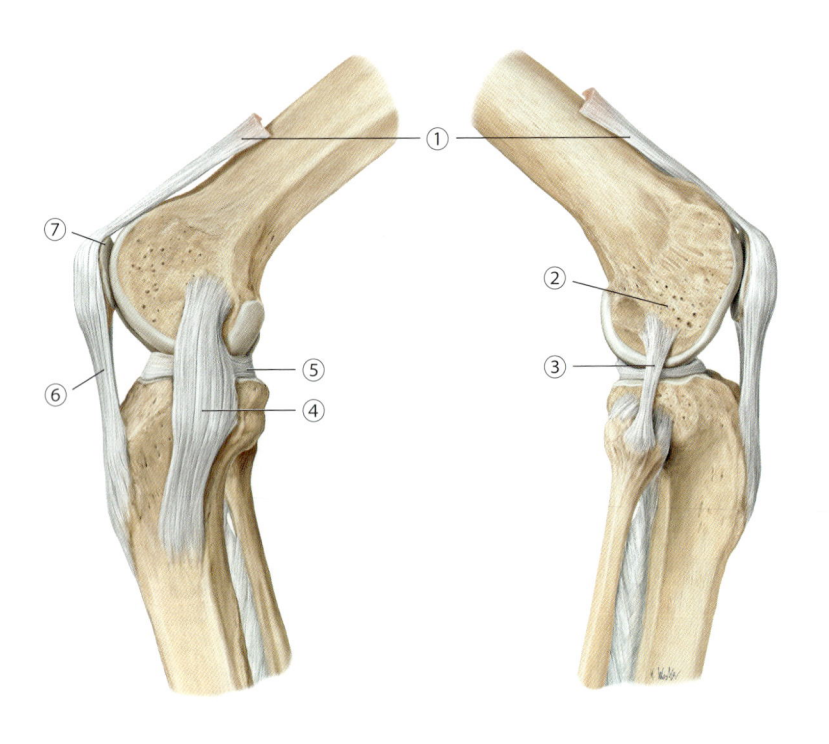

膝関節の靱帯 1

右膝，左：内側面，右：外側面

① □ 大腿四頭筋（腱）　　□ Quadriceps femoris tendon
② □ 外側上顆　　□ Lateral epicondyle
③ □ 外側側副靱帯　　□ Lateral collateral ligament
④ □ 内側側副靱帯　　□ Medial collateral ligament
⑤ □ 内側半月　　□ Medial meniscus
⑥ □ 膝蓋靱帯　　□ Patellar ligament
⑦ □ 膝蓋大腿関節　　□ Femoropatellar joint

解説

膝関節は内側および外側側副靱帯によって補強される．内側側副靱帯は関節包と内側半月に付着するが，外側側副靱帯は関節包と外側半月のどちらとも接触しない．膝関節の伸展位において，側副靱帯は緊張し，冠状断面内で膝関節を安定化する．

Ligaments of the Knee Joint II

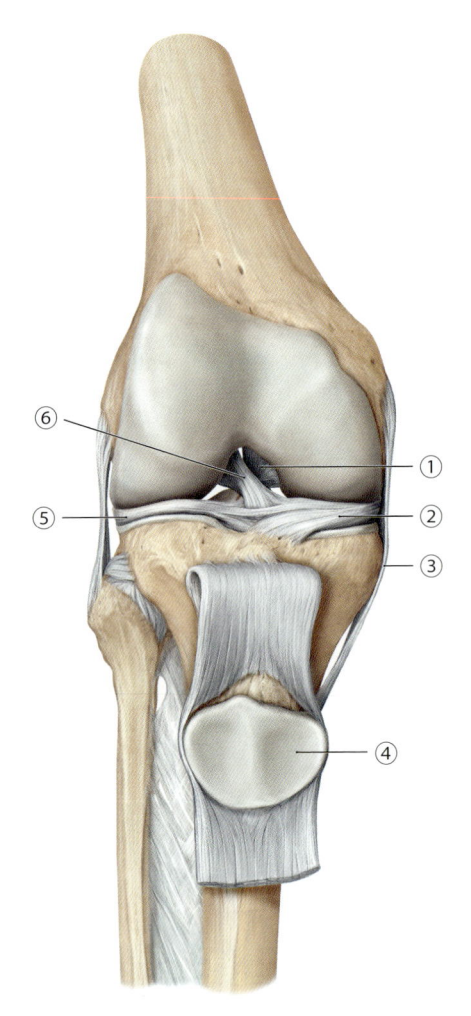

Q 十字靱帯はどのようにして膝関節を安定化するか？

膝関節の靱帯 2

右膝，前面

① □ 後十字靱帯　　□ Posterior cruciate ligament
② □ 内側半月　　　□ Medial meniscus
③ □ 内側側副靱帯　□ Medial collateral ligament
④ □ 膝蓋骨　　　　□ Patella
⑤ □ 外側半月　　　□ Lateral meniscus
⑥ □ 前十字靱帯　　□ Anterior cruciate ligament

A 十字靱帯は，大腿骨が脛骨に対して前方あるいは後方に偏位することを防ぎ，膝関節の安定化をはかっている．すべての肢位において，十字靱帯のどこかが緊張している．

Ligaments of the Knee Joint III

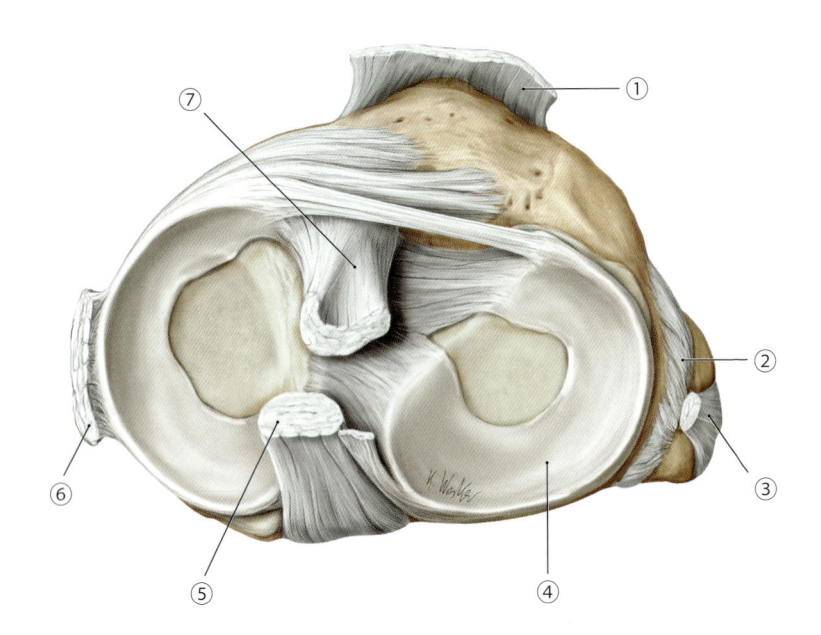

内側半月の外傷性断裂に伴いやすい膝構造の損傷は何か？

膝関節の靭帯 3

右脛骨の上関節面

① □ 膝蓋靭帯　　　　　　□ Patellar ligament
② □ 脛腓関節　　　　　　□ Tibiofibular joint
③ □ 外側側副靭帯　　　　□ Lateral collateral ligament
④ □ 外側半月　　　　　　□ Lateral meniscus
⑤ □ 後十字靭帯　　　　　□ Posterior cruciate ligament
⑥ □ 内側側副靭帯　　　　□ Medial collateral ligament
⑦ □ 前十字靭帯　　　　　□ Anterior cruciate ligament

A 膝関節の外傷時(特に外側からの衝撃を受けた場合)には，内側半月の断裂，内側側副靭帯の断裂，前十字靭帯の断裂の3つがしばしば合併する．

[1] 図 25.8A. p.387　　[2] 図 27.8A. p.411

Muscles of the Anterior Leg

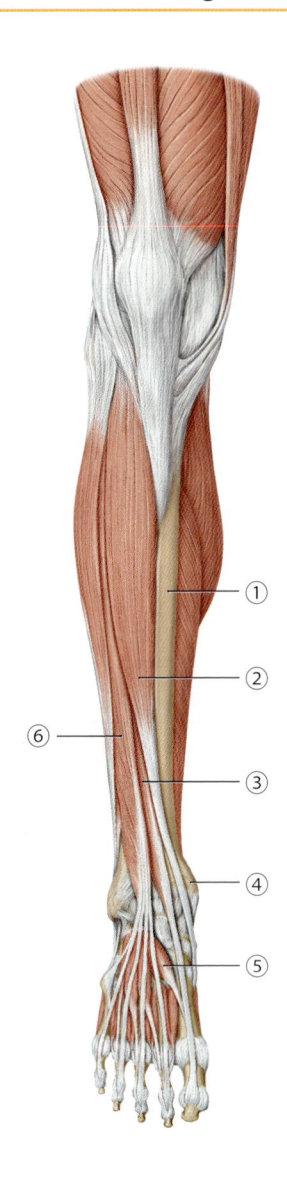

下腿の筋（前面）

右下腿，前面

① □ 脛骨　　　　　　□ Tibia

② □ 前脛骨筋　　　　□ Tibialis anterior

③ □ 長母趾伸筋　　　□ Extensor hallucis longus

④ □ 内果　　　　　　□ Medial malleolus

⑤ □ 短母趾伸筋　　　□ Extensor hallucis brevis

⑥ □ 長趾伸筋　　　　□ Extensor digitorum longus

1 図 25.19A. p.392　2 図 27.19A. p.416

Muscles of the Lateral Leg

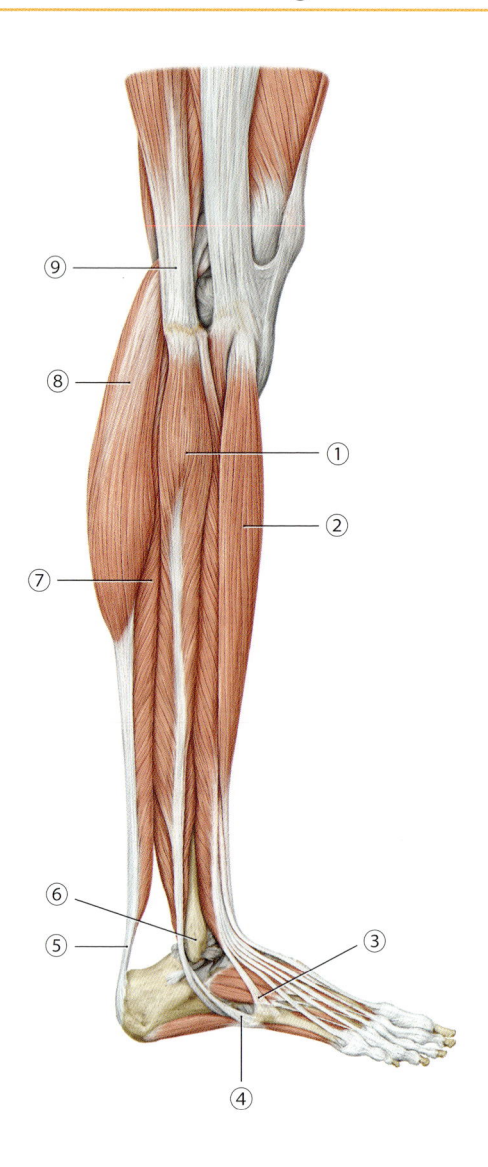

下腿の筋（外側面）

右下腿，外側面

① ☐ 長腓骨筋　　　　　　　　　☐ Fibularis longus
② ☐ 前脛骨筋　　　　　　　　　☐ Tibialis anterior
③ ☐ 第3腓骨筋（欠く場合もある）　☐ Fibularis tertius（variable）
④ ☐ 短腓骨筋　　　　　　　　　☐ Fibularis brevis
⑤ ☐ 踵骨腱（アキレス腱）　　　　☐ Achilles' tendon
⑥ ☐ 外果，腓骨　　　　　　　　☐ Lateral malleolus, fibula
⑦ ☐ ヒラメ筋　　　　　　　　　☐ Soleus
⑧ ☐ 腓腹筋，外側頭　　　　　　☐ Gastrocnemius, lateral head
⑨ ☐ 大腿二頭筋（腱）　　　　　　☐ Biceps femoris tendon

[1] 図 25.20. p.393　[2] 図 27.20. p.417

Muscles of the Posterior Leg I

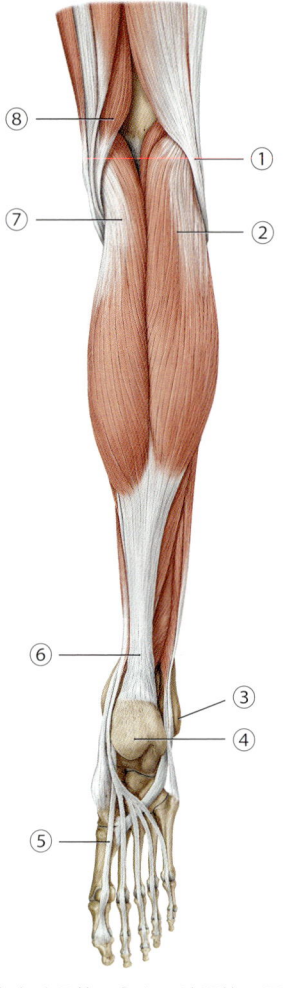

Q 下腿の後区画に存在する筋のうち，膝関節の運動に関与するものはどれか？

下腿の筋（後面）1

右下腿，後面

① □ 大腿二頭筋（腱）　　　□ Biceps femoris tendon
② □ 腓腹筋，外側頭　　　　□ Gastrocnemius, lateral head
③ □ 外果　　　　　　　　　□ Lateral malleolus
④ □ 踵骨　　　　　　　　　□ Calcaneus
⑤ □ 長母趾屈筋（腱）　　　□ Flexor hallucis longus tendon
⑥ □ 踵骨腱（アキレス腱）　□ Achilles' tendon
⑦ □ 腓腹筋，内側頭　　　　□ Gastrocnemius, medial head
⑧ □ 半膜様筋　　　　　　　□ Semimembranosus

A 　腓腹筋は，膝関節を乗り越える筋のうち，膝関節の屈曲作用を有する主要な筋である．足底筋も膝関節を乗り越えるが，小さな筋であるため，関節への影響はほとんど無視できる．

1 図 25.21A. p.394　2 図 27.21A. p.418

Muscles of the Posterior Leg II

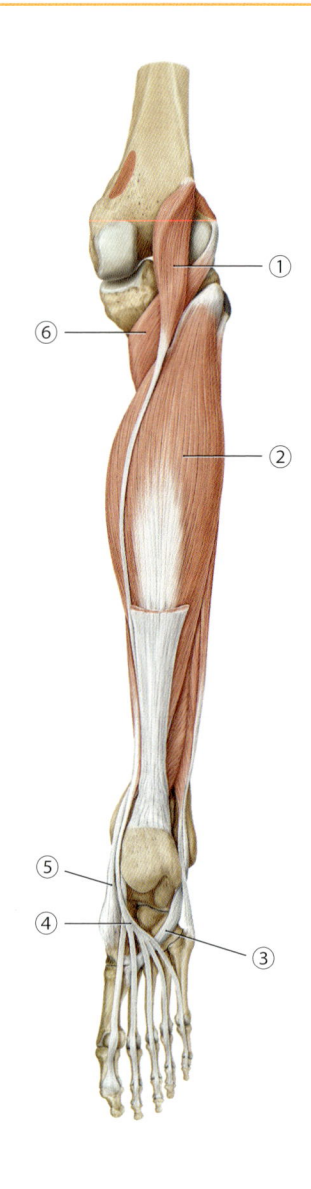

下腿の筋（後面）2

右下腿，後面

① □ 足底筋　　　　　　□ Plantaris

② □ ヒラメ筋　　　　　□ Soleus

③ □ 長腓骨筋（腱）　　□ Fibularis longus tendon

④ □ 長趾屈筋（腱）　　□ Flexor digitorum longus tendon

⑤ □ 後脛骨筋（腱）　　□ Tibialis posterior tendon

⑥ □ 膝窩筋　　　　　　□ Popliteus

Muscles of the Posterior Leg III

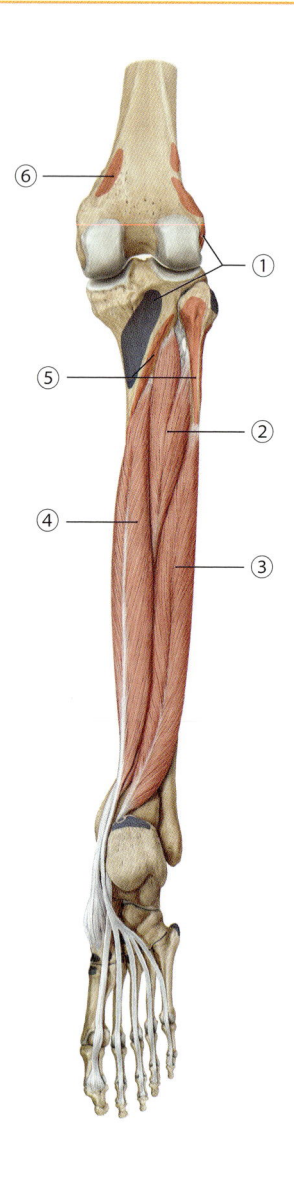

下腿の筋（後面）3

右下腿，後面

① □ 膝窩筋（筋の起始・停止） □ Popliteus（origin and insertion）

② □ 後脛骨筋 □ Tibialis posterior

③ □ 長母趾屈筋 □ Flexor hallucis longus

④ □ 長趾屈筋 □ Flexor digitorum longus

⑤ □ ヒラメ筋（筋の起始） □ Soleus（origin）

⑥ □ 腓腹筋，内側頭（筋の起始） □ Gastrocnemius, medial head（origin）

Bones of the Foot I

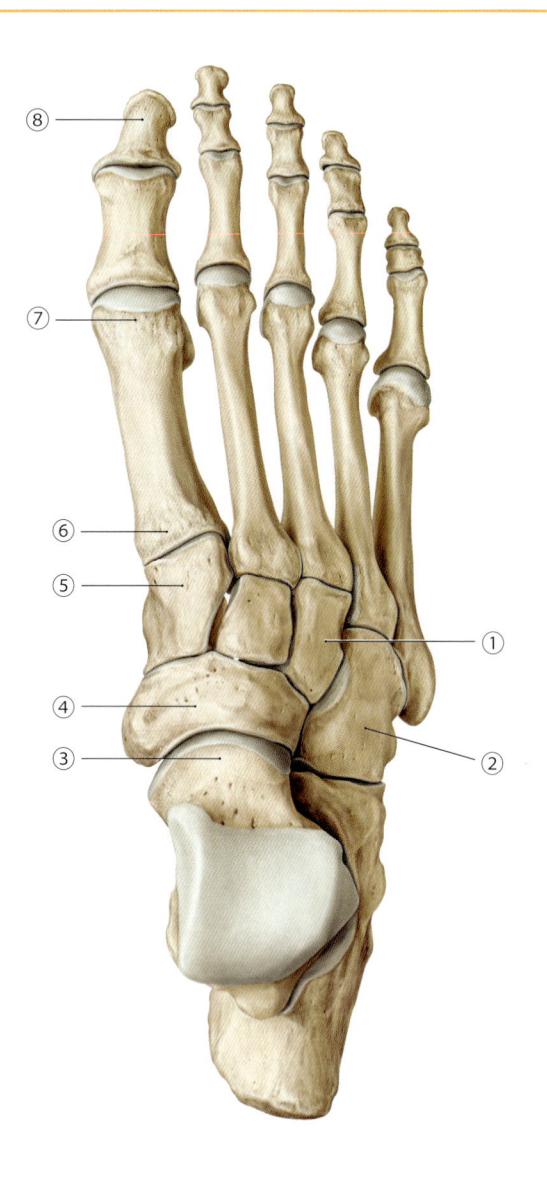

足の骨格 1

右足，背側面（上面）

① ☐ 外側楔状骨　　☐ Lateral cuneiform
② ☐ 立方骨　　☐ Cuboid
③ ☐ 距骨頭　　☐ Head of talus
④ ☐ 舟状骨　　☐ Navicular
⑤ ☐ 内側楔状骨　　☐ Medial cuneiform
⑥ ☐ 第1中足骨底　　☐ Base of 1st metatarsal
⑦ ☐ 第1中足骨頭　　☐ Head of 1st metatarsal
⑧ ☐ 第1末節骨　　☐ 1st distal phalanx

1 図 26.2A. p.400　2 図 28.2A. p.424

Bones of the Foot II

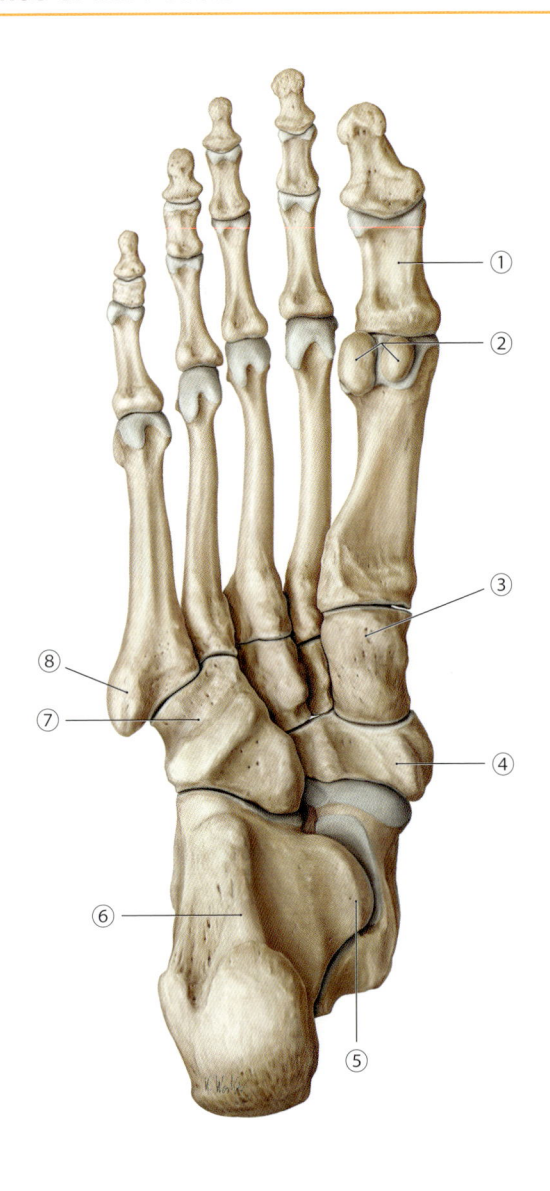

足の骨格 2

右足，足底面（下面）

① □ 第1基節骨　　□ 1st proximal phalanx

② □ 種子骨　　□ Sesamoids

③ □ 内側楔状骨　　□ Medial cuneiform

④ □ 舟状骨　　□ Navicular

⑤ □ 載距突起　　□ Sustentaculum tali

⑥ □ 踵骨　　□ Calcaneus

⑦ □ 長腓骨筋腱溝　　□ Groove for fibularis longus tendon

⑧ □ 第5中足骨粗面　　□ Tuberosity of 5th metatarsal

1 図 26.2C. p.401　2 図 28.2D. p.425

Joints of the Ankle & Foot I

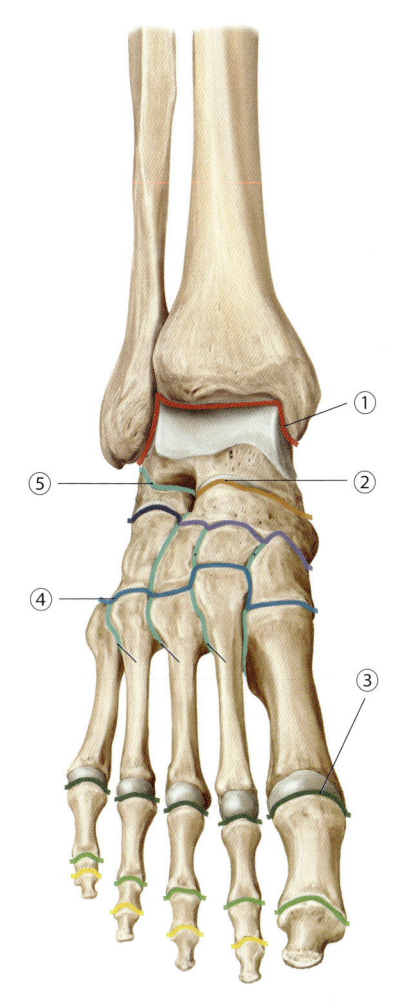

Q 足首が底屈位において損傷を受けやすい理由は何か？

足首と足の関節 1

右足，距腿関節の底屈位，前面

① □ 距腿関節　　　　　　　　□ Talocrural (ankle) joint

② □ 距舟関節　　　　　　　　□ Talonavicular joint

③ □ 中足趾節関節　　　　　　□ Metatarsophalangeal joints

④ □ 足根中足関節　　　　　　□ Tarsometatarsal joints

⑤ □ 距骨下関節　　　　　　　□ Subtalar (talocalcaneal) joint

A 距骨滑車の後部は幅が狭く，底屈位では脛骨と腓骨からなる関節窩の中で距骨滑車の安定性（つまり，距腿関節の安定性）が低下する．このため，距腿関節は，背屈位よりも底屈位において損傷を受けやすい．

[1] 図 26.3A, p.402　[2] 図 28.3A, p.426

Joints of the Ankle & Foot II

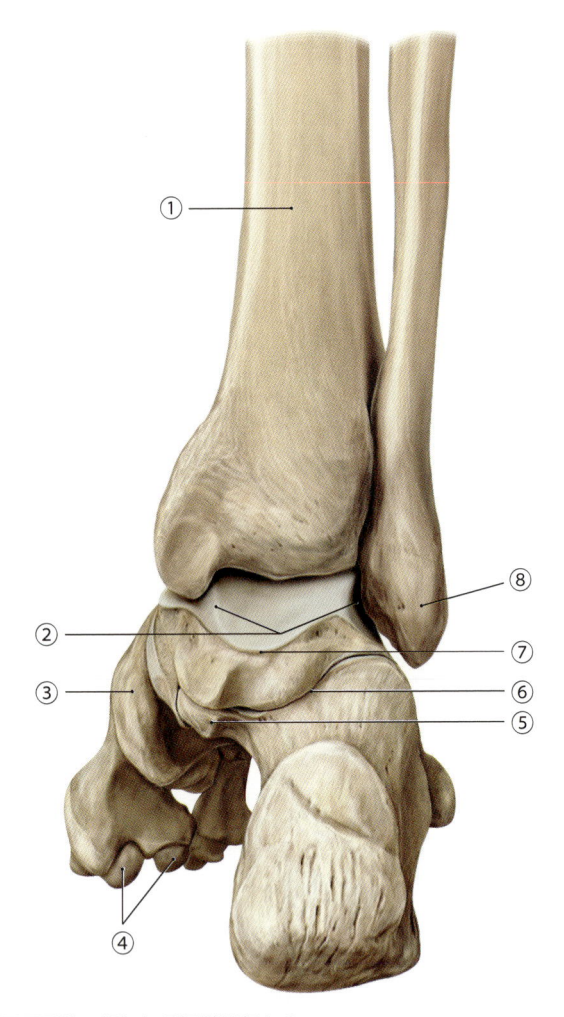

Q 距骨下関節で行われる運動は何か？

足首と足の関節 2

右足，後面

① □ 脛骨　　　　　□ Tibia
② □ 距腿関節　　　□ Talocrural joint
③ □ 舟状骨　　　　□ Navicular
④ □ 種子骨　　　　□ Sesamoids
⑤ □ 載距突起　　　□ Sustentaculum tali
⑥ □ 距骨下関節　　□ Subtaler (talocalcaneal) joint
⑦ □ 距骨　　　　　□ Talus
⑧ □ 外果　　　　　□ Lateral malleolus

A 距骨下関節では，主として足の外反と内反が行われる．

1 図 26.6A. p.404　　2 図 28.6A. p.428

Joints of the Ankle & Foot III

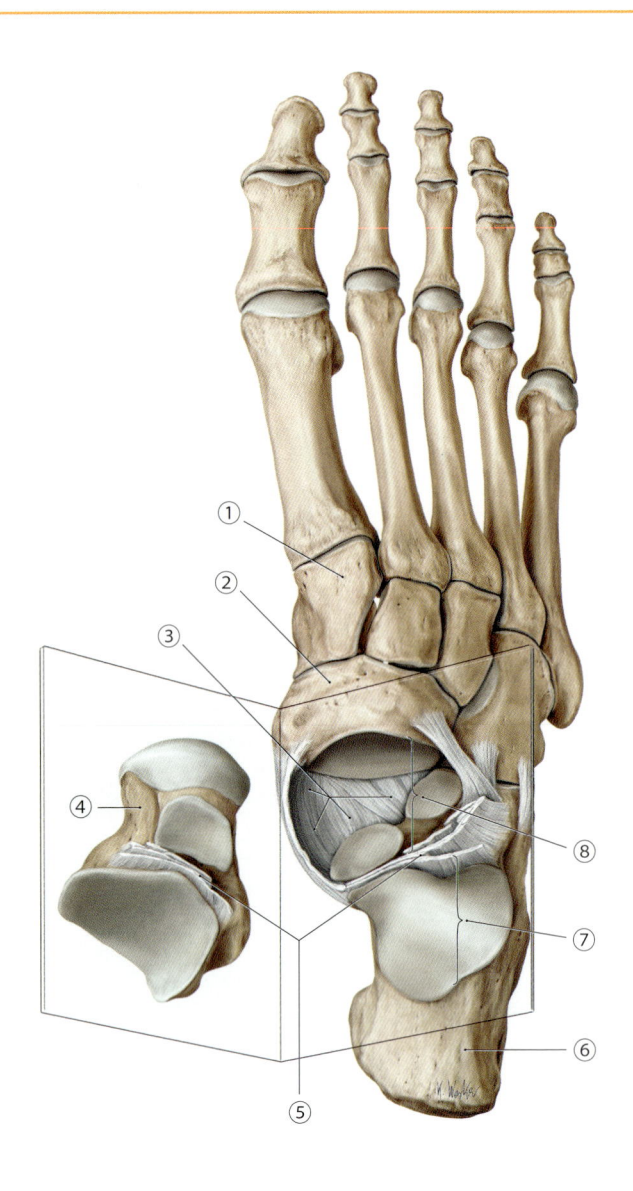

足首と足の関節 3

右足,背側面(上面)

① □ 内側楔状骨　　　　　□ Medial cuneiform
② □ 舟状骨　　　　　　　□ Navicular
③ □ 底側踵舟靱帯　　　　□ Plantar calcaneonavicular ligament
④ □ 距骨　　　　　　　　□ Talus
⑤ □ 骨間距踵靱帯　　　　□ Interosseous talocalcanean ligament
⑥ □ 踵骨　　　　　　　　□ Calcaneus
⑦ □ 距骨下関節,後区　　□ Posterior compartment of subtalar joint
　　（距踵関節）
⑧ □ 距骨下関節,前区　　□ Anterior compartment of subtalar joint
　　（距踵舟関節）

解説

距骨下関節は,骨間距踵靱帯によって分けられた2つの関節(後区の距踵関節と前区の距踵舟関節)からなる.

1 図 26.9A. p.406　2 図 28.9A. p.430

Ligaments of the Ankle & Foot I

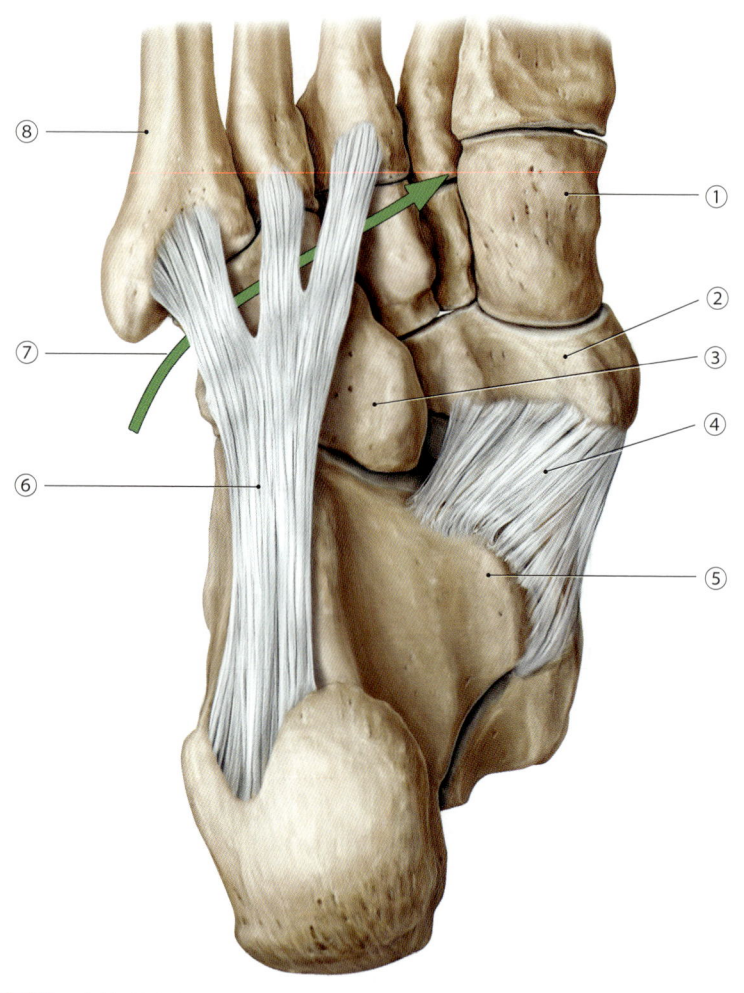

Q 底側踵舟靱帯の機能は何か？

足首と足の靱帯 1

右足，足底面（下面）

① □ 内側楔状骨 □ Medial cuneiform
② □ 舟状骨 □ Navicular
③ □ 立方骨 □ Cuboid
④ □ 底側踵舟靱帯 □ Plantar calcaneonavicular ligament
⑤ □ 載距突起 □ Sustentaculum tali
⑥ □ 長足底靱帯 □ Long plantar ligament
⑦ □ 長腓骨筋（腱）のトンネル □ Tunnel for fibularis longus tendon
⑧ □ 第5中足骨 □ 5th metatarsal

A 底側踵舟靱帯（跳躍靱帯とも呼ばれる）は，距骨頭を下から支えるハンモックのような構造であり，内側縦足弓の最も高い部分を支えている．長足底靱帯は長腓骨筋腱を通すトンネルを形成し，外側縦足弓を支える．

① 図 26.9B, p.406

Ligaments of the Ankle & Foot II

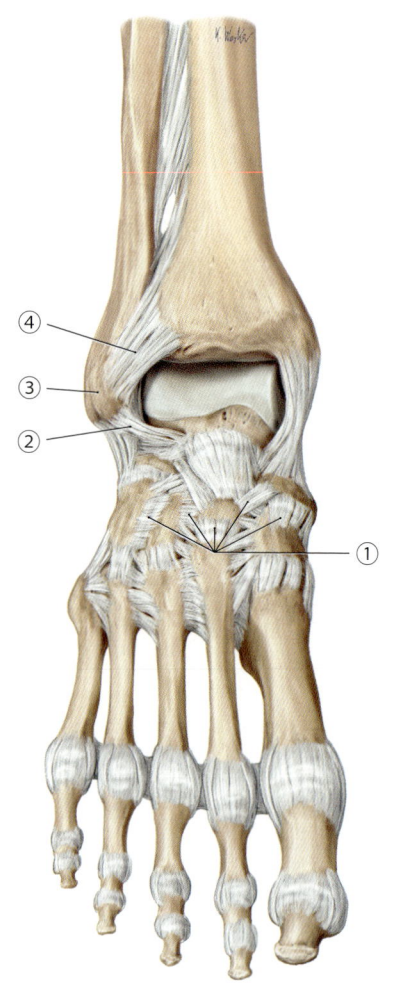

Q 足首の強制的な内反によって引き伸ばされる靱帯はどれか？

足首と足の靱帯 2

右足，前面

① ☐ 背側足根靱帯　　☐ Dorsal tarsal ligaments

② ☐ 前距腓靱帯　　☐ Anterior talofibular ligament

③ ☐ 外果　　☐ Lateral malleolus

④ ☐ 前脛腓靱帯　　☐ Anterior tibiofibular ligament

A 足首の捻挫の大部分は足の強制的な内反によって生じ，外側側副靱帯（特に前距腓靱帯）が損傷を受ける．

1 図 26.11A. p.408　　2 図 28.11A. p.432

Ligaments of the Ankle & Foot III

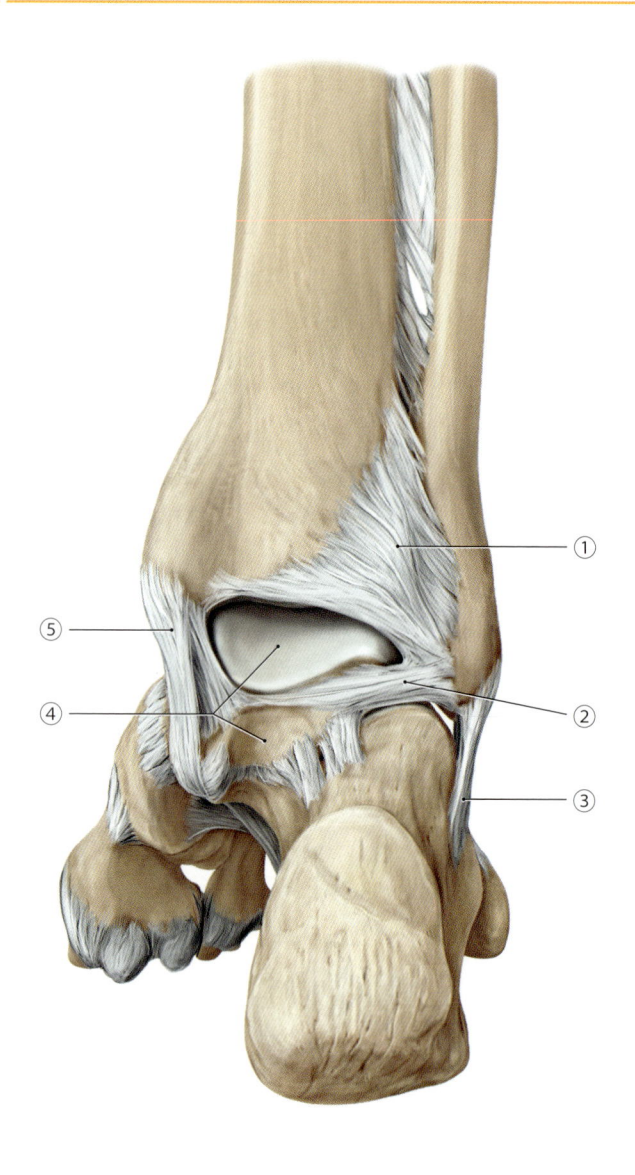

足首と足の靱帯 3

右足，足底を床につけた足位，後面

① □ 後脛腓靱帯　　　　　□ Posterior tibiofibular ligament
② □ 後距腓靱帯　　　　　□ Posterior talofibular ligament
③ □ 踵腓靱帯　　　　　　□ Calcaneofibular ligament
④ □ 距骨　　　　　　　　□ Talus
⑤ □ 三角靱帯　　　　　　□ Deltoid ligament

1 図 26.11C. p.409　2 図 28.11C. p.433

Muscles of the Sole of the Foot I

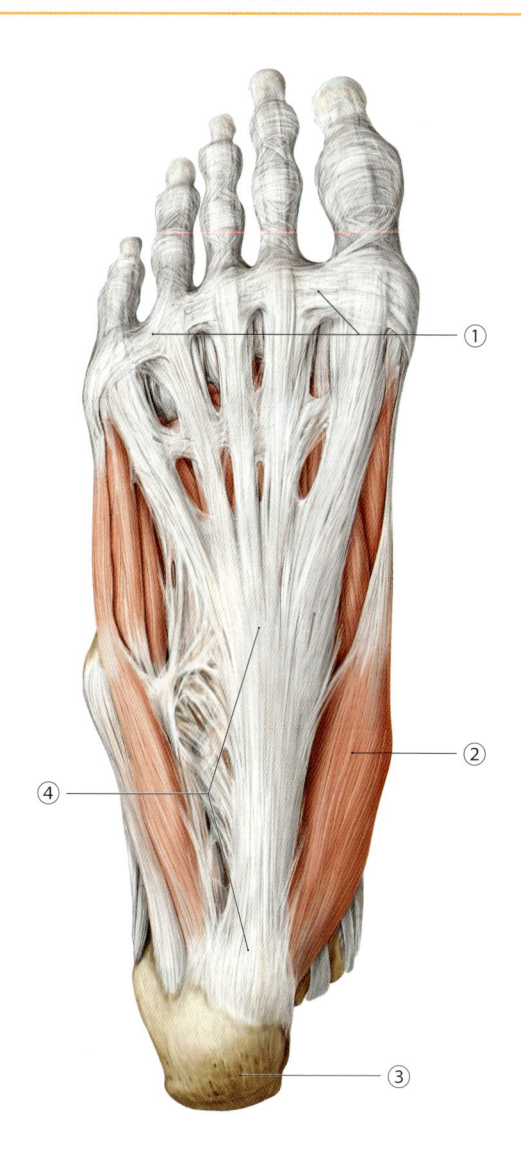

足底の筋 1

右足，足底面（下面）

① □ 浅横中足靱帯　　□ Superficial transverse metacarpal ligament

② □ 母趾外転筋　　□ Abductor hallucis
③ □ 踵骨隆起　　□ Calcaneal tuberosity
④ □ 足底腱膜　　□ Plantar aponeurosis

解説

足底腱膜は頑丈な腱膜であり，中央部が肥厚している．足の縁で足底腱膜は足背筋膜に移行する．

1 図 26.15. p.412　2 図 28.15. p.436

Muscles of the Sole of the Foot II

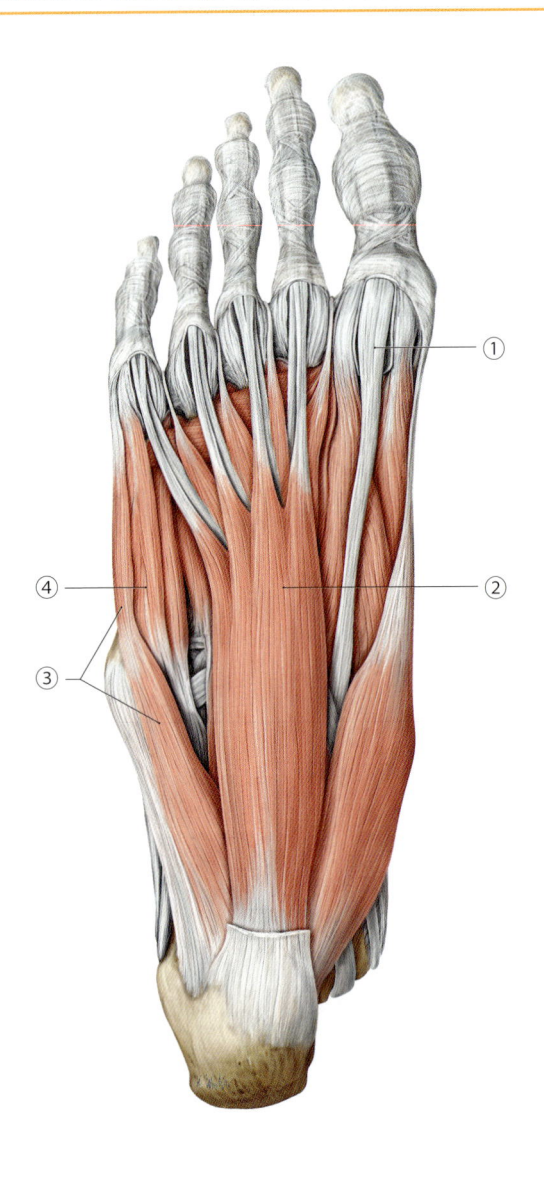

足底の筋 2

右足，足底面（下面）

① □ 長母趾屈筋（腱）　　□ Flexor hallucis longus tendon

② □ 短趾屈筋　　□ Flexor digitorum brevis

③ □ 小趾外転筋　　□ Abductor digiti minimi

④ □ 短小趾屈筋　　□ Flexor digiti minimi brevis

Muscles of the Sole of the Foot III

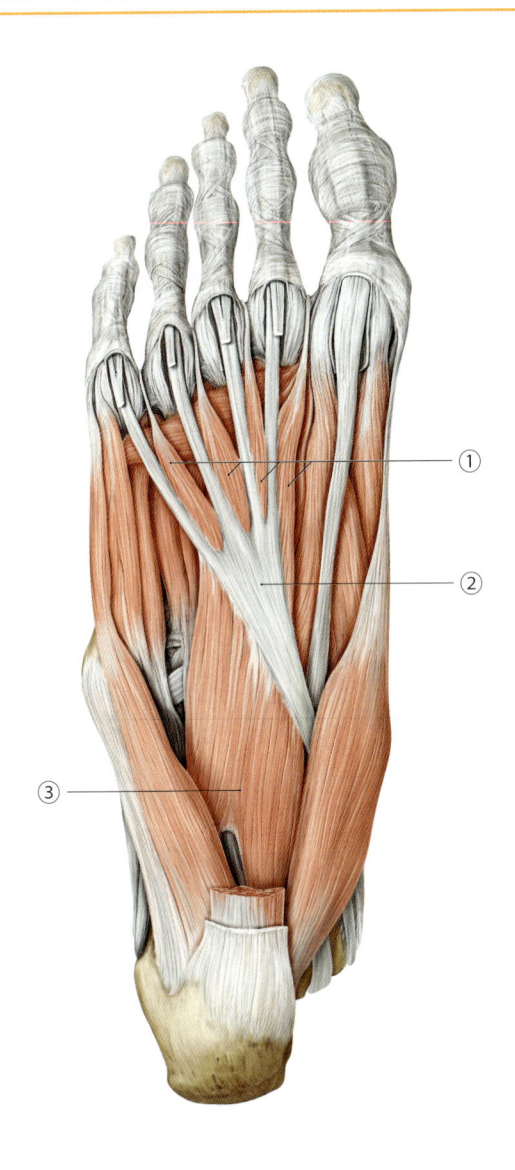

足底の筋 3

右足，足底面（下面）

① ☐ 虫様筋 ☐ Lumbricals
② ☐ 長趾屈筋（腱） ☐ Flexor digitorum longus tendon
③ ☐ 足底方形筋 ☐ Quadratus plantae

Muscles of the Sole of the Foot IV

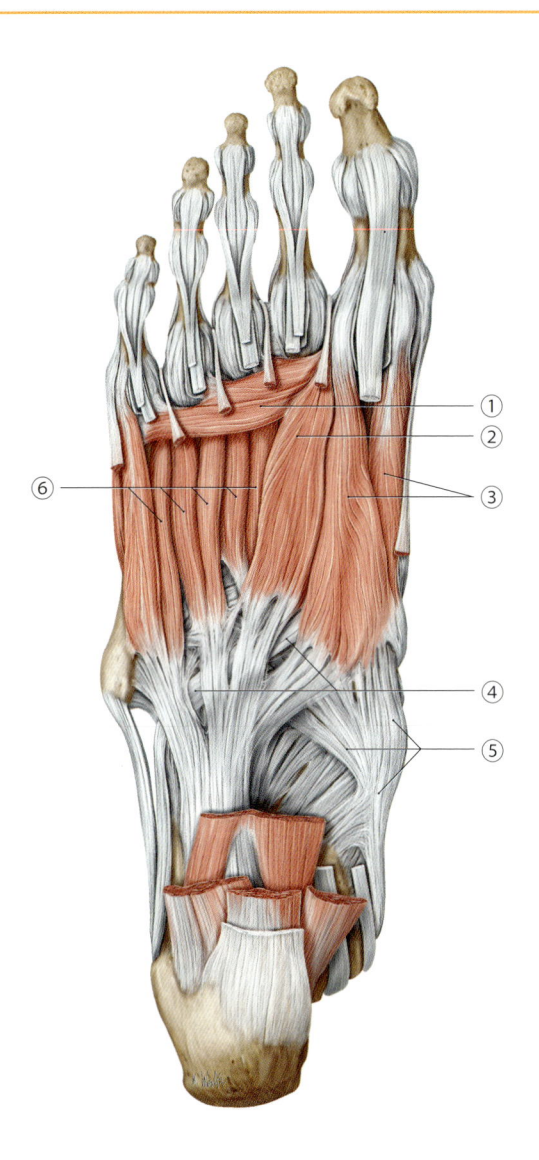

足底の筋 4

右足，足底面（下面）

① □ 母趾内転筋，横頭　　□ Transverse head of adductor hallucis

② □ 母趾内転筋，斜頭　　□ Oblique head of adductor hallucis

③ □ 短母趾屈筋，内側頭と外側頭　　□ Flexor hallucis brevis, medial and lateral heads

④ □ 長腓骨筋（腱）　　□ Fibularis longus tendon

⑤ □ 後脛骨筋（腱）　　□ Tibialis posterior tendon

⑥ □ 底側・背側骨間筋　　□ Plantar and dorsal interossei

1 図 26.16C. p.413　2 図 28.16C. p.437

Anterior Foot & Ankle

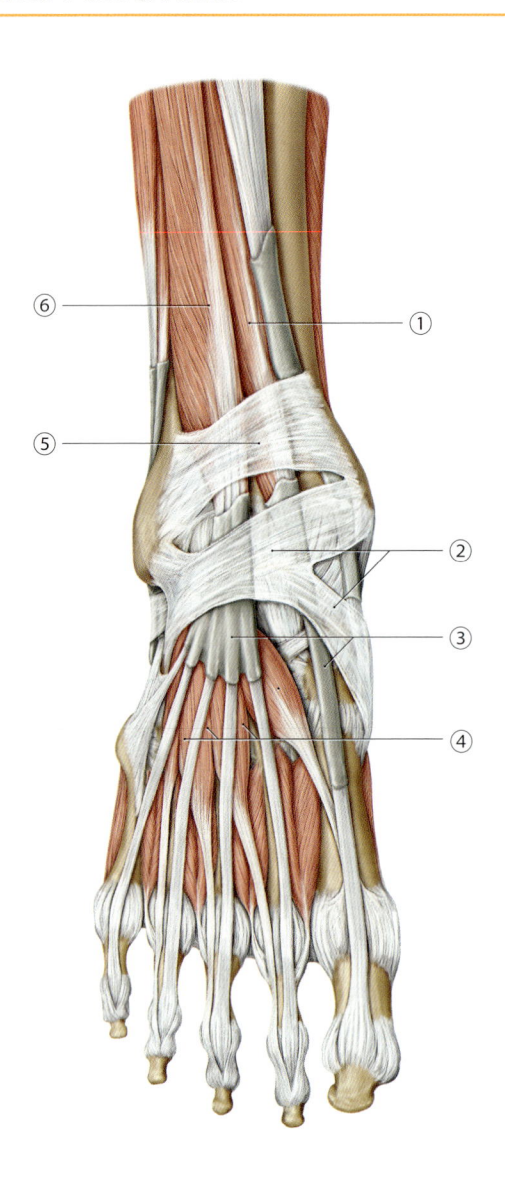

足首と足

右足，前面

① □ 長母趾伸筋　　　　　□ Extensor hallucis longus
② □ 下伸筋支帯　　　　　□ Inferior extensor retinaculum
③ □ 腱鞘　　　　　　　　□ Tendon sheath
④ □ 短趾伸筋　　　　　　□ Extensor digitorum brevis
⑤ □ 上伸筋支帯　　　　　□ Superior extensor retinaculum
⑥ □ 長趾伸筋　　　　　　□ Extensor digitorum longus

解説

支帯は腱を一定の場所に留めておく働きを持つ．伸筋支帯は長い伸筋腱を，腓骨筋支帯は腓骨筋腱を，屈筋支帯は長い屈筋腱をそれぞれ保持する．

1 図 26.18A．p.415　　2 図 28.18A．p.439

Arteries of the Lower Limb I

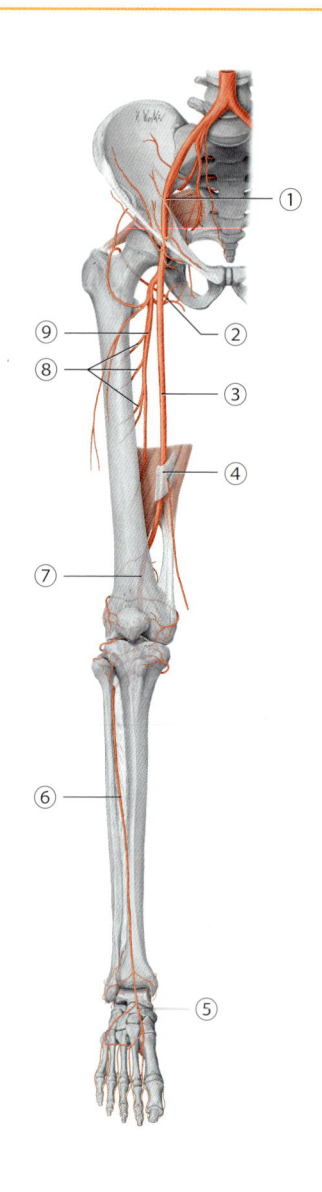

下肢の動脈 1

右下肢，前面

① ☐ 外腸骨動脈　　　　　　　　☐ External iliac artery
② ☐ 内側大腿回旋動脈　　　　　☐ Medial circumflex femoral artery
③ ☐ 大腿動脈　　　　　　　　　☐ Femoral artery
④ ☐ 内転筋管と大内転筋　　　　☐ Adductor canal (with adductor magnus)
⑤ ☐ 足背動脈　　　　　　　　　☐ Dorsal pedal artery
⑥ ☐ 前脛骨動脈　　　　　　　　☐ Anterior tibial artery
⑦ ☐ 膝窩動脈　　　　　　　　　☐ Popliteal artery
⑧ ☐ 第1-3貫通動脈　　　　　　☐ 1st through 3rd perforating arteries
⑨ ☐ 大腿深動脈　　　　　　　　☐ Profunda femoris artery

解説

下肢へ血液を供給する最も主要な動脈は外腸骨動脈であり，鼠径靭帯の遠位で大腿動脈となる．大腿動脈は腱裂孔を通過して膝の後方(膝窩)に入り，膝窩動脈となる．膝窩動脈は下腿に達すると，3本の主要な動脈(前脛骨動脈，後脛骨動脈，腓骨動脈)に分かれる．これらの3本の動脈は足首と足でいくつかの吻合路を形成する．

[1] 図 27.1C, p.420　[2] 図 29.1A, p.444

Arteries of the Lower Limb II

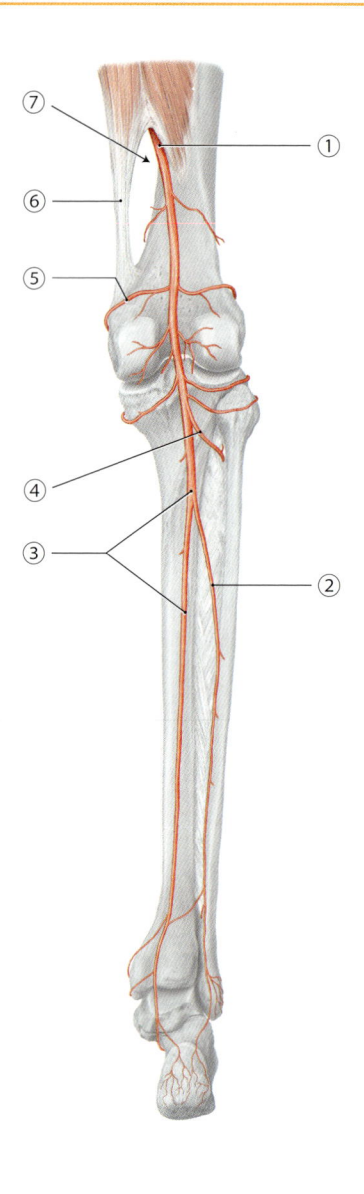

下肢の動脈 2

右下肢，後面

① □ 膝窩動脈　　　　　　□ Popliteal artery
② □ 腓骨動脈　　　　　　□ Fibular artery
③ □ 後脛骨動脈　　　　　□ Posterior tibial artery
④ □ 前脛骨動脈　　　　　□ Anterior tibial artery
⑤ □ 内側上膝動脈　　　　□ Medial superior genicular artery
⑥ □ 大内転筋（腱）　　　□ Adductor magnus tendon
⑦ □ ［内転筋］腱裂孔　　□ Adductor hiatus

Lumbosacral Plexus I

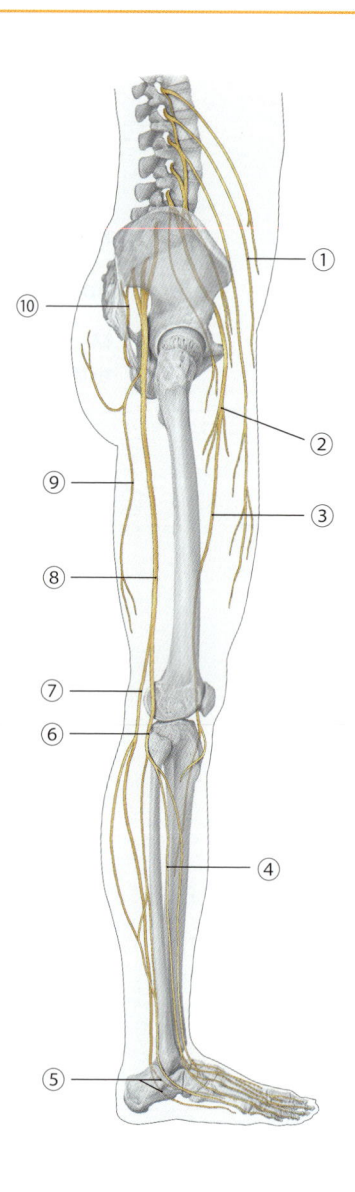

腰仙骨神経叢 1

右側，外側面

① □ 腸骨鼡径神経　　　　　　□ Ilioinguinal nerve
② □ 大腿神経　　　　　　　　□ Femoral nerve
③ □ 伏在神経　　　　　　　　□ Saphenous nerve
④ □ 浅腓骨神経　　　　　　　□ Superficial fibular nerve
⑤ □ 内側・外側足底神経　　　□ Medial and lateral plantar nerves
⑥ □ 総腓骨神経　　　　　　　□ Common fibular nerve
⑦ □ 脛骨神経　　　　　　　　□ Tibial nerve
⑧ □ 坐骨神経　　　　　　　　□ Sciatic nerve
⑨ □ 後大腿皮神経　　　　　　□ Posterior femoral cutaneous nerve
⑩ □ 陰部神経　　　　　　　　□ Pudendal nerve

解説

下肢の筋の多くは仙骨神経叢に由来する神経（坐骨神経など）に支配される．ただし，下肢の前面と内側面の筋は腰神経叢に由来する神経（大腿神経と閉鎖神経）に支配される．

[1] 表27.1, p.424　[2] 表29.1, p.448

Lumbosacral Plexus II

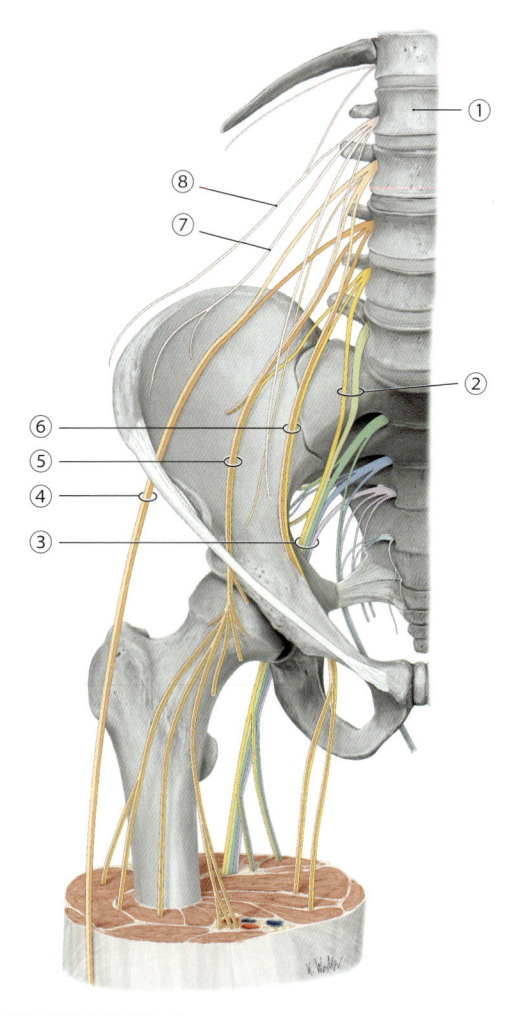

Q 腰仙骨神経幹とは何か？

腰仙骨神経叢 2

右側，前面

① □ 第 1 腰椎　　　　　　　□ L1 vertebra
② □ 腰仙骨神経幹　　　　　□ Lumbosacral trunk
③ □ 坐骨神経　　　　　　　□ Sciatic nerve
④ □ 外側大腿皮神経　　　　□ Lateral femoral cutaneous nerve
⑤ □ 大腿神経　　　　　　　□ Femoral nerve
⑥ □ 閉鎖神経　　　　　　　□ Obturator nerve
⑦ □ 腸骨鼠径神経　　　　　□ Ilioinguinal nerve
⑧ □ 腸骨下腹神経　　　　　□ Iliohypogastric nerve

A 　腰仙骨神経幹は第 4・5 腰神経の前枝からなり，骨盤腔を下行して仙骨神経叢に加わる．

[1] 図 27.11B．p.425　[2] 図 29.11B．p.449

Nerves of the Lumbar Plexus I

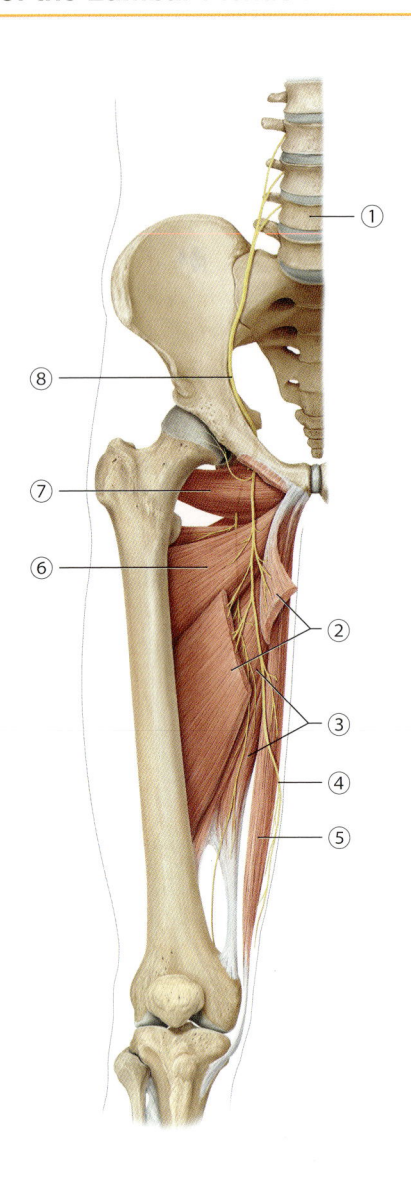

腰神経叢からの神経 1

右側，前面

① □ 第4腰椎　　　　　□ L4 vertebra
② □ 長内転筋　　　　　□ Adductor longus
③ □ 大内転筋　　　　　□ Adductor magnus
④ □ 皮枝　　　　　　　□ Cutaneous branch
⑤ □ 薄筋　　　　　　　□ Gracilis
⑥ □ 短内転筋　　　　　□ Adductor brevis
⑦ □ 外閉鎖筋　　　　　□ Obturator externus
⑧ □ 閉鎖神経　　　　　□ Obturator nerve

1 図 27.15. p.428　2 図 29.15. p.452

Nerves of the Lumbar Plexus II

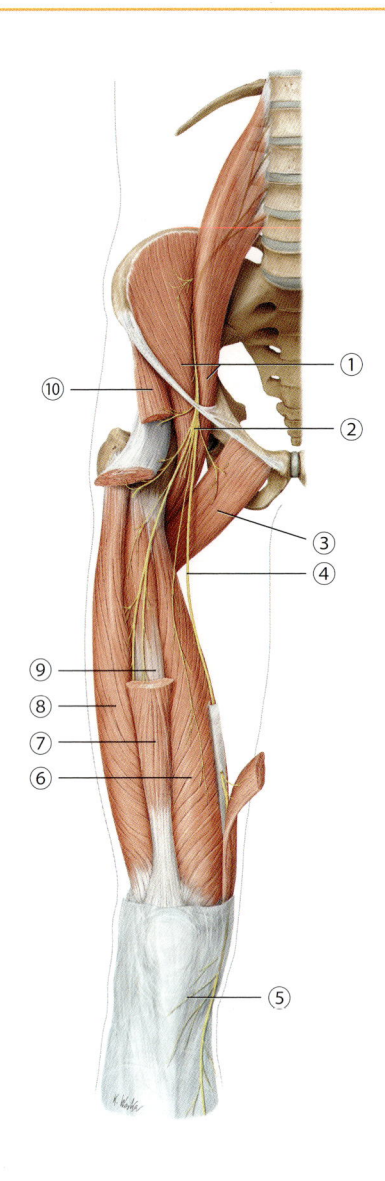

腰神経叢からの神経 2

右側,前面

① ☐ 腸腰筋 ☐ Iliopsoas
② ☐ 大腿神経 ☐ Femoral nerve
③ ☐ 恥骨筋 ☐ Pectineus
④ ☐ 伏在神経 ☐ Saphenous nerve
⑤ ☐ 膝蓋下枝 ☐ Infrapatellar branch
⑥ ☐ 内側広筋 ☐ Vastus medialis
⑦ ☐ 大腿直筋 ☐ Rectus femoris
⑧ ☐ 外側広筋 ☐ Vastus lateralis
⑨ ☐ 中間広筋 ☐ Vastus intermedius
⑩ ☐ 縫工筋 ☐ Sartorius

臨床

大腿四頭筋は膝関節を伸展させる唯一の筋であるため,その支配神経である大腿神経が損傷を受けると膝関節の伸展が行えなくなる.

1 図 27.16. p.429 2 図 29.16. p.453

Nerves of the Sacral Plexus I

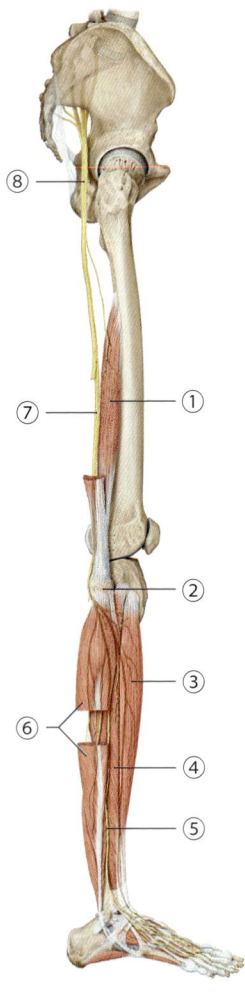

深腓骨神経が損傷を受けると，どのような障害が現れるか？

仙骨神経叢からの神経 1

右下肢，外側面

① ☐ 大腿二頭筋，短頭 　　☐ Biceps femoris, short head
② ☐ 腓骨頭 　　☐ Head of fibula
③ ☐ 前脛骨筋 　　☐ Tibialis anterior
④ ☐ 長趾伸筋 　　☐ Extensor digitorum longus
⑤ ☐ 浅腓骨神経 　　☐ Superficial fibular nerve
⑥ ☐ 長腓骨筋 　　☐ Fibularis longus
⑦ ☐ 総腓骨神経 　　☐ Common fibular nerve
⑧ ☐ 坐骨神経 　　☐ Sciatic nerve

A 　深腓骨神経の損傷では，足首の背屈が行えなくなるとともに，第1趾間の感覚が損なわれる．

1 図 27.23. p.432　　2 図 29.23. p.456

Nerves of the Sacral Plexus II

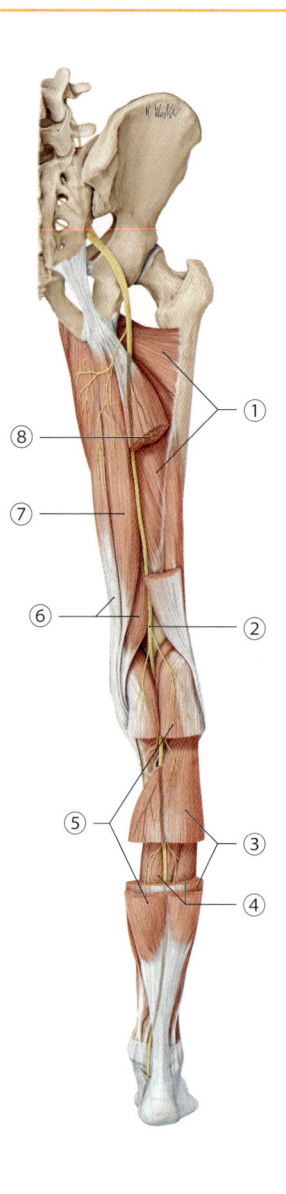

仙骨神経叢からの神経 2

右下肢，後面

① □ 大内転筋，内転筋部　　□ Adductor magnus, adductor part
② □ 脛骨神経　　□ Tibial nerve
③ □ ヒラメ筋　　□ Soleus
④ □ 深層の屈筋群　　□ Deep flexors
⑤ □ 腓腹筋　　□ Gastrocnemius
⑥ □ 半膜様筋　　□ Semimembranosus
⑦ □ 半腱様筋　　□ Semitendinosus
⑧ □ 大腿二頭筋，長頭　　□ Biceps femoris, long head

解説

脛骨神経は坐骨神経の枝であり，大腿後面の筋（大腿二頭筋の短頭を除く），下腿後面の筋，足底の筋を支配する．

Superficial Veins & Nerves

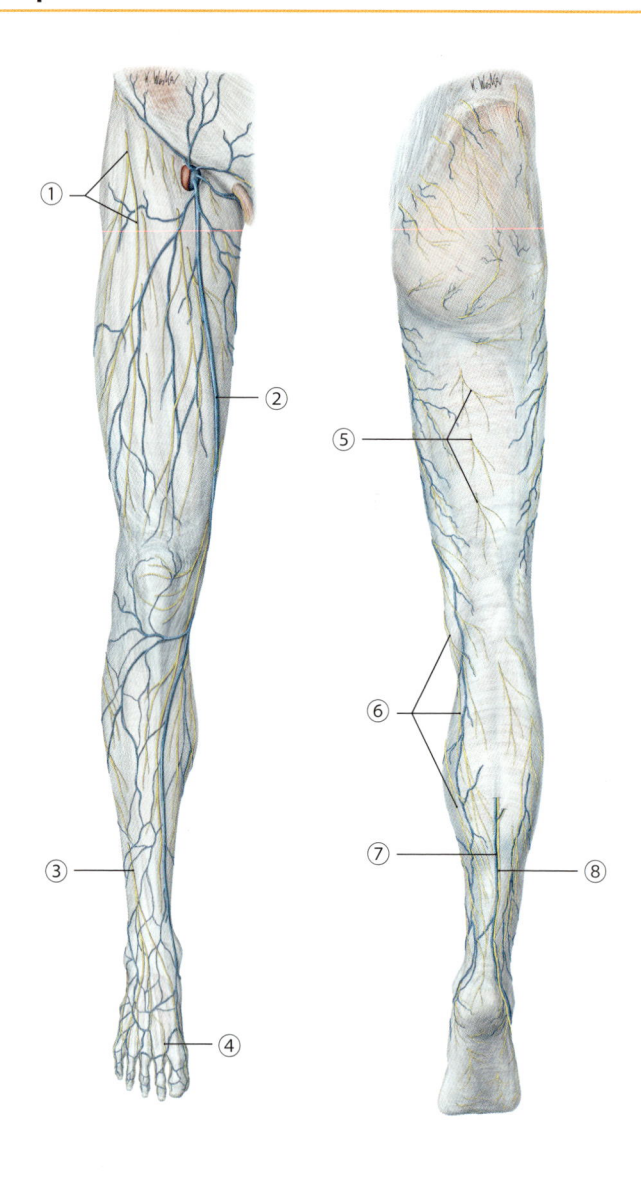

皮静脈と皮神経

右下肢．左：前面，右：後面

① □ 外側大腿皮神経 □ Lateral femoral cutaneous nerve

② □ 大伏在静脈 □ Long saphenous vein

③ □ 浅腓骨神経 □ Superficial fibular nerve

④ □ 深腓骨神経 □ Deep fibular nerve

⑤ □ 後大腿皮神経 □ Posterior femoral cutaneous nerve

⑥ □ 伏在神経（大腿神経の枝） □ Saphenous nerve（femoral nerve）

⑦ □ 小伏在静脈 □ Short saphenous vein

⑧ □ 腓腹神経 □ Sural nerve

解説

皮静脈は深静脈（動脈に伴行する静脈）に流れ込む．皮静脈の流入部は様々な位置に見られるが，特に重要なのが大伏在静脈と小伏在静脈であり，それぞれ大腿静脈と膝窩静脈に流入する．

① 図 27.27A, B. p.434-435　② 図 29.26A, B. p.458

Inguinal Region

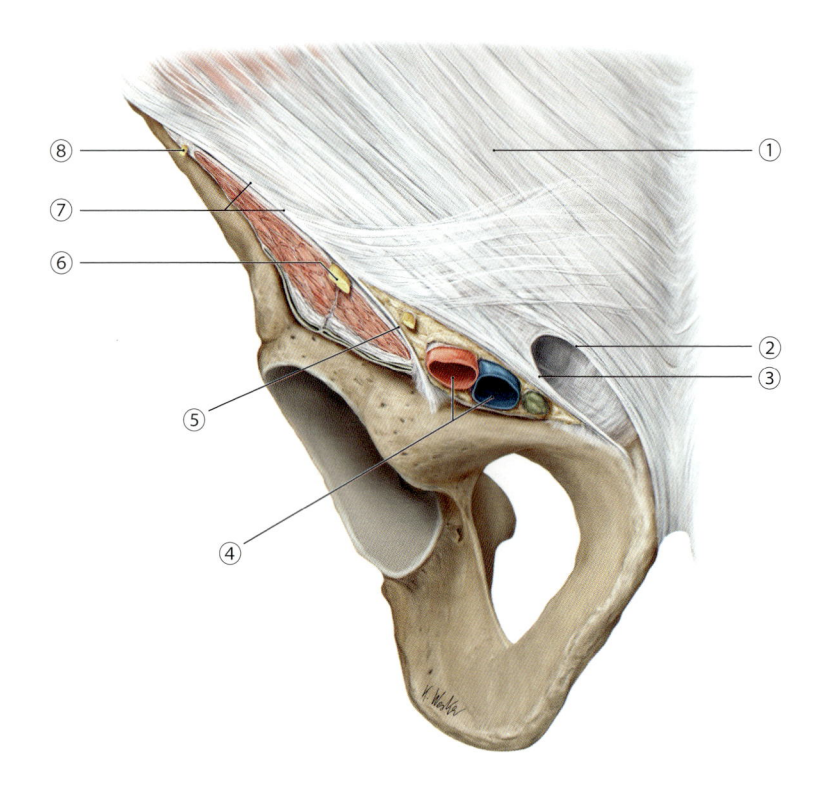

鼡径部

右側，前面

① □ 外腹斜筋腱膜　　　　　　　□ External oblique aponeurosis
② □ 浅鼡径輪，内側脚　　　　　□ Medial crus of external inguinal ring
③ □ 浅鼡径輪，外側脚　　　　　□ Lateral crus of external inguinal ring
④ □ 大腿動脈・静脈　　　　　　□ Femoral artery and vein
⑤ □ 腸恥筋膜弓　　　　　　　　□ Iliopectineal arch
⑥ □ 大腿神経　　　　　　　　　□ Femoral nerve
⑦ □ 鼡径靱帯　　　　　　　　　□ Inguinal ligament
⑧ □ 外側大腿皮神経　　　　　　□ Lateral femoral cutaneous nerve

解説

　鼡径靱帯と鼡径管の後方には，大腿に向かう筋，神経，血管の通路が存在する．筋（腸腰筋）と神経（大腿神経）は筋裂孔を，脈管（大腿動脈・静脈，リンパ管）は血管裂孔を通過する．2つの裂孔は腸恥筋膜弓によって隔てられる．

1 図 27.31, p.437　2 図 29.31, p.461

Sciatic Foramina

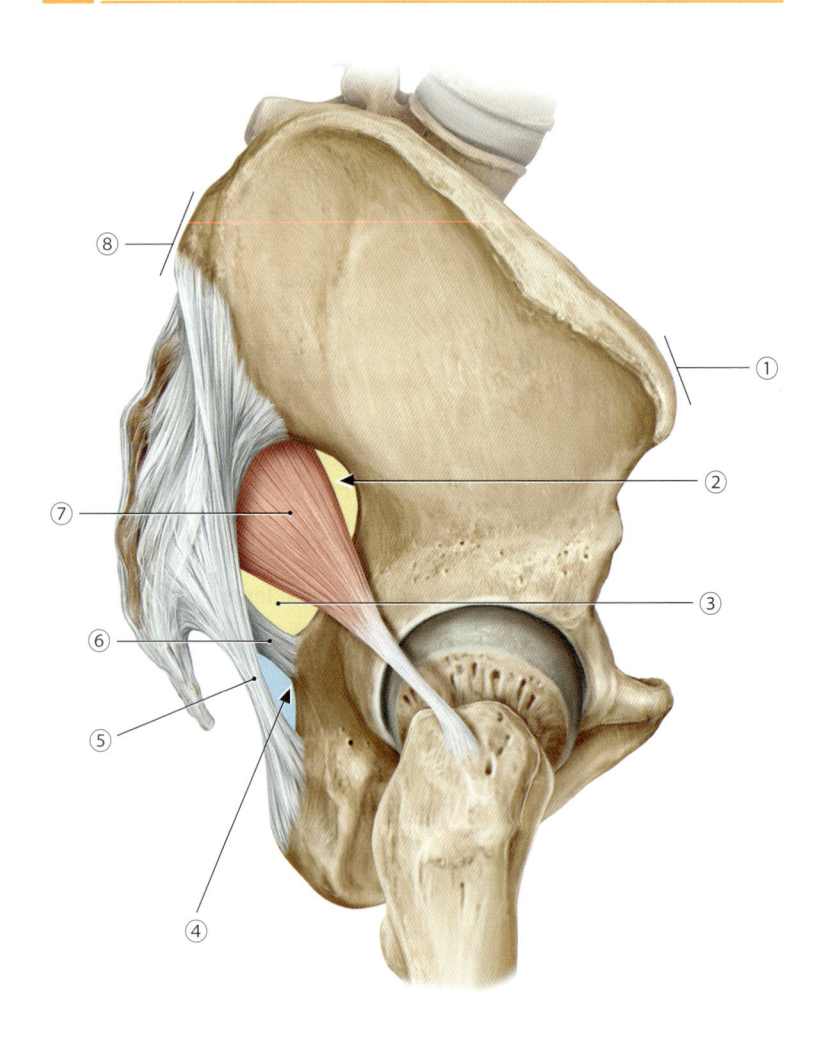

小坐骨孔を通過するものは何か？

坐骨孔

右側,外側面

① ☐ 上前腸骨棘 ☐ Anterior superior iliac spine
② ☐ 大坐骨孔,梨状筋上孔 ☐ Suprapiriform portion of greater sciatic foramen
③ ☐ 大坐骨孔,梨状筋下孔 ☐ Infrapiriform portion of greater sciatic foramen
④ ☐ 小坐骨孔 ☐ Lesser sciatic foramen
⑤ ☐ 仙結節靱帯 ☐ Sacrotuberous ligament
⑥ ☐ 仙棘靱帯 ☐ Sacrospinous ligament
⑦ ☐ 梨状筋 ☐ Piriformis
⑧ ☐ 上後腸骨棘 ☐ Posterior superior iliac spine

A 陰部神経と内陰部動脈・静脈が小坐骨孔を通り,会陰に達する.

Neurovasculature of the Anterior Thigh

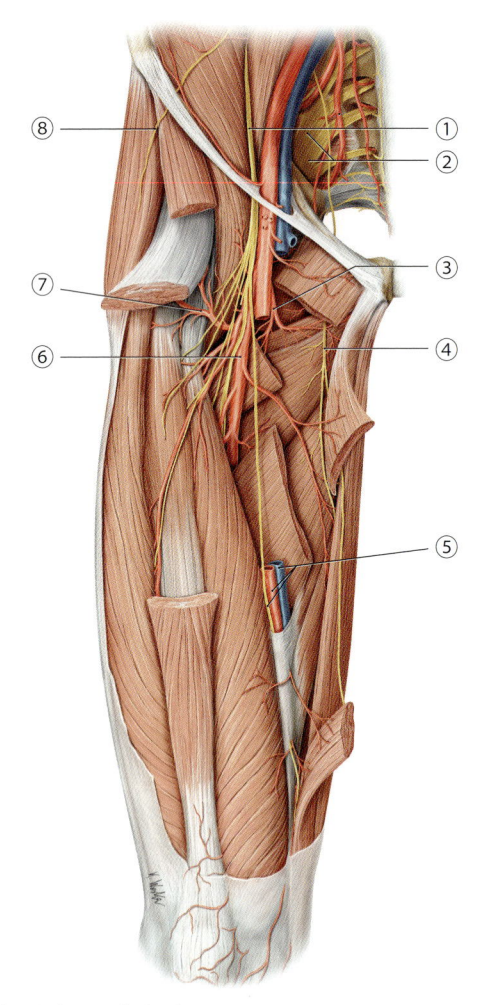

股関節に分布する動脈は何か？

大腿前面の神経・血管

右大腿，前面

① ☐ 大腿神経 　　　　　　　　　　☐ Femoral nerve

② ☐ 仙骨神経叢 　　　　　　　　　☐ Sacral plexus

③ ☐ 内側大腿回旋動脈 　　　　　　☐ Medial circumflex femoral artery

④ ☐ 閉鎖神経 　　　　　　　　　　☐ Obturator nerve

⑤ ☐ 大腿動脈・静脈，伏在神経（広筋内転筋膜の内側にある） ☐ Femoral artery and vein, saphenous nerve (in vastoadductor membrane)

⑥ ☐ 大腿深動脈 　　　　　　　　　☐ Profunda femoris artery

⑦ ☐ 外側大腿回旋動脈，上行枝 　　☐ Lateral circumflex femoral artery, ascending branch

⑧ ☐ 外側大腿皮神経 　　　　　　　☐ Lateral femoral cutaneous nerve

A 　股関節には内側・外側大腿回旋動脈が分布する．さらに，多くの場合，大腿深動脈も分布する．

1 図 27.34B. p.440　　2 図 29.34B. p.464

Neurovasculature of the Posterior Thigh

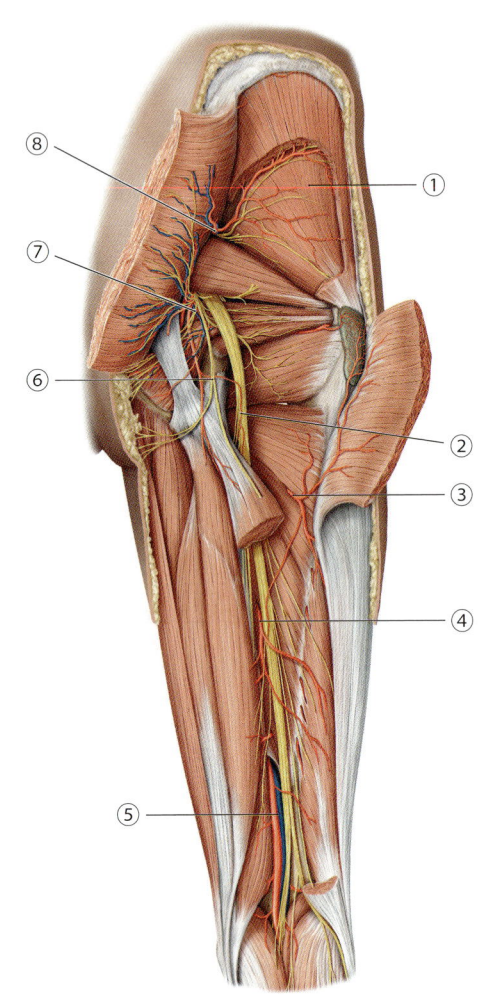

どの神経の損傷によってトレンデレンブルグ試験が陽性となるか？

大腿後面の神経・血管

右大腿，後面

① □ 小殿筋　　　　　　　　□ Gluteus minimus

② □ 坐骨神経，　　　　　　□ Sciatic nerve (with artery)
　　　坐骨神経伴行動脈

③ □ 第1貫通動脈　　　　　□ 1st perforating artery

④ □ 第2貫通動脈　　　　　□ 2nd perforating artery

⑤ □ 膝窩動脈・静脈　　　　□ Popliteal artery and vein

⑥ □ 後大腿皮神経　　　　　□ Posterior femoral cutaneous nerve

⑦ □ 陰部神経　　　　　　　□ Pudendal nerve

⑧ □ 上殿動脈・静脈・神経　□ Superior gluteal artery, vein, and nerve

A 　トレンデレンブルグ試験とは，片足立ちにより，中殿筋と小殿筋（いずれも上殿神経に支配される）の筋力を検査する方法である．上殿神経が損傷され，中殿筋と小殿筋に筋力低下（麻痺）が生じた場合，障害側で片足立ちをすると，骨盤が正常側（遊脚側）へ傾く．この状態をトレンデレンブルグ試験陽性という．

[1] 図 27.35B. p.441　[2] 図 29.35B. p.465

Neurovasculature of the Posterior Leg

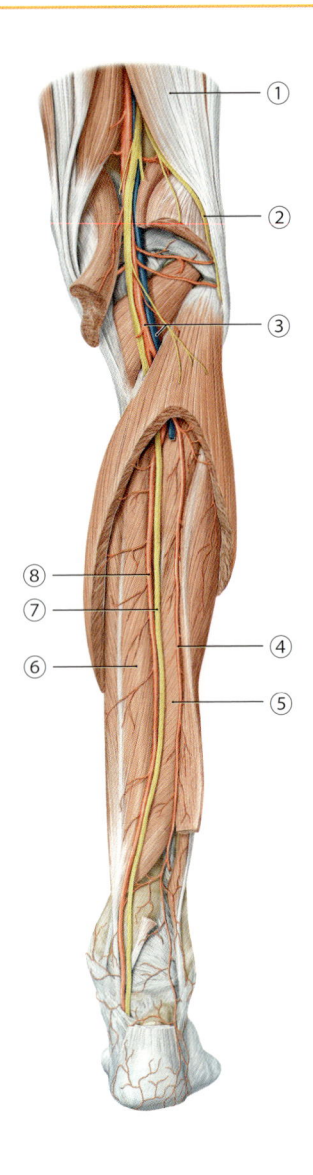

下腿後面の神経・血管

右下腿, 後面

① □ 大腿二頭筋　　　　　□ Biceps femoris
② □ 総腓骨神経　　　　　□ Common fibular nerve
③ □ 膝窩動脈・静脈　　　□ Popliteal artery and vein
④ □ 腓骨動脈　　　　　　□ Fibular artery
⑤ □ 後脛骨筋　　　　　　□ Tibialis posterior
⑥ □ 長趾屈筋　　　　　　□ Flexor digitorum longus
⑦ □ 脛骨神経　　　　　　□ Tibial nerve
⑧ □ 後脛骨動脈　　　　　□ Posterior tibial artery

The Tarsal Tunnel

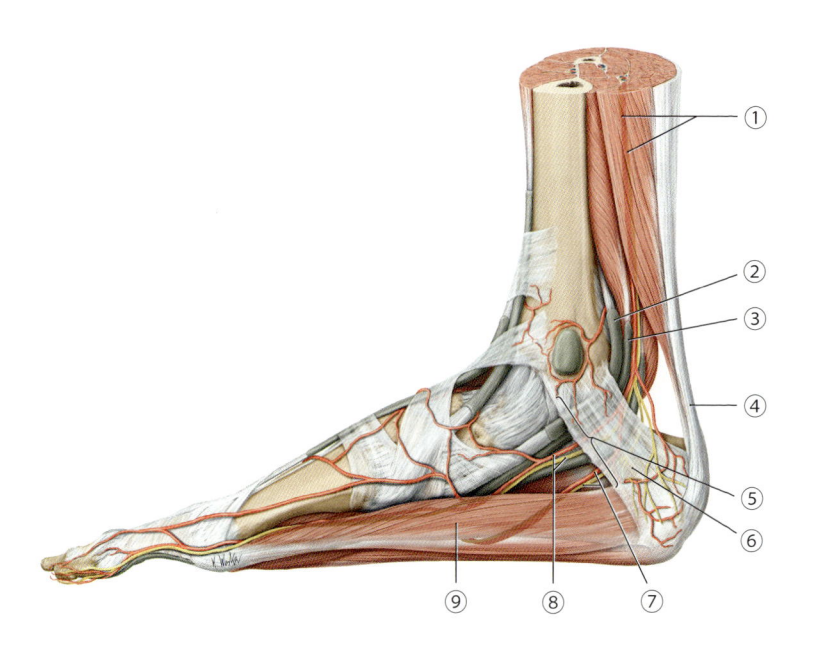

足根管

右足，内側面

① □ 脛骨神経，後脛骨動脈　　□ Tibial nerve, posterior tibial artery

② □ 後脛骨筋　　□ Tibialis posterior
③ □ 長趾屈筋　　□ Flexor digitorum longus
④ □ 踵骨腱（アキレス腱）　　□ Achilles' tendon
⑤ □ 足根管　　□ Tarsal tunnel
⑥ □ 屈筋支帯　　□ Flexor retinaculum
⑦ □ 外側足底動脈・神経　　□ Lateral plantar artery and nerve
⑧ □ 内側足底動脈・神経　　□ Medial plantar artery and nerve
⑨ □ 母趾外転筋　　□ Abductor hallucis

Neurovasculature of the Lateral Leg

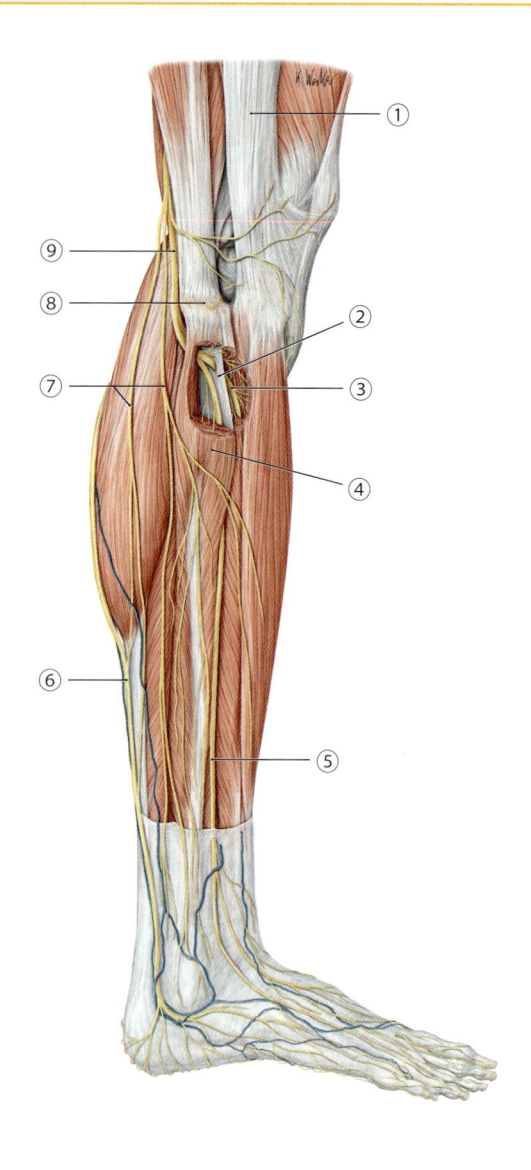

下腿外側の神経・血管

右下腿，外側面

① □ 腸脛靱帯 □ Iliotibial tract
② □ 前下腿筋間中隔 □ Anterior crural intermuscular septum
③ □ 深腓骨神経 □ Deep fibular nerve
④ □ 長腓骨筋 □ Fibularis longus
⑤ □ 浅腓骨神経 □ Superficial fibular nerve
⑥ □ 腓腹神経 □ Sural nerve
⑦ □ 外側腓腹皮神経 □ Lateral sural cutaneous nerve
⑧ □ 腓骨頭 □ Head of fibula
⑨ □ 総腓骨神経 □ Common fibular nerve

解説

総腓骨神経は皮膚の直下で，腓骨頭を取り巻くように走行した後，下腿筋膜を貫いて外側区画に入る．総腓骨神経が腓骨頭の部位で圧迫されると，下腿の前区画と外側区画にある筋に筋力低下（麻痺）が生じる．これらの筋の筋力低下では，下垂足が見られ，足の外反も困難となる．

① 図 27.39. p.444　② 図 29.39. p.468

Neurovasculature of the Anterior Leg

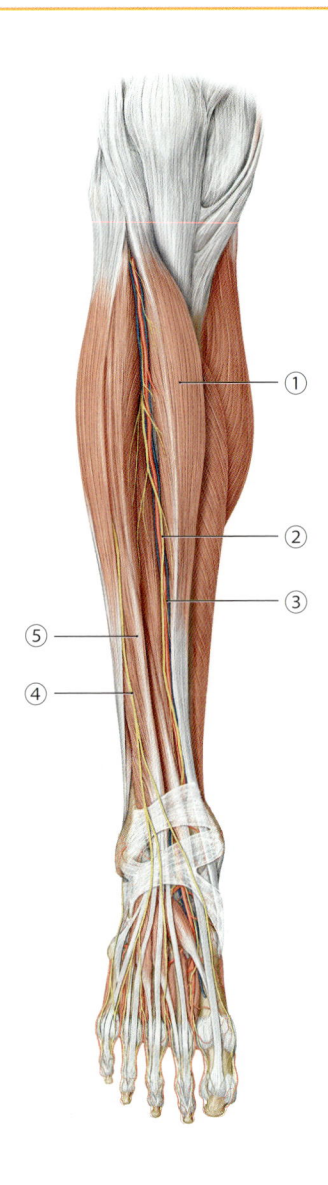

下腿前面の神経・血管

右下腿，前面

① □ 前脛骨筋　　　　　　　□ Tibialis anterior
② □ 深腓骨神経　　　　　　□ Deep fibular nerve
③ □ 前脛骨動脈・静脈　　　□ Anterior tibial artery and vein
④ □ 浅腓骨神経　　　　　　□ Superficial fibular nerve
⑤ □ 長趾伸筋　　　　　　　□ Extensor digitorum longus

臨床

　筋の浮腫や血腫によって下腿の区画（コンパートメント）内の組織圧が異常に高まると，神経や血管が圧迫される．このような状態が長時間続くと，筋や神経が虚血に陥り，不可逆的な障害が残る場合がある．下腿の前区画にこのような状態が生じると，患者は耐えがたい激痛に見舞われ，足趾の背屈が困難となる（前コンパートメント症候群と呼ばれ，コンパートメント症候群の中でも一般的なものである）．このような患者では，下腿筋膜を緊急に切開し，区画内の組織圧を下げなければならない．

1 図 27.40B, p.445　　2 図 29.40B, p.469

Neurovasculature of the Dorsum

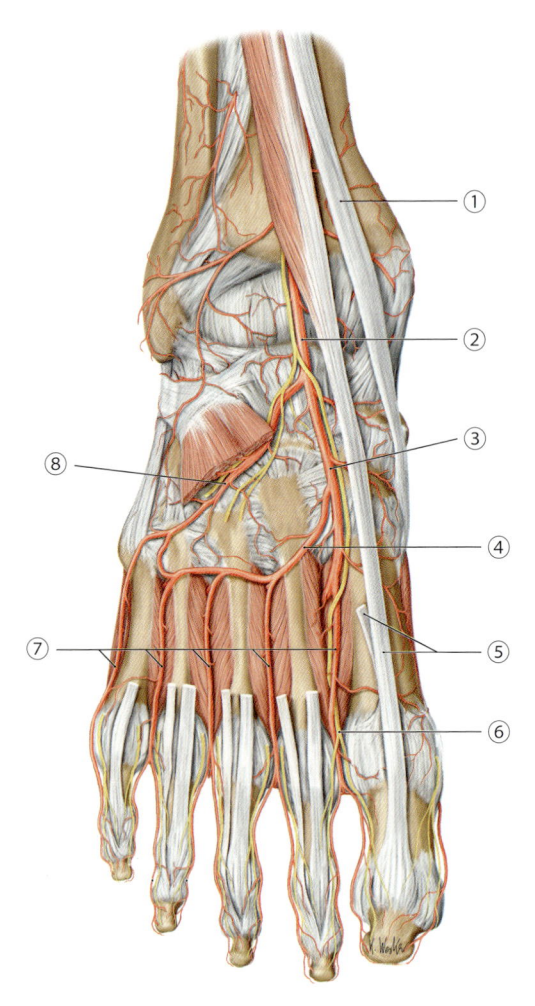

足背動脈はどの動脈から起始するか？

足背の神経・血管

右足，足背面（上面）

① □ 前脛骨筋（腱）　　　　　□ Tibialis anterior tendon
② □ 前脛骨動脈　　　　　　□ Anterior tibial artery
③ □ 足背動脈　　　　　　　□ Dorsal pedal artery
④ □ 弓状動脈　　　　　　　□ Arcuate artery
⑤ □ 長・短母趾伸筋（腱）　　□ Extensors hallucis longus and brevis tendons
⑥ □ 深腓骨神経，皮枝　　　□ Deep fibular nerve, cutaneous branch
⑦ □ 背側中足動脈　　　　　□ Dorsal metatarsal arteries
⑧ □ 外側足根動脈　　　　　□ Lateral tarsal artery

A 足背動脈は前脛骨動脈（膝窩動脈の枝）の延長である．

1 図 27.40A. p.445　　2 図 29.40A. p.469

Neurovasculature of the Sole

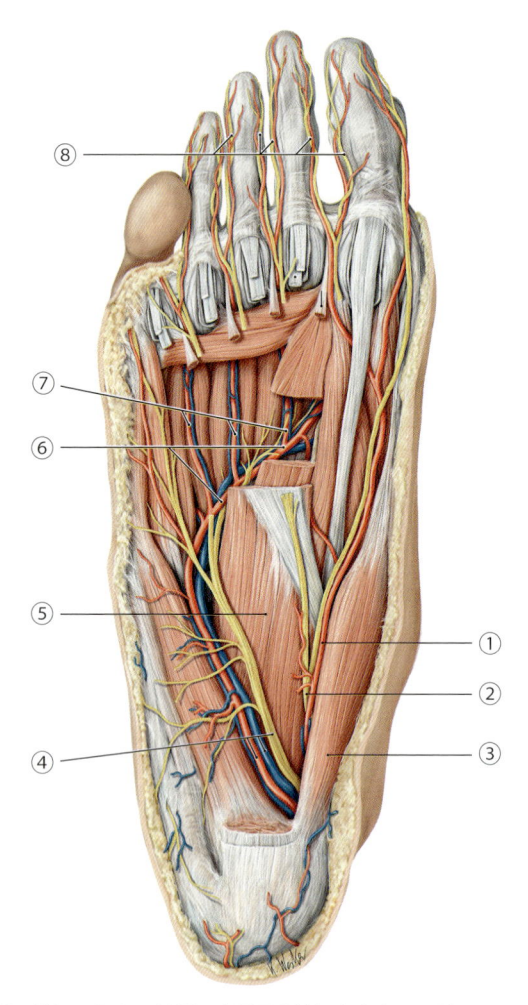

Q 下腿の神経のうち，外側・内側足底神経を出すのはどれか？

足底の神経・血管

右足．足底面（下面）

① ☐ 内側足底動脈　　　　　　　☐ Medial plantar artery

② ☐ 内側足底神経　　　　　　　☐ Medial plantar nerve

③ ☐ 母趾外転筋　　　　　　　　☐ Abductor hallucis

④ ☐ 外側足底動脈・静脈・神経　☐ Lateral plantar artery, vein, and nerve

⑤ ☐ 足底方形筋　　　　　　　　☐ Quadratus plantae

⑥ ☐ 深足底動脈弓　　　　　　　☐ Deep plantar arch

⑦ ☐ 底側中足動脈　　　　　　　☐ Plantar metatarsal arteries

⑧ ☐ 固有底側趾動脈・神経　　　☐ Proper plantar digital arteries and nerves

A 脛骨神経は足に入ると，外側・内側足底神経に分岐し，足底の筋を支配する．深足底動脈弓は足背動脈との間で吻合路を形成する．

[1] 図 27.41C, p.447　[2] 図 29.41C, p.471

Transverse Section of the Thigh

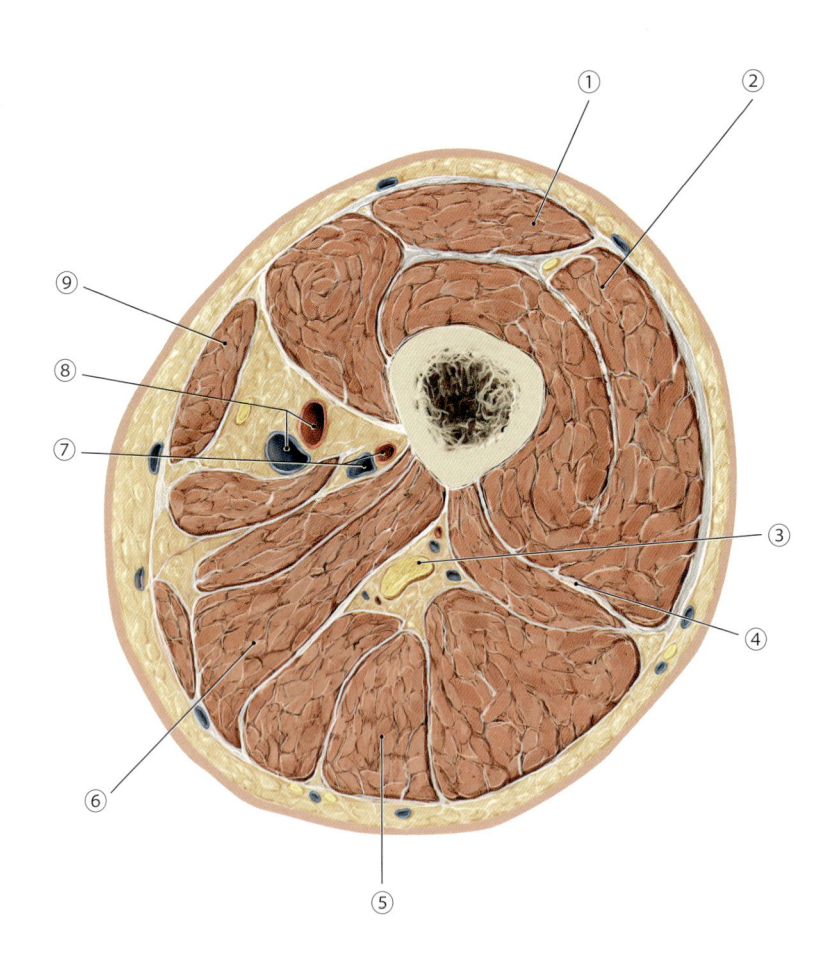

大腿の横断面

右大腿，近位方向（上方）から見たところ

① ☐ 大腿直筋　　　　　　　　☐ Rectus femoris
② ☐ 外側広筋　　　　　　　　☐ Vastus lateralis
③ ☐ 坐骨神経　　　　　　　　☐ Sciatic nerve
④ ☐ 外側大腿筋間中隔　　　　☐ Lateral intermuscular septum
⑤ ☐ 半腱様筋　　　　　　　　☐ Semitendinosus
⑥ ☐ 大内転筋　　　　　　　　☐ Adductor magnus
⑦ ☐ 大腿深動脈・静脈　　　　☐ Profunda femoris artery, deep femoral vein
⑧ ☐ 大腿動脈・静脈　　　　　☐ Femoral artery and vein
⑨ ☐ 縫工筋　　　　　　　　　☐ Sartorius

1 図 27.44A, p.449　2 図 29.44A, p.473

Transverse Section of the Leg

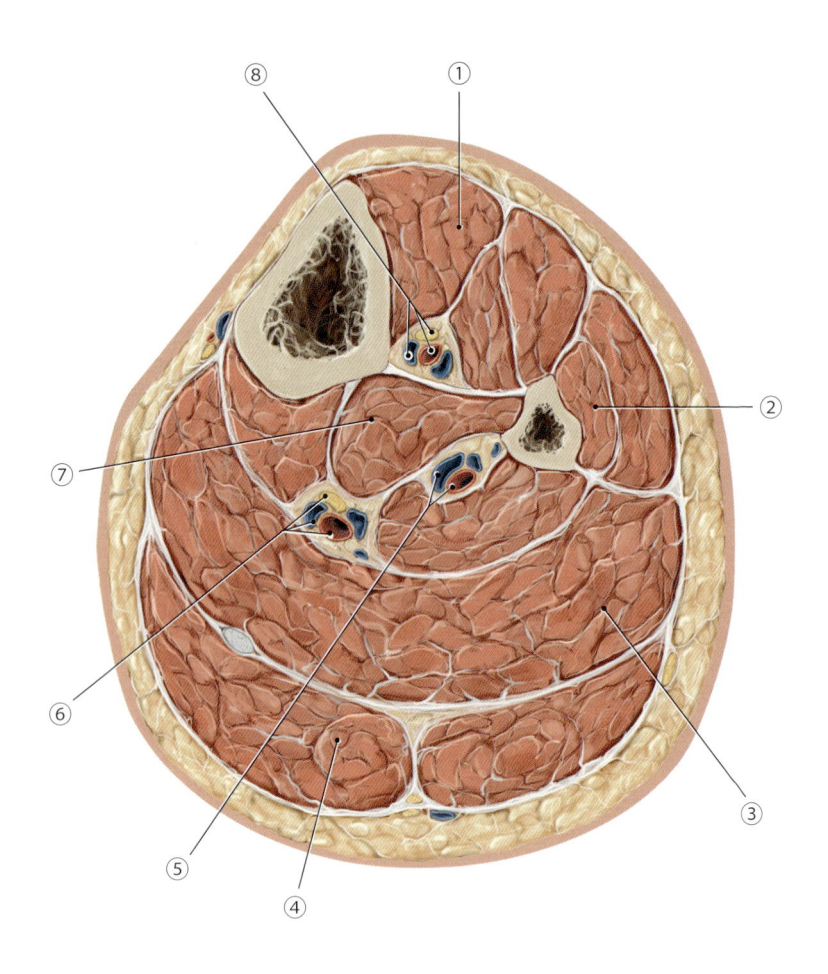

Q 下腿の外側区画に分布する動脈は何か？

下腿の横断面

右下腿，近位面（上面）

① □ 前脛骨筋　　　　　　　□ Tibialis anterior
② □ 短腓骨筋　　　　　　　□ Fibularis brevis
③ □ ヒラメ筋　　　　　　　□ Soleus
④ □ 腓腹筋，内側頭　　　　□ Gastrocnemius, medial head
⑤ □ 腓骨動脈・静脈　　　　□ Fibular artery and vein
⑥ □ 脛骨神経，後脛骨動脈・静脈　□ Tibial nerve, posterior tibial artery and vein
⑦ □ 後脛骨筋　　　　　　　□ Tibialis posterior
⑧ □ 深腓骨神経，前脛骨動脈・静脈　□ Deep fibular nerve, anterior tibial artery and vein

A 外側区画には太い動脈が通過しないため，この区画には前脛骨動脈の枝や腓骨動脈の貫通枝が分布する．

1 図 27.44B. p.449　2 図 29.44B. p.473

536　Lower Limb

Surface Anatomy

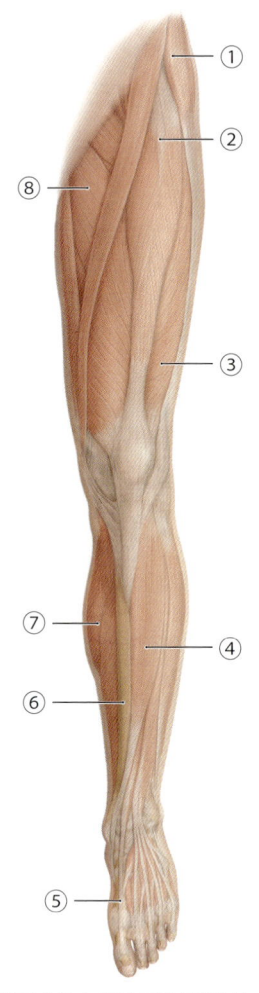

①
②
⑧
③
⑦
④
⑥
⑤

Q 股関節の周囲で触知できる大腿骨の隆起は何か？

下肢の体表解剖

左下肢，前面

① □ 大腿筋膜張筋　　□ Tensor fascia lata
② □ 大腿直筋　　　　□ Rectus femoris
③ □ 外側広筋　　　　□ Vastus lateralis
④ □ 前脛骨筋　　　　□ Tibialis anterior
⑤ □ 長母趾伸筋（腱）□ Extensor hallucis longus tendon
⑥ □ 脛骨　　　　　　□ Tibia
⑦ □ 腓腹筋　　　　　□ Gastrocnemius
⑧ □ 長内転筋　　　　□ Adductor longus

A 大腿骨の近位部で体表から触知できるのは大転子だけである．

① 図 28.1B. p.450　② 図 25.3A. p.381

頭頸部 Head & Neck

頭蓋の骨 1 …… 540	鼻腔の骨 1 …… 618
頭蓋の骨 2 …… 542	鼻腔の骨 2 …… 620
頭蓋の骨 3 …… 544	鼻腔の骨 3 …… 622
頭蓋底 1 …… 546	鼻腔の神経・血管 1 …… 624
頭蓋底 2 …… 548	鼻腔の神経・血管 2 …… 626
頭蓋底 3 …… 550	外耳 …… 628
表情筋 …… 552	耳介の構造 …… 630
脳神経 1 …… 554	鼓室 …… 632
脳神経 2 …… 556	耳小骨連鎖 …… 634
脳神経 3 …… 558	内耳 …… 636
脳神経 4 …… 560	下顎骨 …… 638
脳神経 5 …… 562	口腔の三叉神経 …… 640
脳神経 6 …… 564	舌背 …… 642
脳神経 7 …… 566	舌の筋肉 …… 644
脳神経 8 …… 568	舌の感覚性神経支配 …… 646
脳神経 9 …… 570	舌の神経と血管 …… 648
脳神経10 …… 572	口腔の区分 1 …… 650
感覚神経支配 …… 574	口腔の区分 2 …… 652
頭蓋と顔面の動脈 1 …… 576	唾液腺 1 …… 654
頭蓋と顔面の動脈 2 …… 578	唾液腺 2 …… 656
頭頸部の静脈 1 …… 580	咽頭筋 1 …… 658
頭頸部の静脈 2 …… 582	咽頭筋 2 …… 660
顔面浅層の神経・血管 1 …… 584	咽頭の神経・血管 …… 662
顔面浅層の神経・血管 2 …… 586	頸部の筋 …… 664
耳下腺咬筋部 1 …… 588	頸部の動脈 …… 666
耳下腺咬筋部 2 …… 590	頸部の神経 …… 668
側頭下窩 1 …… 592	甲状腺 …… 670
側頭下窩 2 …… 594	甲状腺の関係 …… 672
側頭下窩 3 …… 596	喉頭の構造 …… 674
翼口蓋窩 …… 598	喉頭腔 …… 676
眼窩の骨 …… 600	喉頭の神経・血管 1 …… 678
眼窩の筋 …… 602	喉頭の神経・血管 2 …… 680
眼窩の神経 1 …… 604	頸部の部位 …… 682
眼窩の神経 2 …… 606	胸郭上口 1 …… 684
眼窩の局所解剖 1 …… 608	胸郭上口 2 …… 686
眼窩の局所解剖 2 …… 610	外側頸三角部の局所解剖 1 …… 688
眼瞼と結膜 …… 612	外側頸三角部の局所解剖 2 …… 690
涙器 …… 614	頭頸部の体表解剖 …… 692
眼球の構造 …… 616	

Bones of the Skull I

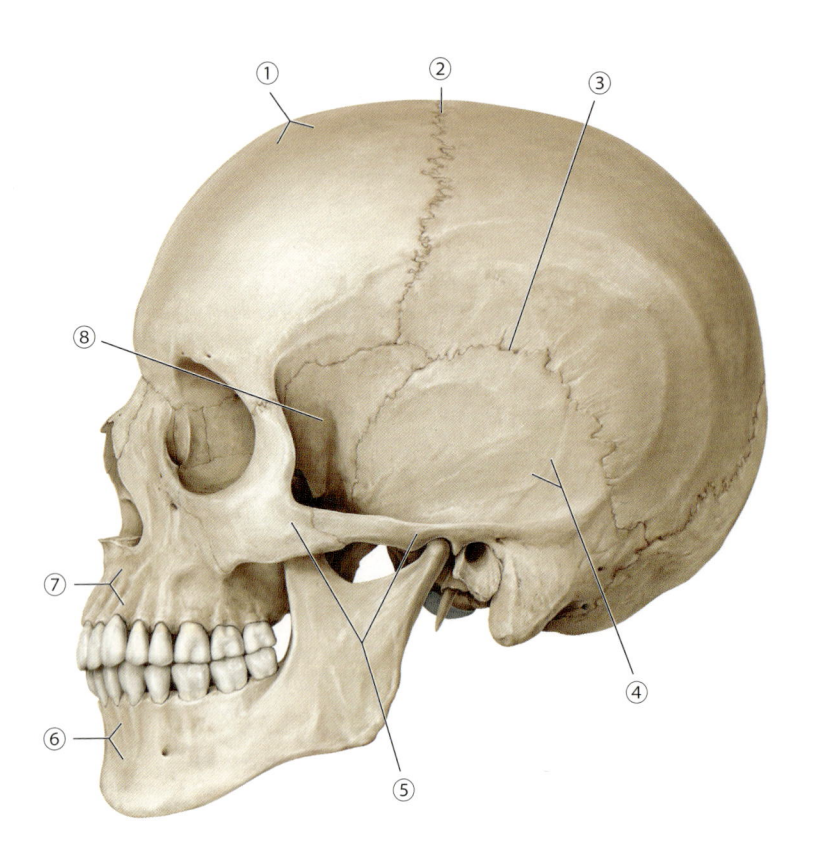

頭蓋の骨 1

左外側面

① □ 前頭骨　　　　　　　　□ Frontal bone
② □ 冠状縫合　　　　　　　□ Coronal suture
③ □ 鱗状縫合　　　　　　　□ Squamous suture
④ □ 側頭骨，鱗部　　　　　□ Temporal bone, squamous part
⑤ □ 頬骨弓　　　　　　　　□ Zygomatic arch
⑥ □ 下顎骨　　　　　　　　□ Mandible
⑦ □ 上顎骨　　　　　　　　□ Maxilla
⑧ □ 蝶形骨，大翼　　　　　□ Sphenoid bone, greater wing

解説

頭蓋は脳頭蓋と顔面頭蓋に分けられる．脳頭蓋は脳を保護し，顔面頭蓋は顔面の諸部分を収容して，保護する．

1 図 29.1. p.454　 2 図 31.1. p.478

Bones of the Skull II

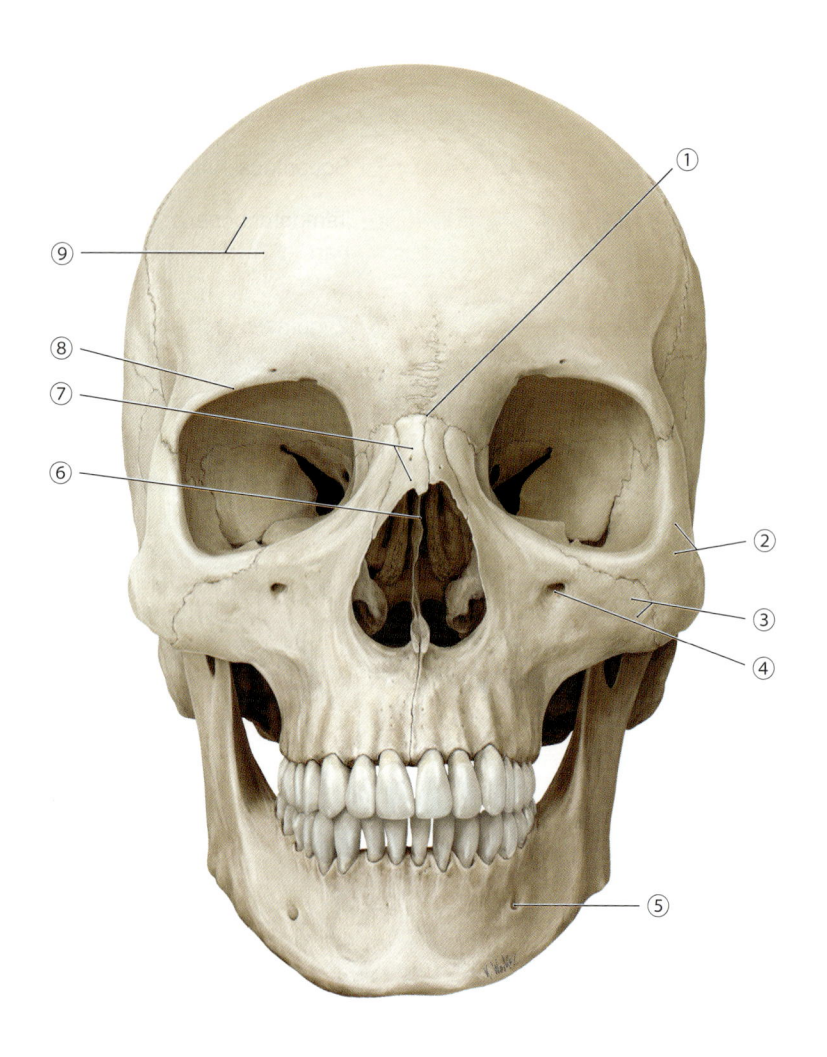

頭蓋の骨 2

前面

① □ 鼻根点　　　　　　　□ Nasion
② □ 頬骨　　　　　　　　□ Zygomatic bone
③ □ 上顎骨　　　　　　　□ Maxilla
④ □ 眼窩下孔　　　　　　□ Infraorbital foramen
⑤ □ オトガイ孔　　　　　□ Mental foramen
⑥ □ 篩骨，垂直板　　　　□ Ethmoid bone, perpendicular plate
⑦ □ 鼻骨　　　　　　　　□ Nasal bone
⑧ □ 眼窩上縁　　　　　　□ Supraorbital margin
⑨ □ 前頭骨　　　　　　　□ Frontal bone

臨床

　顔面骨格は枠状の構造であるために骨折線は特徴的なパターンを示し，ル・フォールⅠ～Ⅲ型に分類される．

1 図 29.2. p.455　　2 図 31.2. p.479

Bones of the Skull III

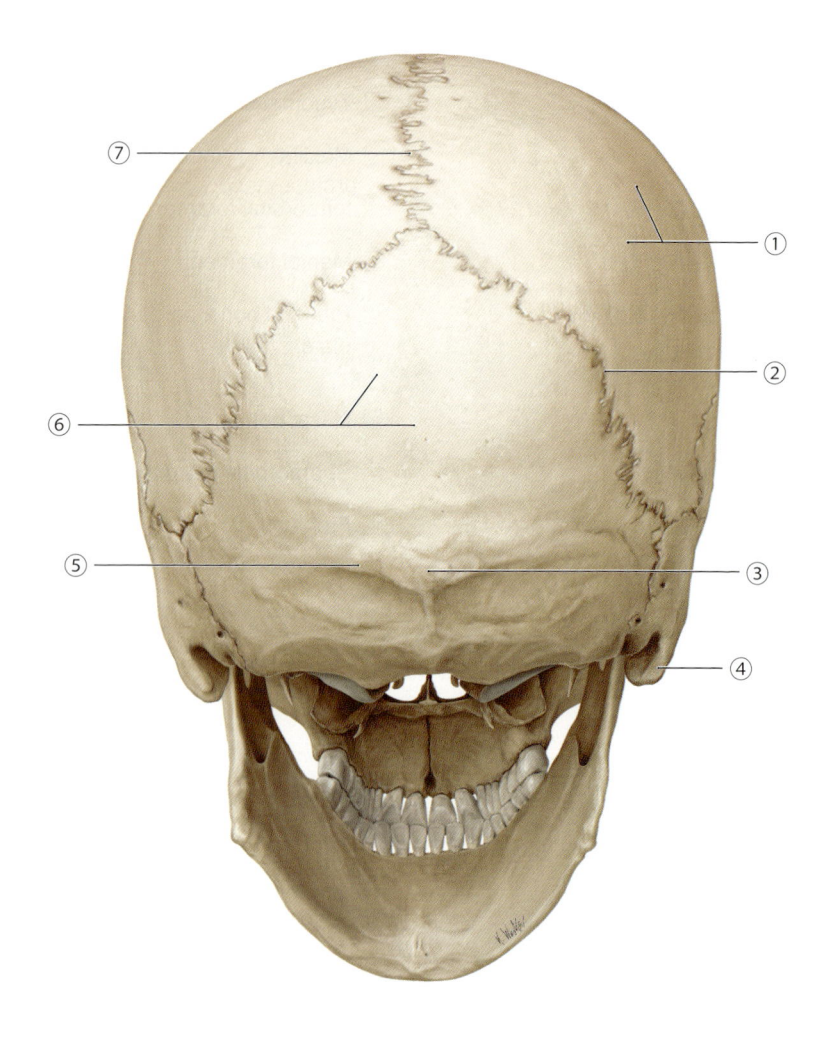

頭蓋の骨 3

後面

① □ 頭頂骨 　　　　　□ Parietal bone
② □ ラムダ縫合 　　　□ Lambdoid suture
③ □ 外後頭隆起 　　　□ External occipital protuberance
④ □ 乳様突起 　　　　□ Mastoid process
⑤ □ 上項線 　　　　　□ Superior nuchal line
⑥ □ 後頭骨 　　　　　□ Occipital bone
⑦ □ 矢状縫合 　　　　□ Sagittal suture

Base of the Skull I

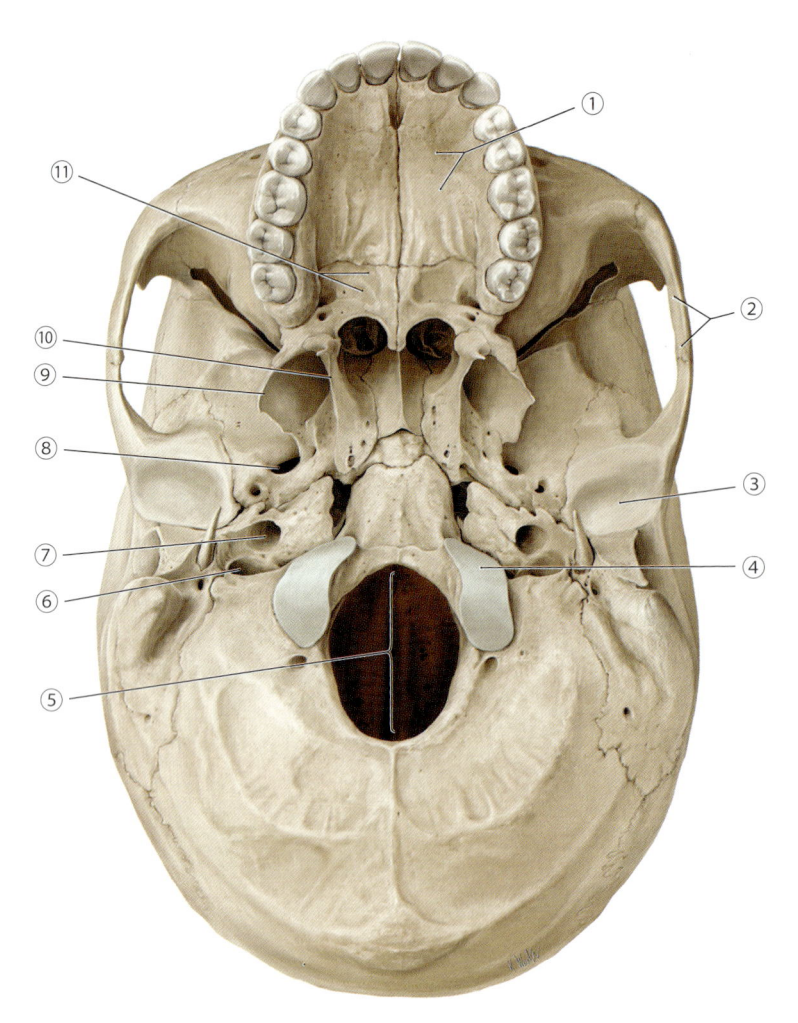

外側板と内側板があるのはどの頭蓋骨か？

頭蓋底 1

下面

① ☐ 上顎骨，口蓋突起 ☐ Palatine process of maxilla
② ☐ 頬骨弓 ☐ Zygomatic arch
③ ☐ 下顎窩 ☐ Mandibular fossa
④ ☐ 後頭顆 ☐ Occipital condyle
⑤ ☐ 大後頭孔 ☐ Foramen magnum
⑥ ☐ 頸静脈孔 ☐ Jugular foramen
⑦ ☐ 頸動脈管 ☐ Carotid canal
⑧ ☐ 卵円孔 ☐ Foramen ovale
⑨ ☐ 翼状突起，外側板 ☐ Lateral plate of pterygoid process
⑩ ☐ 翼状突起，内側板 ☐ Medial plate of pterygoid process
⑪ ☐ 口蓋骨 ☐ Palatine bone

外側板と内側板は蝶形骨の翼状突起にある．

1 図 29.6. p.458　2 図 31.6. p.482

Base of the Skull II

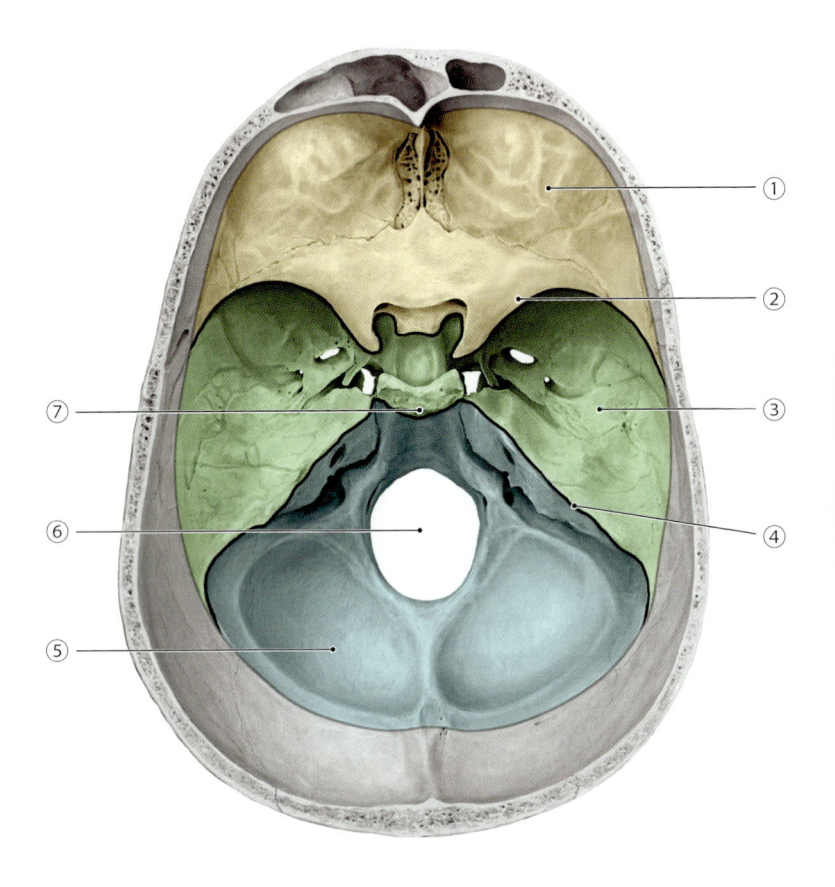

頭蓋底 2

上面

① □ 前頭蓋窩 □ Anterior cranial fossa
② □ 蝶形骨の小翼 □ Lesser wing of sphenoid bone
③ □ 中頭蓋窩 □ Middle cranial fossa
④ □ 錐体上縁 □ Petrous ridge
⑤ □ 後頭蓋窩 □ Posterior cranial fossa
⑥ □ 大後頭孔 □ Foramen magnum
⑦ □ 鞍背 □ Dorsum sellae

解説

頭蓋底の内面は連続する3つの窩からなる．これらの窩は前方から後方に向かって段階的に深くなる．

1 図 29.7B. p.459　2 図 31.7B. p.483

550   Head & Neck

Base of the Skull III

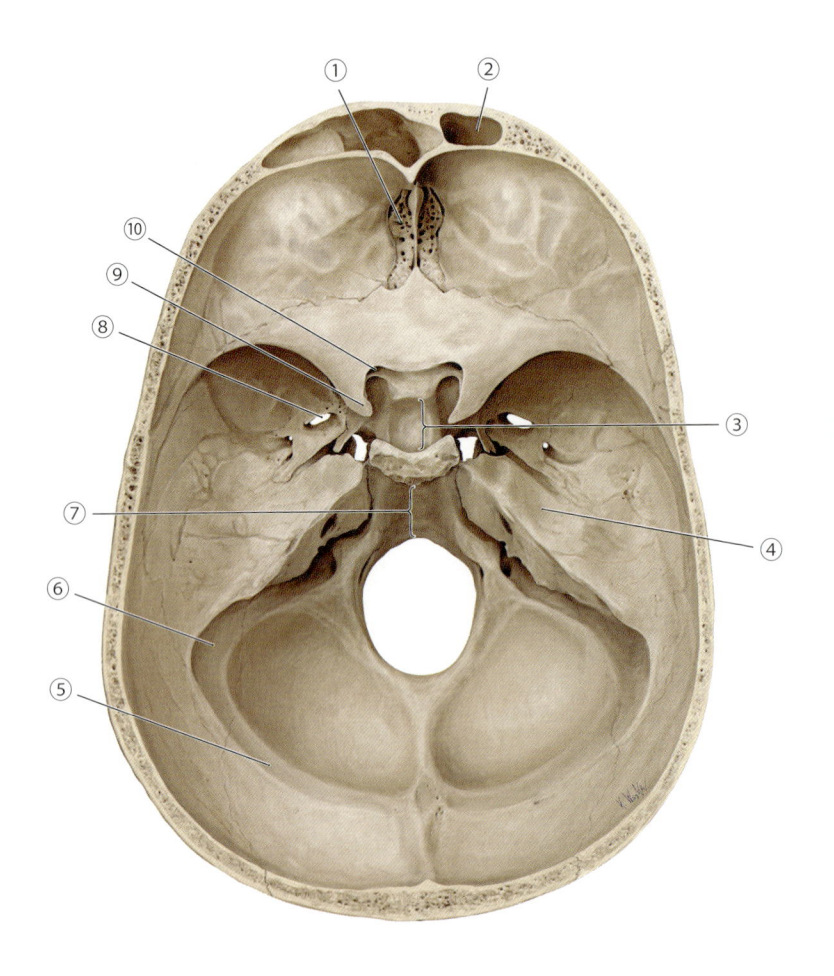

頭蓋底 3

上面

① ☐ 篩板　　　　　　　　　☐ Cribriform plate

② ☐ 前頭洞　　　　　　　　☐ Frontal sinus

③ ☐ 下垂体窩（トルコ鞍）　　☐ Hypophyseal fossa (sella turcica)

④ ☐ 側頭骨，岩様部　　　　☐ Temporal bone, petrous part

⑤ ☐ 横洞溝　　　　　　　　☐ Groove for transverse sinus

⑥ ☐ S状洞溝　　　　　　　 ☐ Groove for sigmoid sinus

⑦ ☐ 斜台　　　　　　　　　☐ Clivus

⑧ ☐ 卵円孔　　　　　　　　☐ Foramen ovale

⑨ ☐ 前床突起　　　　　　　☐ Anterior clinoid process

⑩ ☐ 視神経管　　　　　　　☐ Optic canal

1 図 29.8. p.459　　2 図 31.8. p.483

552 Head & Neck

Muscles of Facial Expression

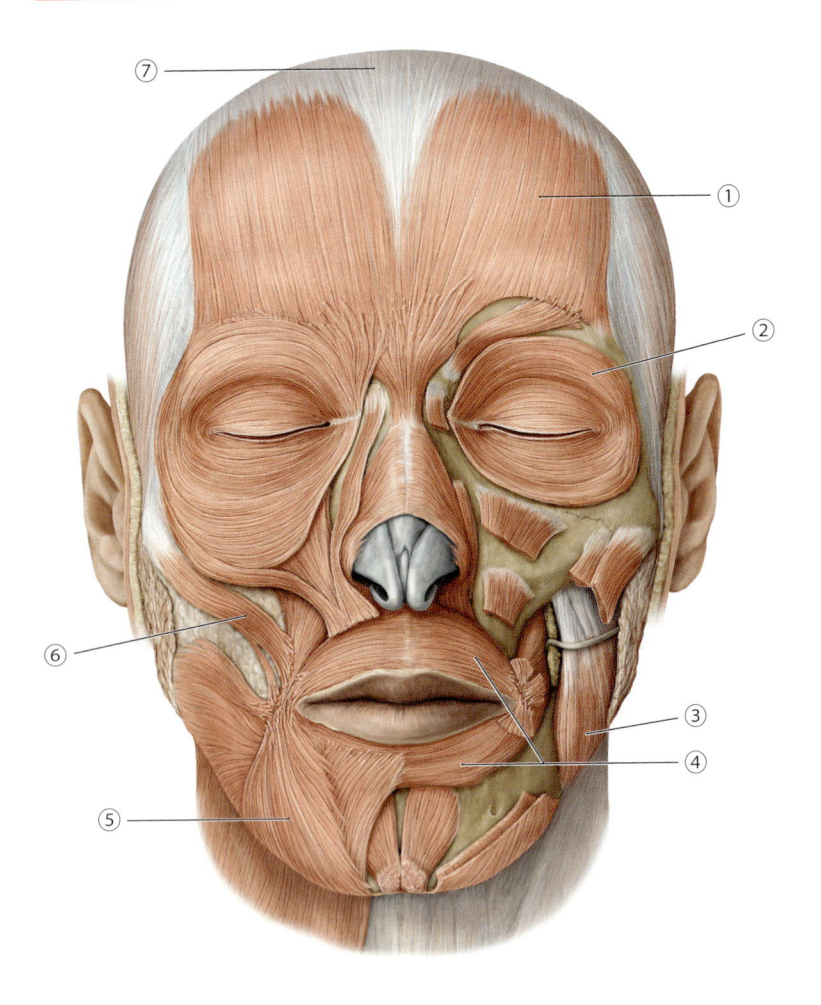

Q 表情筋と咀嚼筋の支配神経は何か？

表情筋

前面

① ☐ 前頭筋（後頭前頭筋）　　☐ Occipitofrontalis, frontal belly

② ☐ 眼輪筋　　☐ Orbicularis oculi

③ ☐ 咬筋　　☐ Masseter

④ ☐ 口輪筋　　☐ Orbicularis oris

⑤ ☐ 口角下制筋　　☐ Depressor anguli oris

⑥ ☐ 大頬骨筋　　☐ Zygomaticus major

⑦ ☐ 帽状腱膜　　☐ Galea aponeurotica (epicranial aponeurosis)

A 顔面神経は表情筋の運動を支配する．咀嚼筋は下顎神経に支配される．

1 図 30.1A. p.462　　2 図 32.1A. p.488

Cranial Nerves I

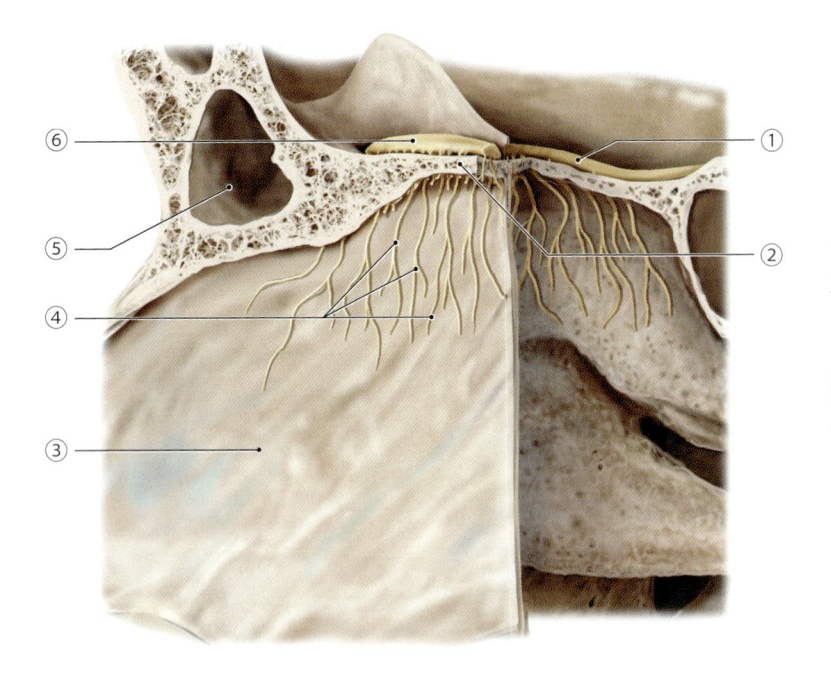

脳神経 1

左鼻中隔の一部と右鼻腔の外壁，左外側面

① ☐ 嗅索　　　　　　　　　　☐ Olfactory tract
② ☐ 篩板　　　　　　　　　　☐ Cribriform plate
③ ☐ 鼻中隔（篩骨の垂直板）　　☐ Nasal septum (perpendicular plate of ethmoid bone)
④ ☐ 嗅神経糸　　　　　　　　☐ Olfactory fibers
⑤ ☐ 前頭洞　　　　　　　　　☐ Frontal sinus
⑥ ☐ 嗅球　　　　　　　　　　☐ Olfactory bulb

1 図 31.3C. p.472　2 図 33.3C. p.498

Cranial Nerves II

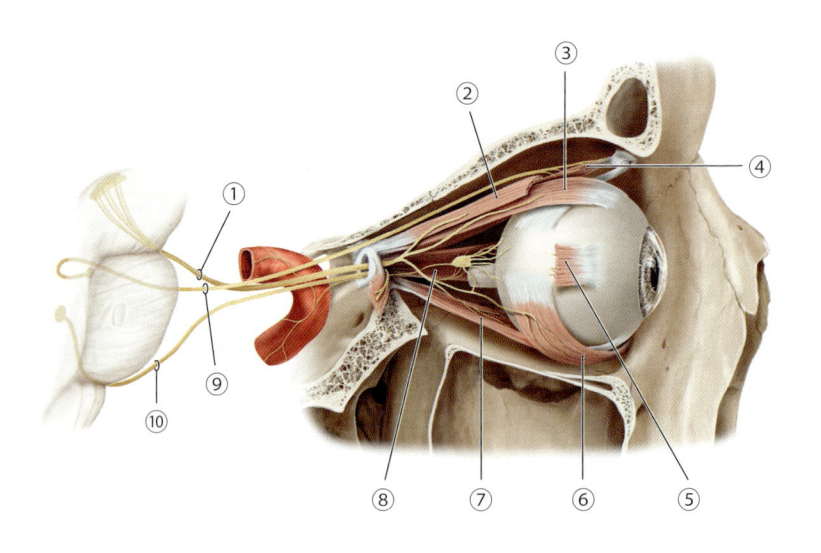

脳神経 2

右眼窩，外側面

① □ 動眼神経　　　　　　　□ Oculomotor nerve (CN III)

② □ 上眼瞼挙筋　　　　　　□ Levator palpebrae superioris

③ □ 上直筋　　　　　　　　□ Superior rectus

④ □ 上斜筋　　　　　　　　□ Superior oblique

⑤ □ 外側直筋（断端）　　　　□ Lateral rectus (cut)

⑥ □ 下斜筋　　　　　　　　□ Inferior oblique

⑦ □ 下直筋　　　　　　　　□ Inferior rectus

⑧ □ 内側直筋　　　　　　　□ Medial rectus

⑨ □ 滑車神経　　　　　　　□ Trochlear nerve (CN IV)

⑩ □ 外転神経　　　　　　　□ Abducent nerve (CN VI)

臨床

　動眼神経は内眼筋を副交感性に支配し，外眼筋の大部分と上眼瞼挙筋を体性運動性に支配する．動眼神経の副交感性線維は毛様体神経節でシナプスを形成する．動眼神経麻痺が起こると，その影響が副交感性線維だけに現れる場合や体性線維だけに現れる場合，さらに両方に現れる場合がある．

① 図 31.6A. p.475　② 図 33.6A. p.501

Cranial Nerves III

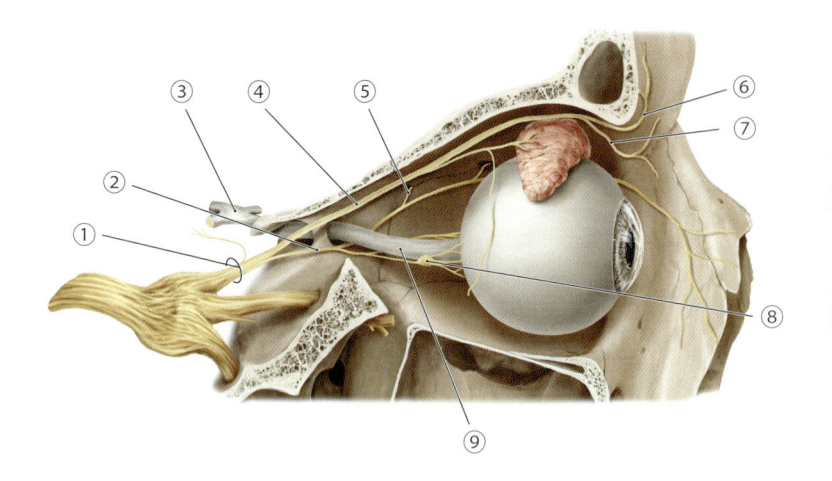

脳神経 3

右眼窩, 外側面

① □ 眼神経　　　　　□ Ophthalmic division (CN V₁)
② □ 鼻毛様体神経　　□ Nasociliary nerve
③ □ 視交叉　　　　　□ Optic chiasm
④ □ 前頭神経　　　　□ Frontal nerve
⑤ □ 後篩骨神経　　　□ Posterior ethmoidal nerve
⑥ □ 眼窩上神経　　　□ Supraorbital nerve
⑦ □ 滑車上神経　　　□ Supratrochlear nerve
⑧ □ 毛様体神経節　　□ Ciliary ganglion
⑨ □ 視神経　　　　　□ Optic nerve (CN II)

解説

視神経は視神経管を通って眼窩に至り, 他の脳神経は上眼窩裂を通って眼窩に入る.

1 図 31.9A. p.477　2 図 33.9A. p.503

Cranial Nerves IV

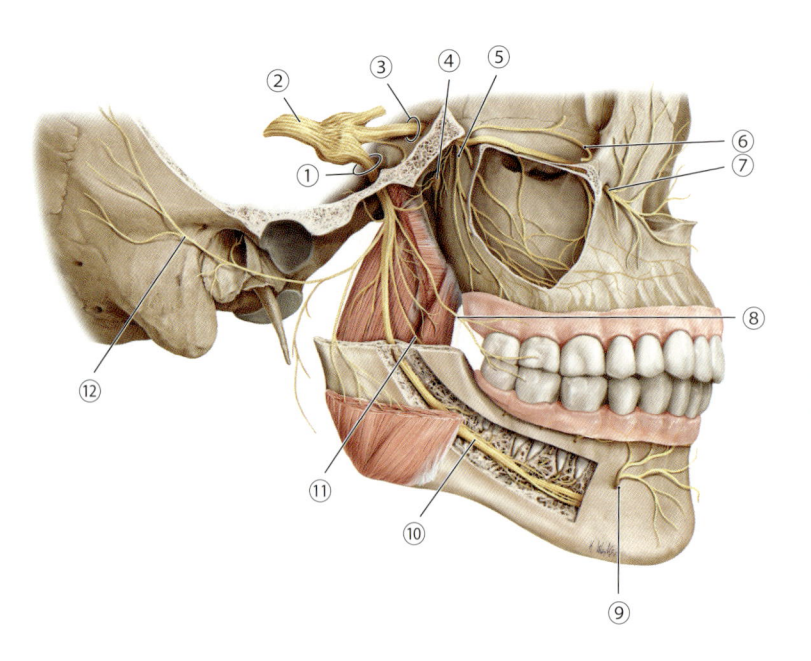

脳神経 4

右外側面

① ☐ 下顎神経(卵円孔を通る) ☐ Mandibular division (CN V_3, via foramen ovale)

② ☐ 三叉神経 ☐ Trigeminal nerve (CN V)

③ ☐ 上顎神経(正円孔を通る) ☐ Maxillary division (CN V_2, via foramen rotundum)

④ ☐ 翼口蓋神経節 ☐ Pterygopalatine ganglion

⑤ ☐ 上歯槽神経，後上歯槽枝 ☐ Posterior superior alveolar nerves

⑥ ☐ 頬骨神経 ☐ Zygomatic nerve

⑦ ☐ 眼窩下神経と眼窩下孔 ☐ Infraorbital nerve (and foramen)

⑧ ☐ 頬神経 ☐ Buccal nerve

⑨ ☐ オトガイ神経とオトガイ孔 ☐ Mental nerve (and foramen)

⑩ ☐ 下歯槽神経(下顎管にある) ☐ Inferior alveolar nerve (in mandibular canal)

⑪ ☐ 舌神経 ☐ Lingual nerve

⑫ ☐ 耳介側頭神経 ☐ Auriculotemporal nerve

1 図 36.17. p.546   2 図 33.9C. p.503

Cranial Nerves V

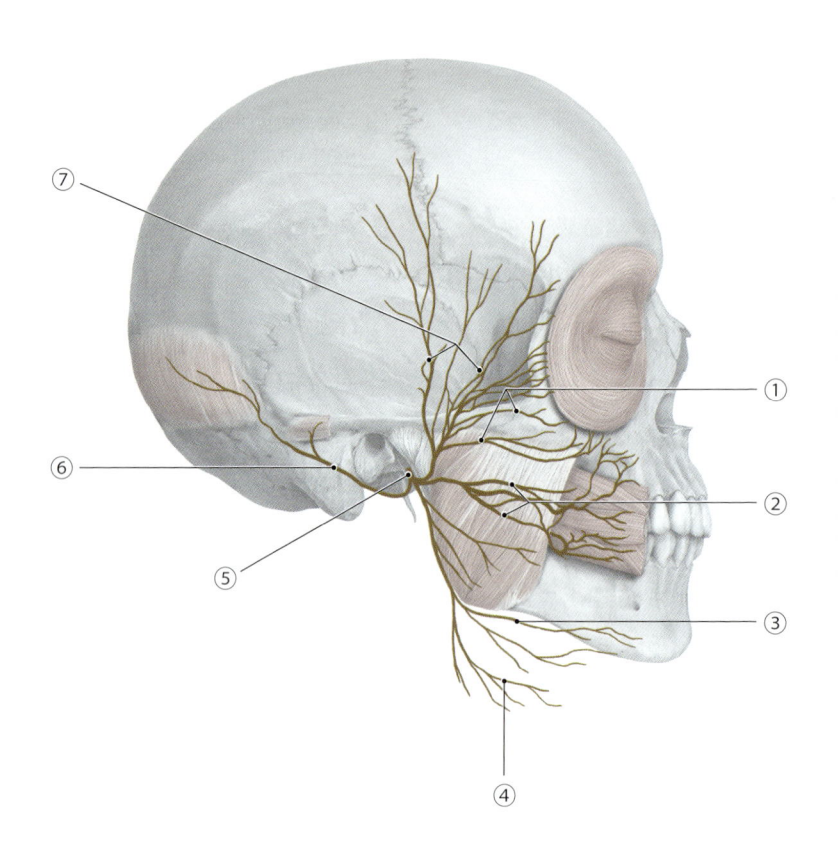

脳神経 5

右外側面

① ☐ 頬骨枝 　　　　　☐ Zygomatic branches

② ☐ 頬筋枝 　　　　　☐ Buccal branches

③ ☐ 下顎縁枝 　　　　☐ Marginal mandibular branch

④ ☐ 頸枝 　　　　　　☐ Cervical branch

⑤ ☐ 顔面神経 　　　　☐ Facial nerve

⑥ ☐ 後耳介神経 　　　☐ Posterior auricular nerve

⑦ ☐ 側頭枝 　　　　　☐ Temporal branches

解説

顔面神経は表情筋を支配する．

Cranial Nerves VI

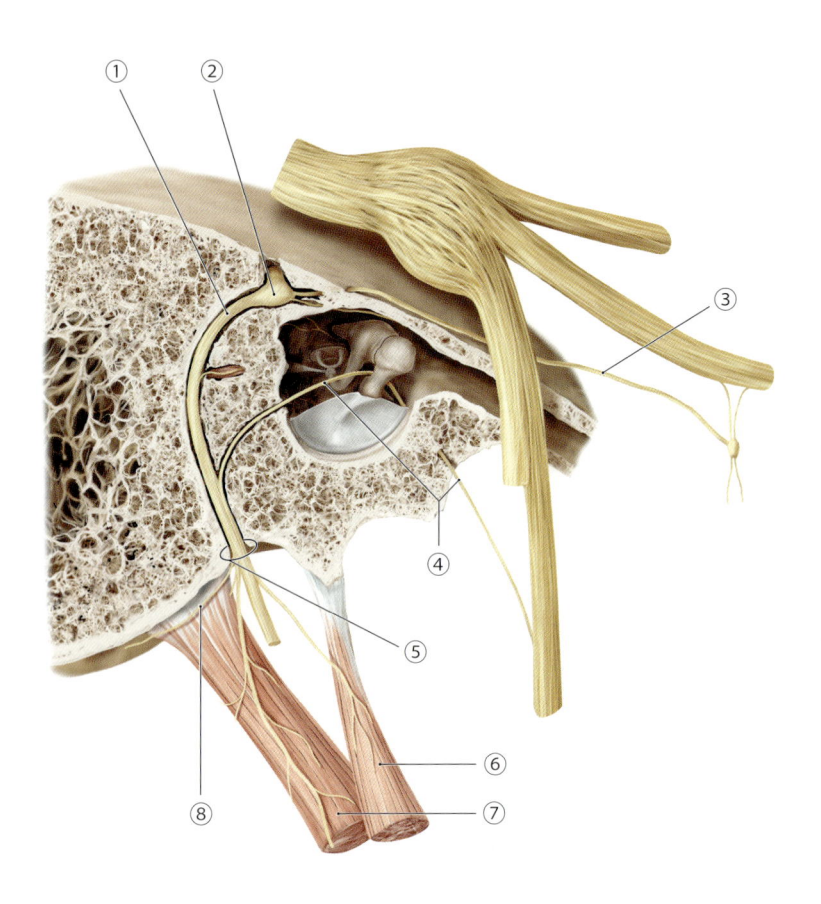

鼓索神経に運ばれるのはどのような線維か？

脳神経 6

右外側面

① ☐ 顔面神経　　　　　　　　☐ Facial nerve (CN VII)

② ☐ 膝神経節　　　　　　　　☐ Geniculate ganglion

③ ☐ 大錐体神経　　　　　　　☐ Greater petrosal nerve

④ ☐ 鼓索神経　　　　　　　　☐ Chorda tympani

⑤ ☐ 茎乳突孔　　　　　　　　☐ Stylomastoid foramen

⑥ ☐ 茎突舌骨筋　　　　　　　☐ Stylohyoid

⑦ ☐ 顎二腹筋（後腹）　　　　☐ Digastric (posterior belly)

⑧ ☐ 後耳介神経　　　　　　　☐ Posterior auricular nerve

A 鼓索神経は，舌と軟口蓋に味覚線維を，また顎下神経節でシナプスを形成して顎下腺と舌下腺に分布する分泌神経を運ぶ．

1 図 31.11A, p.478　　2 図 33.11A, p.504

Cranial Nerves VII

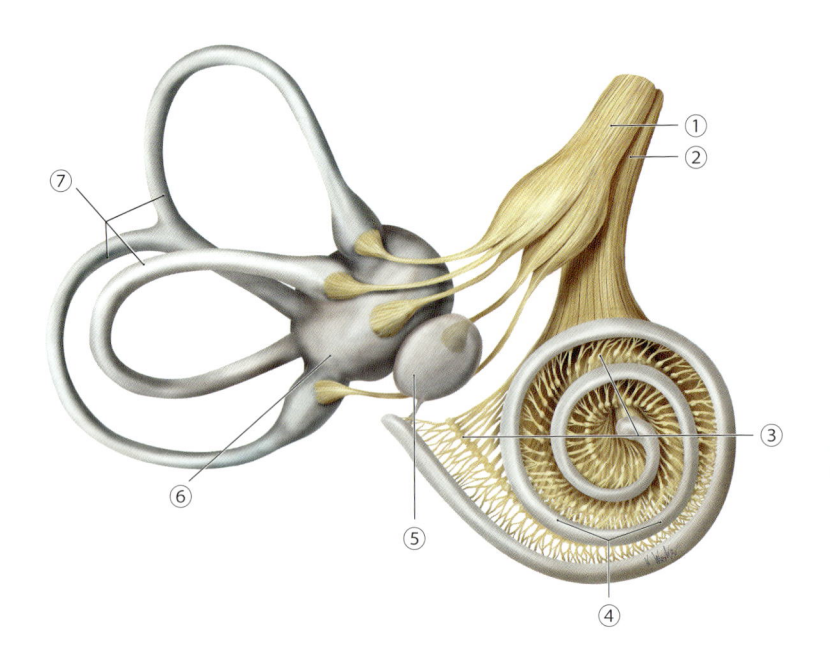

①
②
③
④
⑤
⑥
⑦

Q 内耳神経の前庭神経の損傷による影響は？

脳神経 7

前庭神経節と蝸牛神経節（ラセン神経節）
Vestibular and cochlear (spiral) ganglia

① □ 前庭神経　　　　　□ Vestibular root
② □ 蝸牛神経　　　　　□ Cochlear root
③ □ ラセン神経節　　　□ Spiral ganglia
④ □ 蝸牛　　　　　　　□ Cochlea
⑤ □ 球形嚢　　　　　　□ Saccule
⑥ □ 卵形嚢　　　　　　□ Utricle
⑦ □ 半規管　　　　　　□ Semicircular ducts

A 内耳神経は2つの根からなる特殊体性求心性神経である．前庭神経は骨半規管，球形嚢，卵形嚢からの情報を受け取り，空間内の方向に関する情報を伝える．前庭神経が障害されると眩暈が起こる．蝸牛神経は蝸牛のコルチ器からの情報を伝える．蝸牛神経が障害されると聴覚障害が起こる．

１ 図 31.15. p.481　２ 図 33.15. p.507

Cranial Nerves VIII

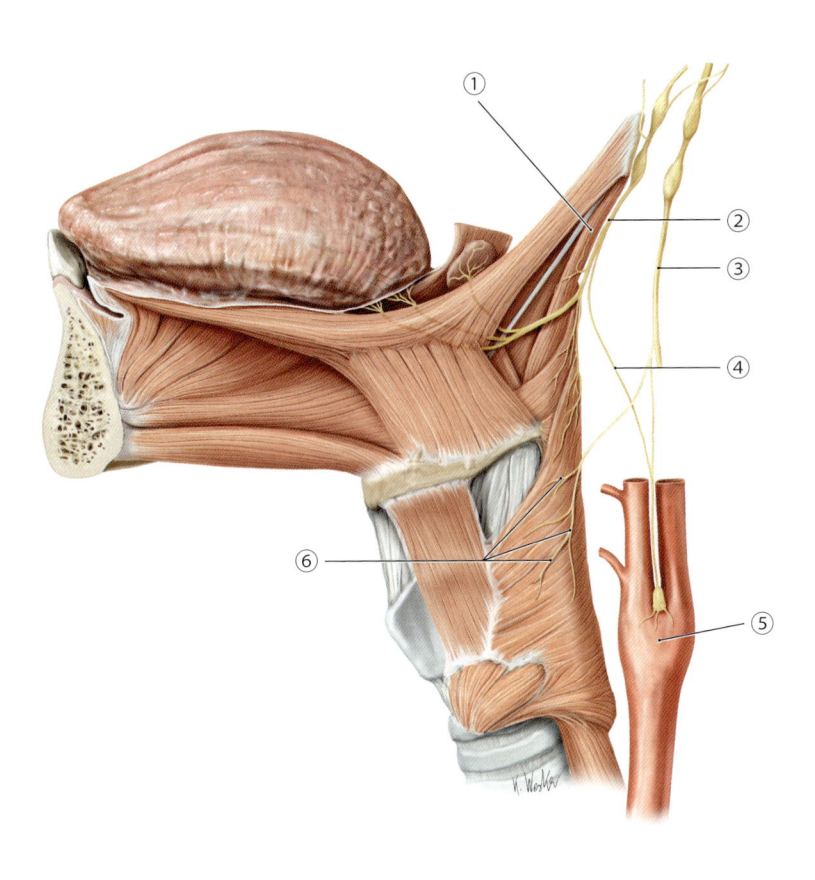

脳神経 8

左外側面

① ☐ 茎突咽頭筋 ☐ Stylopharyngeus
② ☐ 舌咽神経 ☐ Glossopharyngeal nerve (CN IX)
③ ☐ 迷走神経 ☐ Vagus nerve (CN X)
④ ☐ 頸動脈洞枝 ☐ Branch to carotid sinus
⑤ ☐ 頸動脈洞 ☐ Carotid sinus
⑥ ☐ 咽頭神経叢 ☐ Pharyngeal plexus

解説

迷走神経(CN X)の線維と舌咽神経(CN IX)の線維は咽頭神経叢を形成して，頸動脈洞に分布する．

① 図 31.18. p.482　② 図 33.18. p.508

Cranial Nerves IX

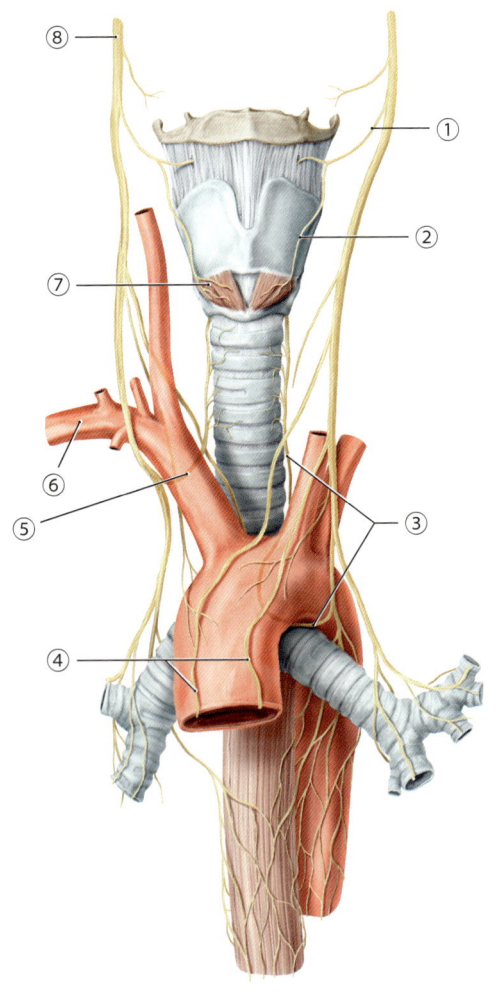

甲状腺の手術の後に嗄声が起こることがあるのはなぜか？

脳神経 9

前面

① ☐ 上喉頭神経 ☐ Superior laryngeal nerve
② ☐ 外枝 ☐ External branch (external laryngeal nerve)
③ ☐ 左反回神経 ☐ Left recurrent laryngeal nerve
④ ☐ 頸心臓枝 ☐ Cervical cardiac branches
⑤ ☐ 右反回神経 ☐ Right recurrent laryngeal nerve
⑥ ☐ 鎖骨下動脈 ☐ Subclavian artery
⑦ ☐ 輪状甲状筋 ☐ Cricothyroid muscle
⑧ ☐ 迷走神経 ☐ Vagus nerve (CN X)

A 反回神経は甲状腺の後面に接している．外科手術時に反回神経の障害によって同側の声帯と喉頭筋が麻痺することがあり，嗄声を引き起こす．

1 図 31.22A. p.485 2 図 33.22A. p.511

572 Head & Neck

Cranial Nerves X

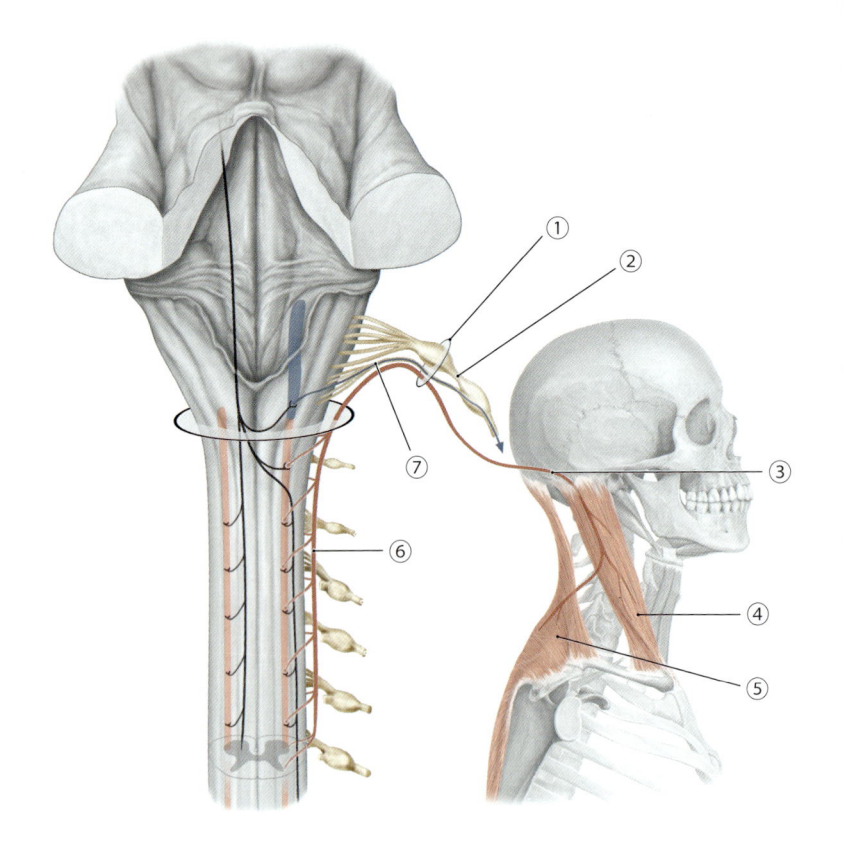

脳神経 10

脳幹の後面

① □ 頸静脈孔　　　　　□ Jugular foramen
② □ 迷走神経　　　　　□ Vagus nerve (CN X)
③ □ 副神経　　　　　　□ (Spinal) accessory nerve
④ □ 胸鎖乳突筋　　　　□ Sternocleidomastoid
⑤ □ 僧帽筋　　　　　　□ Trapezius
⑥ □ 脊髄根　　　　　　□ Spinal root
⑦ □ 延髄根　　　　　　□ Cranial root

解説

伝統的に副神経（CN XI）の延髄根とされてきたものは，現在では迷走神経（CN X）の一部として考えられ，脊髄根と短い距離だけ合流しているが，すぐに分離する．延髄根の線維は迷走神経を介して分配されるが，脊髄根の線維は副神経（CN XI）として伸びていく．

1 図 31.23. p.486　2 図 33.23. p.512

574 Head & Neck

Sensory Innervation

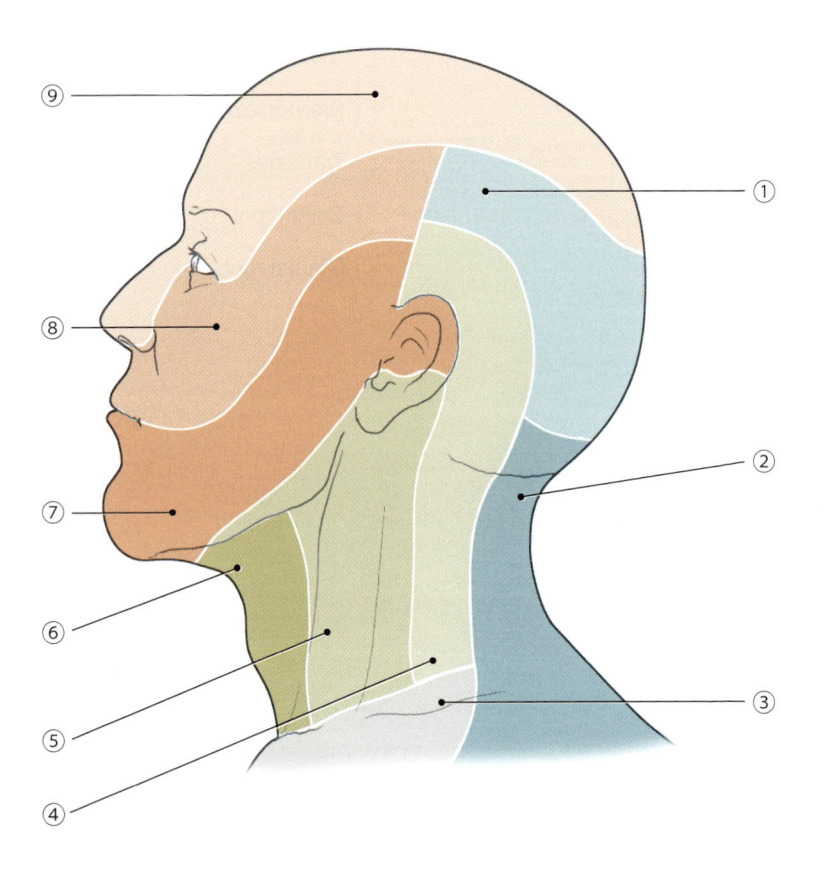

感覚神経支配

左外側面

① ☐ 大後頭神経 — ☐ Greater occipital nerve (C2)

② ☐ 脊髄神経, 後枝 — ☐ Spinal nerves, dorsal rami

③ ☐ 鎖骨上神経 — ☐ Supraclavicular nerves

④ ☐ 小後頭神経 — ☐ Lesser occipital nerve

⑤ ☐ 大耳介神経 — ☐ Great auricular nerve

⑥ ☐ 頸横神経 — ☐ Transverse cervical nerve

⑦ ☐ 三叉神経, 下顎神経 — ☐ Mandibular division of trigeminal nerve

⑧ ☐ 三叉神経, 上顎神経 — ☐ Maxillary division of trigeminal nerve

⑨ ☐ 三叉神経, 眼神経 — ☐ Ophthalmic division of trigeminal nerve

[1] 図 32.2B. p.489　[2] 34.2B. p.515

Arteries of the Skull & Face I

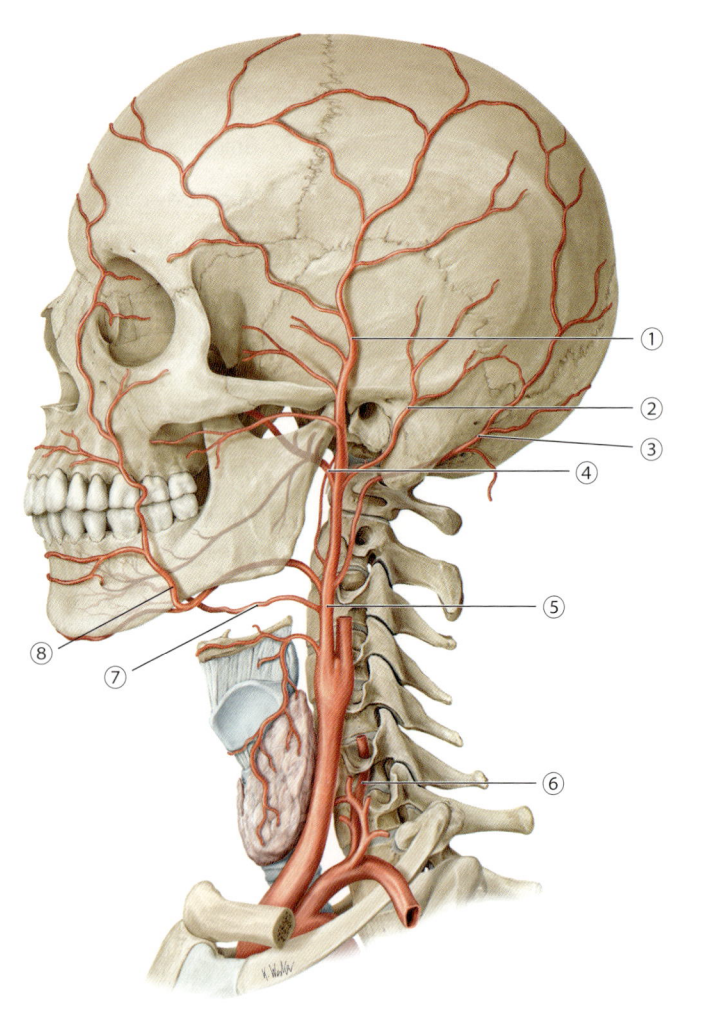

①
②
③
④
⑤
⑥
⑦
⑧

Q 左右どちらかの外頸動脈を結紮すると，顔面の組織にどのような影響が出るか？

頭蓋と顔面の動脈 1

左外側面

① □ 浅側頭動脈　　□ Superficial temporal artery
② □ 後耳介動脈　　□ Posterior auricular artery
③ □ 後頭動脈　　　□ Occipital artery
④ □ 顎動脈　　　　□ Maxillary artery
⑤ □ 外頸動脈　　　□ External carotid artery
⑥ □ 椎骨動脈　　　□ Vertebral artery
⑦ □ 舌動脈　　　　□ Lingual artery
⑧ □ 顔面動脈　　　□ Facial artery

A 左右の外頸動脈の枝の間には吻合が多数あるため，片方の外頸動脈を結紮しても顔面の組織の血液供給にはほとんど影響はない．さらに，特に眼窩と鼻腔には外頸動脈と内頸動脈の間の吻合路がある．

1 図 32.4B. p.491　2 図 34.4B. p.517

Arteries of the Skull & Face II

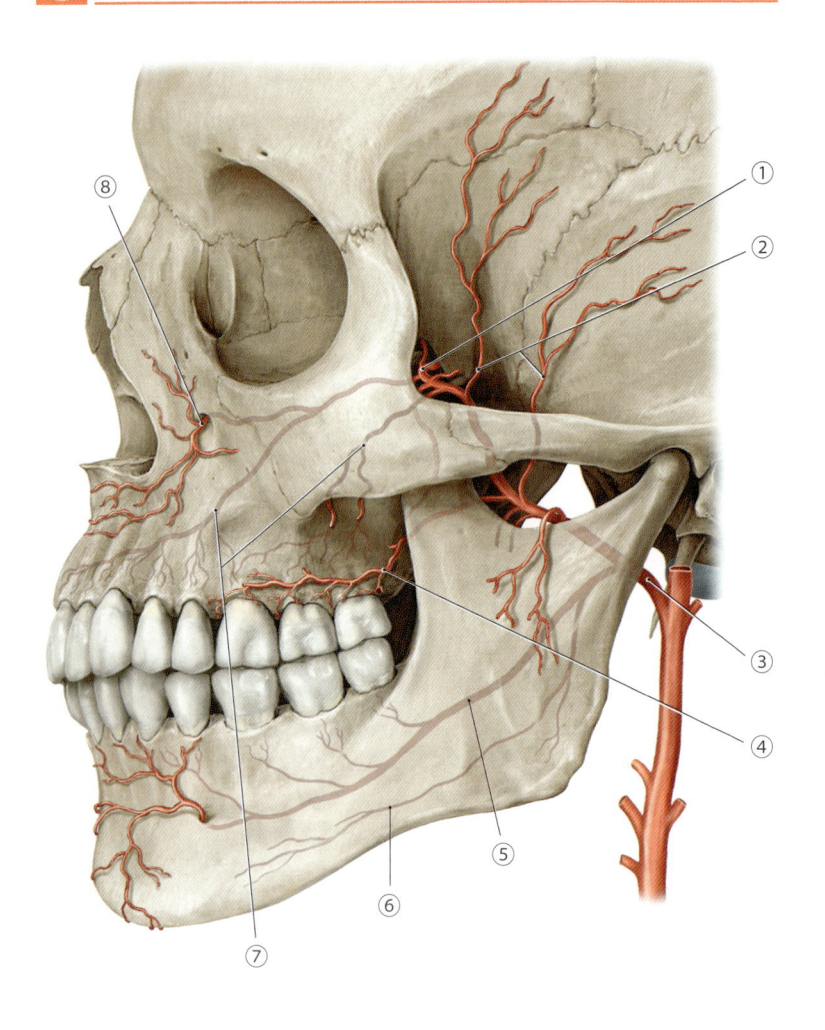

Q 頭蓋のプテリオンの外傷が特に危険であるのはなぜか？

頭蓋と顔面の動脈 2

左外側面

① ☐ 蝶口蓋動脈　　☐ Sphenopalatine artery
② ☐ 深側頭動脈　　☐ Deep temporal arteries
③ ☐ 顎動脈　　☐ Maxillary artery
④ ☐ 頬動脈　　☐ Buccal artery
⑤ ☐ 下歯槽動脈　　☐ Inferior alveolar artery
⑥ ☐ 顎舌骨筋枝　　☐ Mylohyoid branch
⑦ ☐ 前・後上歯槽動脈　　☐ Anterior and posterior superior alveolar arteries
⑧ ☐ 眼窩下動脈　　☐ Infraorbital artery

A　顎動脈の枝の1つである中硬膜動脈は，髄膜とその上にある頭蓋冠に分布し，プテリオンの領域の内側面を通過する．一般に外傷によって動脈が破裂すると硬膜外血腫が生じる．

1 図32.8B. p.495　2 図34.8B. p.521

Veins of the Head & Neck I

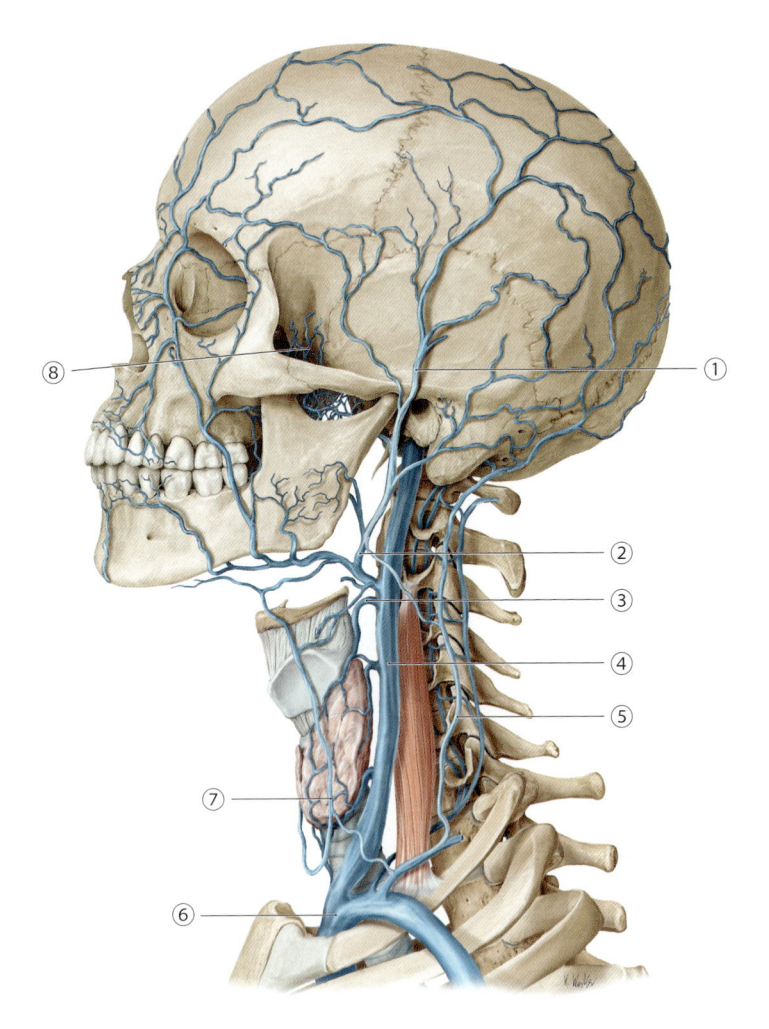

頭頸部の３本の主要な浅静脈は何か？

頭頸部の静脈 1

左外側面

① □ 浅側頭静脈　　　　　□ Superficial temporal vein
② □ 下顎後静脈　　　　　□ Retromandibular vein
③ □ 上甲状腺静脈　　　　□ Superior thyroid vein
④ □ 内頸静脈　　　　　　□ Internal jugular vein
⑤ □ 外頸静脈　　　　　　□ External jugular vein
⑥ □ 左腕頭静脈　　　　　□ Left brachiocephalic vein
⑦ □ 前頸静脈　　　　　　□ Anterior jugular vein
⑧ □ 翼突筋静脈叢（深側頭静脈）　□ Pterygoid plexus (deep temporal veins)

A 　内頸静脈，外頸静脈，前頸静脈．これらの浅静脈は頭頸部から腕頭静脈へと注ぐ．

1 図 32.9B. p.496　　2 図 34.9B. p.522

Veins of the Head & Neck II

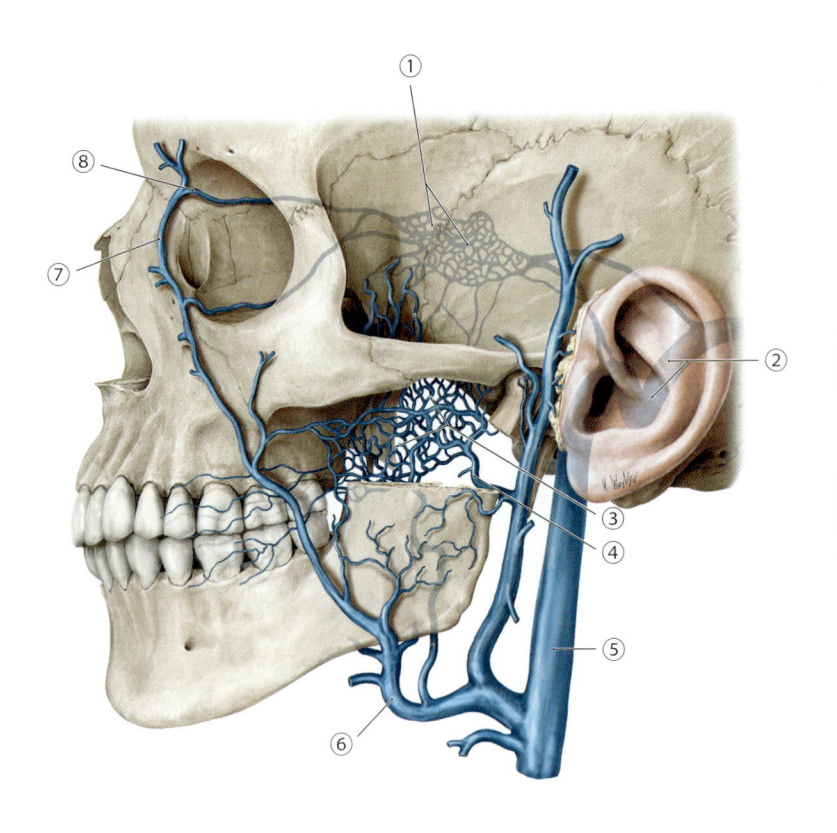

頭頸部の静脈 2

左外側面

① □ 海綿静脈洞　　　　　□ Cavernous sinus

② □ S状静脈洞　　　　　□ Sigmoid sinus

③ □ 翼突筋静脈叢　　　　□ Pterygoid plexus

④ □ 顎静脈　　　　　　　□ Maxillary vein

⑤ □ 内頸静脈　　　　　　□ Internal jugular vein

⑥ □ 顔面静脈　　　　　　□ Facial vein

⑦ □ 眼角静脈　　　　　　□ Angular vein

⑧ □ 上眼静脈　　　　　　□ Superior ophthalmic vein

解説

翼突筋静脈叢は下顎枝と咀嚼筋の間にある静脈網である．海綿静脈洞は顔面静脈の枝をS状静脈洞に連絡する．

[1] 図 32.10. p.497　[2] 図 34.10. p.523

Superficial Neurovasculature I

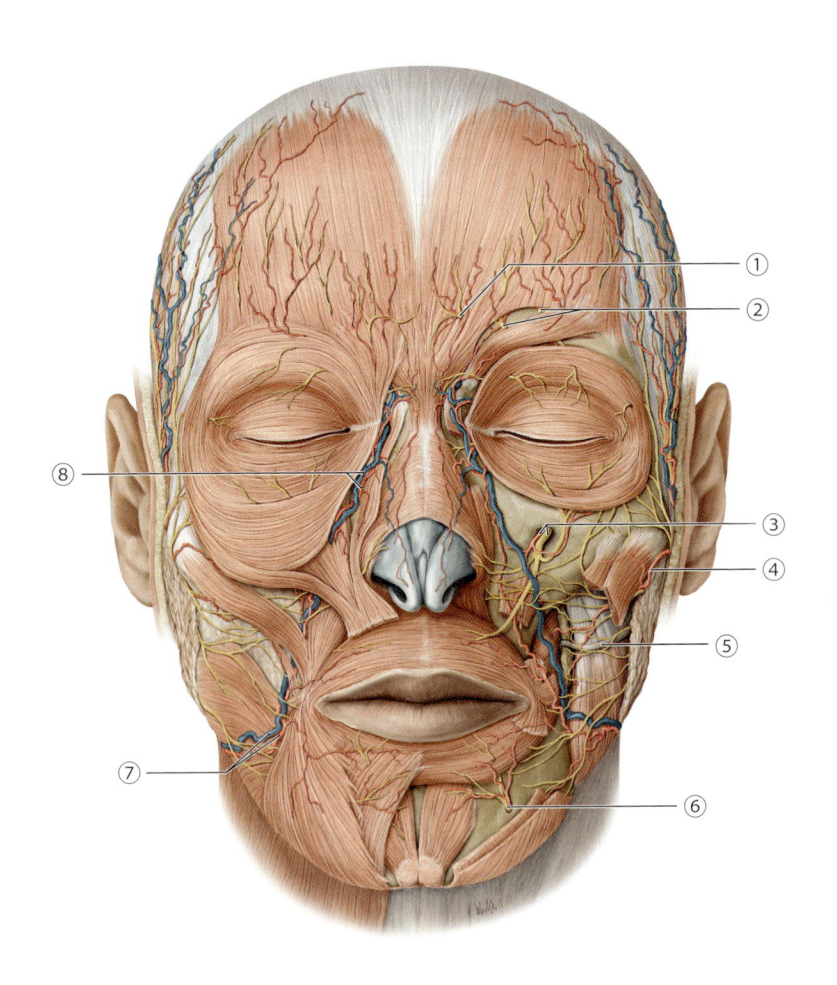

鼻根と左右の唇交連によってできる三角形の領域の血管系に潜在的に存在する危険性は何か？

顔面浅層の神経・血管 1

前面

① ☐ 滑車上神経 ☐ Supratrochlear nerve

② ☐ 眼窩上神経, 内・外側枝 ☐ Supraorbital nerve, medial and lateral branches

③ ☐ 眼窩下動脈・神経（眼窩下孔にある） ☐ Infraorbital artery and nerve (in infraorbital foramen)

④ ☐ 顔面横動脈 ☐ Transverse facial artery

⑤ ☐ 耳下腺管 ☐ Parotid duct

⑥ ☐ オトガイ神経（オトガイ孔にある） ☐ Mental nerve (in mental foramen)

⑦ ☐ 顔面動脈・静脈 ☐ Facial artery and vein

⑧ ☐ 眼角動脈・静脈 ☐ Angular artery and vein

A この領域は顔面の静脈と硬膜静脈洞との連絡部位を含む．この領域の静脈には弁がないので，顔面領域の細菌感染が頭蓋腔内にまで広がる危険性が高い．

1 図 32.12. p.498 2 図 34.20. p.528

Superficial Neurovasculature II

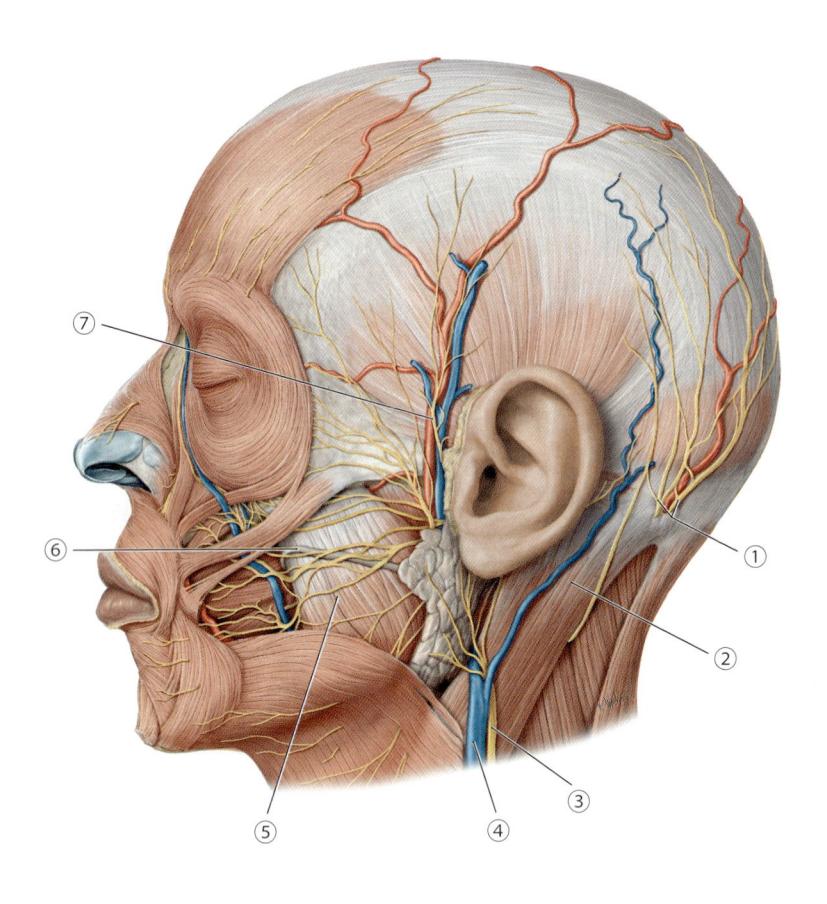

顔面浅層の神経・血管 2

左外側面

① □ 大後頭神経　　　□ Greater occipital nerve
② □ 胸鎖乳突筋　　　□ Sternocleidomastoid
③ □ 大耳介神経　　　□ Great auricular nerve
④ □ 外頸静脈　　　　□ External jugular vein
⑤ □ 咬筋　　　　　　□ Masseter
⑥ □ 耳下腺管　　　　□ Parotid duct
⑦ □ 耳介側頭神経　　□ Auriculotemporal nerve

1 図 32.13. p.499　2 図 34.21. p.529

Parotid Region I

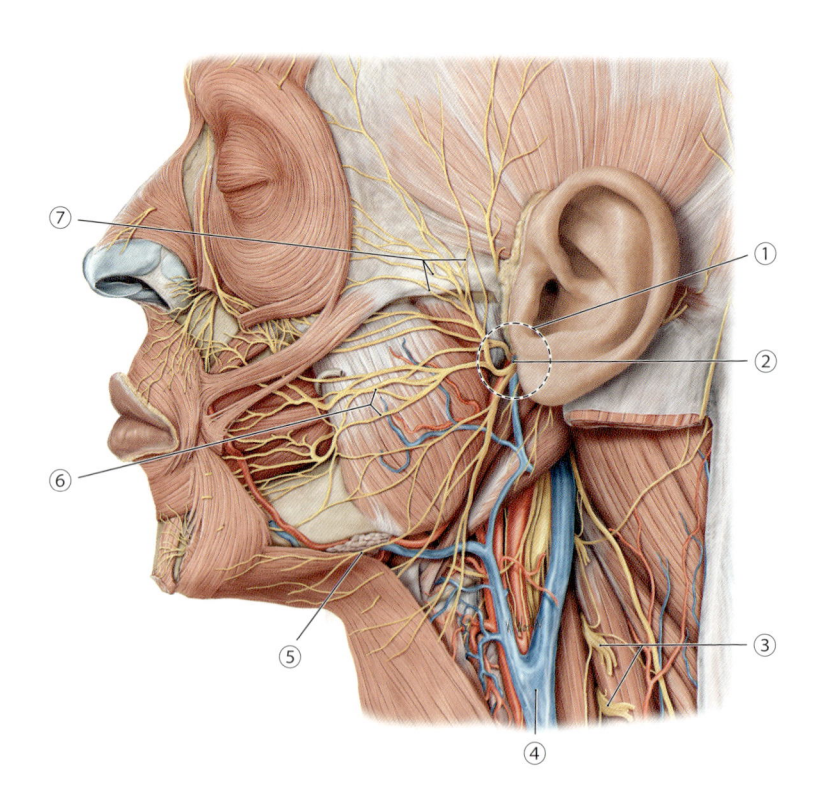

顔面神経が頭蓋外に出るときに通過する孔は何か？

耳下腺咬筋部 1

左外側面

① ☐ 顔面神経の耳下腺神経叢 ☐ Parotid plexus of facial nerve (CN VII)

② ☐ 顔面神経 ☐ Facial nerve (CN VII)

③ ☐ 頸神経叢 ☐ Cervical plexus

④ ☐ 内頸静脈 ☐ Internal jugular vein

⑤ ☐ 顔面神経，下顎縁枝 ☐ Facial nerve, marginal mandibular branch

⑥ ☐ 顔面神経，頬筋枝 ☐ Facial nerve, buccal branches

⑦ ☐ 顔面神経，側頭枝 ☐ Facial nerve, temporal branches

A 顔面神経は茎乳突孔から頭蓋外に出る．

1 図 32.14. p.500　2 図 34.22. p.530

Parotid Region II

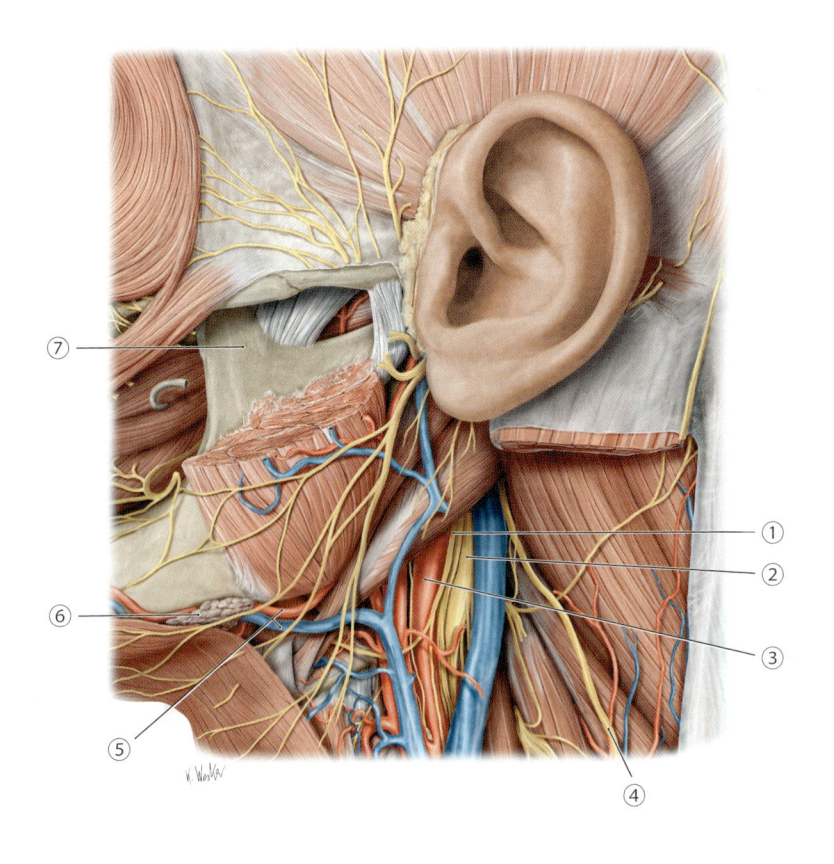

耳下腺咬筋部 2

左外側面

① ☐ 舌下神経　　　　　　　☐ Hypoglossal nerve
② ☐ 上頸神経節　　　　　　☐ Superior cervical ganglion
③ ☐ 内頸動脈　　　　　　　☐ Internal carotid artery
④ ☐ 副神経　　　　　　　　☐ Accessory nerve
⑤ ☐ 顔面動脈・静脈　　　　☐ Facial artery and vein
⑥ ☐ 顎下腺　　　　　　　　☐ Submandibular gland
⑦ ☐ 筋突起　　　　　　　　☐ Coronoid process

Infratemporal Fossa I

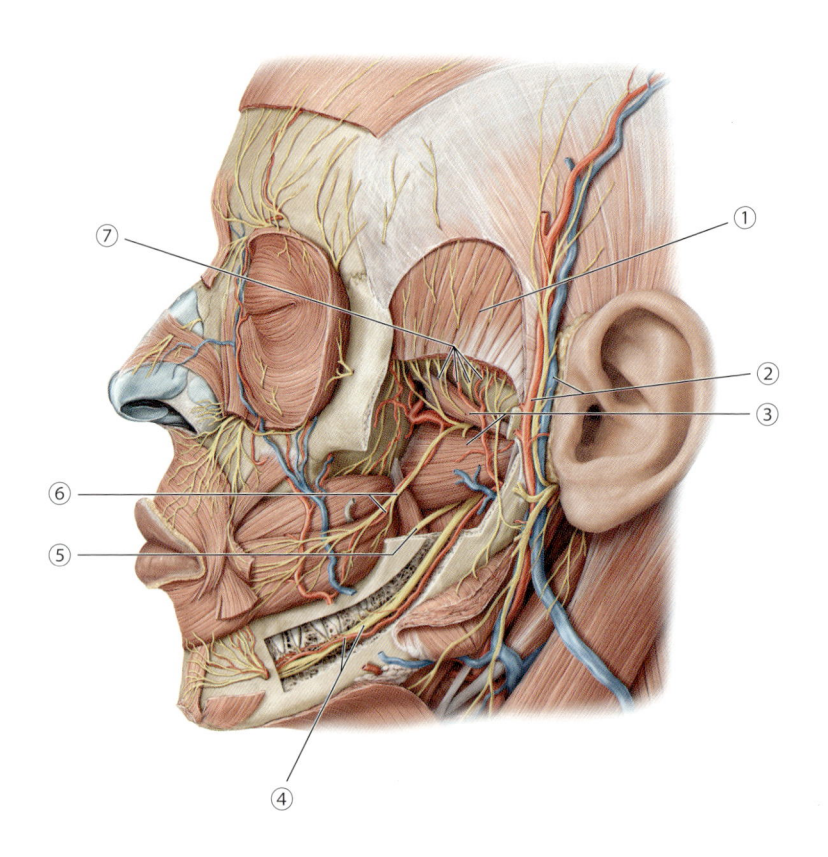

外側翼突筋の機能は何か？

側頭下窩 1

左外側面

① □ 側頭筋 □ Temporalis
② □ 浅側頭動脈・静脈 □ Superficial temporal artery and vein
③ □ 外側翼突筋 □ Lateral pterygoid
④ □ 下歯槽動脈・神経（下顎管にある） □ Inferior alveolar artery and nerve (in mandibular canal)
⑤ □ 舌神経 □ Lingual nerve
⑥ □ 頬動脈・神経 □ Buccal artery and nerve
⑦ □ 深側頭動脈・神経 □ Deep temporal arteries and nerves

A 外側翼突筋は，両側が収縮したときには下顎を前方に突き出し，片側のみが収縮したときには咀嚼時に下顎を横方向に動かす．

[1] 図 32.16. p.502　[2] 図 34.24. p.532

Infratemporal Fossa II

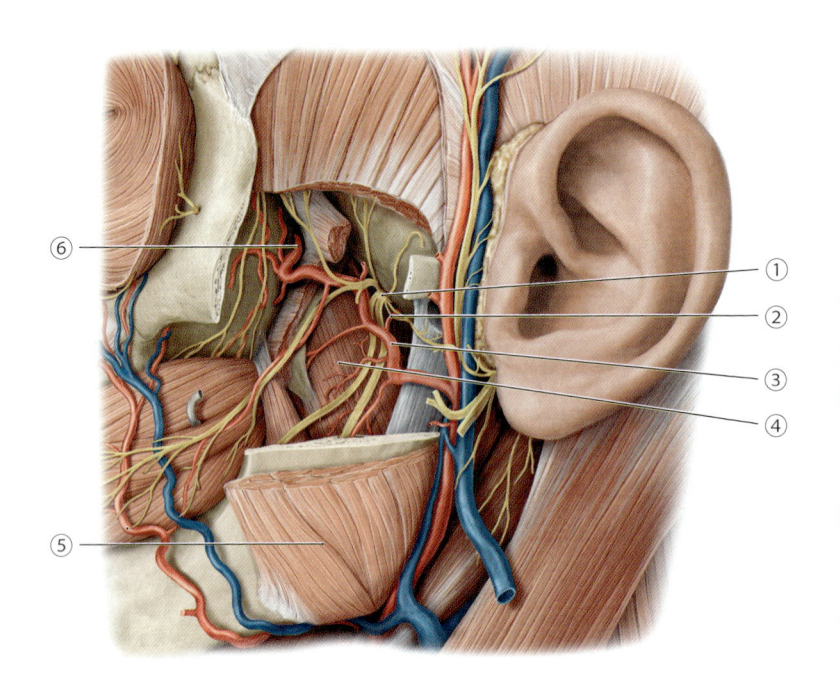

側頭下窩にある主要な神経と動脈は何か？

側頭下窩 2

左外側面

① □ 下顎神経 □ Mandibular nerve (CN V$_3$)
② □ 中硬膜動脈 □ Middle meningeal artery
③ □ 顎動脈 □ Maxillary artery
④ □ 内側翼突筋 □ Medial pterygoid
⑤ □ 咬筋 □ Masseter
⑥ □ 蝶口蓋動脈 □ Sphenopalatine artery

A 側頭下窩には下顎神経があり，側頭部の深部の筋と咀嚼筋に分布する．外頸動脈の枝である顎動脈は側頭下窩を横断する間に，側頭部の深部と下部の筋肉や口腔と下顎の諸構造に枝を出す．

1 図 32.17. p.503 2 図 34.25. p.533

Infratemporal Fossa III

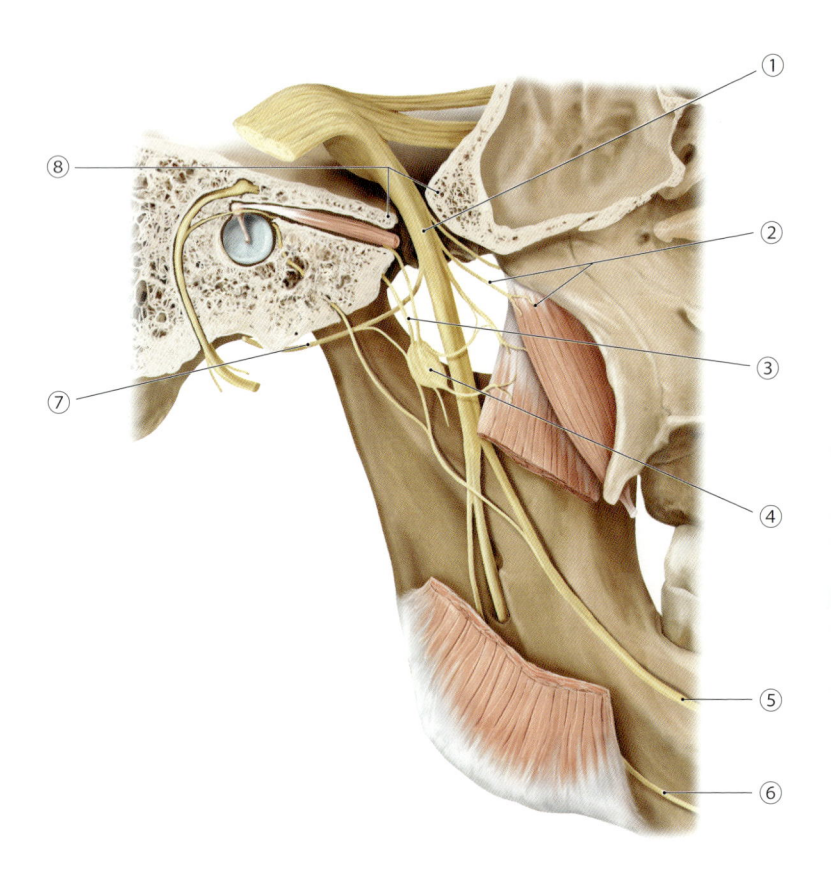

Q 耳神経節でシナプスを形成する副交感神経性の節後線維はどこに分布するか？

側頭下窩 3

内側面

① ☐ 下顎神経 — ☐ Mandibular division (CN V$_3$)

② ☐ 口蓋帆張筋神経と口蓋帆張筋 — ☐ Nerve of tensor veli palatini (with muscle)

③ ☐ 小錐体神経 — ☐ Lesser petrosal nerve

④ ☐ 耳神経節 — ☐ Otic ganglion

⑤ ☐ 舌神経 — ☐ Lingual nerve

⑥ ☐ 顎舌骨筋神経 — ☐ Mylohyoid nerve

⑦ ☐ 耳介側頭神経 — ☐ Auriculotemporal nerve

⑧ ☐ 卵円孔 — ☐ Foramen ovale

A 耳神経節でシナプスを形成した副交感神経性の節後線維は耳下腺に分布する.

1 図 32.18B. p.503　2 図 34.26B. p.533

Pterygopalatine Fossa

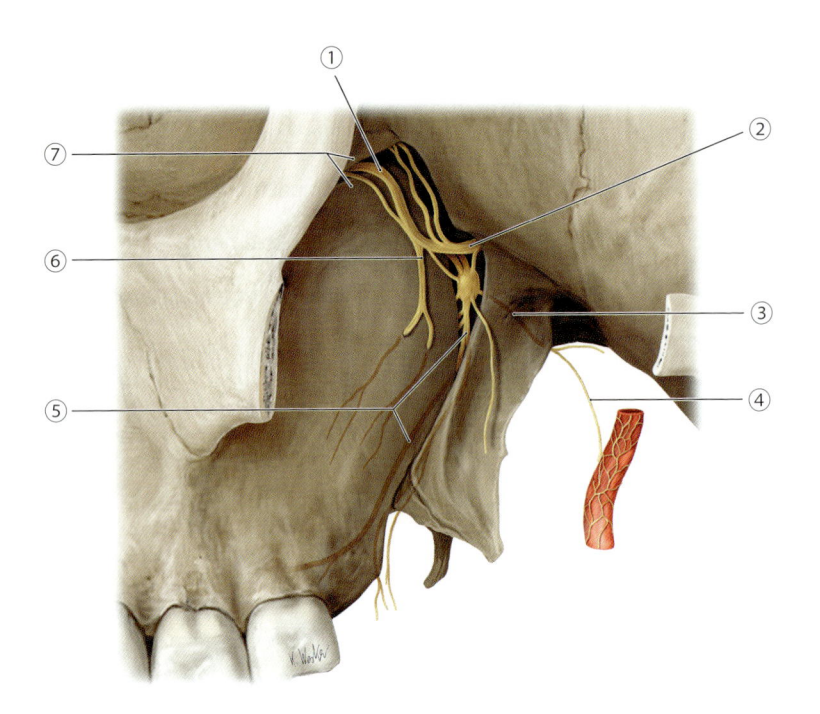

翼口蓋窩

左外側面

① ☐ 眼窩下神経 — ☐ Infraorbital nerve

② ☐ 上顎神経 — ☐ Maxillary nerve

③ ☐ 翼突管神経（大錐体神経，深錐体神経） — ☐ Nerve of pterygoid canal (greater and deep petrosal nerves)

④ ☐ 深錐体神経 — ☐ Deep petrosal nerve

⑤ ☐ 大口蓋神経 — ☐ Greater palatine nerve

⑥ ☐ 上歯槽神経，後上歯槽枝 — ☐ Superior alveolar nerves, posterior superior alveolar branches

⑦ ☐ 下眼窩裂 — ☐ Inferior orbital fissure

解説

小さなピラミッド状の翼口蓋窩は上顎神経やその枝などの中頭蓋窩，眼窩，鼻腔，口腔を進む神経・血管が交差する場所である．深錐体神経の交感性線維はシナプスを形成せずに翼口蓋窩を通過するが，大錐体神経の副交感性線維は翼口蓋神経節でシナプスを形成する．

1 図 32.20. p.505 2 図 34.28. p.535

Bones of the Orbit

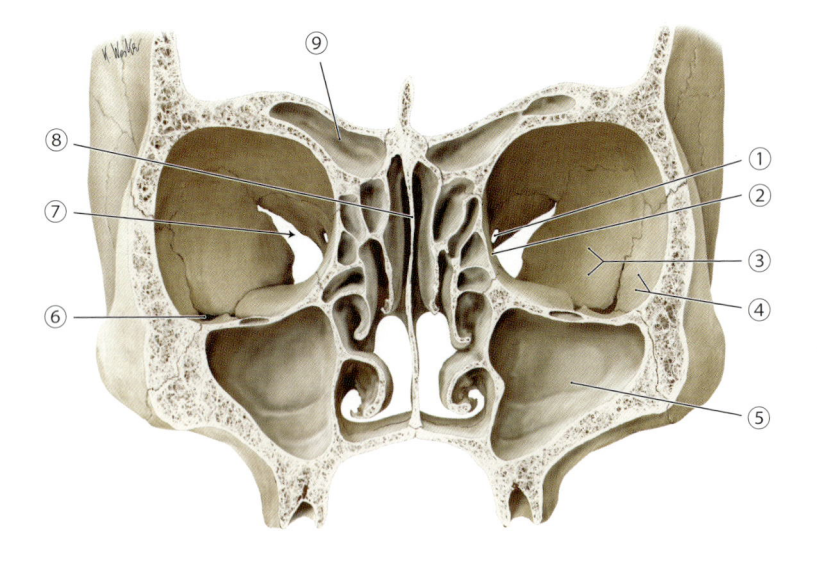

眼窩の骨

冠状断面，前面

① □ 視神経管　　　　　　　　□ Optic canal
② □ 篩骨，眼窩板（紙様板）　　□ Ethmoid bone, orbital plate (lamina papyracea)
③ □ 蝶形骨，大翼　　　　　　□ Sphenoid bone, greater wing
④ □ 頬骨，眼窩面　　　　　　□ Zygomatic bone, orbital surface
⑤ □ 上顎洞　　　　　　　　　□ Maxillary sinus
⑥ □ 下眼窩裂　　　　　　　　□ Inferior orbital fissure
⑦ □ 上眼窩裂　　　　　　　　□ Superior orbital fissure
⑧ □ 篩骨，垂直板　　　　　　□ Ethmoid bone, perpendicular plate
⑨ □ 前頭洞　　　　　　　　　□ Frontal sinus

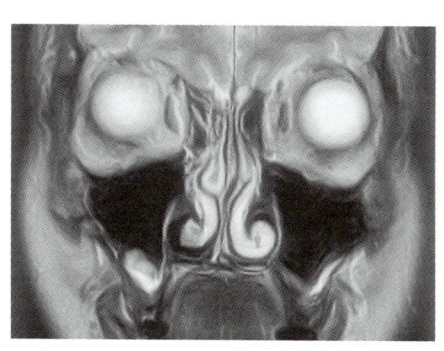

副鼻腔の MR 像

1 図 33.1D，図 34.5C. p.507, 523　2 図 36.5A, C. p.553

Muscles of the Orbit

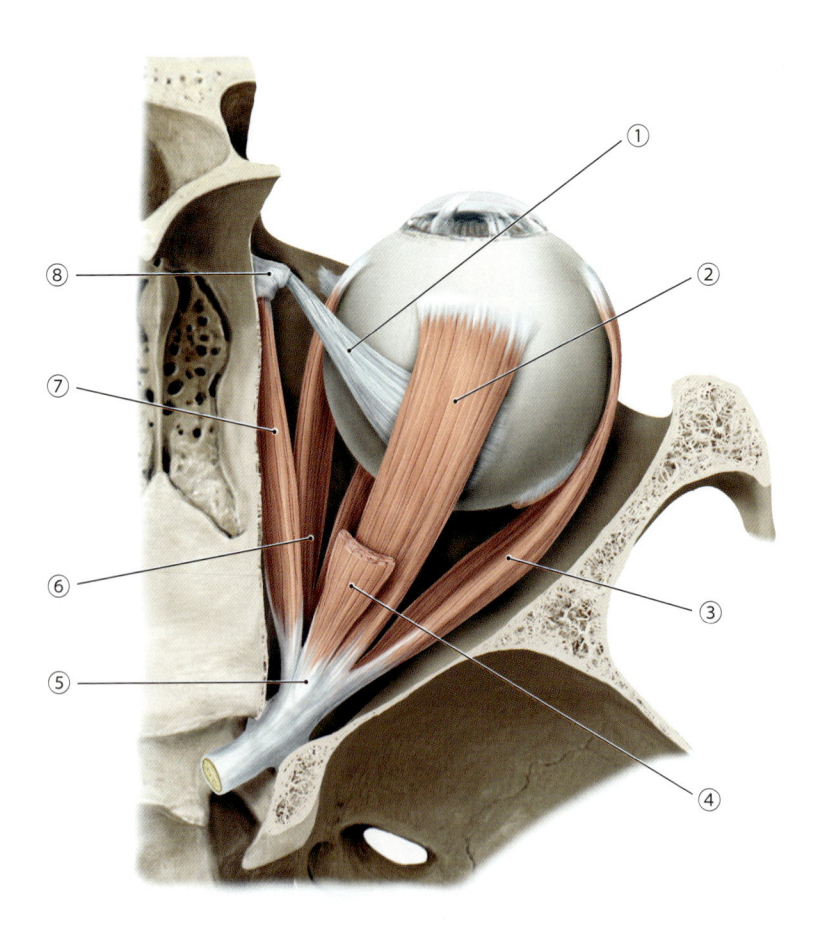

Q 上右方の視野にある対象を見るときに，眼球を回転させる外眼筋は何か？

眼窩の筋

開かれた眼窩,上面

① □ 上斜筋(腱)　　　　　　□ Tendon of superior oblique
② □ 上直筋　　　　　　　　□ Superior rectus
③ □ 外側直筋　　　　　　　□ Lateral rectus
④ □ 上眼瞼挙筋　　　　　　□ Levator palpebrae superioris
⑤ □ 総腱輪　　　　　　　　□ Common tendinous ring
⑥ □ 内側直筋　　　　　　　□ Medial rectus
⑦ □ 上斜筋　　　　　　　　□ Superior oblique
⑧ □ 滑車　　　　　　　　　□ Trochlea

A 上右方の視野を見るときには,右の下斜筋と左の上直筋が働く.

1 図 33.2B. p.508　2 図 35.2B. p.538

Nerves of the Orbit I

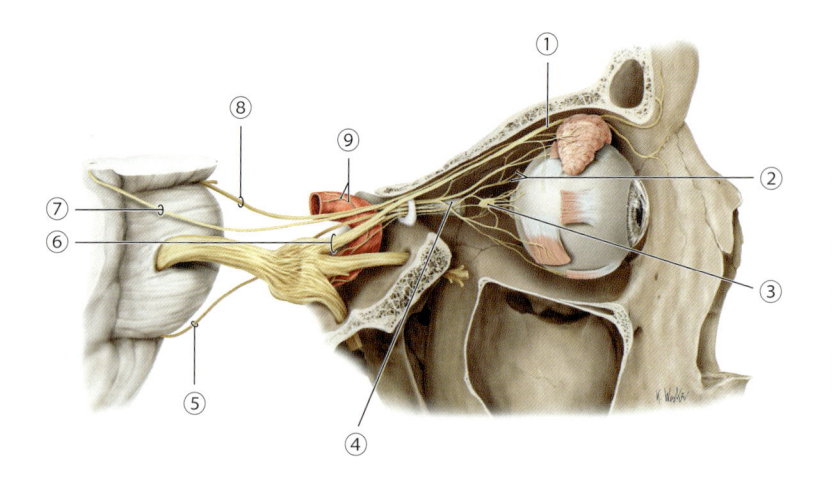

Q 瞳孔の光反射に関わる神経は何か？

眼窩の神経 1

右眼窩，外側面

① □ 前頭神経 □ Frontal nerve
② □ 長毛様体神経 □ Long ciliary nerves
③ □ 毛様体神経節 □ Ciliary ganglion
④ □ 視神経 □ Optic nerve (CN II)
⑤ □ 外転神経 □ Abducent nerve (CN VI)
⑥ □ 眼神経 □ Ophthalmic division (CN V_1)
⑦ □ 滑車神経 □ Trochlear nerve (CN IV)
⑧ □ 動眼神経 □ Oculomotor nerve (CN III)
⑨ □ 内頸動脈と内頸動脈神経叢 □ Internal carotid artery with internal carotid plexus

A 光が入ったときに瞳孔を急速に小さくする反射には，視神経（CN II）が求心性神経，動眼神経（CN III）が遠心性神経として関与する．

1 図 33.7. p.511　2 図 35.8. p.541

Nerves of the Orbit II

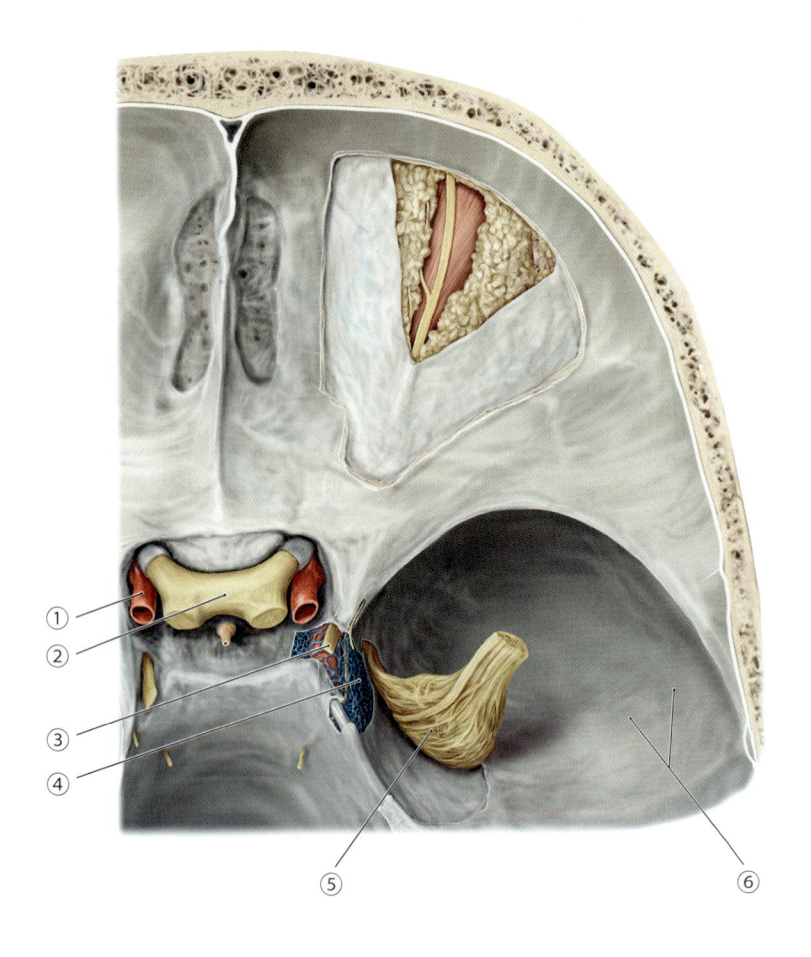

眼窩の神経 2

右側，上面

① □ 内頸動脈　　　　　　　　□ Internal carotid artery
② □ 視交叉（視神経）　　　　□ Optic chiasm (optic nerve, CN II)
③ □ 動眼神経　　　　　　　　□ Oculomotor nerve (CN III)
④ □ 海綿静脈洞　　　　　　　□ Cavernous sinus
⑤ □ 三叉神経節　　　　　　　□ Trigeminal ganglion
⑥ □ 中頭蓋窩　　　　　　　　□ Middle cranial fossa

臨床

眼窩に入る視神経以外の脳神経は，海綿静脈洞を通過する．動眼神経・滑車神経・眼神経は海綿静脈洞の外壁に沿うが，外転神経は内頸動脈に接近しながら海綿静脈洞の中心を通るので，海綿静脈洞内動脈瘤の影響を受ける恐れがある．

1 図 33.8. p.511　2 図 35.9. p.541

Topography of the Orbit I

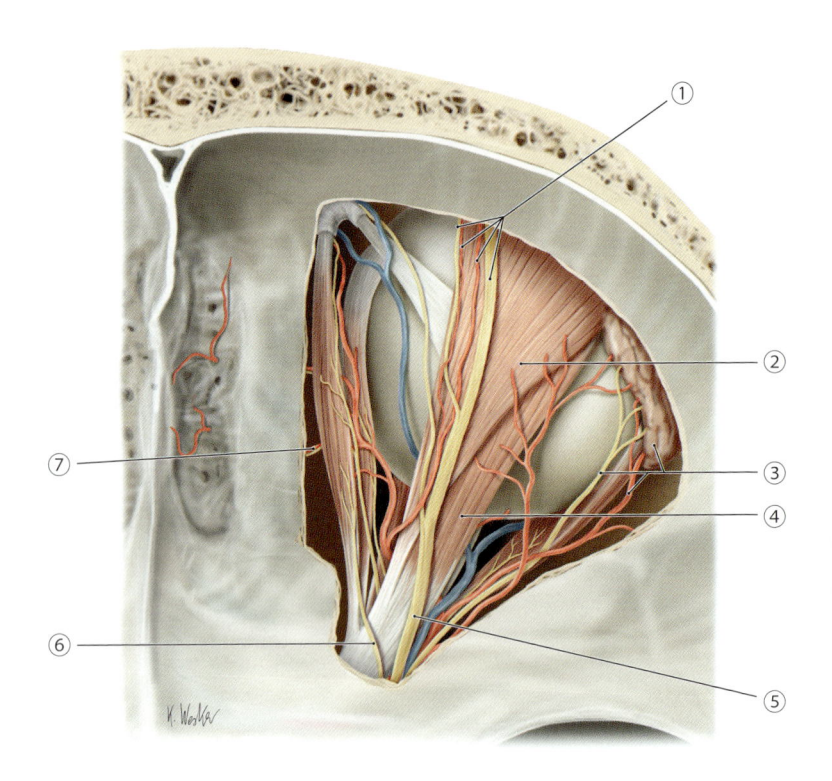

①
②
③
④
⑤
⑥
⑦

Q 上眼瞼挙筋の機能と支配神経は何か？

眼窩の局所解剖 1

上面

① □ 眼窩上動脈・神経　　　□ Supraorbital arteries and nerves

② □ 上眼瞼挙筋　　　□ Levator palpebrae superioris

③ □ 涙腺動脈・神経と涙腺　　　□ Lacrimal artery and nerve (with gland)

④ □ 上直筋　　　□ Superior rectus

⑤ □ 前頭神経　　　□ Frontal nerve

⑥ □ 滑車神経　　　□ Trochlear nerve (CN IV)

⑦ □ 後篩骨動脈・神経　　　□ Posterior ethmoidal artery and nerve

A 　上眼瞼挙筋は上眼瞼を挙上し，動眼神経によって支配される．下面の平滑筋線維は交感神経性の刺激にも反応する．

1 図 33.11A. p.513　2 図 35.12A. p.543

Topography of the Orbit II

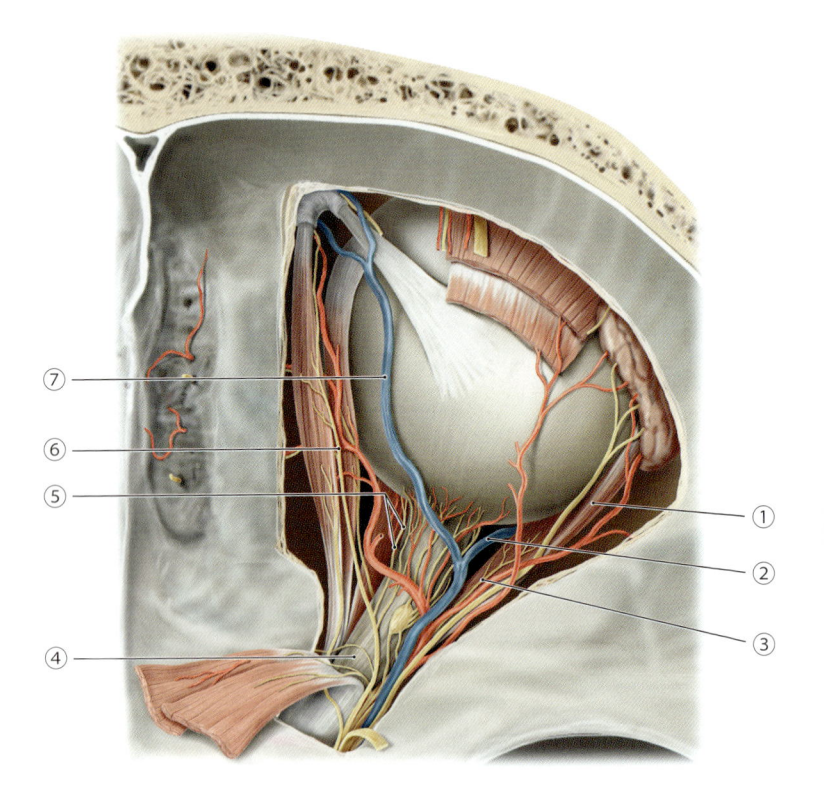

眼窩の局所解剖 2

右側，上面

①	☐ 外側直筋	☐ Lateral rectus
②	☐ 下眼静脈	☐ Inferior ophthalmic vein
③	☐ 外転神経	☐ Abducent nerve (CN VI)
④	☐ 視神経	☐ Optic nerve (CN II)
⑤	☐ 長毛様体神経	☐ Long ciliary nerves
⑥	☐ 鼻毛様体神経	☐ Nasociliary nerve
⑦	☐ 上眼静脈	☐ Superior ophthalmic vein

[1] 図 33.11B. p.513　[2] 図 35.12B. p.543

Eyelid & Conjunctiva

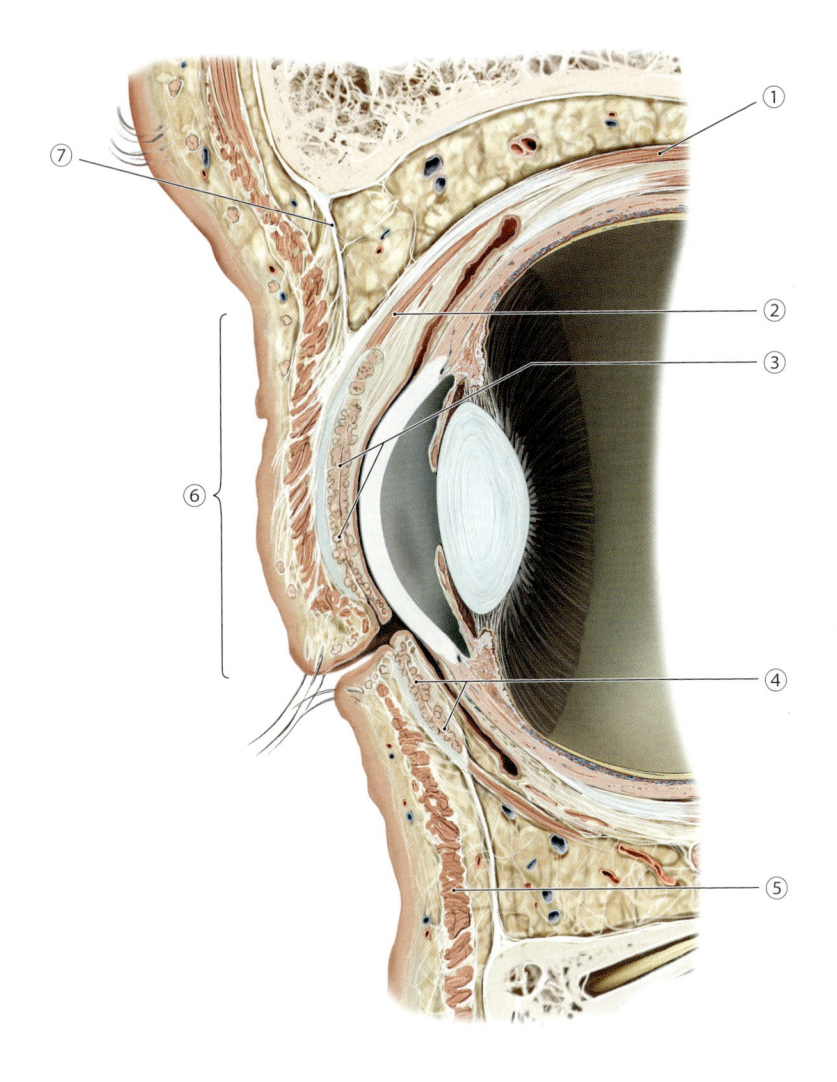

眼瞼と結膜

矢状断面

① □ 上眼瞼挙筋 □ Levator palpebrae superioris
② □ 上瞼板筋 □ Superior tarsal muscle
③ □ 上瞼板と瞼板腺（マイボーム腺） □ Superior tarsus (with tarsal glands)
④ □ 下瞼板 □ Inferior tarsus
⑤ □ 眼輪筋, 眼瞼部 □ Orbicularis oculi, palpebral part
⑥ □ 上眼瞼 □ Upper eyelid
⑦ □ 眼窩隔膜 □ Orbital septum

臨床

閉経後の女性は涙腺での涙液産生不足のため，しばしば慢性的にドライアイ（乾性角結膜炎）になる．（細菌による）急性の涙腺炎症は一般的ではないが，激しい炎症を起こし，触診するときわめて柔らかいのが特徴である．上眼瞼は特徴的なS字カーブを描く．

[1] 図 33.13. p.514   [2] 図 35.14. p.544

Lacrimal Apparatus

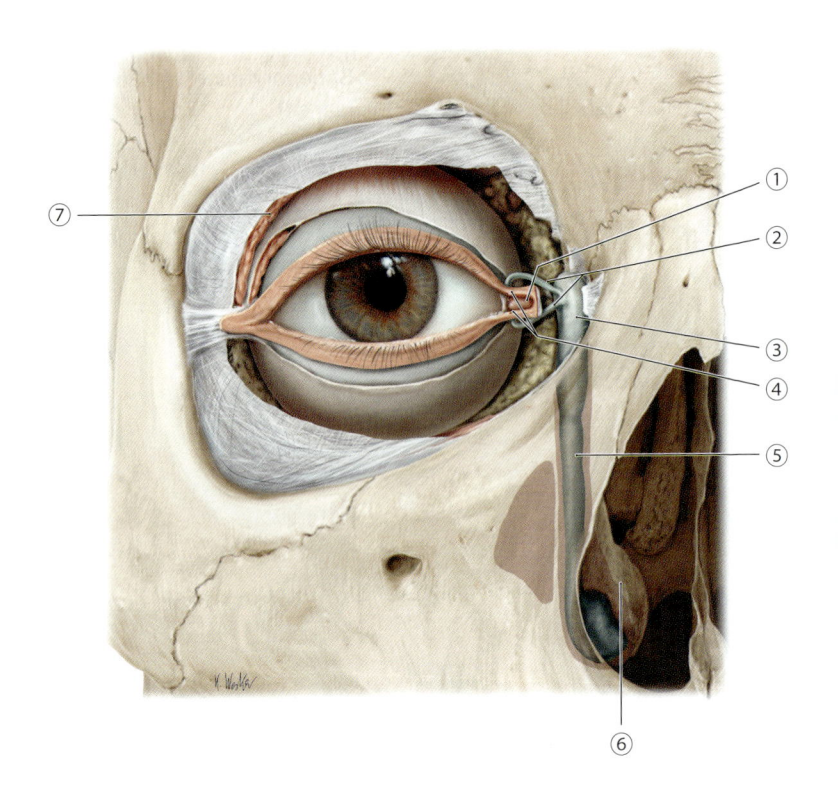

涙腺の支配神経は何か？

涙器

前面

① □ 涙丘 — □ Lacrimal caruncle
② □ 上・下涙小管 — □ Superior and inferior lacrimal canaliculi
③ □ 涙嚢 — □ Lacrimal sac
④ □ 上・下涙点 — □ Superior and inferior puncta
⑤ □ 鼻涙管 — □ Nasolacrimal duct
⑥ □ 下鼻甲介 — □ Inferior nasal concha
⑦ □ 涙腺，眼窩部 — □ Lacrimal gland, orbital part

A 節前線維は顔面神経から起こり，大錐体神経を通って翼口蓋神経節でシナプスを形成する．節後線維は上顎神経を通って涙腺に至る．

Structure of the Eyeball

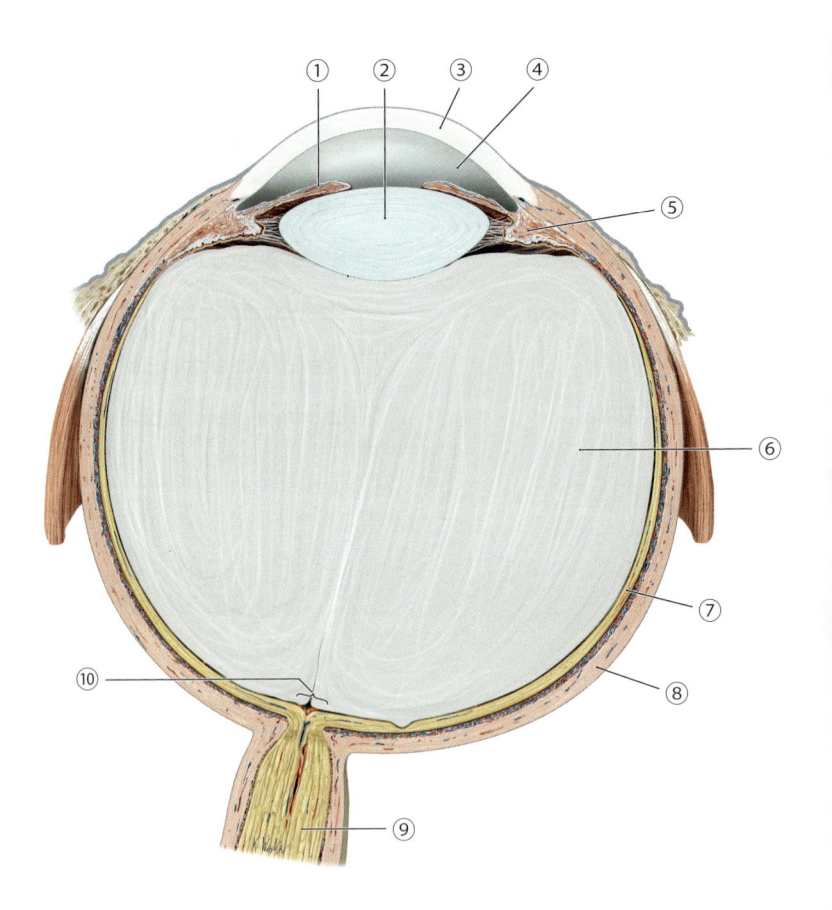

Q 緑内障とは何か？

眼球の構造

上面

① ☐ 虹彩 ☐ Iris
② ☐ 水晶体 ☐ Lens
③ ☐ 角膜 ☐ Cornea
④ ☐ 前眼房 ☐ Anterior chamber
⑤ ☐ 毛様体，毛様体筋 ☐ Ciliary body, ciliary muscle
⑥ ☐ 硝子体 ☐ Vitreous body
⑦ ☐ 網膜 ☐ Retina
⑧ ☐ 強膜 ☐ Sclera
⑨ ☐ 視神経 ☐ Optic nerve (CN II)
⑩ ☐ 視神経乳頭（視神経円板） ☐ Optic disk

A 　前眼房での眼房水の産生および排出の障害によって起こる眼内圧亢進状態を緑内障という．亢進した圧は眼球の強膜に付着するところで視神経を圧迫することがあり，失明する場合もある．

[1] 図 33.15. p.516　　[2] 図 35.16. p.546

Bones of the Nasal Cavity I

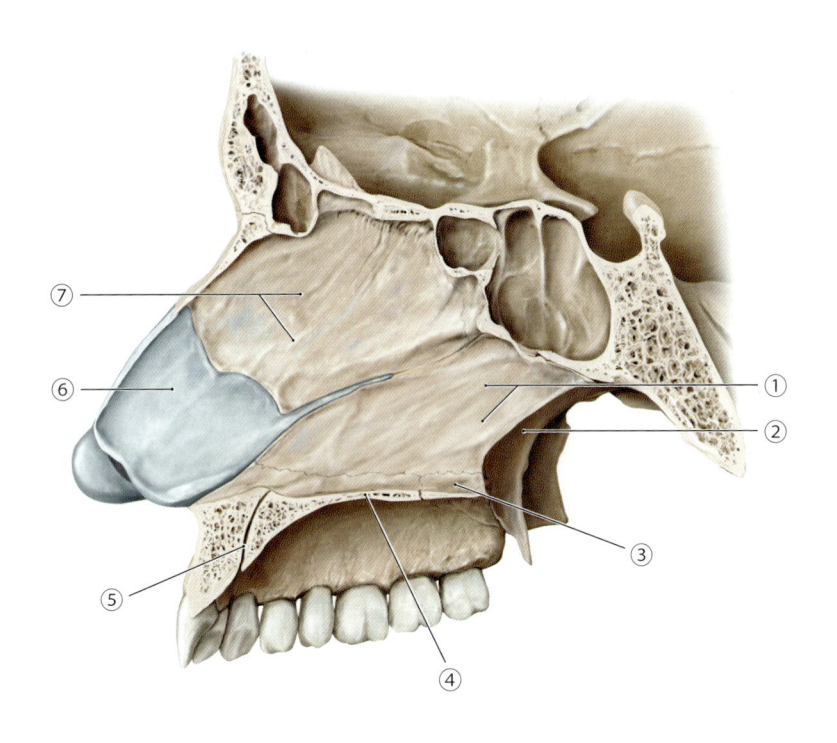

鼻腔の骨 1

傍矢状断面，左外側面

① ☐ 鋤骨   ☐ Vomer

② ☐ 後鼻孔   ☐ Choana

③ ☐ 口蓋骨，水平板   ☐ Palatine bone, horizontal plate

④ ☐ 上顎骨，口蓋突起   ☐ Maxilla, palatine process

⑤ ☐ 切歯管   ☐ Incisive canal

⑥ ☐ 鼻中隔軟骨   ☐ Septal cartilage

⑦ ☐ 篩骨，垂直板   ☐ Ethmoid bone, perpendicular plate

臨床

正常位の鼻中隔は鼻腔をほぼ対称に隔てている．鼻中隔が極端に外側に偏位すると鼻腔が閉塞されるが，軟骨を除去すること（鼻中隔形成術）で解消される．

1 図 34.2A. p.520   2 図 36.2A. p.550

Bones of the Nasal Cavity II

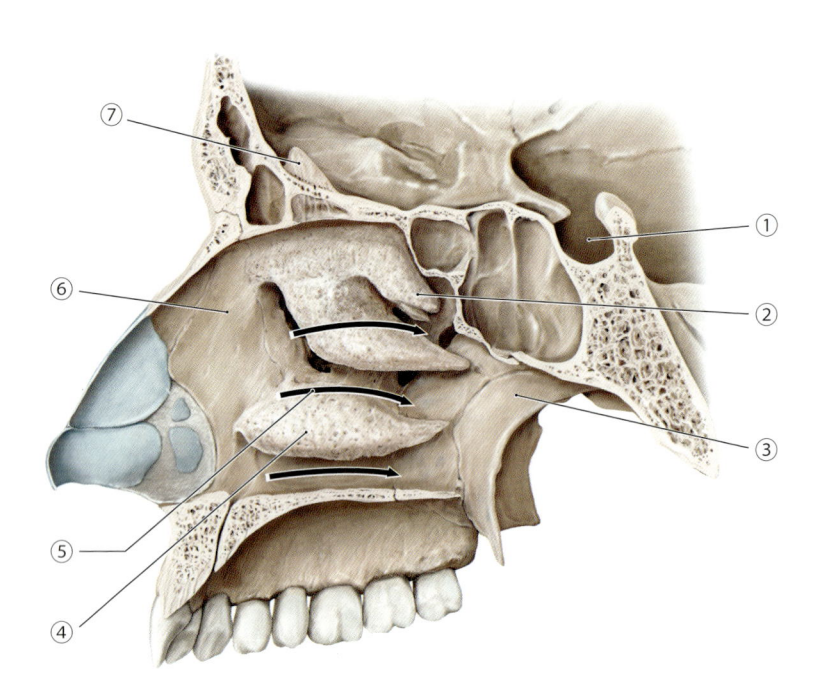

中鼻道に通じる副鼻腔はどれか？

鼻腔の骨 2

正中断面，右側内側面

① □ 下垂体窩 　　　　　　　□ Hypophyseal fossa
② □ 上鼻甲介（篩骨）　　　　□ Superior nasal concha (ethmoid bone)
③ □ 翼状突起，内側板　　　　□ Pterygoid process, medial plate
④ □ 下鼻甲介 　　　　　　　□ Inferior nasal concha
⑤ □ 中鼻道 　　　　　　　　□ Middle meatus
⑥ □ 上顎骨，前頭突起　　　　□ Maxilla, frontal process
⑦ □ 鶏冠 　　　　　　　　　□ Crista galli

A 前頭洞，上顎洞，前篩骨蜂巣と中篩骨蜂巣は中鼻道に通じる．

1 図 34.2B. p.521　　2 図 36.2B. p.551

Bones of the Nasal Cavity III

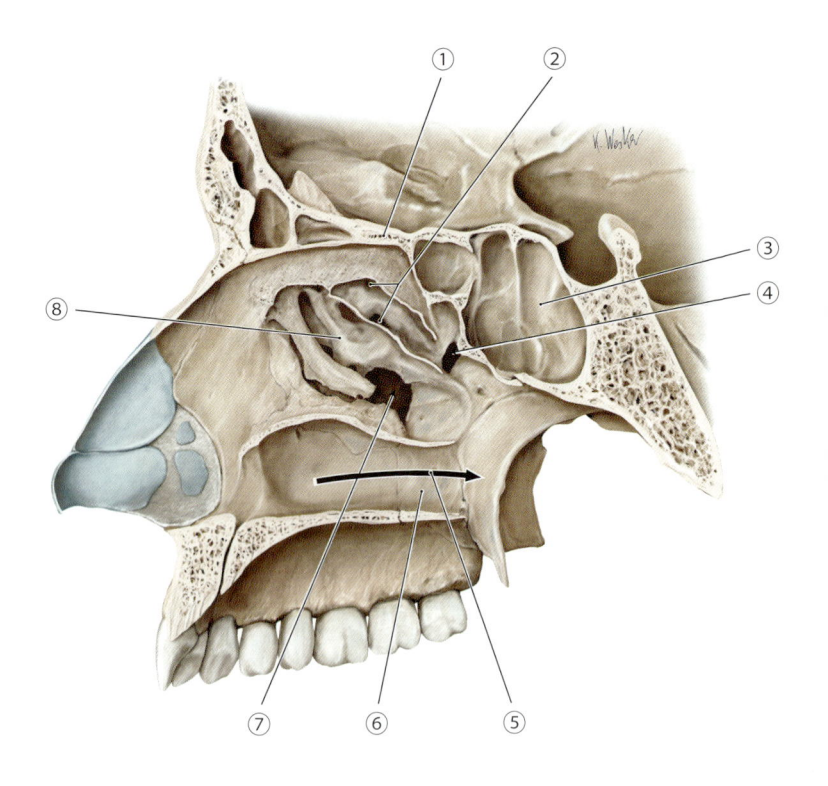

鼻腔の骨 3

正中断面, 右側内側面

① □ 篩板 □ Cribriform plate
② □ 後篩骨洞の開口部 □ Orifices of posterior ethmoid sinus
③ □ 蝶形骨洞 □ Sphenoid sinus
④ □ 蝶口蓋孔 □ Sphenopalatine foramen
⑤ □ 下鼻道 □ Inferior meatus
⑥ □ 口蓋骨, 垂直板 □ Palatine bone, perpendicular plate
⑦ □ 上顎洞裂孔 □ Maxillary hiatus
⑧ □ 篩骨胞 □ Ethmoid bulla

解説

前頭洞, 上顎洞, 前篩骨蜂巣と中篩骨蜂巣は中鼻道に, 蝶形骨洞は蝶篩陥凹に, 後篩骨蜂巣は上鼻道に, 鼻涙管は下鼻道に通じる.

① 図 34.2C. p.521　② 図 36.2C. p.551

Neurovasculature of the Nasal Cavity I

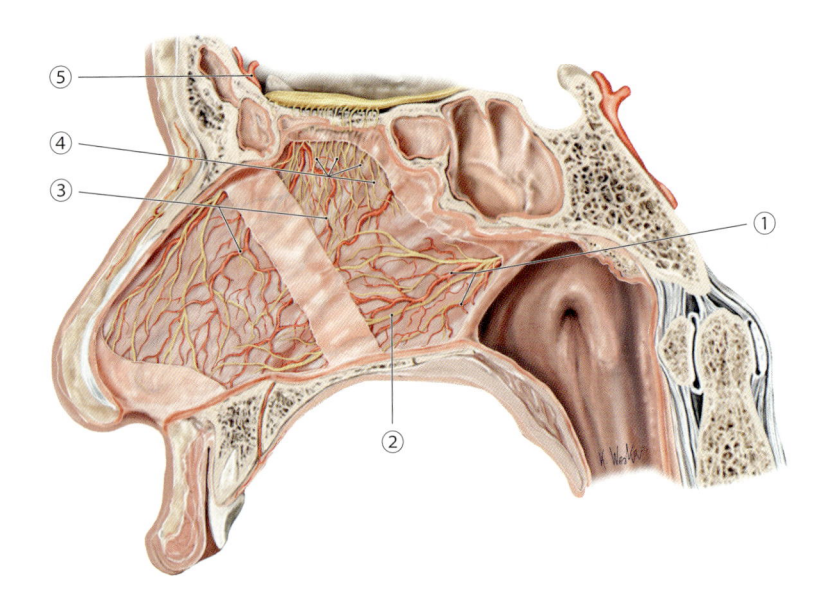

通常の鼻出血に関係する鼻腔の動脈は何か？

鼻腔の神経・血管 1

左外側面

① ☐ 中隔後鼻枝 ☐ Posterior septal branches (from sphenopalatine artery)

② ☐ 鼻口蓋神経 ☐ Nasopalatine nerve

③ ☐ 中隔前鼻枝 ☐ Anterior septal branches (from ophthalmic artery)

④ ☐ 嗅神経糸 ☐ Olfactory fibers

⑤ ☐ 前篩骨動脈 ☐ Anterior ethmoidal artery

A 通常鼻出血は鼻中隔の前部のキーゼルバッハ部位で起こり，この部位には内頸動脈の枝の前篩骨動脈と外頸動脈の枝の蝶口蓋動脈の両方からの血管が高密度で分布する．

1 図 34.6B. p.524 　2 図 36.6B. p.554

Neurovasculature of the Nasal Cavity II

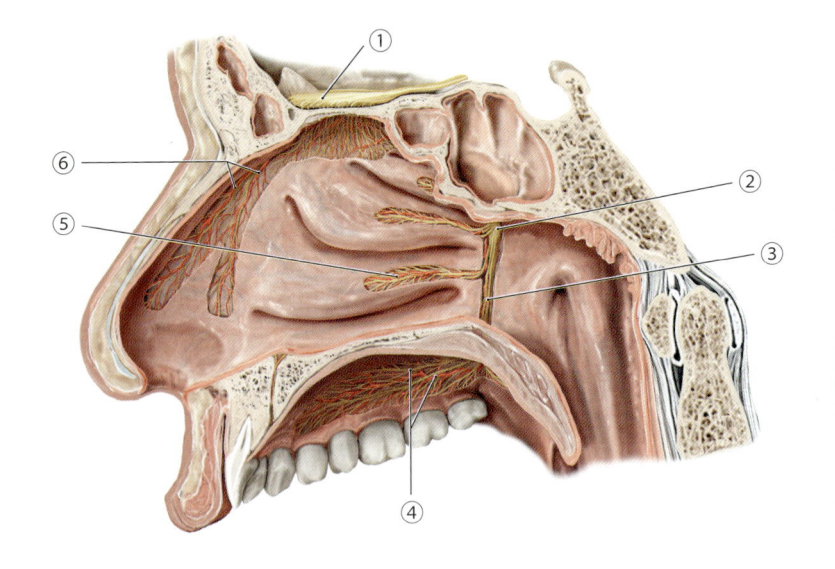

鼻腔の神経・血管 2

左外側面

① ☐ 嗅球 — ☐ Olfactory bulb (CN I)

② ☐ 翼口蓋神経節 — ☐ Pterygopalatine ganglion

③ ☐ 下行口蓋動脈, 大・小口蓋神経 — ☐ Descending palatine artery, greater and lesser palatine nerves

④ ☐ 大口蓋動脈・神経 — ☐ Greater palatine artery and nerve

⑤ ☐ 下後鼻枝, 外側後鼻枝 — ☐ Inferior posterior nasal branches, lateral posterior nasal arteries

⑥ ☐ 前篩骨動脈 — ☐ Anterior ethmoidal artery

1 図 34.8B. p.525　2 図 36.8B. p.555

External Ear

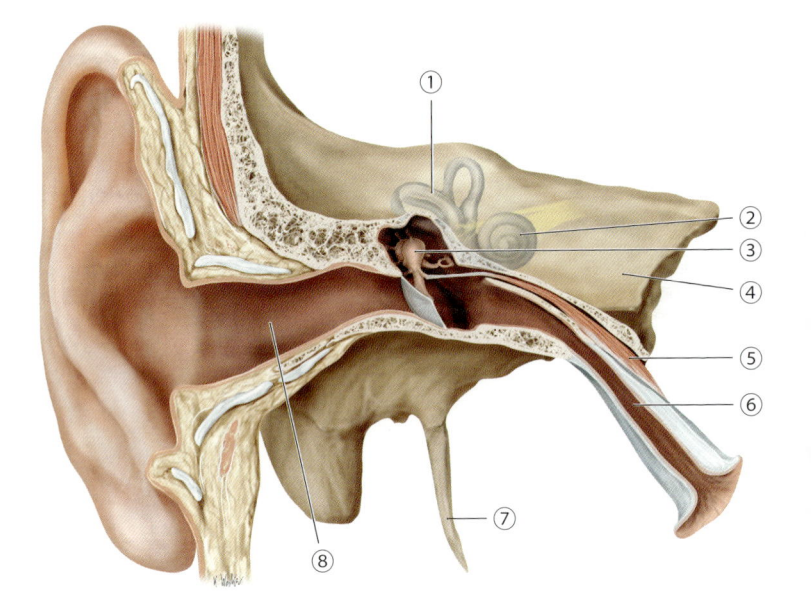

外耳

右耳の冠状断面，前面

① □ 外側骨半規管　　□ Lateral semicircular canal
② □ 蝸牛　　□ Cochlea
③ □ ツチ骨　　□ Malleus
④ □ 側頭骨，岩様部　　□ Temporal bone, petrous part
⑤ □ 鼓膜張筋　　□ Tensor tympani
⑥ □ 耳管　　□ Pharyngotympanic (auditory) tube
⑦ □ 茎状突起　　□ Styloid process
⑧ □ 外耳道　　□ External auditory canal

> **臨床**
>
> 外耳道は軟骨性部で大きく弯曲している．オトスコープ(耳鏡)を挿入するときは，耳介を後上方に引くと外耳道がまっすぐになり，耳鏡を挿入することができる．

1 図 35.3, p.528　2 図 37.3, p.558

Structure of the Auricle

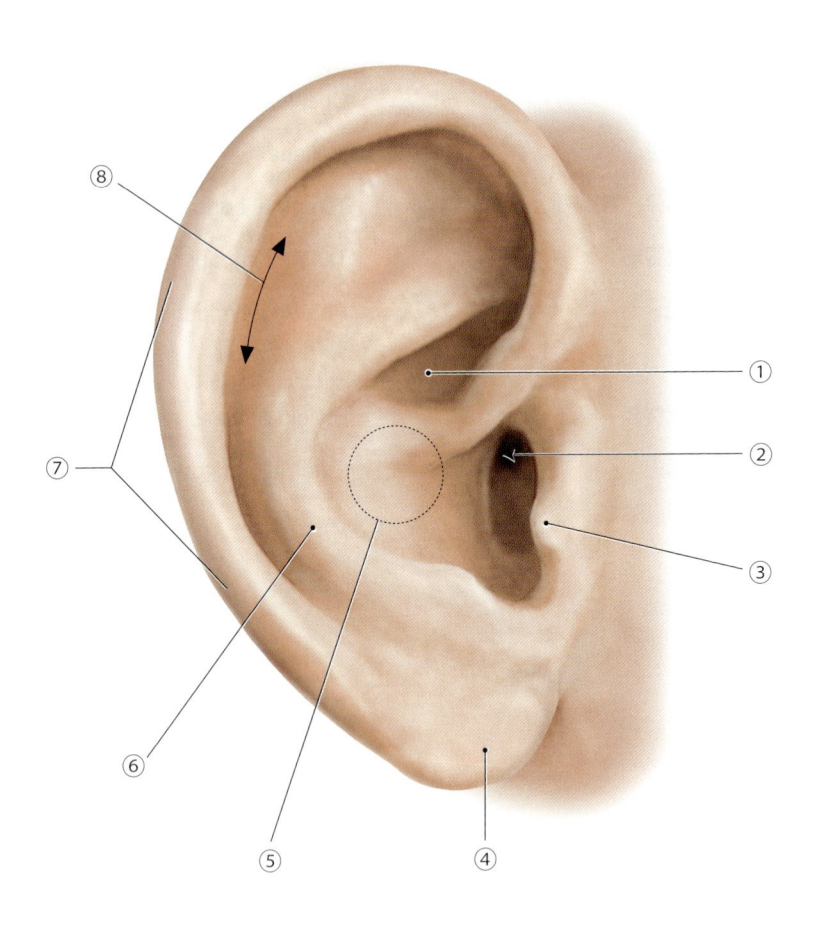

耳介に分布する神経は何か？

耳介の構造

右外側面

① ☐ 耳甲介舟 ☐ Cymba conchae
② ☐ 外耳道 ☐ External auditory canal
③ ☐ 耳珠 ☐ Tragus
④ ☐ 耳垂 ☐ Earlobe
⑤ ☐ 耳甲介 ☐ Concha
⑥ ☐ 対輪 ☐ Antihelix
⑦ ☐ 耳輪 ☐ Helix
⑧ ☐ 舟状窩 ☐ Scaphoid fossa

A 耳介の神経は三叉神経(CN V), 顔面神経(CN Ⅶ), 迷走神経(CN X), 舌咽神経(CN Ⅸ)から起こる. 頸神経叢からの小後頭神経と大耳介神経も耳介に分布する.

1 図 35.5A. p.529　2 図 37.5A. p.559

Tympanic Cavity

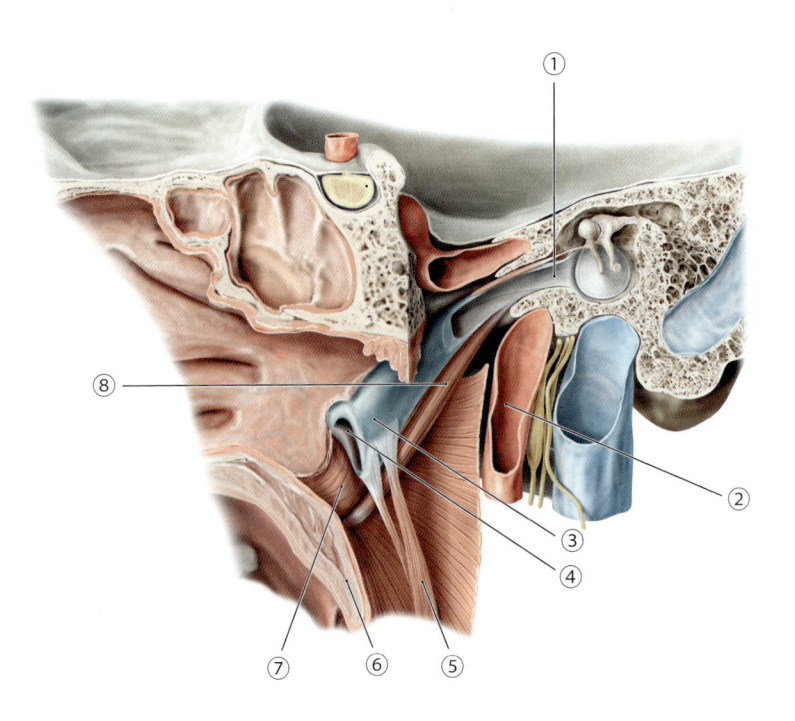

Q 嚥下や欠伸時に鼓膜の両側の圧を等しくさせるために働く筋肉は何か？

鼓室

内側面

① ☐ 耳管骨部 ☐ Pharyngotympanic tube, bony part
② ☐ 内頸動脈 ☐ Internal carotid artery
③ ☐ 耳管，軟骨部 ☐ Pharyngotympanic tube, cartilaginous part
④ ☐ 咽頭口 ☐ Pharyngeal orifice
⑤ ☐ 耳管咽頭筋 ☐ Salpingopharyngeus
⑥ ☐ 口蓋垂 ☐ Uvula
⑦ ☐ 口蓋帆挙筋 ☐ Levator veli palatini
⑧ ☐ 口蓋帆張筋 ☐ Tensor veli palatini

A 軟口蓋の口蓋帆張筋と口蓋帆挙筋，および上咽頭収縮筋の耳管咽頭筋は耳管を開口させる．

Ossicular Chain

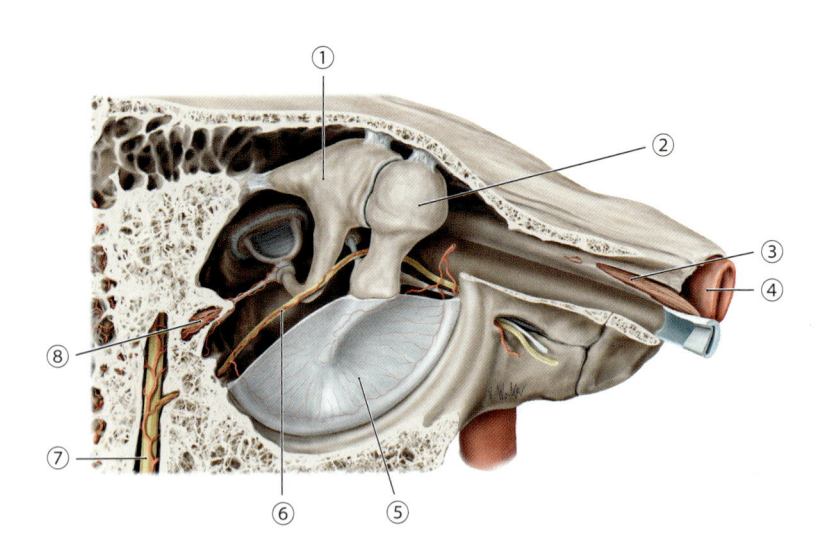

アブミ骨筋と鼓膜張筋の機能は何か？

耳小骨連鎖

外側面

① □ キヌタ骨　　　□ Incus
② □ ツチ骨　　　　□ Malleus
③ □ 鼓膜張筋　　　□ Tensor tympani
④ □ 内頸動脈　　　□ Internal carotid artery
⑤ □ 鼓膜　　　　　□ Tympanic membrane
⑥ □ 鼓索神経　　　□ Chorda tympani
⑦ □ 顔面神経　　　□ Facial nerve(CN Ⅶ)
⑧ □ アブミ骨筋　　□ Stapedius

A 　アブミ骨筋と鼓膜張筋は中耳の音伝導を減衰させるように働く．どちらの筋も大きな音刺激に対して反射収縮する．

Inner Ear

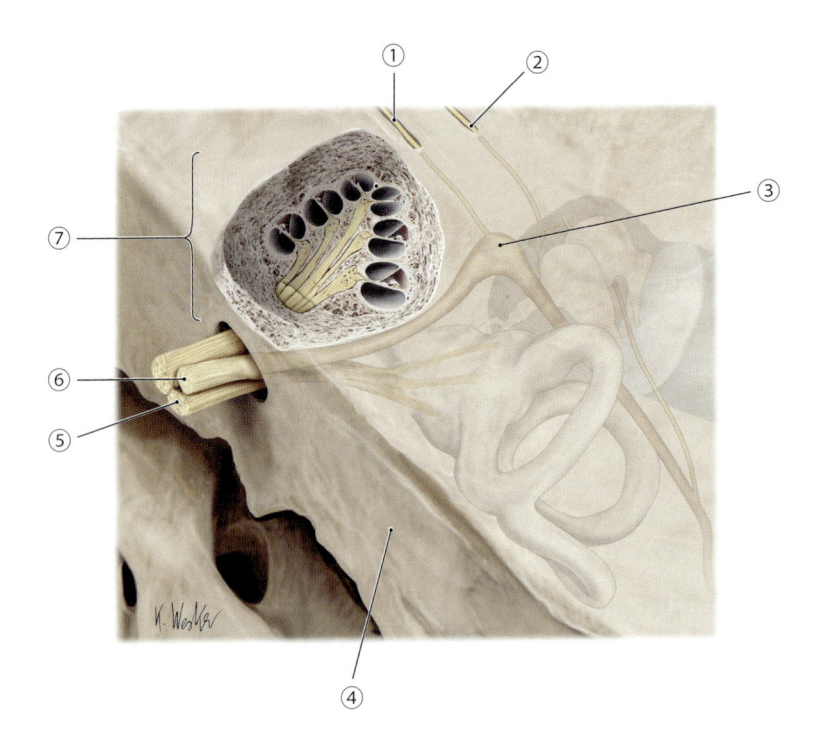

内耳

上面

① □ 大錐体神経 □ Greater petrosal nerve

② □ 小錐体神経 □ Lesser petrosal nerve

③ □ 膝神経節 □ Geniculate ganglion

④ □ 側頭骨，岩様部 □ Temporal bone, petrous part

⑤ □ 前庭神経 □ Vestibulocochlear nerve (CN VIII), vestibular part

⑥ □ 顔面神経 □ Facial nerve (CN VII)

⑦ □ 蝸牛 □ Cochlea

1 図 35.20C. p.536　2 図 37.20C. p.566

Mandible

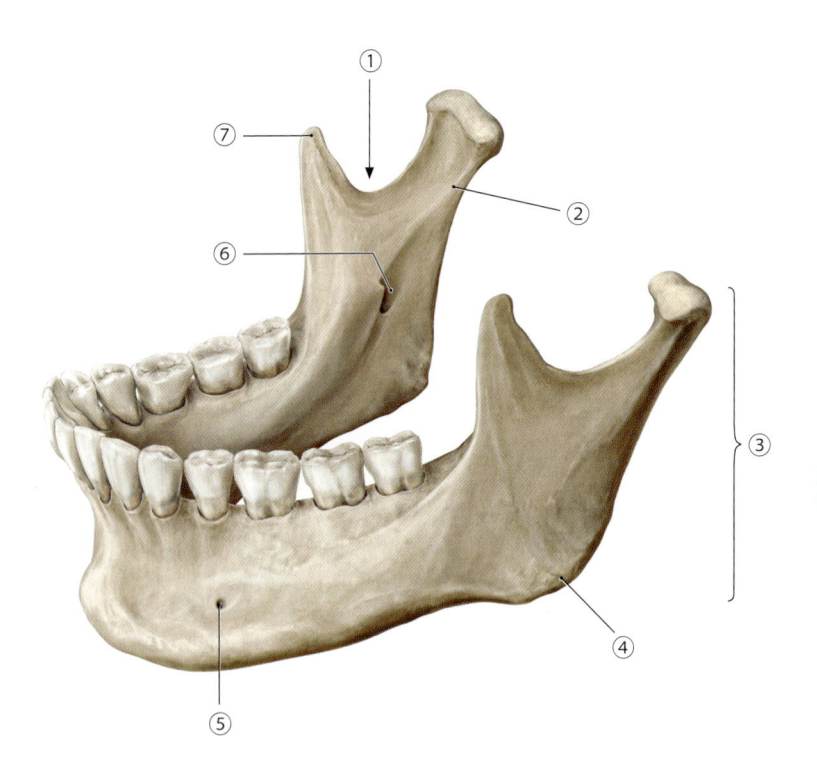

下顎骨

左斜外側面

① □ 下顎切痕 □ Mandibular notch
② □ 関節突起 □ Condylar process
③ □ 下顎枝 □ Ramus
④ □ 下顎角 □ Mandibular angle
⑤ □ オトガイ孔 □ Mental foramen
⑥ □ 下顎孔 □ Mandibular foramen
⑦ □ 筋突起 □ Coronoid process

1 図 36.4C. p.539　2 図 38.4C. p.569

Trigeminal Nerve in the Oral Cavity

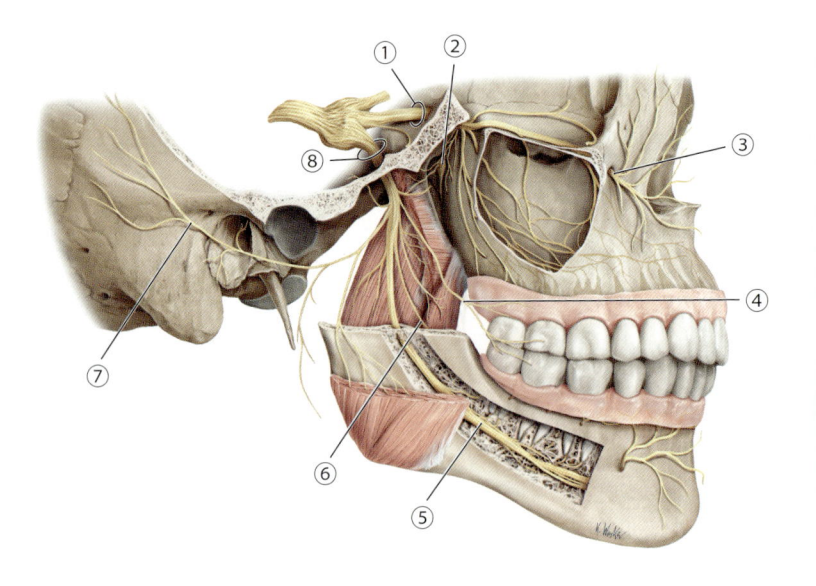

口腔の三叉神経

右外側面

① □ 上顎神経（正円孔を通る） □ Maxillary division (CN V_2, via foramen rotundum)

② □ 翼口蓋神経節 □ Pterygopalatine ganglion

③ □ 眼窩下神経と眼窩下孔 □ Infraorbital nerve (and foramen)

④ □ 頬神経 □ Buccal nerve

⑤ □ 下歯槽神経（下顎管にある） □ Inferior alveolar nerve (in mandibular canal)

⑥ □ 舌神経 □ Lingual nerve

⑦ □ 耳介側頭神経 □ Auriculotemporal nerve

⑧ □ 下顎神経（卵円孔を通る） □ Mandibular division (CN V_3, via foramen ovale)

642　Head & Neck

Dorsum of the Tongue

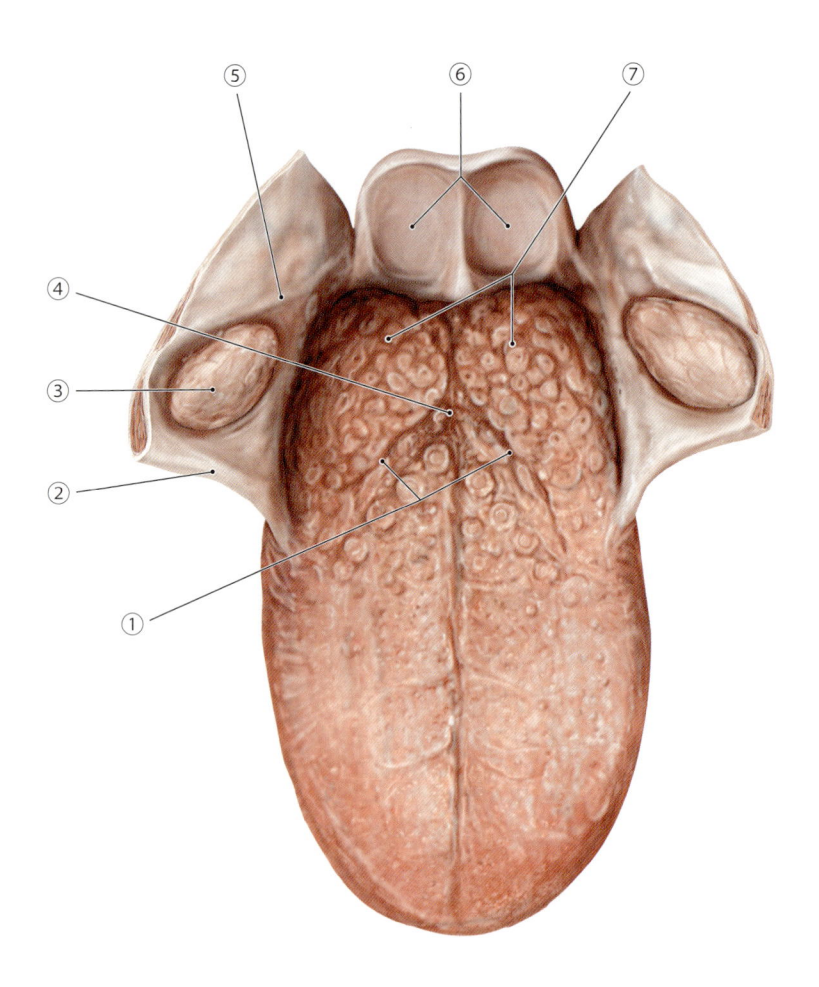

Q 舌の分界溝とは何か？

舌背

上面

① □ 分界溝 □ Sulcus terminalis

② □ 口蓋舌弓 □ Palatoglossal arch

③ □ 口蓋扁桃 □ Palatine tonsil

④ □ 舌盲孔 □ Foramen cecum

⑤ □ 口蓋咽頭弓 □ Palatopharyngeal arch

⑥ □ 喉頭蓋 □ Epiglottis

⑦ □ 舌扁桃 □ Lingual tonsil

A V字形の分界溝によって，舌は前2/3と後ろ1/3に分けられる．これは発生期に異なる鰓弓から生じたことの名残である．

① 図36.20A. p.548 ② 図38.20. p.578

Muscles of the Tongue

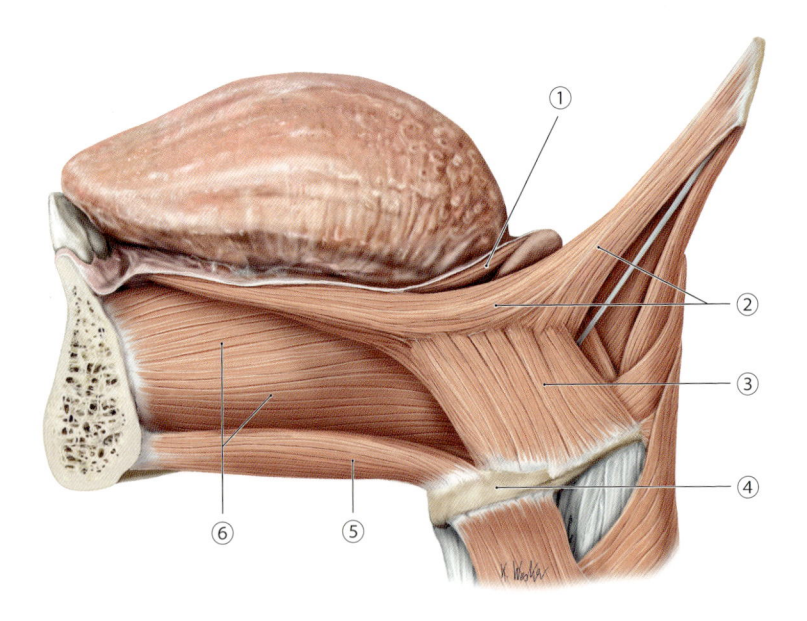

舌の筋肉

左外側面

① □ 口蓋舌筋　　□ Palatoglossus

② □ 茎突舌筋　　□ Styloglossus

③ □ 舌骨舌筋　　□ Hyoglossus

④ □ 舌骨　　　　□ Hyoid bone

⑤ □ オトガイ舌骨筋　□ Geniohyoid

⑥ □ オトガイ舌筋　□ Genioglossus

解説

　外舌筋（オトガイ舌筋，舌骨舌筋，口蓋舌筋，茎突舌筋）は骨に付着し，舌全体を動かす．内舌筋（上縦舌筋，下縦舌筋，横舌筋，垂直舌筋）は骨に付着せず，舌の形を変える．

① 図 36.21A. p.548　② 図 38.21A. p.578

Sensory Innervation of the Tongue

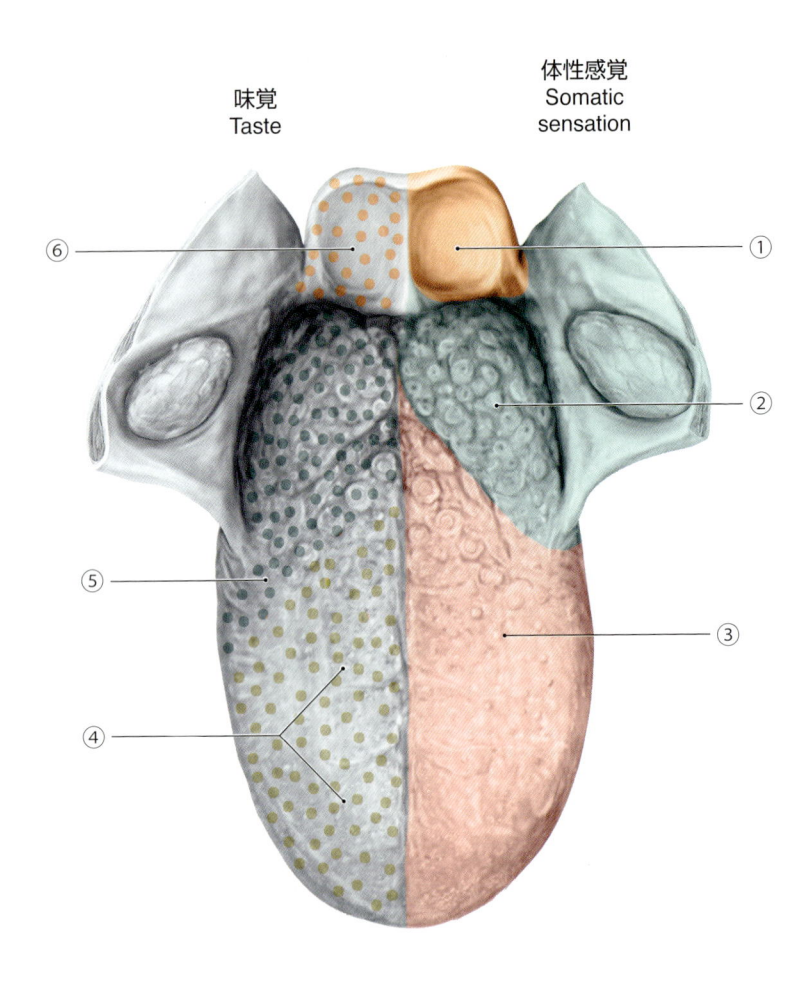

味覚
Taste

体性感覚
Somatic sensation

舌の感覚性神経支配

上面

① □ 迷走神経　　　　　　　　□ Vagus nerve (CN X)

② □ 舌咽神経　　　　　　　　□ Glossopharyngeal nerve (CN IX)

③ □ 舌神経(下顎神経)　　　　□ Lingual nerve (from mandibular nerve, CN V₃)

④ □ 顔面神経(鼓索神経経由)　□ Facial nerve (CN VII, via chorda tympani)

⑤ □ 舌咽神経　　　　　　　　□ Glossopharyngeal nerve (CN IX)

⑥ □ 迷走神経　　　　　　　　□ Vagus nerve (CN X)

解説

口蓋舌筋は迷走神経(CN X)の神経支配を受ける．他の舌筋は舌下神経(CN XII)に体性運動性に支配される．

[1] 図 36.22. p.549　[2] 図 38.22. p.578

Neurovasculature of the Tongue

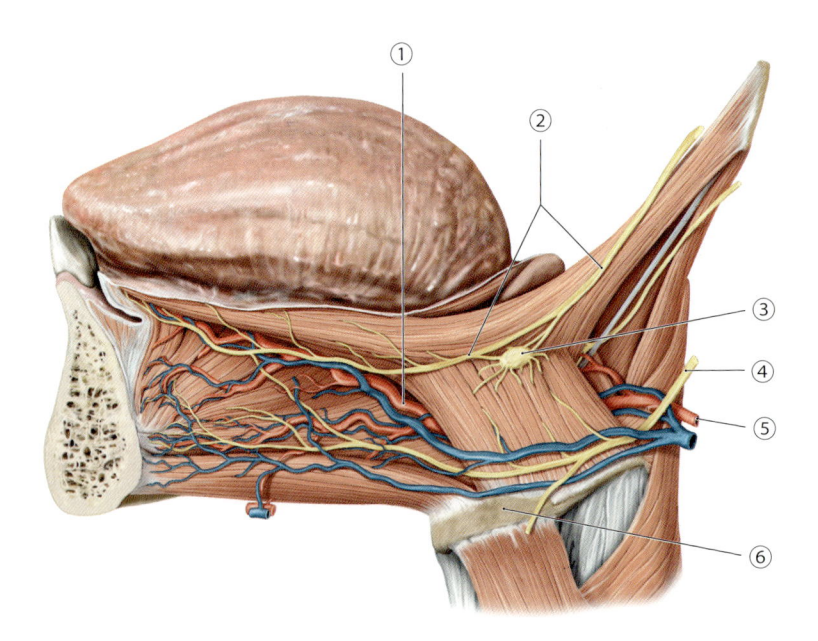

Q 片側の舌下神経の障害によって前方に突出した舌はどのような形になるか？

舌の神経と血管

左外側面

① ☐ 舌深動脈 ☐ Deep lingual artery
② ☐ 舌神経 ☐ Lingual nerve（CN V₃）
③ ☐ 顎下神経節 ☐ Submandibular ganglion
④ ☐ 舌下神経 ☐ Hypoglossal nerve（CN XII）
⑤ ☐ 舌動脈（外頸動脈から） ☐ Lingual artery（from external carotid artery）
⑥ ☐ 舌骨 ☐ Hyoid bone

A 　片側の舌下神経が障害を受けると，障害を受けていない側のオトガイ舌筋が優位になり，舌を前方に突出させると麻痺側へ偏位する．

Boundaries of the Oral Cavity I

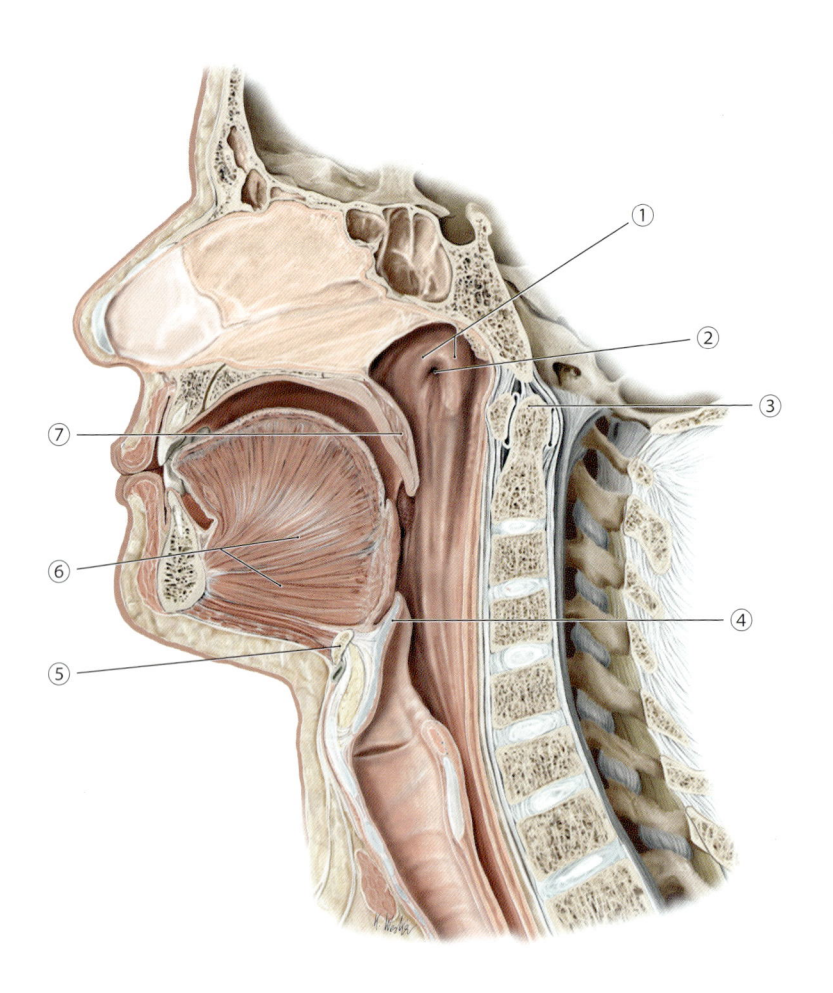

口腔の区分 1

正中断面，左外側面

① □ リンパ組織（耳管扁桃）を伴う耳管隆起　　□ Torus tubarius with lymphatic tissue (tonsilla tubaria)

② □ 耳管咽頭口　　□ Pharyngeal orifice of pharyngotympanic tube

③ □ 軸椎の歯突起　　□ Dens of axis (C2)

④ □ 喉頭蓋　　□ Epiglottis

⑤ □ 舌骨　　□ Hyoid bone

⑥ □ オトガイ舌筋　　□ Genioglossus

⑦ □ 軟口蓋（口蓋帆）　　□ Soft palate

1 図 36.24B. p.550　2 図 38.25B. p.580

Boundaries of the Oral Cavity II

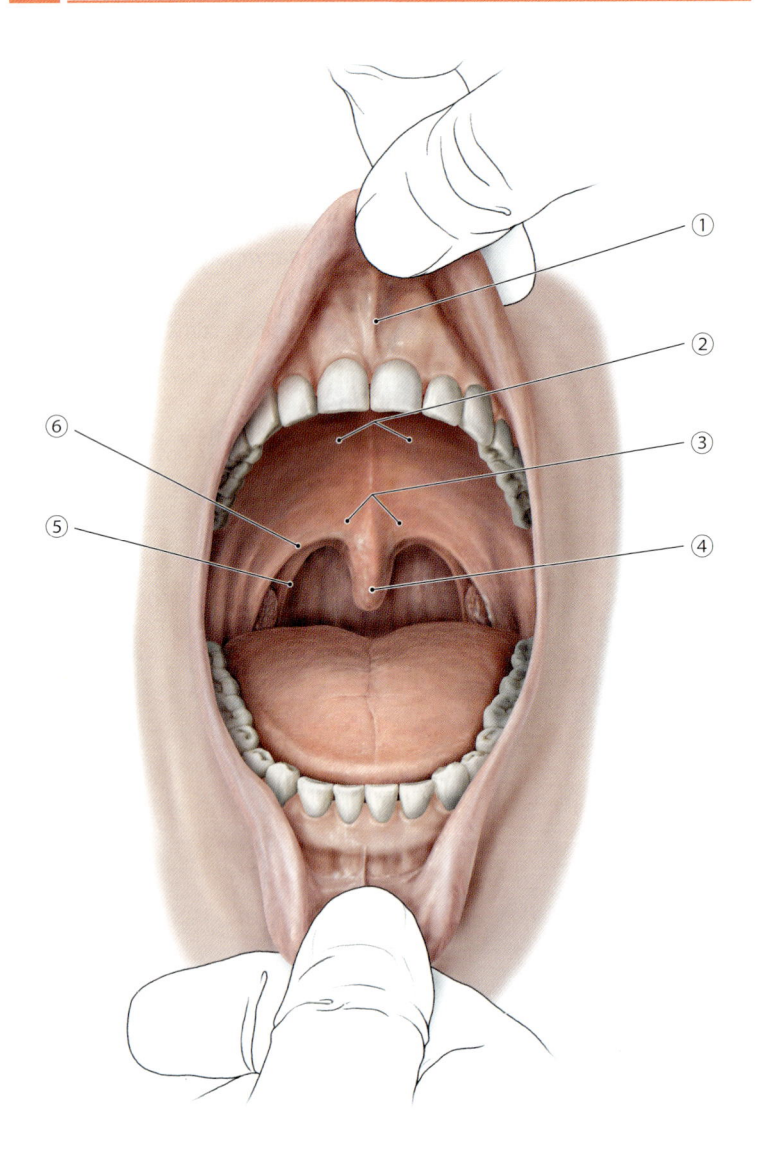

口腔の区分 2

前面

① □ 上唇小帯　　　　　　　□ Frenulum of upper lip
② □ 硬口蓋　　　　　　　　□ Hard palate
③ □ 軟口蓋(口蓋帆)　　　　□ Soft palate
④ □ 口蓋垂　　　　　　　　□ Uvula
⑤ □ 口蓋咽頭弓　　　　　　□ Palatopharyngeal arch
⑥ □ 口蓋舌弓　　　　　　　□ Palatoglossal arch

654 Head & Neck

Salivary Glands I

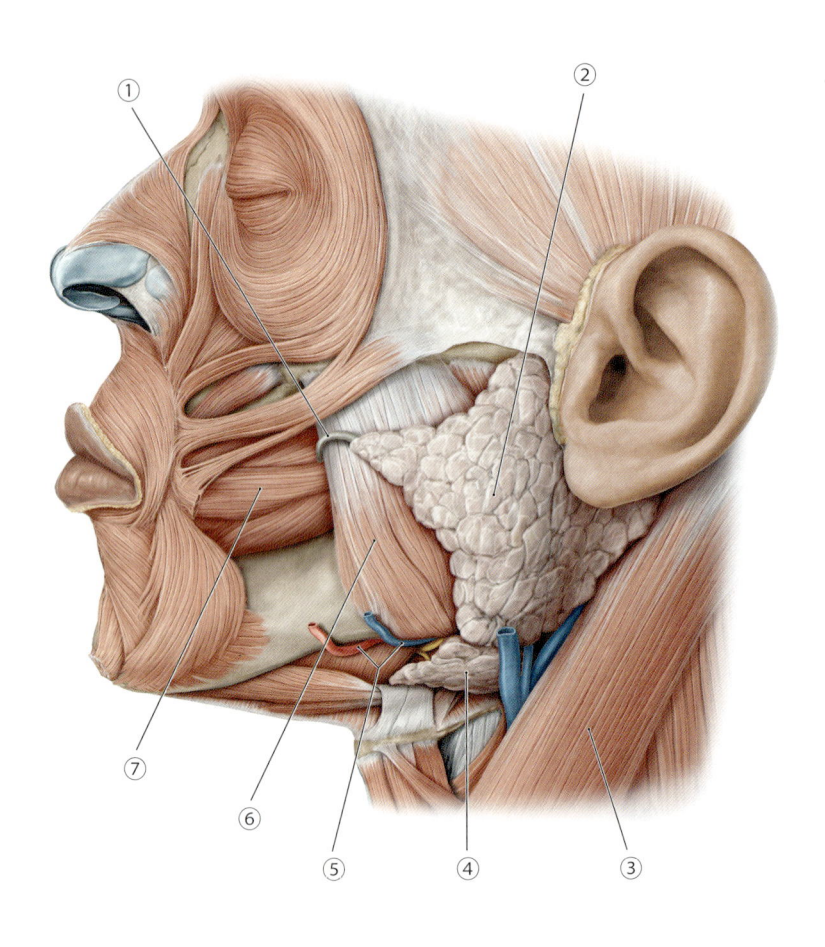

唾液腺 1

左外側面

① □ 耳下腺管　　　　　□ Parotid duct

② □ 耳下腺　　　　　　□ Parotid gland

③ □ 胸鎖乳突筋　　　　□ Sternocleidomastoid

④ □ 顎下腺　　　　　　□ Submandibular gland

⑤ □ 顔面動脈・静脈　　□ Facial artery and vein

⑥ □ 咬筋　　　　　　　□ Masseter

⑦ □ 頬筋　　　　　　　□ Buccinator

解説

耳下腺管は頬筋を貫通して上顎第2大臼歯に対向するところに開口する．

1 図 36.26A. p.551　2 図 38.27A. p.581

Salivary Glands II

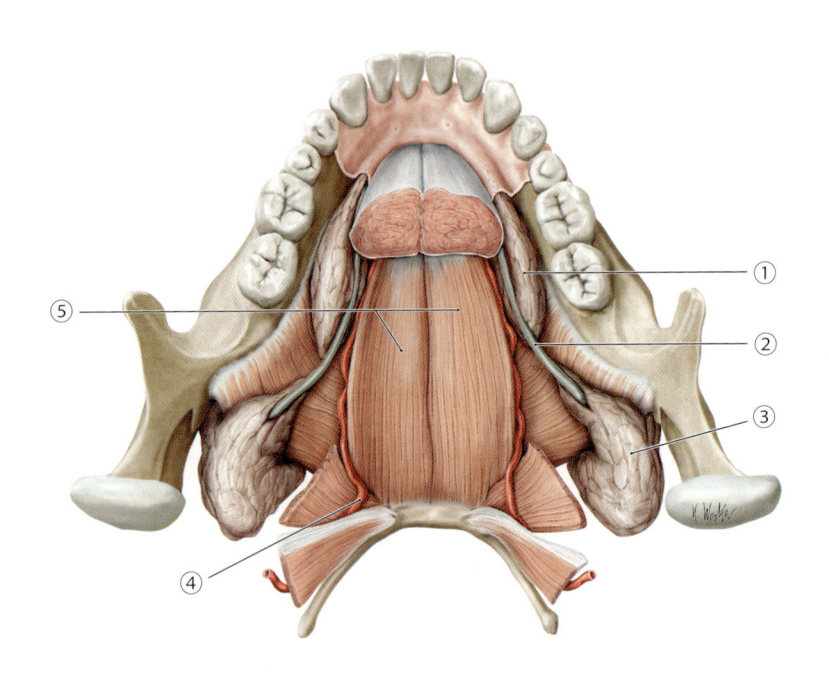

① ② ③ ④ ⑤

Q 三対の唾液腺それぞれからの分泌液の特徴は何か？

唾液腺 2

上面

① □ 舌下腺　　　　　　　□ Sublingual gland
② □ 顎下腺管　　　　　　□ Submandibular duct
③ □ 顎下腺　　　　　　　□ Submandibular gland
④ □ 舌動脈　　　　　　　□ Lingual artery
⑤ □ オトガイ舌骨筋　　　□ Geniohyoid

A 　耳下腺の分泌液は純粋な漿液，舌下腺は主に粘液，顎下腺は漿粘液である．

1 図 36.26C. p.551　　2 図 38.27C. p.581

Pharyngeal Muscles I

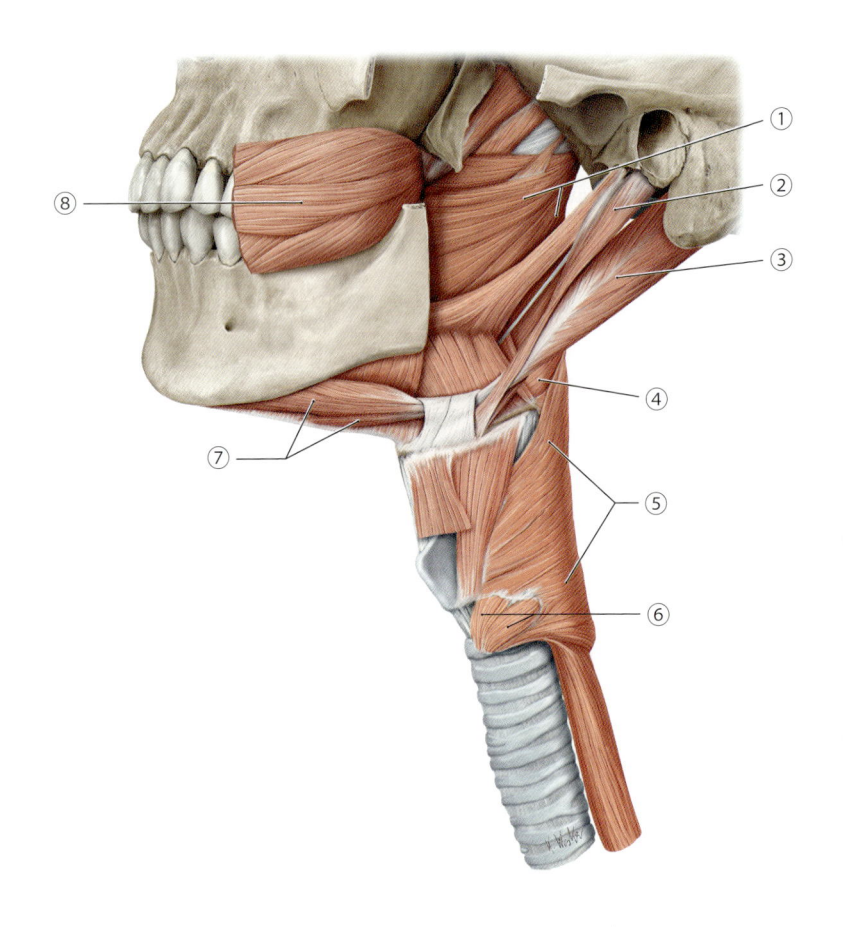

咽頭筋 1

左外側面

① ☐ 上咽頭収縮筋　　　　☐ Superior pharyngeal constrictor

② ☐ 茎突舌骨筋　　　　　☐ Stylohyoid

③ ☐ 顎二腹筋（後腹）　　☐ Digastric muscle (posterior belly)

④ ☐ 中咽頭収縮筋　　　　☐ Middle pharyngeal constrictor

⑤ ☐ 下咽頭収縮筋　　　　☐ Inferior pharyngeal constrictor

⑥ ☐ 輪状甲状筋　　　　　☐ Cricothyroid

⑦ ☐ 顎二腹筋（前腹）　　☐ Digastric muscle (anterior belly)

⑧ ☐ 頬筋　　　　　　　　☐ Buccinator

解説

咽頭の筋系は咽頭収縮筋と比較的弱い咽頭挙筋からなる．

1 図36.29A, p.554　 2 図38.30A, p.584

Pharyngeal Muscles II

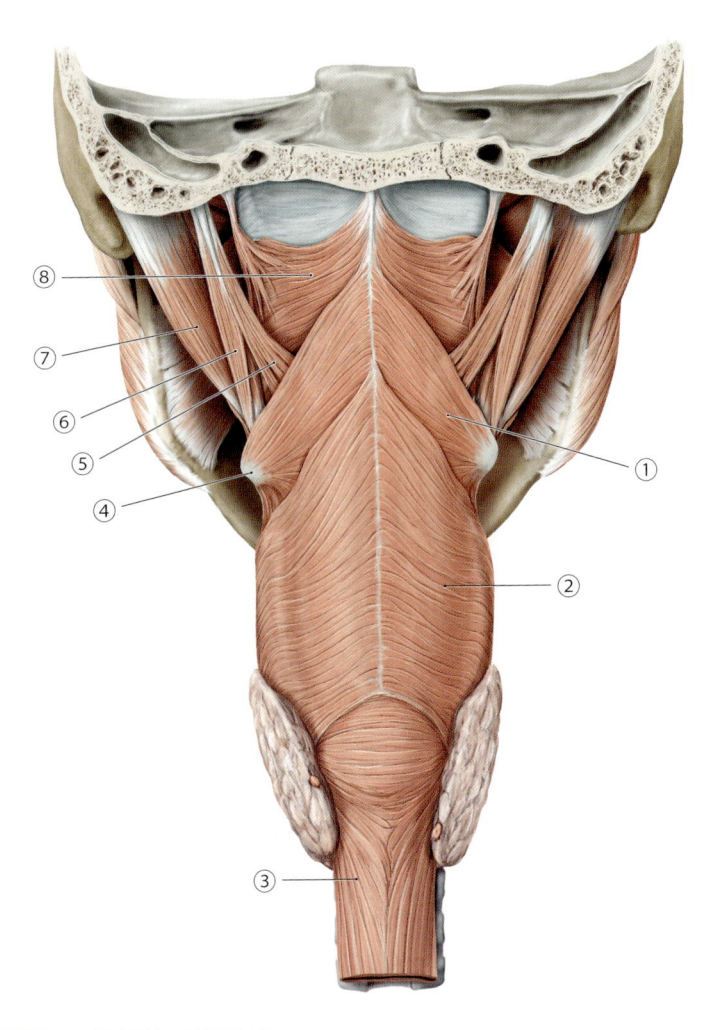

Q 咽頭収縮筋の機能は？

咽頭筋 2

後面

① □ 中咽頭収縮筋　　　　　□ Middle pharyngeal constrictor

② □ 下咽頭収縮筋　　　　　□ Inferior pharyngeal constrictor

③ □ 食道　　　　　　　　　□ Esophagus

④ □ 舌骨，大角　　　　　　□ Hyoid bone, greater horn

⑤ □ 茎突咽頭筋　　　　　　□ Stylopharyngeus

⑥ □ 茎突舌骨筋　　　　　　□ Stylohyoid

⑦ □ 顎二腹筋，後腹　　　　□ Digastric muscle, posterior belly

⑧ □ 上咽頭収縮筋　　　　　□ Superior pharyngeal constrictor

A 　上・中・下咽頭収縮筋は，嚥下時に順に収縮して咽頭から食道への食塊の移動を助ける．

1 図 36.30A, p.555　　2 図 38.31A, p.585

Neurovasculature of the Pharynx

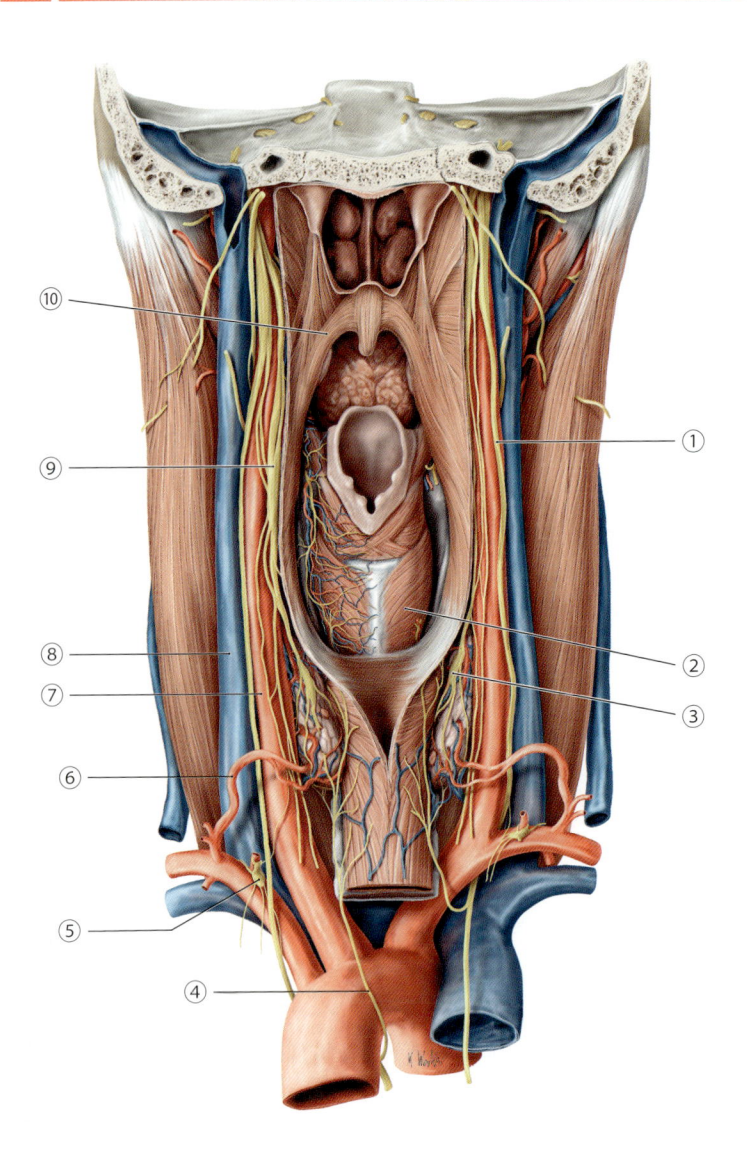

咽頭の神経・血管

後面

① □ 迷走神経 □ Vagus nerve (CN X)
② □ 後輪状披裂筋 □ Posterior cricoarytenoid
③ □ 中頸神経節 □ Middle cervical ganglion
④ □ 左反回神経 □ Left recurrent laryngeal nerve
⑤ □ 星状神経節 □ Stellate ganglion
⑥ □ 下甲状腺動脈 □ Inferior thyroid artery
⑦ □ 総頸動脈 □ Common carotid artery
⑧ □ 内頸静脈 □ Internal jugular vein
⑨ □ 交感神経幹 □ Sympathetic trunk
⑩ □ 口蓋咽頭筋 □ Palatopharyngeus

1 図 36.33. p.557　2 図 38.34. p.587

Muscles of the Neck

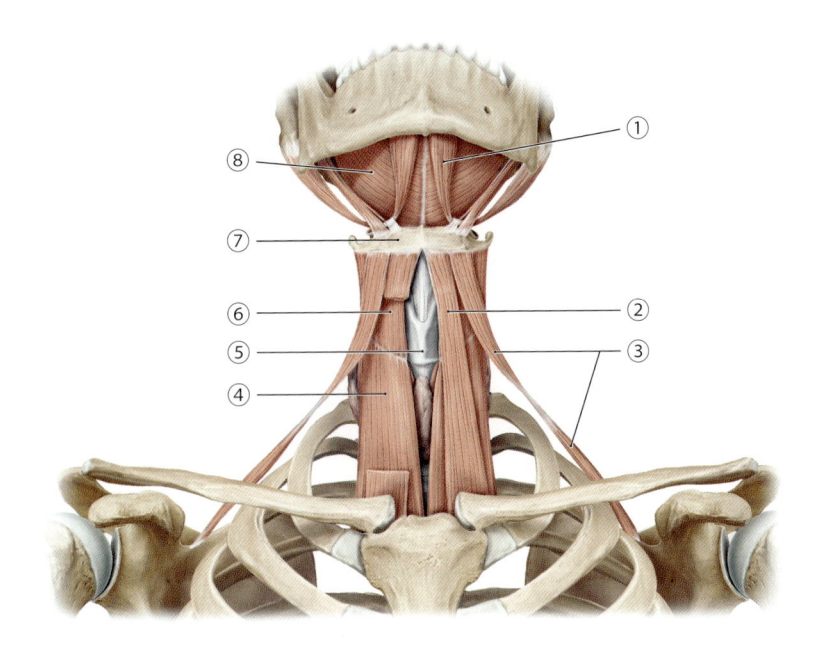

頸部の筋

前面

① □ 顎二腹筋，前腹　　□ Digastric, anterior belly
② □ 胸骨舌骨筋　　□ Sternohyoid
③ □ 肩甲舌骨筋，上腹・下腹　　□ Omohyoid, superior and inferior belly
④ □ 胸骨甲状筋　　□ Sternothyroid
⑤ □ 甲状軟骨　　□ Thyroid cartilage
⑥ □ 甲状舌骨筋　　□ Thyrohyoid
⑦ □ 舌骨　　□ Hyoid bone
⑧ □ 顎舌骨筋　　□ Mylohyoid

1 図 37.8C. p.563　2 図 39.5C. p.591

666 Head & Neck

Arteries of the Neck

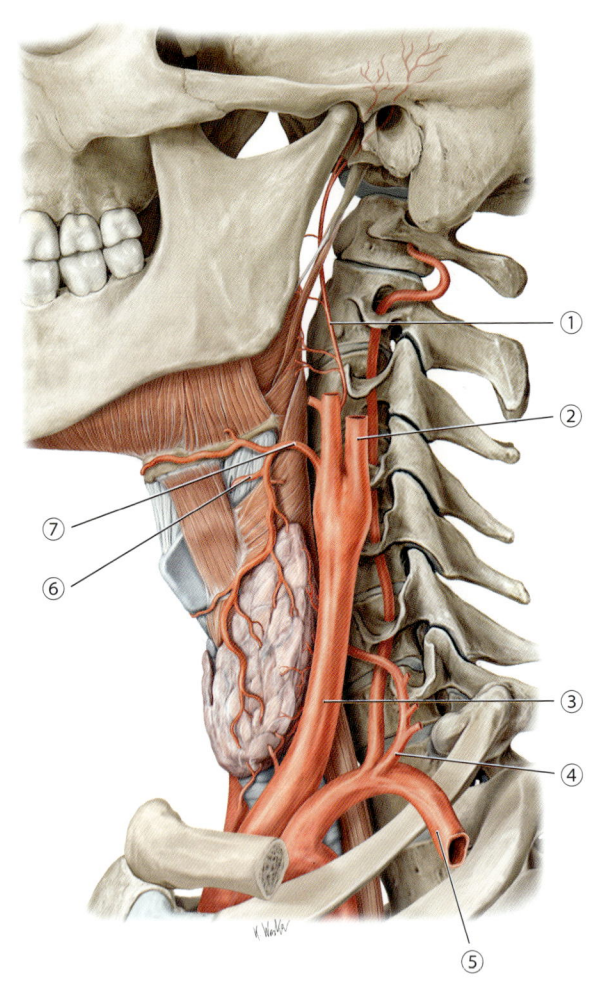

Q 内頸動脈の枝が分布する頸部の構造は何か？

頸部の動脈

左外側面

① ☐ 上行咽頭動脈　　　　　☐ Ascending pharyngeal artery
② ☐ 内頸動脈　　　　　　　☐ Internal carotid artery
③ ☐ 総頸動脈　　　　　　　☐ Common carotid artery
④ ☐ 甲状頸動脈　　　　　　☐ Thyrocervical trunk
⑤ ☐ 左鎖骨下動脈　　　　　☐ Left subclavian artery
⑥ ☐ 上喉頭動脈　　　　　　☐ Superior laryngeal artery
⑦ ☐ 上甲状腺動脈　　　　　☐ Superior thyroid artery

A 内頸動脈は頸部では枝を出さないため，この領域のどの構造にも分布しない．

1 図 37.11. p.566　　2 図 39.8. p.594

Nerves of the Neck

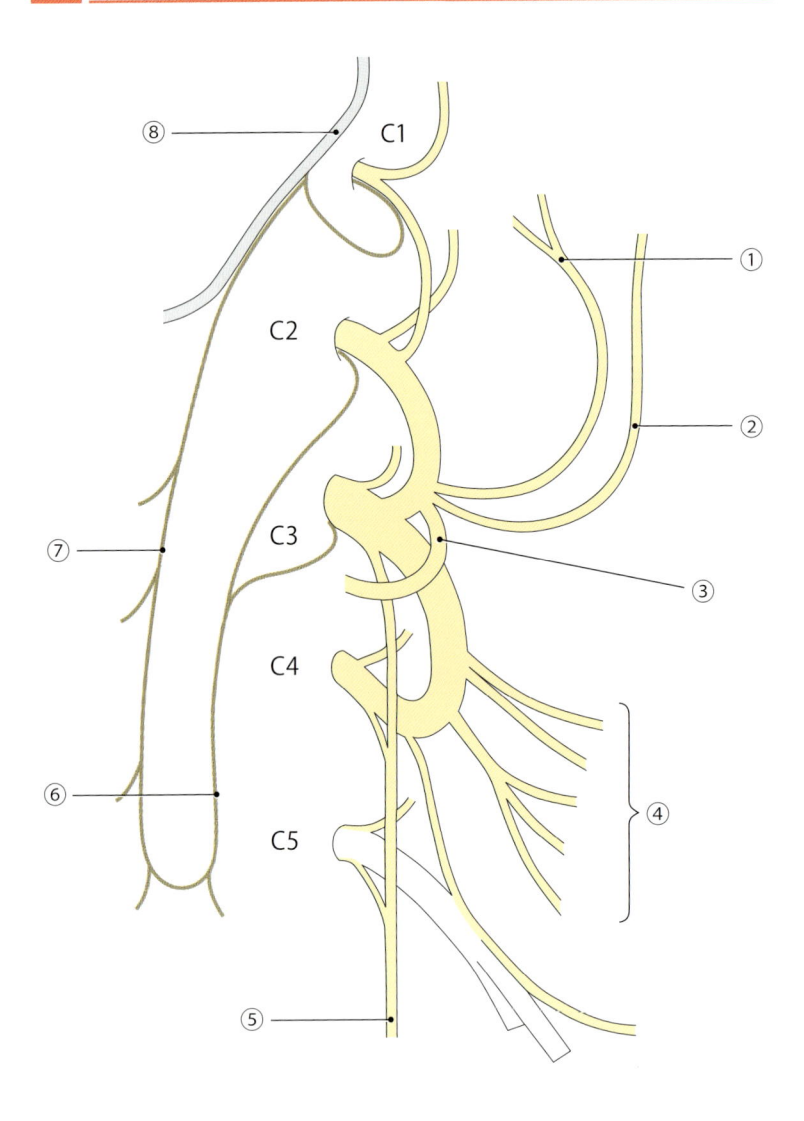

頸部の神経

① ☐ 小後頭神経　　　　☐ Lesser occipital nerve
② ☐ 大耳介神経　　　　☐ Great auricular nerve
③ ☐ 頸横神経　　　　　☐ Transverse cervical nerve
④ ☐ 鎖骨上神経　　　　☐ Supraclavicular nerves
⑤ ☐ 横隔神経　　　　　☐ Phrenic nerve
⑥ ☐ 頸神経ワナ，下根　☐ Inferior root of ansa cervicalis
⑦ ☐ 頸神経ワナ，上根　☐ Superior root of ansa cervicalis
⑧ ☐ 舌下神経　　　　　☐ Hypoglossal nerve (CN XII)

1 表37.8. p.568　2 表39.6. p.596

Thyroid Gland

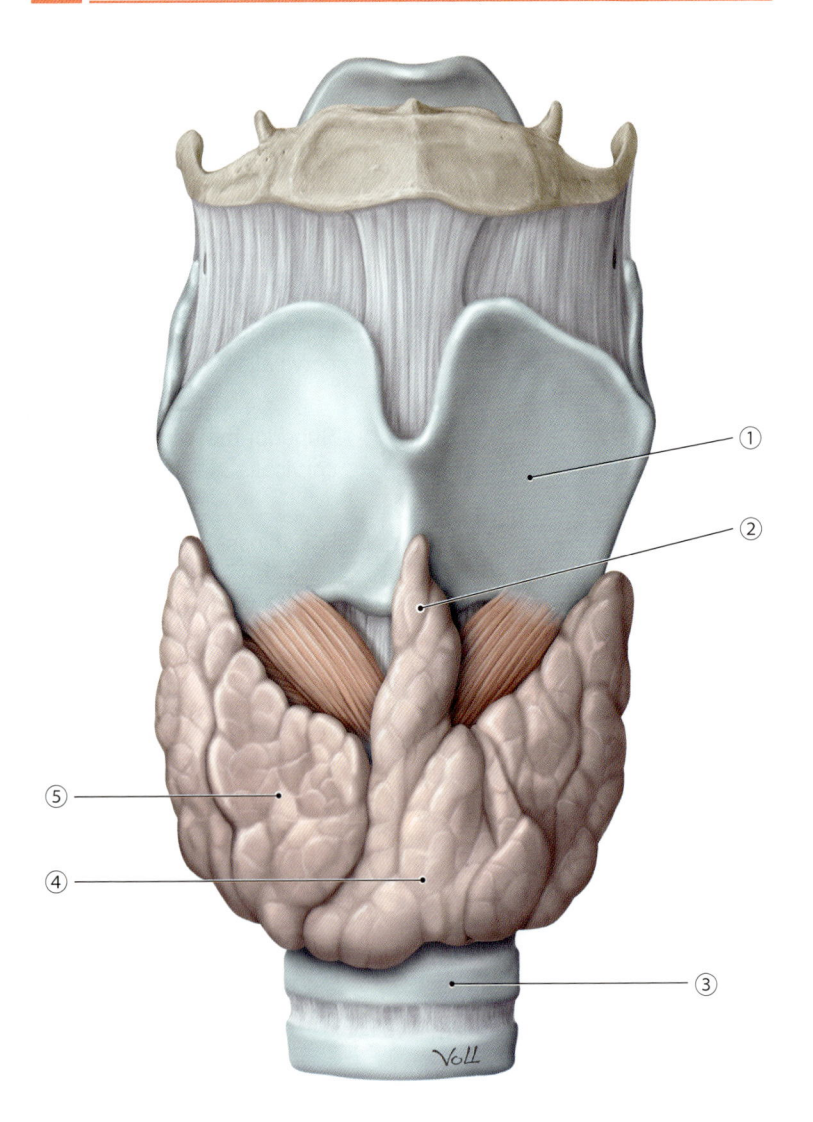

甲状腺

前面

① □ 甲状軟骨　　　　　　□ Thyroid cartilage

② □ 甲状腺，錐体葉　　　□ Thyroid gland, pyramidal lobe

③ □ 気管　　　　　　　　□ Trachea

④ □ 甲状腺峡部　　　　　□ Isthmus of thyroid gland

⑤ □ 甲状腺，右葉　　　　□ Thyroid gland, right lobe

1 図 37.25A. p.574　　2 図 39.22A. p.602

Relations of the Thyroid

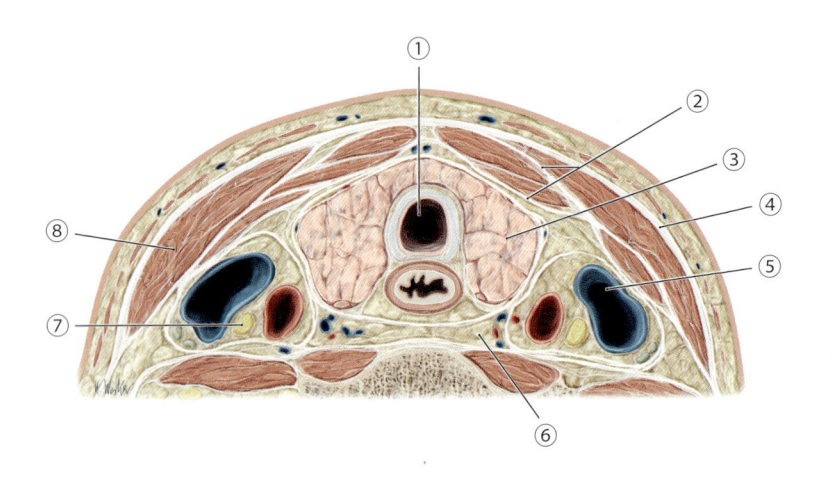

甲状腺の関係

横断面

① □ 気管 □ Trachea
② □ 頸筋膜（筋部），気管前葉 □ Pretracheal layer of cervical fascia, muscular portion
③ □ 甲状腺 □ Thyroid gland
④ □ 頸筋膜，浅葉 □ Investing layer of cervical fascia
⑤ □ 内頸静脈 □ Internal jugular vein
⑥ □ 咽頭後隙 □ Retropharyngeal space
⑦ □ 迷走神経 □ Vagus nerve (CN X)
⑧ □ 胸鎖乳突筋 □ Sternocleidomastoid

1 図 37.25C. p.574　2 図 39.22C. p.602

Structure of the Larynx

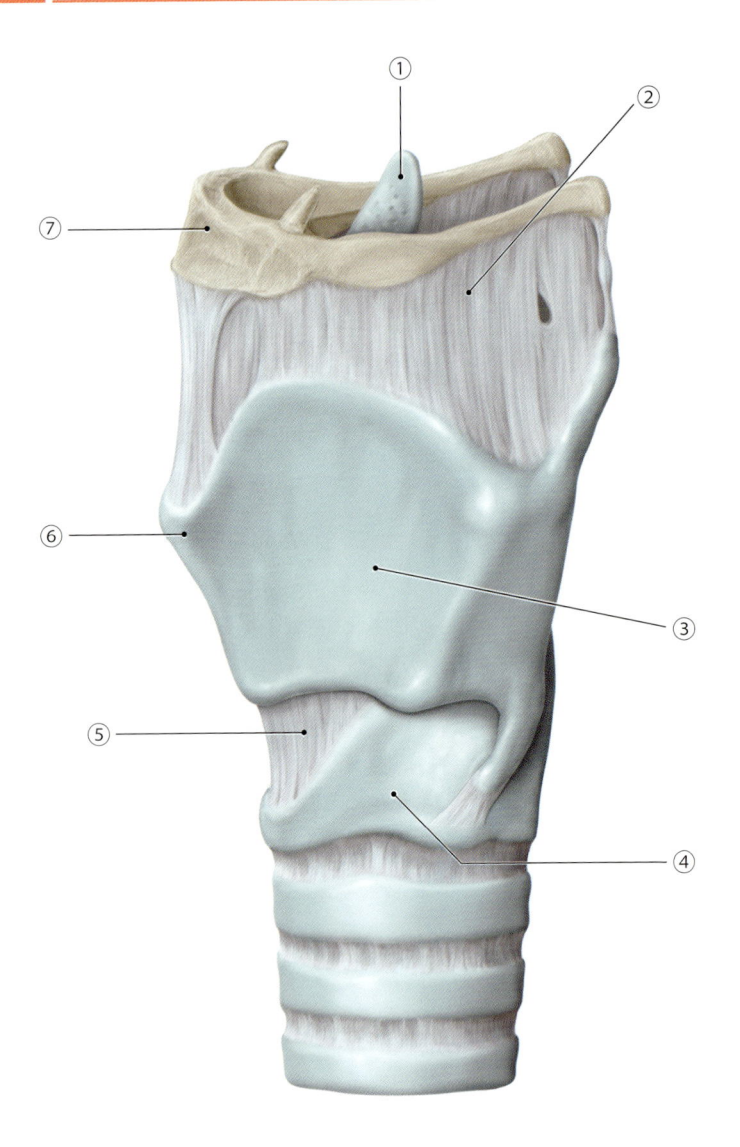

喉頭の構造

左前斜面

① ☐ 喉頭蓋 ☐ Epiglottis
② ☐ 甲状舌骨膜 ☐ Thyrohyoid membrane
③ ☐ 甲状軟骨 ☐ Thyroid cartilage
④ ☐ 輪状軟骨 ☐ Cricoid cartilage
⑤ ☐ 輪状甲状靱帯 ☐ Cricothyroid ligament
⑥ ☐ 喉頭隆起 ☐ Laryngeal prominence of thyroid cartilage
⑦ ☐ 舌骨体 ☐ Hyoid bone

Cavity of the Larynx

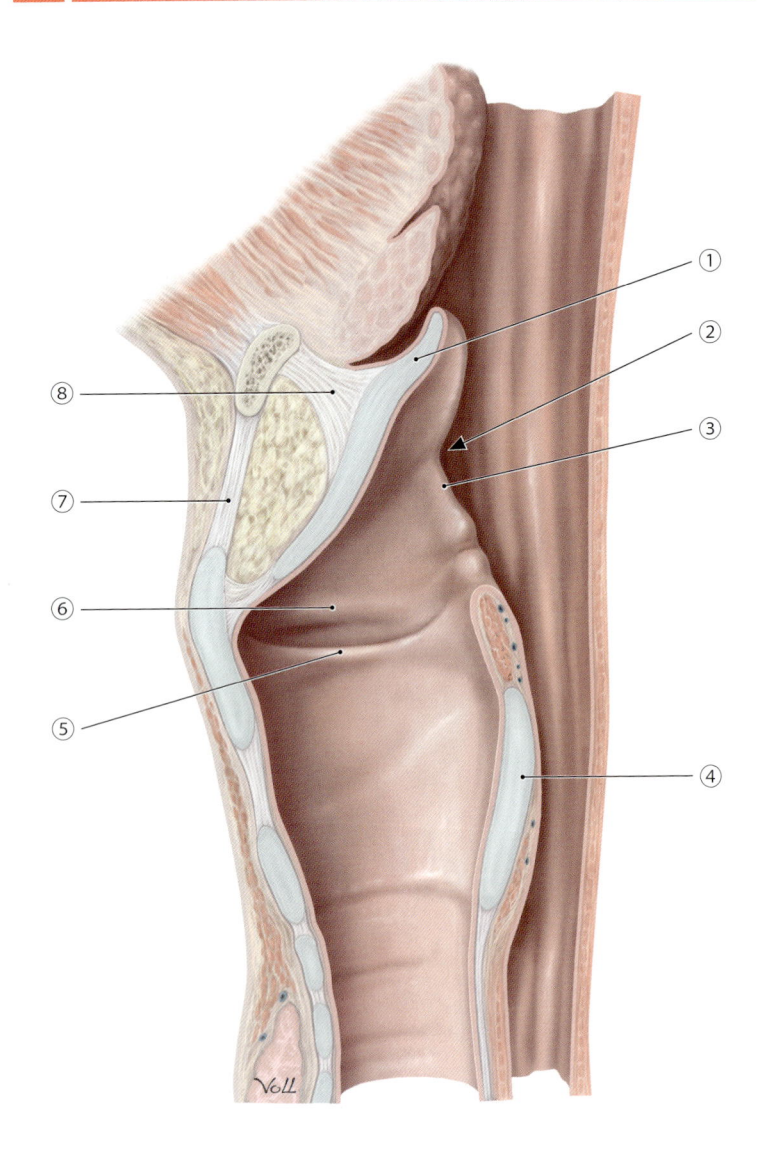

喉頭腔

正中矢状断面，右内側面

① ☐ 喉頭蓋　　　　　　　☐ Epiglottis
② ☐ 梨状陥凹　　　　　　☐ Piriform recess
③ ☐ 披裂喉頭蓋ヒダ　　　☐ Aryepiglottic fold
④ ☐ 輪状軟骨　　　　　　☐ Cricoid cartilage
⑤ ☐ 声帯ヒダ　　　　　　☐ Vocal fold
⑥ ☐ 前庭ヒダ　　　　　　☐ Vestibular fold
⑦ ☐ 甲状舌骨靱帯　　　　☐ Thyrohyoid ligament
⑧ ☐ 舌骨喉頭蓋靱帯　　　☐ Hyoepiglottic ligament

1 図 37.23B. p.573　2 図 39.20B. p.601

678 Head & Neck

Neurovasculature of the Larynx I

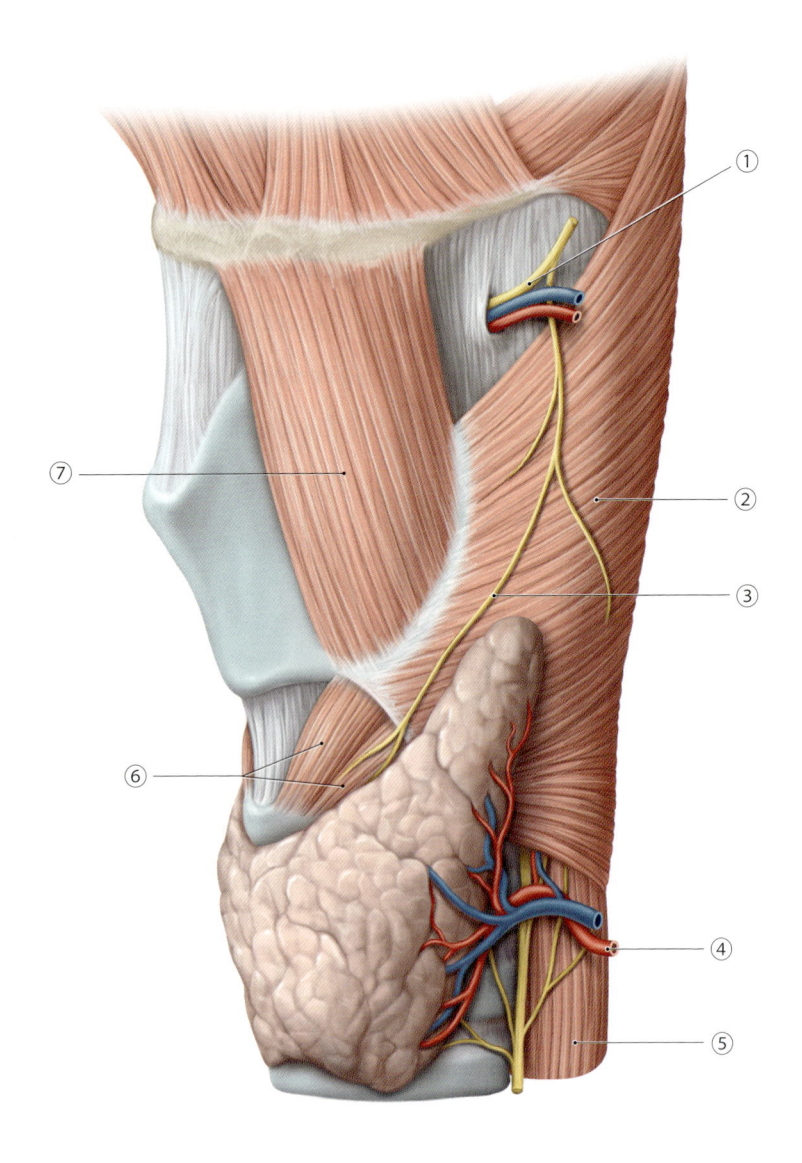

喉頭の神経・血管 1

左外側面

① □ 上喉頭神経，内枝 　　　　□ Superior laryngeal nerve, internal branch

② □ 舌咽頭収縮筋 　　　　□ Inferior pharyngeal constrictor

③ □ 上喉頭神経，外枝 　　　　□ Superior laryngeal nerve, external branch

④ □ 下甲状腺動脈 　　　　□ Inferior thyroid artery

⑤ □ 食道 　　　　□ Esophagus

⑥ □ 輪状甲状筋 　　　　□ Cricothyroid

⑦ □ 甲状舌骨筋 　　　　□ Thyrohyoid

解説

喉頭は迷走神経の枝によって支配される．声帯ヒダより上方は上喉頭神経の内枝によって支配され，声帯ヒダより下方は下喉頭神経に支配される．上喉頭神経の外枝に支配される輪状甲状筋以外のすべての喉頭筋は下喉頭神経に支配される．

1 図 37.28A, p.575　　2 図 39.25A, p.603

Neurovasculature of the Larynx II

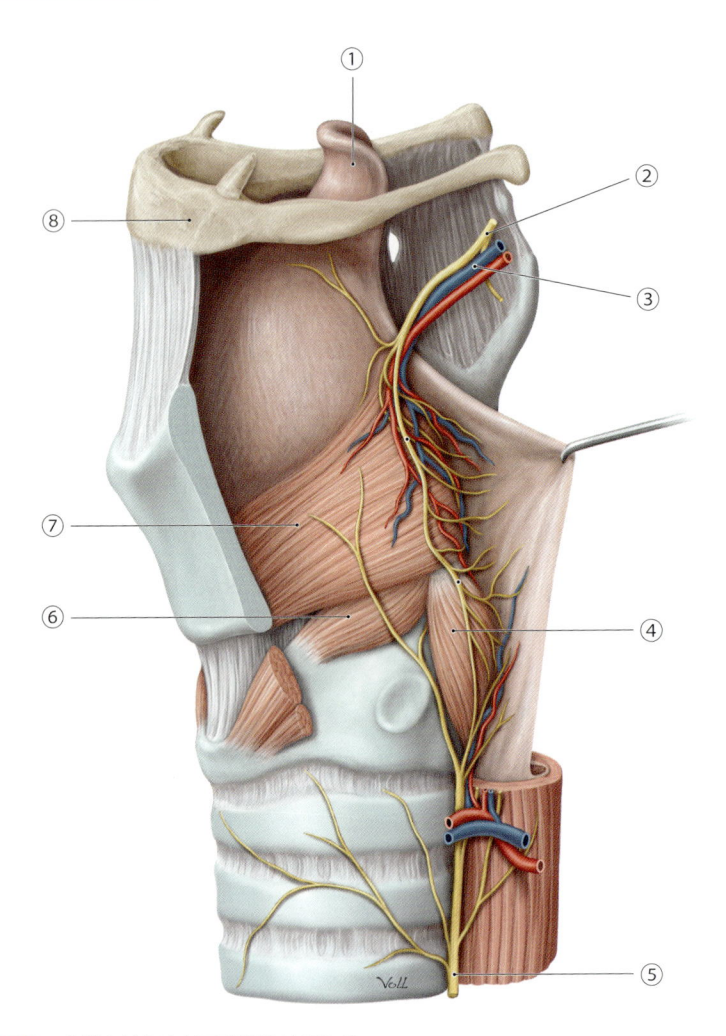

Q 声帯を外転させる喉頭筋は何か？

喉頭の神経・血管 2

左外側面

① □ 喉頭蓋 — □ Epiglottis
② □ 上喉頭神経，内枝 — □ Superior laryngeal nerve, internal branch
③ □ 上喉頭動脈・静脈 — □ Superior laryngeal artery and vein
④ □ 後輪状披裂筋 — □ Posterior cricoarytenoid
⑤ □ 舌喉頭神経 — □ Inferior laryngeal nerve
⑥ □ 外側輪状甲状筋 — □ Lateral cricothyroid
⑦ □ 甲状披裂筋 — □ Thyroarytenoid
⑧ □ 舌骨 — □ Hyoid bone

A 後輪状披裂筋は声帯を外転させる唯一の喉頭筋である．

Cervical Regions

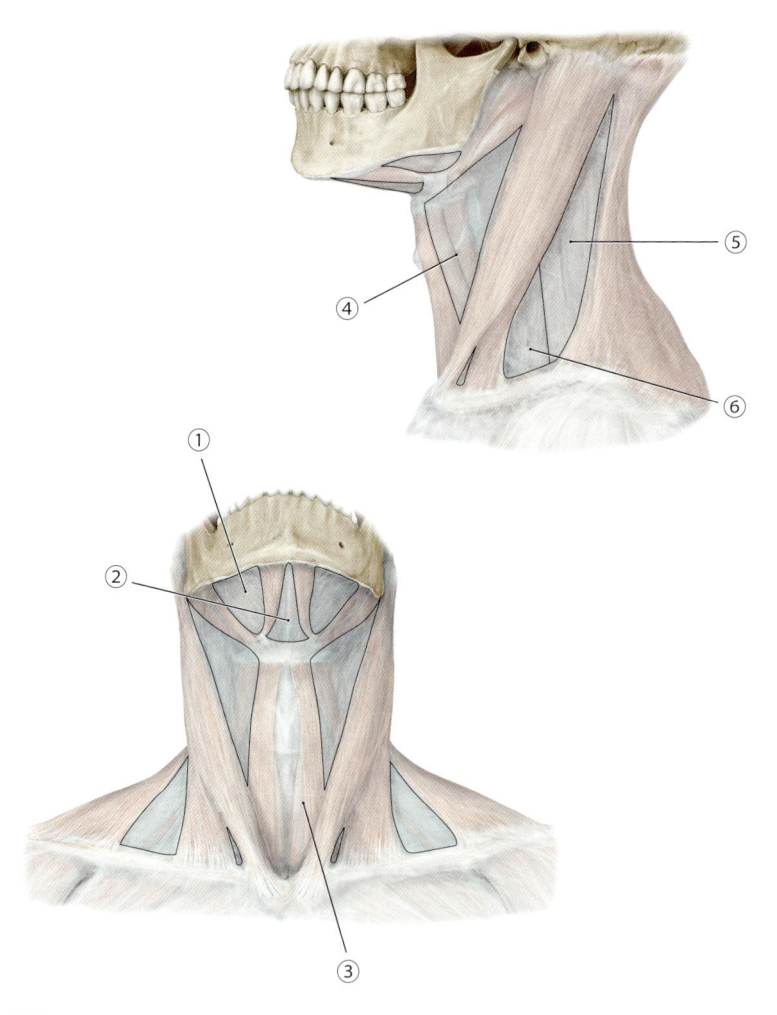

Q 頸部にある三角のうち，腕神経叢はどこにあるか，また内頸静脈はどこにあるか？

頸部の部位

上：左外側面，下：前面

① □ 顎下三角　　　　　□ Submandibular (digastric) triangle

② □ オトガイ下三角　　□ Submental triangle

③ □ 筋三角　　　　　　□ Muscular triangle

④ □ 頸動脈三角　　　　□ Carotid triangle

⑤ □ 後頭三角　　　　　□ Occipital triangle

⑥ □ 肩甲鎖骨三角　　　□ Omoclavicular triangle

A 　腕神経叢は外側頸三角部の後頸三角にあり，内頸静脈は総頸動脈とともに頸動脈三角を通過する．

1 図 37.29A, B. p.576　2 図 37.26A, B. p.604

Thoracic Inlet I

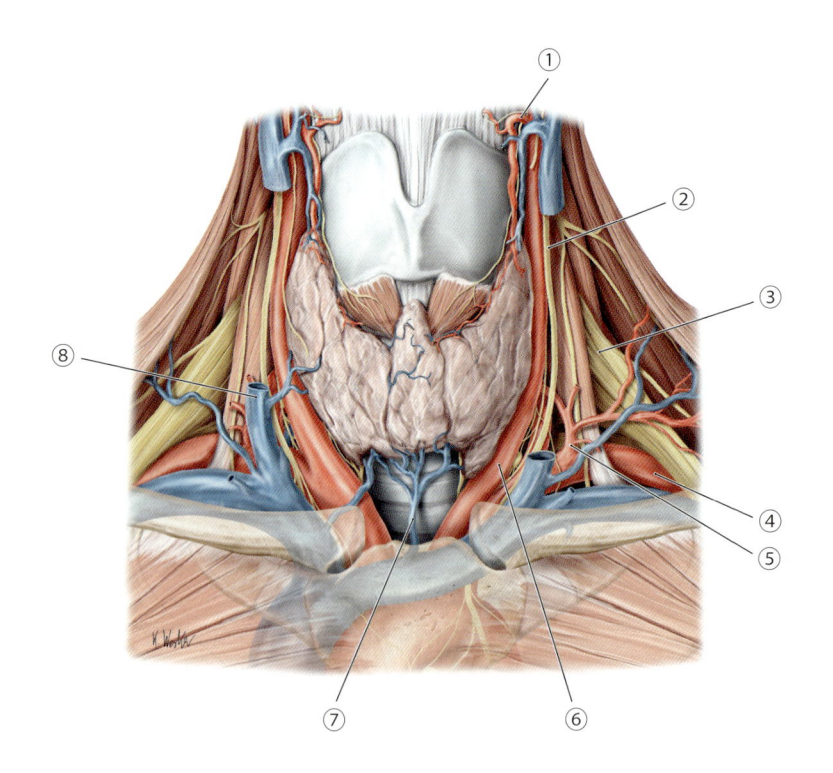

胸郭上口 1

前面

① □ 上甲状腺動脈　　　□ Superior thyroid artery
② □ 迷走神経　　　　　□ Vagus nerve (CN X)
③ □ 腕神経叢　　　　　□ Brachial plexus
④ □ 鎖骨下動脈　　　　□ Subclavian artery
⑤ □ 甲状頸動脈　　　　□ Thyrocervical trunk
⑥ □ 総頸動脈　　　　　□ Common carotid artery
⑦ □ 下甲状腺静脈　　　□ Inferior thyroid vein
⑧ □ 内頸静脈　　　　　□ Internal jugular vein

1 図 37.31C. p.579　　2 図 39.28C. p.607

Thoracic Inlet II

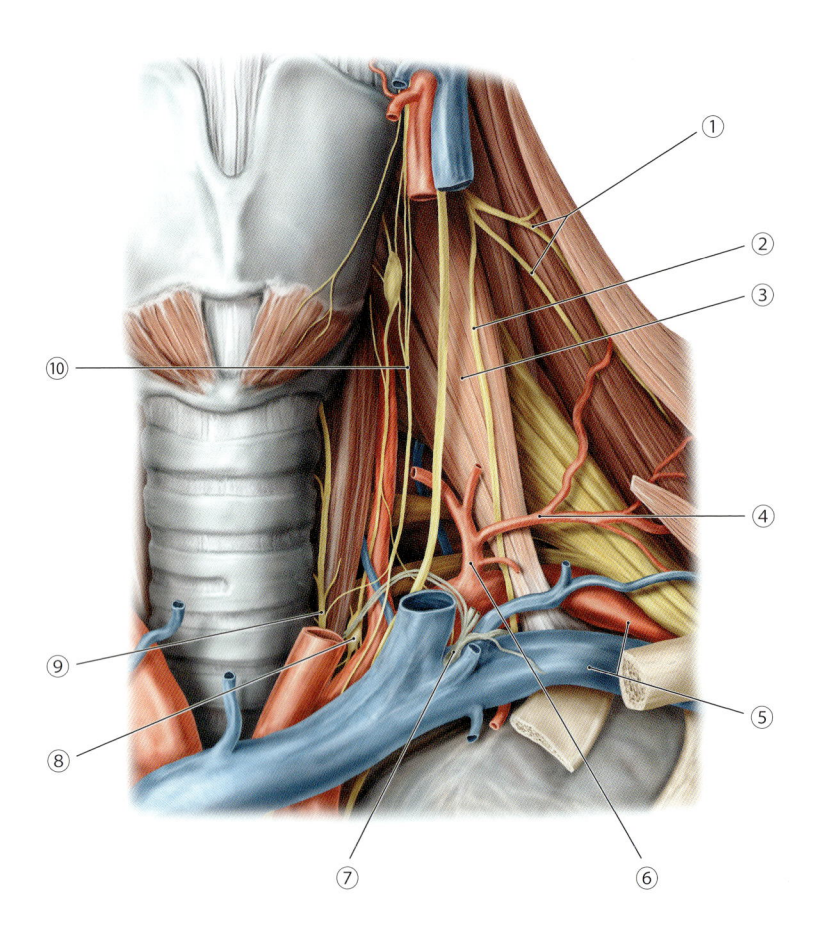

胸郭上口 2

前面

① ☐ 副神経   ☐ (Spinal) accessory nerve (CN XI)

② ☐ 横隔神経   ☐ Phrenic nerve

③ ☐ 前斜角筋   ☐ Anterior scalene

④ ☐ 頸横動脈   ☐ Transverse cervical artery

⑤ ☐ 鎖骨下動脈・静脈   ☐ Subclavian artery and vein

⑥ ☐ 甲状頸動脈   ☐ Thyrocervical trunk

⑦ ☐ 胸管   ☐ Thoracic duct

⑧ ☐ 星状神経節   ☐ Stellate ganglion

⑨ ☐ 反回神経   ☐ Recurrent laryngeal nerve

⑩ ☐ 交感神経幹   ☐ Sympathetic trunk

1 図 37.31D. p.579   2 図 39.28D. p.607

Lateral Cervical Topography I

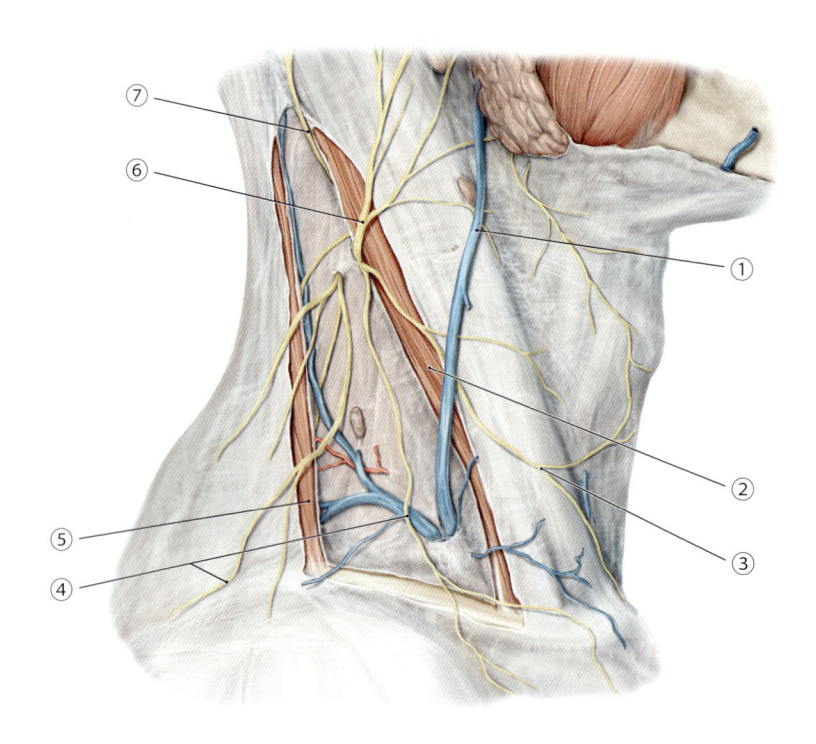

Q 神経点（エルプ点）として知られている頸の標識構造は何か？

外側頸三角部の局所解剖 1

右外側面

① ☐ 外頸静脈　　　　　　　　☐ External jugular vein
② ☐ 胸鎖乳突筋　　　　　　　☐ Sternocleidomastoid
③ ☐ 頸横神経　　　　　　　　☐ Transverse cervical nerve
④ ☐ 鎖骨上神経　　　　　　　☐ Supraclavicular nerves
⑤ ☐ 僧帽筋　　　　　　　　　☐ Trapezius
⑥ ☐ 大耳介神経　　　　　　　☐ Great auricular nerve
⑦ ☐ 小後頭神経　　　　　　　☐ Lesser occipital nerve

A 　頸部の神経点(エルプ点)は，胸鎖乳突筋後縁のほぼ中点にある標識構造で，頸筋膜を貫いてくる頸神経叢の皮枝がある．

[1] 図 37.34B. p.582　　[2] 図 39.32B. p.610

Lateral Cervical Topography II

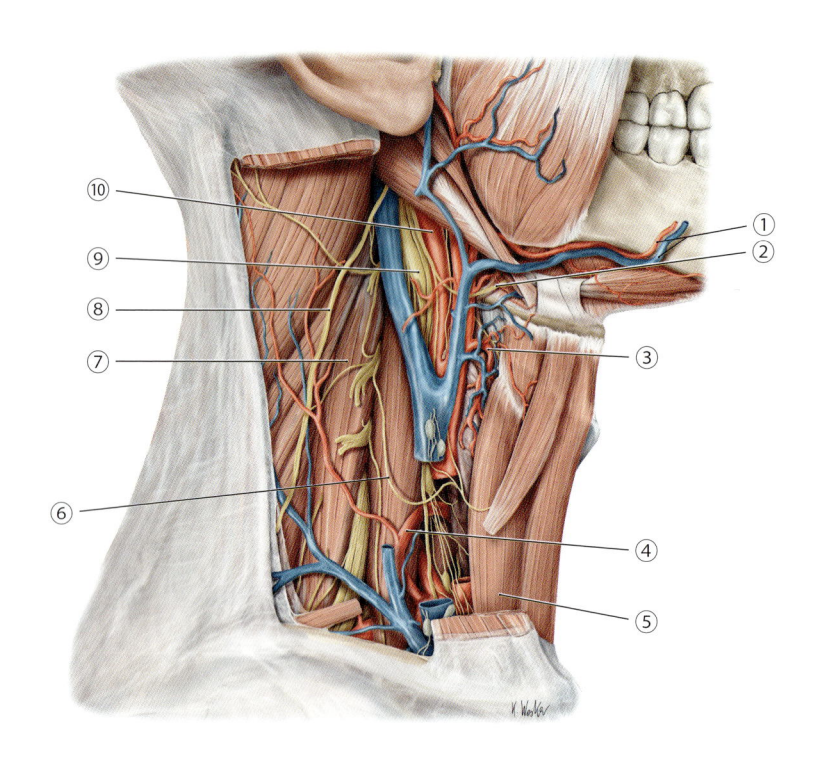

斜角筋隙の重要性は何か？

外側頸三角部の局所解剖 2

右外側面

① ☐ 顔面動脈・静脈　　　　　☐ Facial artery and vein

② ☐ 舌下神経　　　　　　　☐ Hypoglossal nerve (CN XII)

③ ☐ 上甲状腺動脈　　　　　☐ Superior thyroid artery

④ ☐ 下甲状腺動脈　　　　　☐ Inferior thyroid artery

⑤ ☐ 胸骨甲状筋　　　　　　☐ Sternothyroid

⑥ ☐ 頸神経ワナ　　　　　　☐ Ansa cervicalis

⑦ ☐ 中斜角筋　　　　　　　☐ Middle scalene

⑧ ☐ 副神経，外枝　　　　　☐ (Spinal) accessory nerve (CN XI), external branch

⑨ ☐ 上頸神経節　　　　　　☐ Superior cervical ganglion

⑩ ☐ 内頸動脈　　　　　　　☐ Internal carotid artery

A 　斜角筋隙は，頸神経叢と腕神経叢の前枝が脊柱から出て，前斜角筋と中斜角筋の間を通過する冠状面と一致している．斜角筋隙の底部では鎖骨下動脈が腕神経叢の根部とともにある．

1 図 37.33. p.581　2 図 39.31. p.609

692 Head & Neck

Surface Anatomy

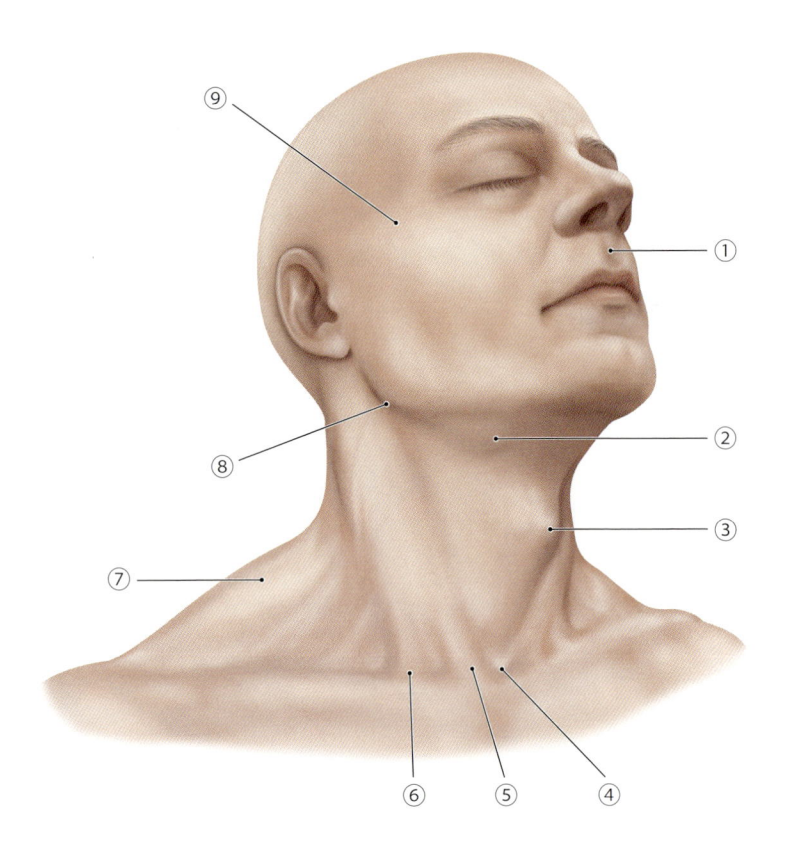

頭頸部の体表解剖

右前外側面

① ☐ 人中 — ☐ Philtrum
② ☐ 顎下腺 — ☐ Submandibular gland
③ ☐ 甲状軟骨 — ☐ Thyroid cartilage
④ ☐ 頸切痕 — ☐ Jugular notch
⑤ ☐ 胸鎖乳突筋，胸骨頭 — ☐ Sternal head of sternocleidomastoid
⑥ ☐ 胸鎖乳突筋，鎖骨頭 — ☐ Clavicular head of sternocleidomastoid
⑦ ☐ 僧帽筋 — ☐ Trapezius
⑧ ☐ 下顎角 — ☐ Mandibular angle
⑨ ☐ 頬骨 — ☐ Zygomatic bone

1 図38.2A. p.589 2 図30.2A. p.476

神経解剖 Neuroanatomy

- 成人の脳1 ················· 696
- 成人の脳2 ················· 698
- 大脳白質 ················· 700
- 海馬とその関連構造 ················· 702
- 間脳 ················· 704
- 脳の内部構造1 ················· 706
- 脳の内部構造2 ················· 708
- 脳の内部構造3 ················· 710
- 脳幹1 ················· 712
- 脳幹2 ················· 714
- 脊髄 ················· 716
- 脊髄の横断面 ················· 718
- 髄膜1 ················· 720
- 髄膜2 ················· 722
- 硬膜中隔 ················· 724
- 脳脊髄液の循環 ················· 726
- 脳室系 ················· 728
- 静脈洞交会 ················· 730
- 頭蓋底にある硬膜静脈洞 ················· 732
- 脳の動脈 ················· 734
- 脊髄の動脈 ················· 736
- 感覚系と運動系 ················· 738
- 脊髄の上行路 ················· 740
- 脊髄の下行路 ················· 742
- 視覚系 ················· 744
- 自律神経系 ················· 746

Adult Brain I

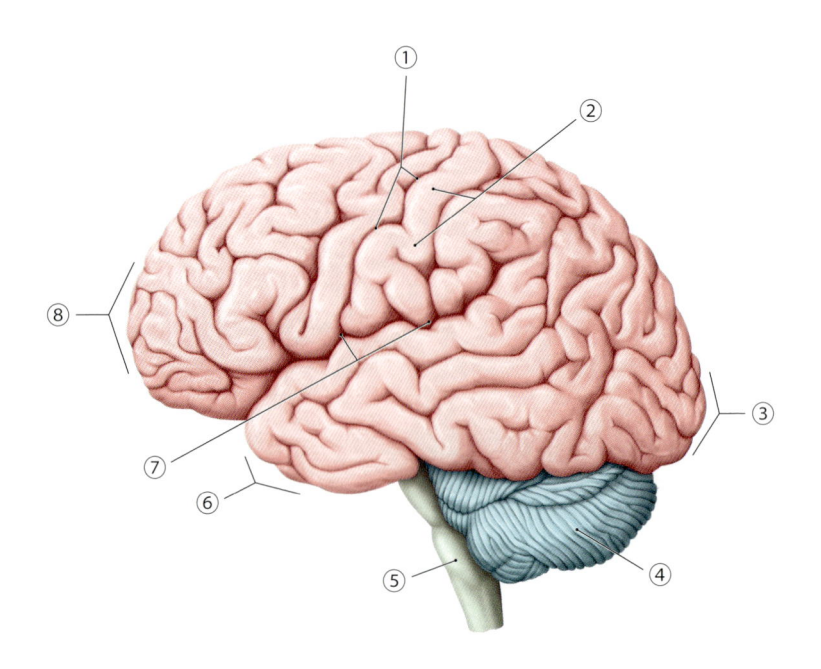

中心溝によって分けられる 2 つの葉は何か？

成人の脳 1

左外側面

① □ 中心溝　　　　　　□ Central sulcus
② □ 中心後回　　　　　□ Postcentral gyrus
③ □ 後頭葉　　　　　　□ Occipital lobe
④ □ 小脳　　　　　　　□ Cerebellum
⑤ □ 延髄　　　　　　　□ Medulla oblongata
⑥ □ 側頭葉　　　　　　□ Temporal lobe
⑦ □ 外側溝　　　　　　□ Lateral sulcus
⑧ □ 前頭葉　　　　　　□ Frontal lobe

A 前頭葉と頭頂葉が中心溝によって分けられる．

1 図 39.6A. p.593　 2 図 40.6A. p.625

Adult Brain II

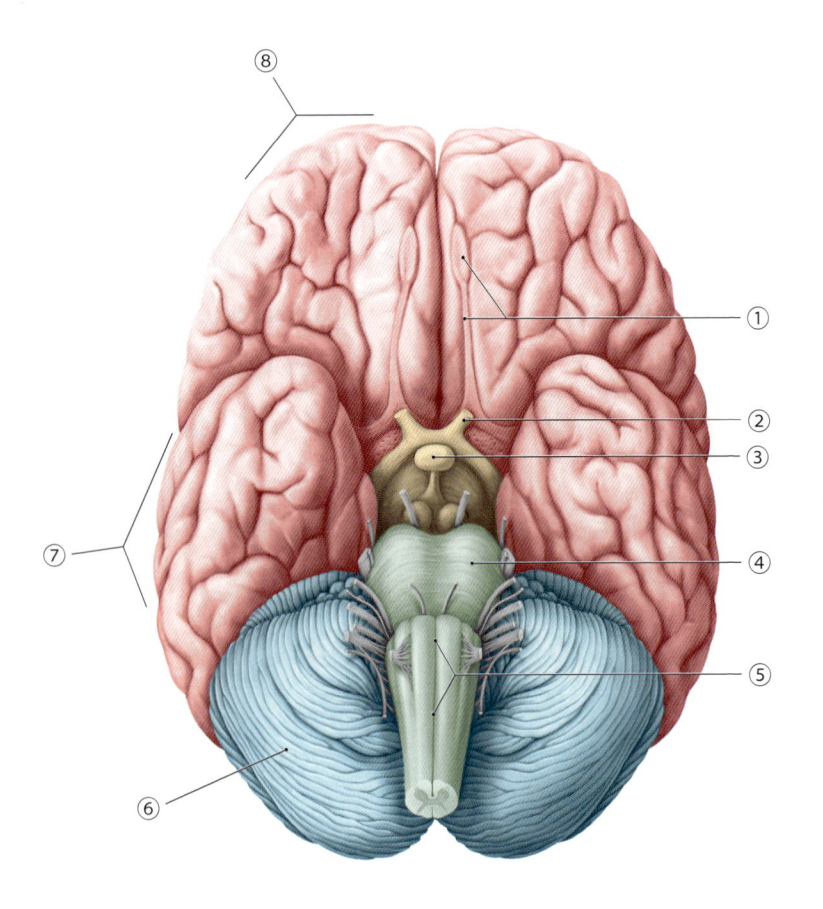

成人の脳 2

底面

① □ 嗅球, 嗅索 　　　　□ Olfactory bulb and tract
② □ 視神経 　　　　　　□ Optic nerve (CN II)
③ □ 下垂体 　　　　　　□ Hypophysis
④ □ 橋 　　　　　　　　□ Pons
⑤ □ 延髄 　　　　　　　□ Medulla oblongata
⑥ □ 小脳 　　　　　　　□ Cerebellum
⑦ □ 側頭葉 　　　　　　□ Temporal lobe
⑧ □ 前頭葉 　　　　　　□ Frontal lobe

1 図 39.6B. p.593　2 図 40.6B. p.625

White Matter of the Telencephalon

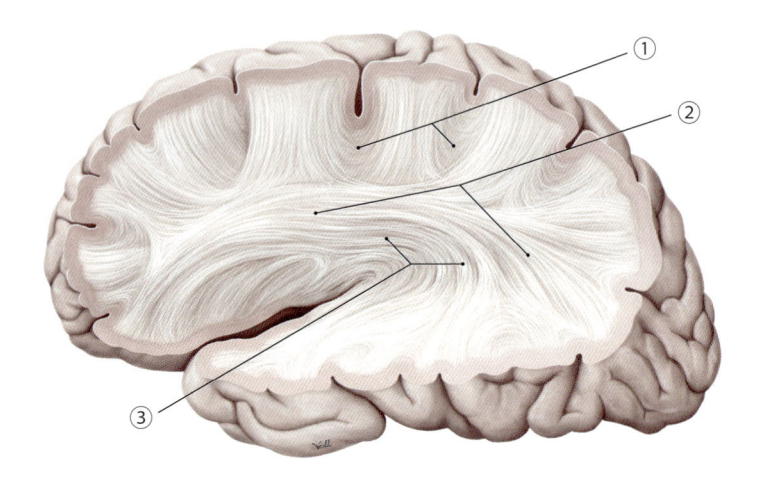

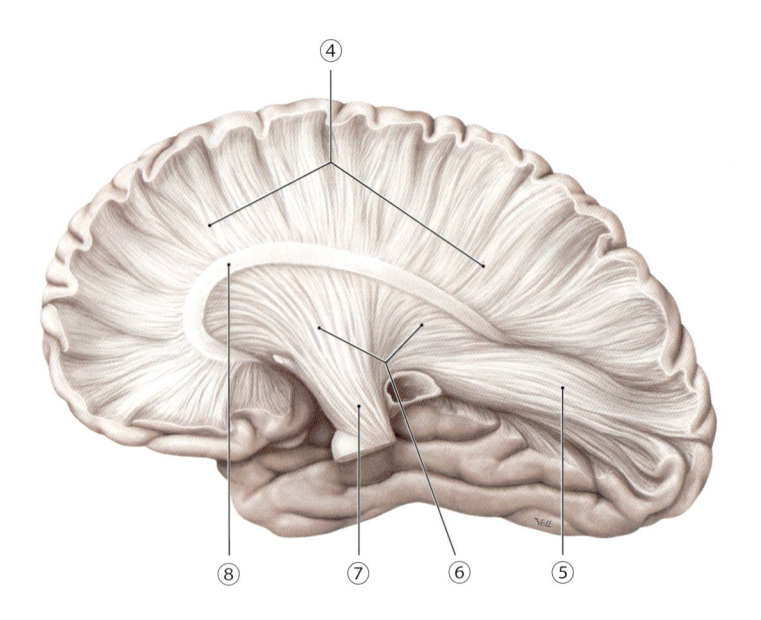

大脳白質

上：左大脳半球の外側面，下：右大脳半球の内側面

① ☐ 大脳弓状線維　　　　　☐ Cerebral arcuate fibers (U fibers)

② ☐ 上縦束　　　　　　　　☐ Superior longitudinal fasciculus

③ ☐ 前頭側頭束　　　　　　☐ Frontotemporal fasciculus

④ ☐ 放線冠　　　　　　　　☐ Corona radiata

⑤ ☐ 視放線　　　　　　　　☐ Optic radiation

⑥ ☐ 内包　　　　　　　　　☐ Internal capsule

⑦ ☐ 大脳脚　　　　　　　　☐ Cerebral peduncle

⑧ ☐ 脳梁　　　　　　　　　☐ Corpus callosum

解説

肉眼では，神経細胞の細胞体が集まった部位は灰白色に，軸索（髄鞘が取り巻いている）が集まった部位は白色に見える．

1 図39.8A, B. p.594　2 図40.8A, B. p.626

Hippocampal Formation

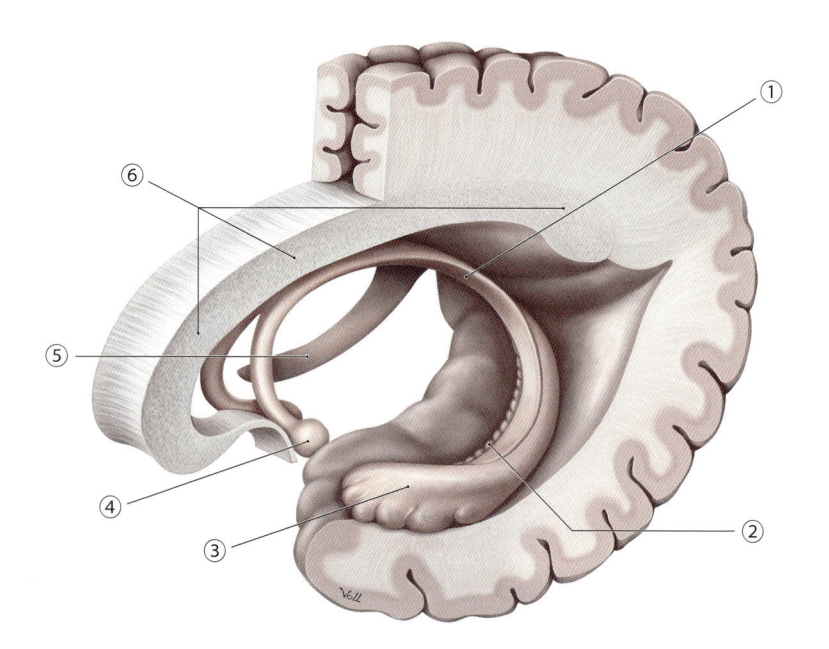

海馬とその関連構造

左前上面

① □ 脳弓体　　　　　　　　□ Body of fornix

② □ 歯状回　　　　　　　　□ Dentate gyrus

③ □ 海馬　　　　　　　　　□ Hippocampus

④ □ 乳頭体　　　　　　　　□ Mammillary body

⑤ □ 脳弓脚　　　　　　　　□ Crus of fornix

⑥ □ 脳梁　　　　　　　　　□ Corpus callosum

解説

海馬，脳弓，扁桃体は辺縁系の主要な構成要素である．

1 図 39.13B. p.596　　2 図 40.13B. p.628

Diencephalon

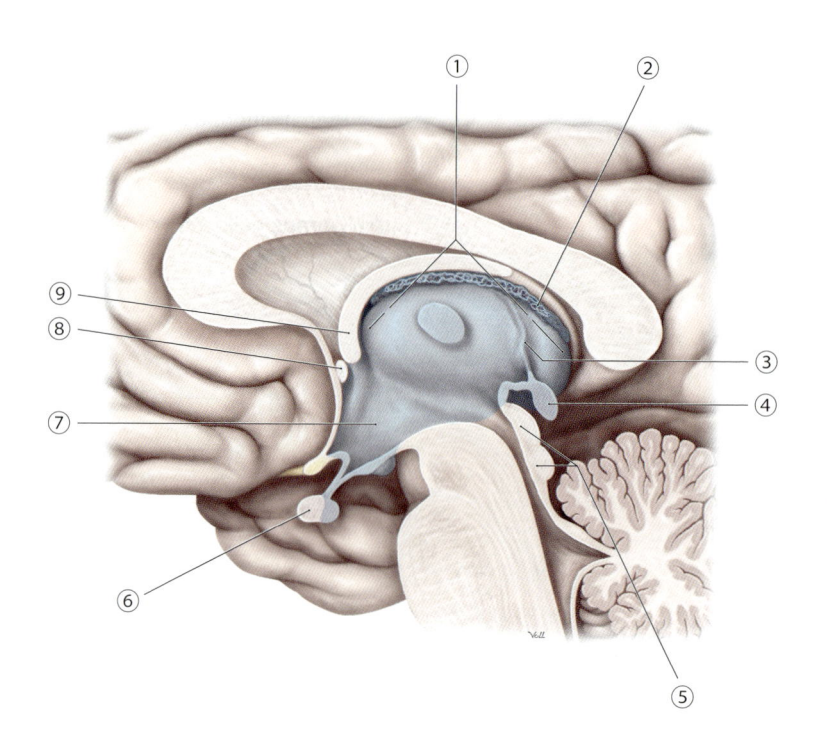

Q 下垂体前葉（腺下垂体）は胎児期にどこから形成されるか？

● 間脳

正中矢状断面

① □ 視床　　　　　　　　　□ Thalamus
② □ 脈絡叢　　　　　　　　□ Choroid plexus
③ □ 視床髄条　　　　　　　□ Stria medullaris thalami
④ □ 松果体　　　　　　　　□ Pineal gland
⑤ □ 四丘体板　　　　　　　□ Quadrigeminal plate
⑥ □ 下垂体，前葉（腺下垂体）□ Hypophysis, anterior lobe (adenohypophysis)
⑦ □ 視床下部　　　　　　　□ Hypothalamus
⑧ □ 前交連　　　　　　　　□ Anterior commissure
⑨ □ 脳弓　　　　　　　　　□ Fornix

A 下垂体前葉（腺下垂体）は，口咽頭の上皮の突出部であるラトケ嚢に由来する．

1 図 39.14. p.596　2 図 40.14. p.628

Internal Structures I

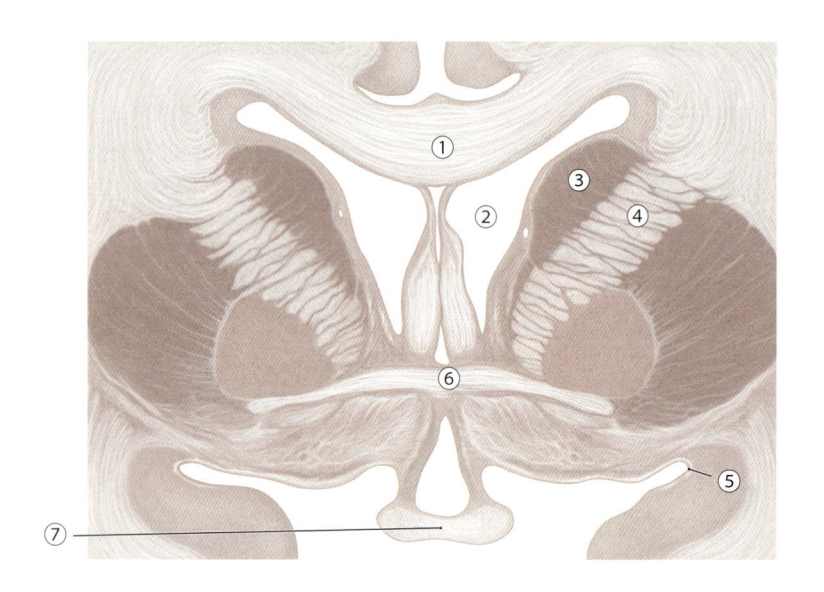

Q 左右の大脳半球をつなぐ2つの構造は何か？

脳の内部構造 1

前額断面(視神経交叉を通る断面)

① ☐ 脳梁　　　　　☐ Corpus callosum
② ☐ 側脳室　　　　☐ Lateral ventricle
③ ☐ 尾状核　　　　☐ Caudate nucleus
④ ☐ 内包　　　　　☐ Internal capsule
⑤ ☐ 外側嗅条　　　☐ Lateral olfactory stria
⑥ ☐ 前交連　　　　☐ Anterior commissure
⑦ ☐ 視交叉　　　　☐ Optic chiasm (CN II)

A 左右の大脳半球は，脳梁と前交連によって連結している．

Internal Structures II

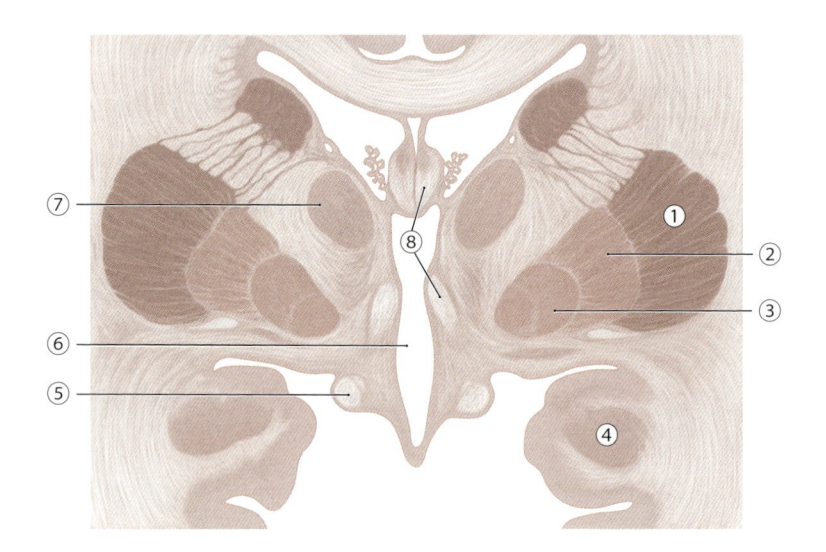

Q 扁桃体が属する機能系は何か？

脳の内部構造 2

前額断面(灰白隆起を通る断面)

① □ 被殻 　　　　　　　　□ Putamen

② □ 淡蒼球の外節 　　　　□ Lateral segment of globus pallidus

③ □ 淡蒼球の内節 　　　　□ Medial segment of globus pallidus

④ □ 扁桃体 　　　　　　　□ Amygdala

⑤ □ 視索 　　　　　　　　□ Optic tract

⑥ □ 第三脳室 　　　　　　□ 3rd ventricle

⑦ □ 視床(視床核) 　　　　□ Thalamus

⑧ □ 脳弓 　　　　　　　　□ Fornix

A 扁桃体は辺縁系の構成要素である.

1 図39.15B, p.597　2 図40.15B, p.629

Internal Structures III

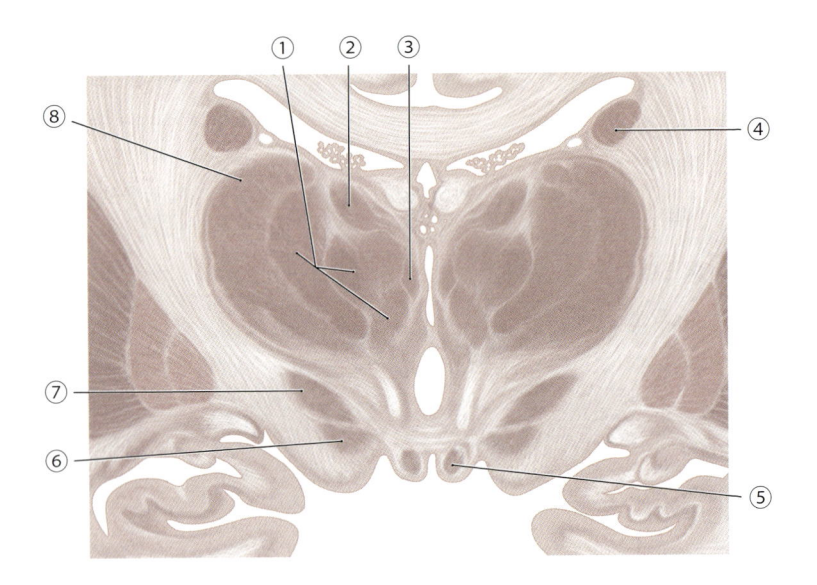

Q 視床核のうち，意識にのぼる固有覚（位置覚や運動覚）を中継するのはどれか？

脳の内部構造 3

前額断面(乳頭体を通る断面)

① ☐ 視床内側核群　　☐ Medial thalamic nuclei
② ☐ 視床前核群　　　☐ Anterior thalamic nuclei
③ ☐ 視床室傍核群　　☐ Paraventricular nuclei
④ ☐ 尾状核　　　　　☐ Caudate nucleus
⑤ ☐ 乳頭体　　　　　☐ Mammillary body
⑥ ☐ 黒質　　　　　　☐ Substantia nigra
⑦ ☐ 視床下核　　　　☐ Subthalamic nucleus
⑧ ☐ 視床外側腹側核群　☐ Ventrolateral thalamic nuclei

A 意識にのぼる固有覚は後外側腹側核を中継し，大脳皮質へ伝えられる．

1 図 39.15C, p.597　2 図 40.15C, p.629

Brainstem I

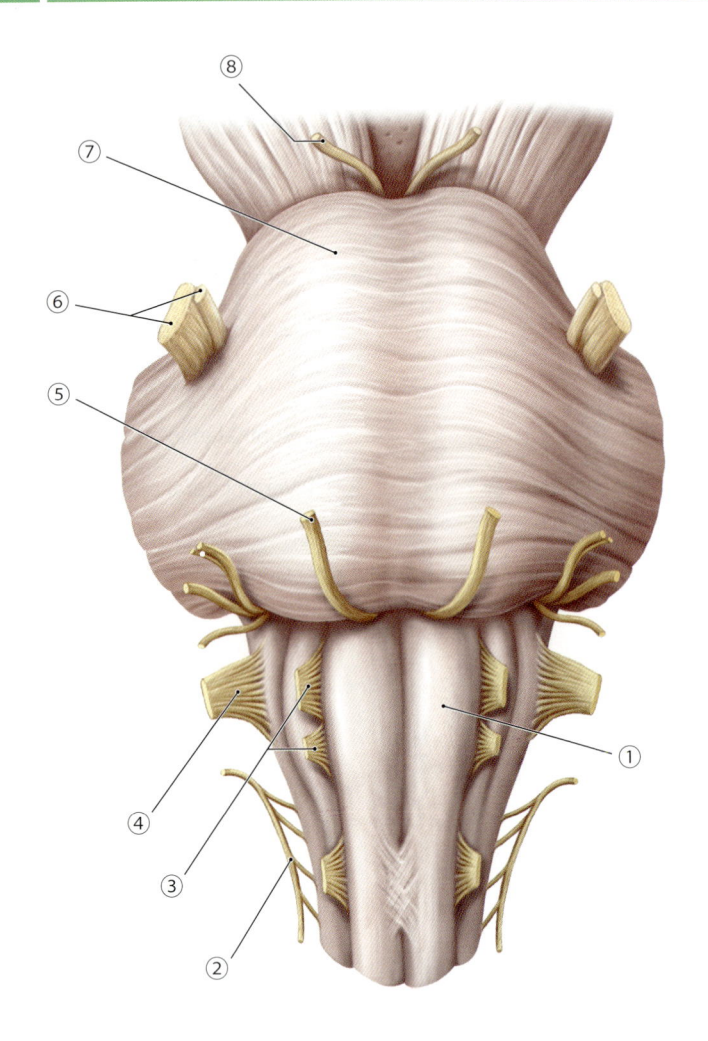

Q 橋に存在する脳神経核は何か？

脳幹 1

前面

① □ 延髄錐体 □ Pyramid of medulla oblongata

② □ 副神経 □ Accessory nerve (CN XI)

③ □ 舌下神経 □ Hypoglossal nerve (CN XII)

④ □ 迷走神経 □ Vagus nerve (CN X)

⑤ □ 外転神経 □ Abducent nerve (CN VI)

⑥ □ 三叉神経 □ Trigeminal nerve (CN V)

⑦ □ 橋 □ Pons

⑧ □ 動眼神経 □ Oculomotor nerve (CN III)

A 　三叉神経(V)，外転神経(VI)，顔面神経(VII)，内耳神経(VIII)に関する神経核が橋に存在する．ただし，前庭神経核は延髄にまで，三叉神経脊髄路核は脊髄にまで伸び出している．

[1] 図 39.19B, p.599 　 [2] 図 40.19B, p.631

714　Neuroanatomy

Brainstem II

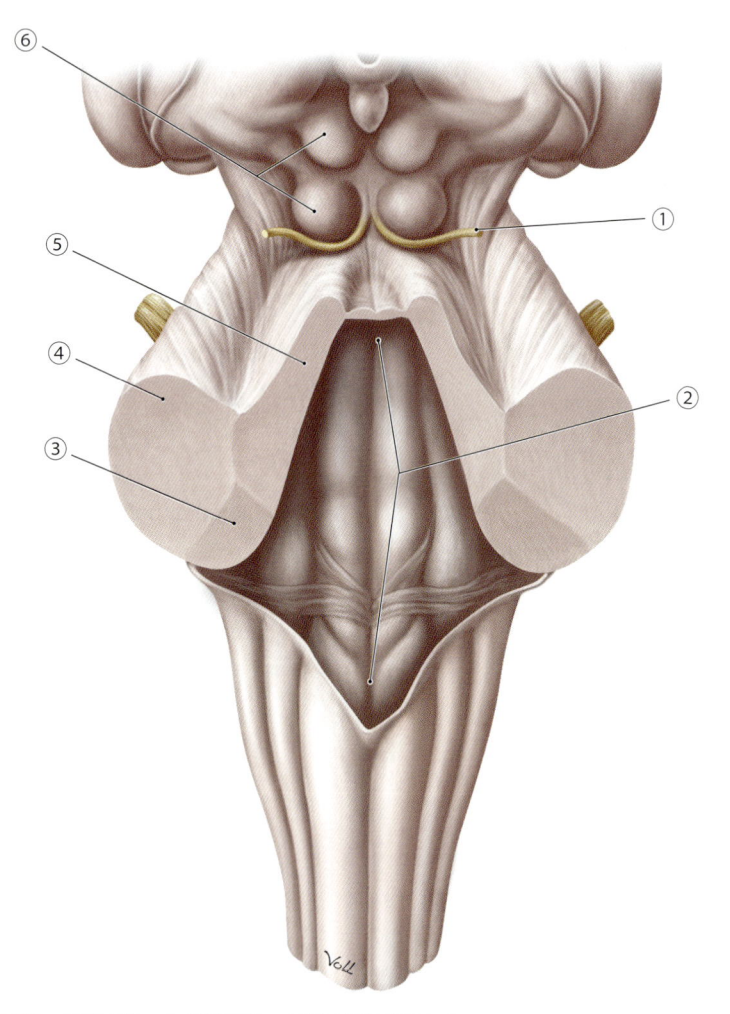

脳幹の後方から出る唯一の脳神経はどれか？

脳幹 2

後面

① □ 滑車神経 □ Trochlear nerve (CN IV)

② □ 菱形窩 □ Rhomboid fossa

③ □ 下小脳脚 □ Inferior cerebellar peduncle

④ □ 中小脳脚 □ Middle cerebellar peduncle

⑤ □ 上小脳脚 □ Superior cerebellar peduncle

⑥ □ 蓋板(四丘体板)の上丘と下丘 □ Superior and inferior colliculi of quadrigeminal plate

A 　滑車神経(Ⅳ)は，脳幹(中脳)の後面にある下丘の遠位から現れる．脳幹から出るその他の脳神経は，すべてが脳幹の前面から現れる．

1 図 39.19D. p.599　2 図 40.19D. p.631

Spinal Cord

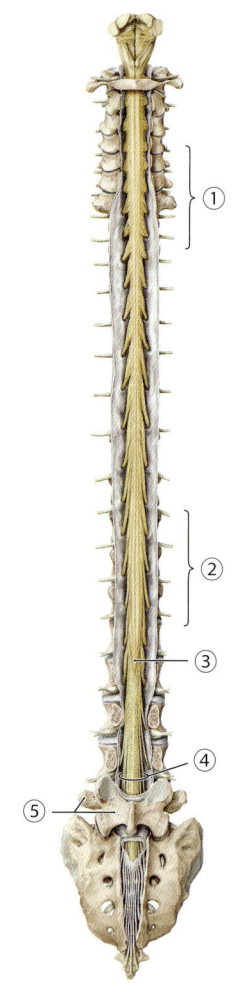

①
②
③
④
⑤

Q 成人では脊髄の下端はおよそどの高さに位置するか？

脊髄

後面

① ☐ 頸膨大 　　　　　☐ Cervical enlargement

② ☐ 腰膨大 　　　　　☐ Lumbosacral enlargement

③ ☐ 脊髄円錐 　　　　☐ Conus medullaris

④ ☐ 馬尾 　　　　　　☐ Cauda equina

⑤ ☐ 第5腰椎 　　　　☐ L5 vertebra

A 成人では，脊髄の下端はL1の高さに位置する．これは，脊髄の成長が停止した後も，脊柱の成長が進行することによる．第1腰神経よりも下位の脊髄神経は，脊柱管内を馬尾となって下行する．

1 図39.21. p.600　2 図4.6. p.40

Transverse section of the Spinal Cord

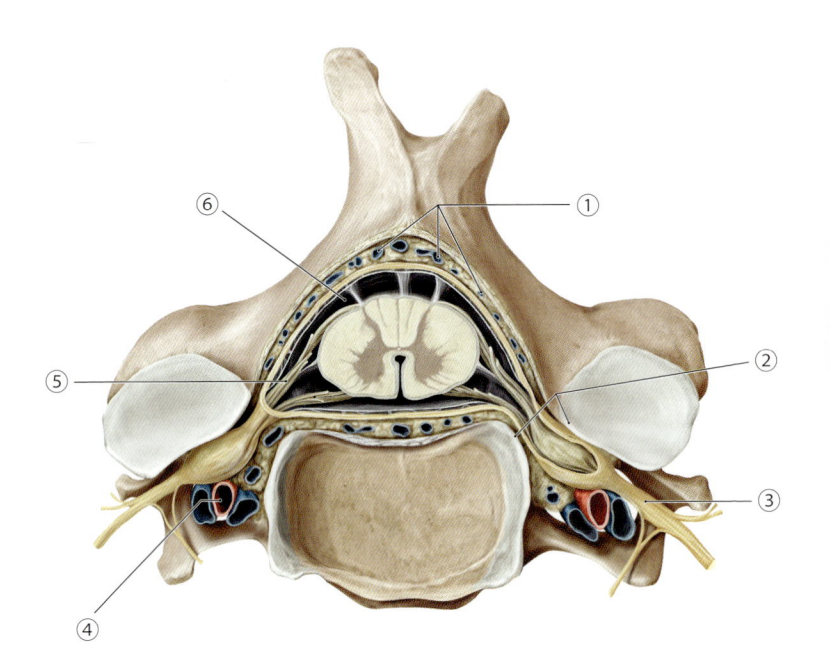

Q 脳脊髄液によって満たされるのはどこか？

脊髄の横断面

横断面,上面

① □ 後内椎骨静脈叢 　　　□ Posterior internal vertebral venous plexus
② □ 椎間孔 　　　□ Intervertebral foramen
③ □ 脊髄神経 　　　□ Spinal nerve
④ □ 椎骨動脈 　　　□ Vertebral artery
⑤ □ 後根 　　　□ Dorsal root
⑥ □ クモ膜下腔 　　　□ Subarachnoid space

A 脳脊髄液はクモ膜下腔を満たしている.

Meninges I

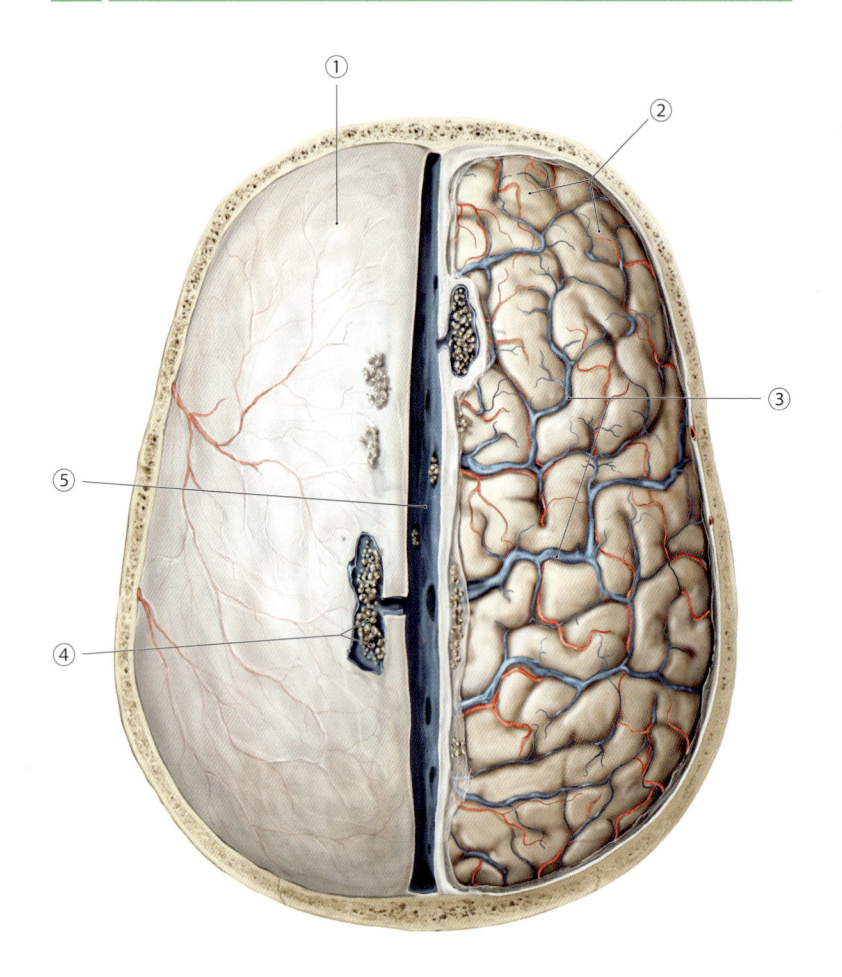

クモ膜顆粒の機能は何か？

髄膜 1

上面

① ☐ 硬膜 ☐ Dura mater
② ☐ 軟膜（大脳表面にある） ☐ Pia mater (on cerebral surface)
③ ☐ 上大脳静脈 ☐ Superior cerebral veins
④ ☐ クモ膜顆粒 ☐ Arachnoid granulations
　　（クモ膜絨毛） 　　(arachnoid villi)
⑤ ☐ 上矢状静脈洞 ☐ Superior sagittal sinus

A クモ膜顆粒は，脳脊髄液をクモ膜下腔から上矢状静脈洞へ再吸収している．

[1] 図39.25A. p.602　[2] 図34.16B. p.526

Meninges II

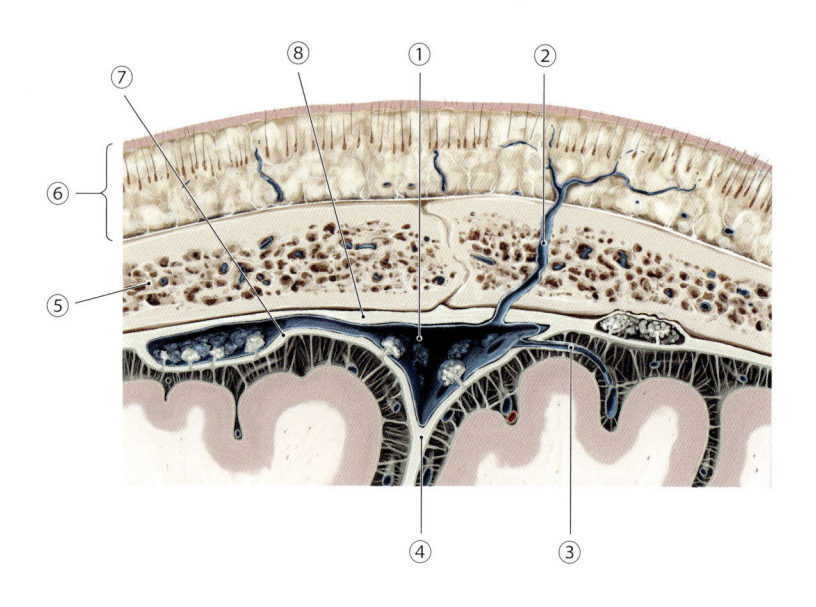

髄膜 2

冠状断面，前面

① ☐ 上矢状静脈洞　　　　　☐ Superior sagittal sinus

② ☐ 導出静脈　　　　　　　☐ Emissary vein

③ ☐ 架橋静脈　　　　　　　☐ Bridging vein

④ ☐ 大脳鎌　　　　　　　　☐ Falx cerebri

⑤ ☐ 板間層　　　　　　　　☐ Diploë of cranial bone

⑥ ☐ 頭皮　　　　　　　　　☐ Scalp

⑦ ☐ 硬膜，髄膜性の内層　　☐ Meningeal layer of dura mater

⑧ ☐ 硬膜，骨膜性の外層　　☐ Periosteal layer of dura mater

臨床

　頭蓋内出血は脳硬膜との位置関係により3つのタイプ（硬膜外出血，硬膜下出血，クモ膜下出血）に分けられる．硬膜外出血や硬膜下出血は，放置すると大きくなった血腫により脳が圧迫を受ける．血腫がさらに大きくなると，頭蓋内圧の上昇により，脳の直接圧迫を受けている部位だけでなく，離れた部位にも損傷が及ぶ．

1 図 39.25D. p.602　2 図 34.16A. p.526

Dural Septa

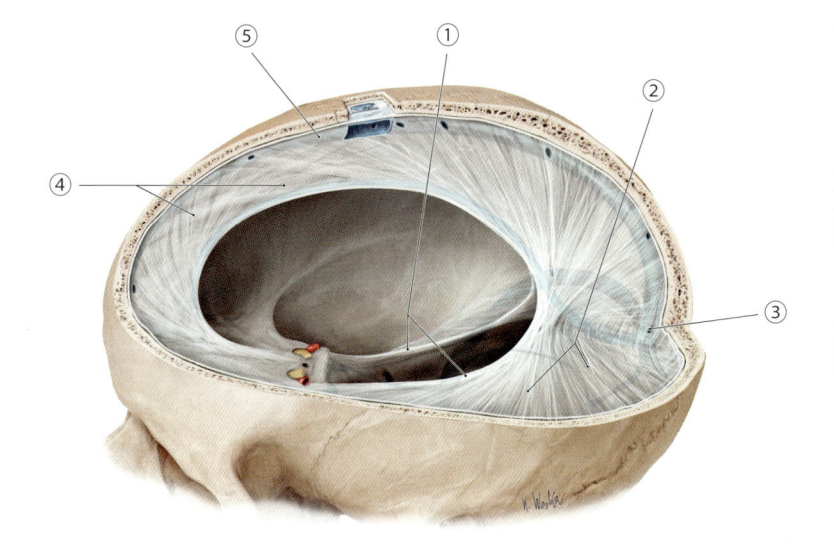

硬膜中隔

左前上外側面

① □ テント切痕　　　　　　　　□ Tentorial notch

② □ 小脳テント　　　　　　　　□ Tentorium cerebelli

③ □ 静脈洞交会　　　　　　　　□ Confluence of the sinuses

④ □ 大脳鎌　　　　　　　　　　□ Falx cerebri

⑤ □ 上矢状静脈洞　　　　　　　□ Superior sagittal sinus

解説

硬膜の反転部によってできる中隔のうち，主要なものには大脳鎌，小脳テント，小脳鎌がある．このような中隔は脳の特定の部位に入り込み，脳のいくつかの部位を隔てている．

1 図 39.26. p.603　　2 図 34.13. p.524

CSF Circulation

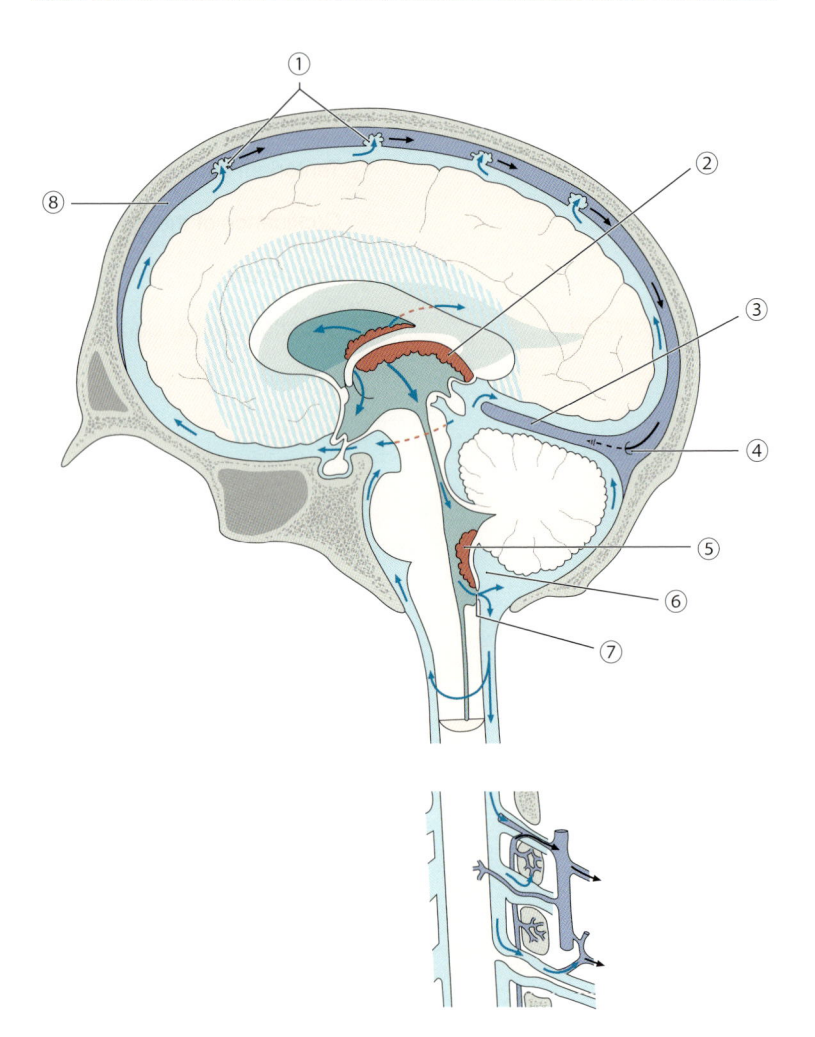

Q 第三脳室と第四脳室を連結する構造は何か？

脳脊髄液の循環

左外側面

① ☐ クモ膜顆粒　　　　　　　　☐ Arachnoid granulations

② ☐ 第三脳室脈絡叢　　　　　　☐ Choroid plexus (3rd ventricle)

③ ☐ 直静脈洞　　　　　　　　　☐ Straight sinus

④ ☐ 静脈洞交会　　　　　　　　☐ Confluence of the sinuses

⑤ ☐ 第四脳室脈絡叢　　　　　　☐ Choroid plexus (4th ventricle)

⑥ ☐ 小脳延髄槽（大槽）　　　　☐ Cerebellomedullary cistern (cisterna magna)

⑦ ☐ 第四脳室正中口　　　　　　☐ Median aperture

⑧ ☐ 上矢状静脈洞　　　　　　　☐ Superior sagittal sinus

A 中脳水道が第三脳室と第四脳室を連結する.

1 図 39.29. p.604　　2 図 40.20. p.632

Ventricular System

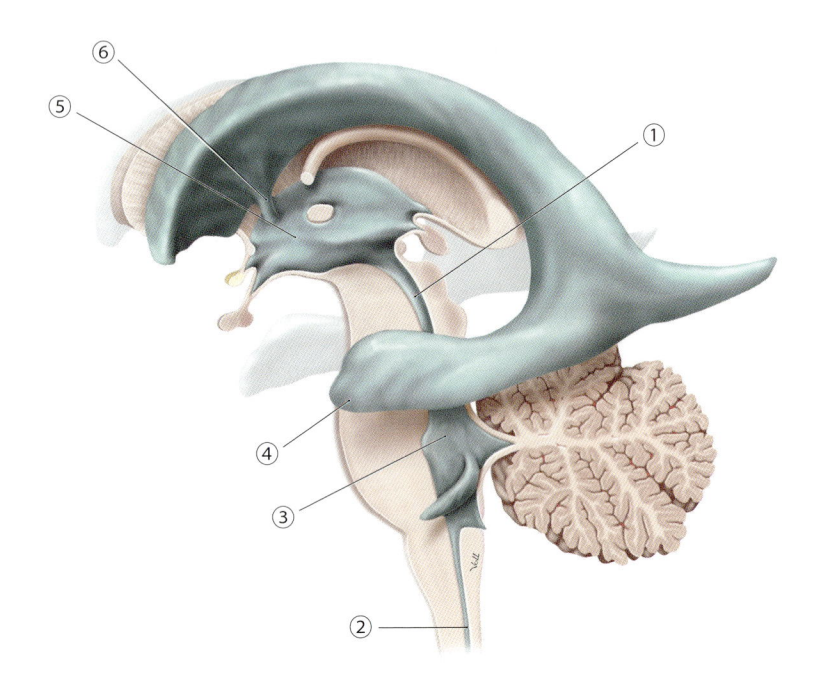

Q 水頭症とは何か？

脳室系

左外側面

① ☐ 中脳水道　　　　　　　　☐ Cerebral aqueduct

② ☐ 中心管　　　　　　　　　☐ Central canal

③ ☐ 第四脳室　　　　　　　　☐ 4th ventricle

④ ☐ 側脳室（下角）　　　　　☐ Lateral ventricle (inferior horn)

⑤ ☐ 第三脳室　　　　　　　　☐ 3rd ventricle

⑥ ☐ 室間孔　　　　　　　　　☐ Interventricular foramen

A 水頭症は脳脊髄液が異常に溜まった状態を指す．

Confluence of the Sinuses

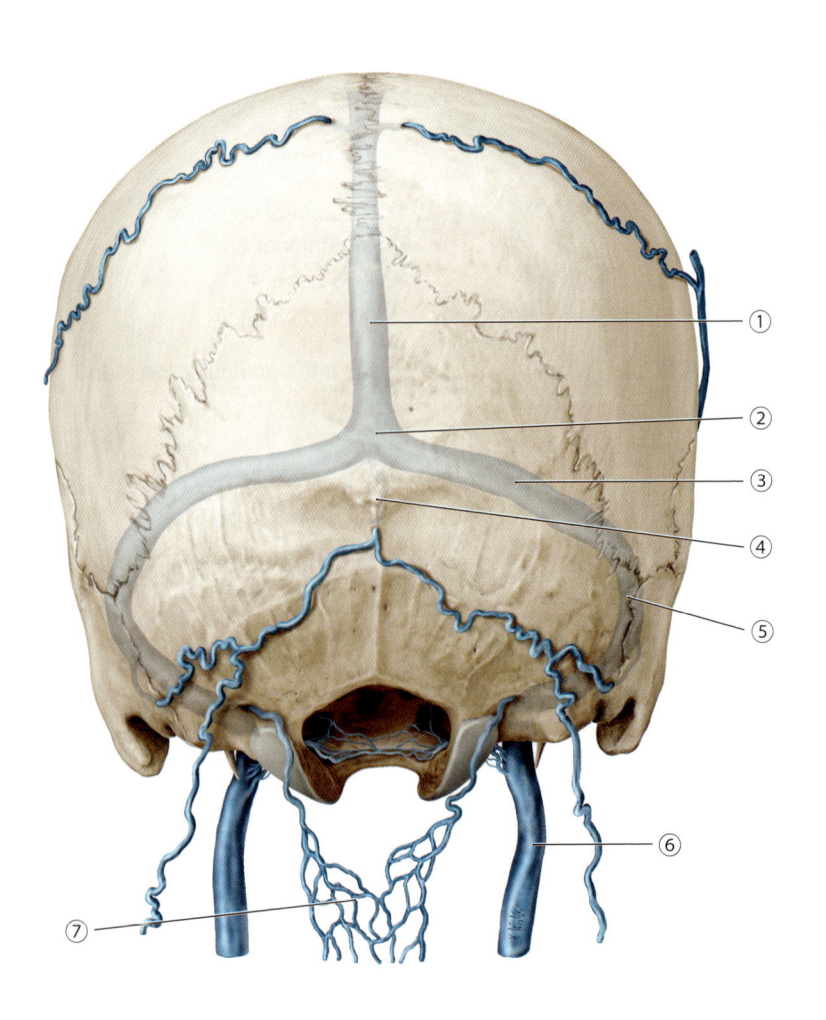

静脈洞交会

後面

① □ 上矢状静脈洞 □ Superior sagittal sinus
② □ 静脈洞交会 □ Confluence of the sinuses
③ □ 横静脈洞 □ Transverse sinus
④ □ 外後頭隆起 □ External occipital protuberance
⑤ □ S状静脈洞 □ Sigmoid sinus
⑥ □ 内頸静脈 □ Internal jugular vein
⑦ □ 外椎骨静脈叢 □ External vertebral venous plexus

Dural Sinuses in the Skull Base

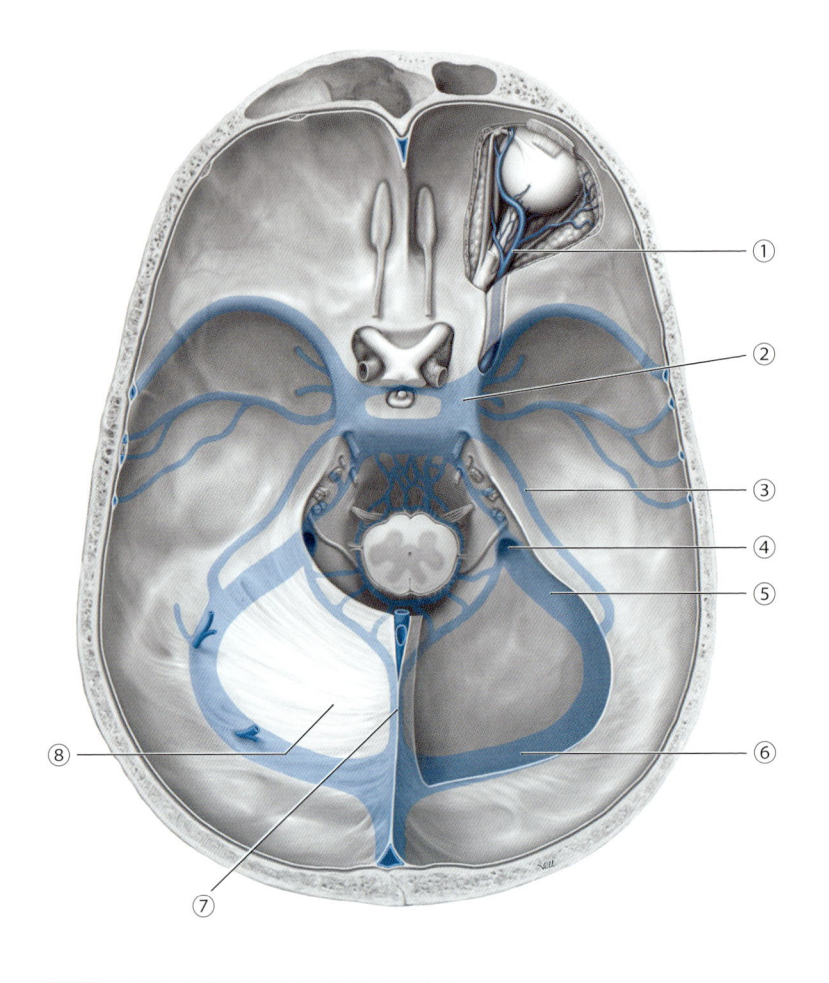

①
②
③
④
⑤
⑥
⑦
⑧

Q 小脳と大脳半球を隔てる構造は何か？

頭蓋底にある硬膜静脈洞

上面

① □ 上眼静脈　　　　　□ Superior ophthalmic vein
② □ 海綿静脈洞　　　　□ Cavernous sinus
③ □ 上錐体静脈洞　　　□ Superior petrosal sinus
④ □ 頸静脈孔　　　　　□ Jugular foramen
⑤ □ S状静脈洞　　　　□ Sigmoid sinus
⑥ □ 横静脈洞　　　　　□ Transverse sinus
⑦ □ 直静脈洞　　　　　□ Straight sinus
⑧ □ 小脳テント　　　　□ Tentorium cerebelli

A 　小脳と大脳半球は小脳テントによって隔てられる．小脳テントは，小脳が入っている後頭蓋窩を覆う屋根を形成する．また，小脳テントは大脳鎌に連なっている．

1 図 40.5, p.607　2 図 34.17, p.526

Arteries of the Brain

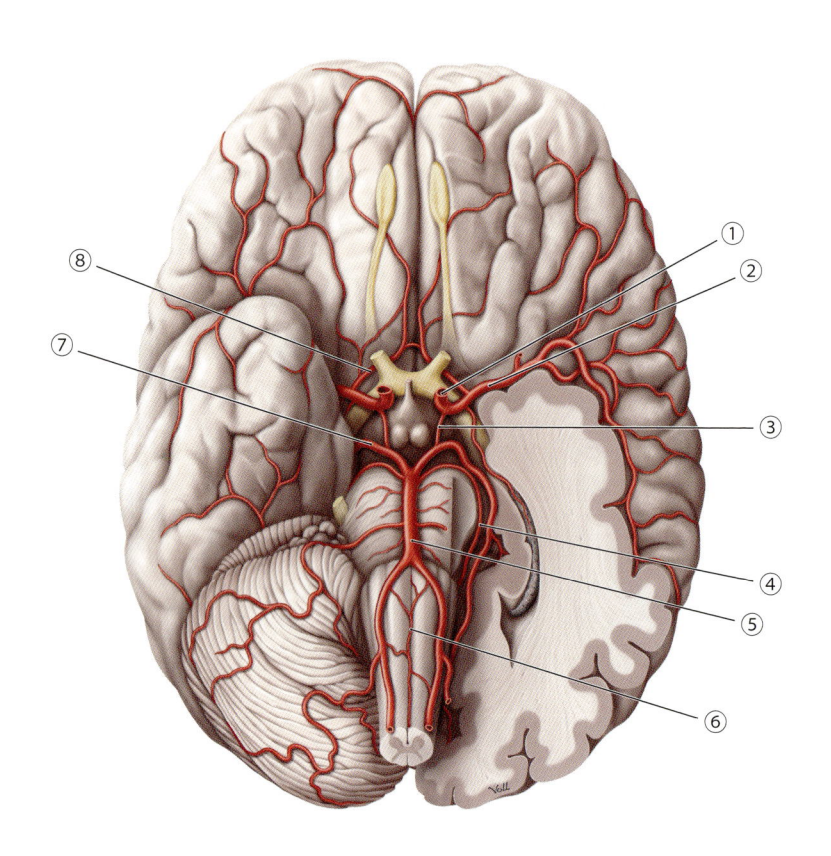

Q 前大脳動脈が分布する構造は何か？

脳の動脈

下面（底面）

① □ 内頸動脈　　　　　□ Internal carotid artery
② □ 中大脳動脈　　　　□ Middle cerebral artery
③ □ 後交通動脈　　　　□ Posterior communicating artery
④ □ 上小脳動脈　　　　□ Superior cerebellar artery
⑤ □ 脳底動脈　　　　　□ Basilar artery
⑥ □ 前脊髄動脈　　　　□ Anterior spinal artery
⑦ □ 後大脳動脈　　　　□ Posterior cerebral artery
⑧ □ 前大脳動脈　　　　□ Anterior cerebral artery

A 前大脳動脈は前頭葉の全体と頭頂葉の一部に分布する．

1 図 40.8, p.608　 2 図 41.6, p.636

Arteries of the Spinal Cord

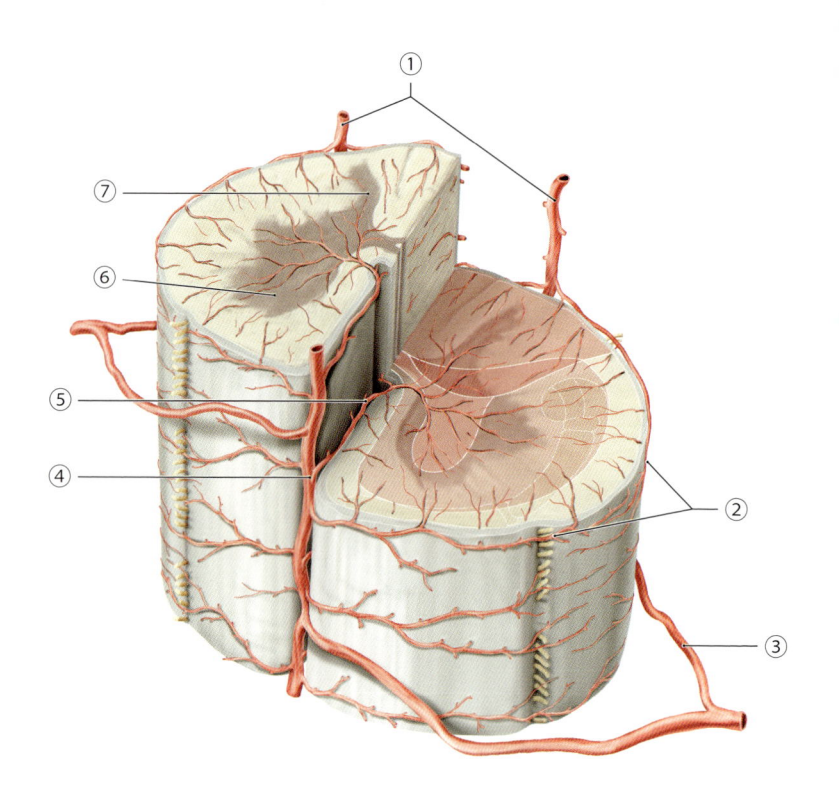

脊髄の大部分に分布する動脈は何か？

脊髄の動脈

左前上面

① □ 後脊髄動脈　　□ Posterior spinal arteries
② □ 血管冠　　□ Vasocorona
③ □ 後髄節動脈　　□ Posterior segmental medullary artery
④ □ 前脊髄動脈　　□ Anterior spinal artery
⑤ □ 溝動脈　　□ Sulcal artery
⑥ □ 前角　　□ Anterior horn
⑦ □ 後角　　□ Posterior horn

A 脊髄への血流の75%は前脊髄動脈から供給される．この動脈は椎骨動脈の枝であるが，様々な高さで前髄節動脈と吻合する．

1 図40.11A. p.610

Sensory & Motor System

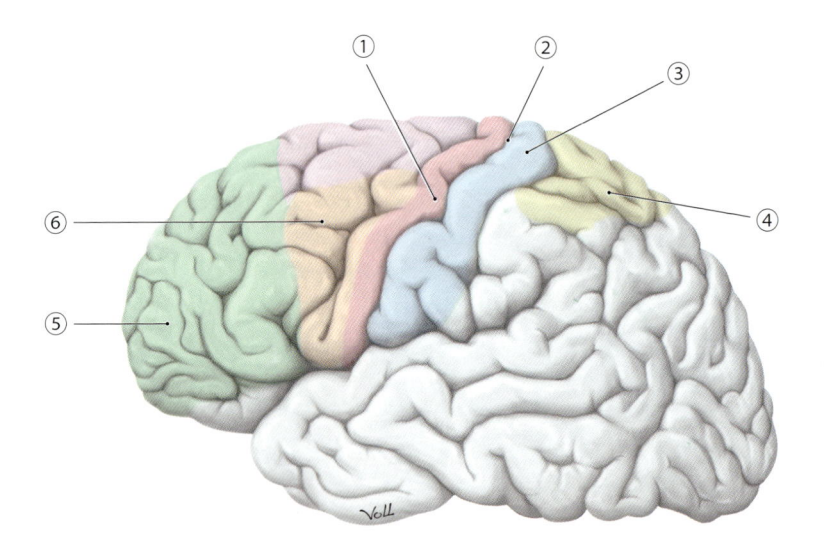

感覚系と運動系

左外側面

① ☐ 中心前回(一次運動野) ☐ Precentral gyrus (primary motor cortex)

② ☐ 中心溝 ☐ Central sulcus

③ ☐ 中心後回(一次体性感覚野) ☐ Postcentral gyrus (primary somatosensory cortex)

④ ☐ 後頭頂野 ☐ Posterior parietal cortex

⑤ ☐ 前頭前野 ☐ Prefrontal cortex

⑥ ☐ 運動前野 ☐ Premotor cortex

1 図 41.5A. p.613   2 図 42.5A. p.639

Ascending Tracts of the Spinal Cord

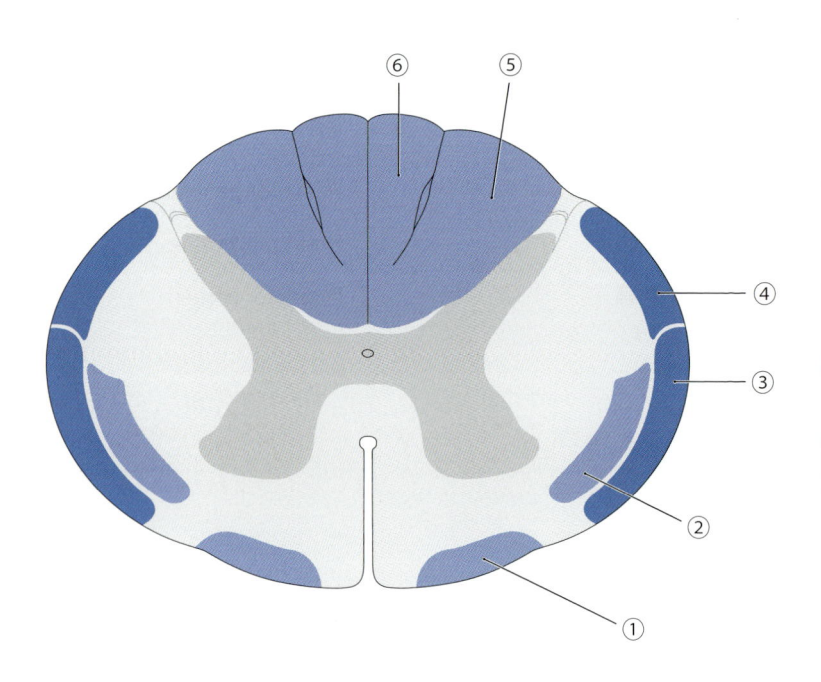

Q 温痛覚の伝導路は何か？

脊髄の上行路

上面

① □ 前脊髄視床路　　□ Anterior spinothalamic tract
② □ 外側脊髄視床路　□ Lateral spinothalamic tract
③ □ 前脊髄小脳路　　□ Anterior spinocerebellar tract
④ □ 後脊髄小脳路　　□ Posterior spinocerebellar tract
⑤ □ 楔状束　　　　　□ Fasciculus cuneatus
⑥ □ 薄束　　　　　　□ Fasciculus gracilis

A 温痛覚は外側脊髄視床路によって伝達される．

[1] 表 41.1, p.614　[2] 表 42.1, p.640

Descending Tracts of the Spinal Cord

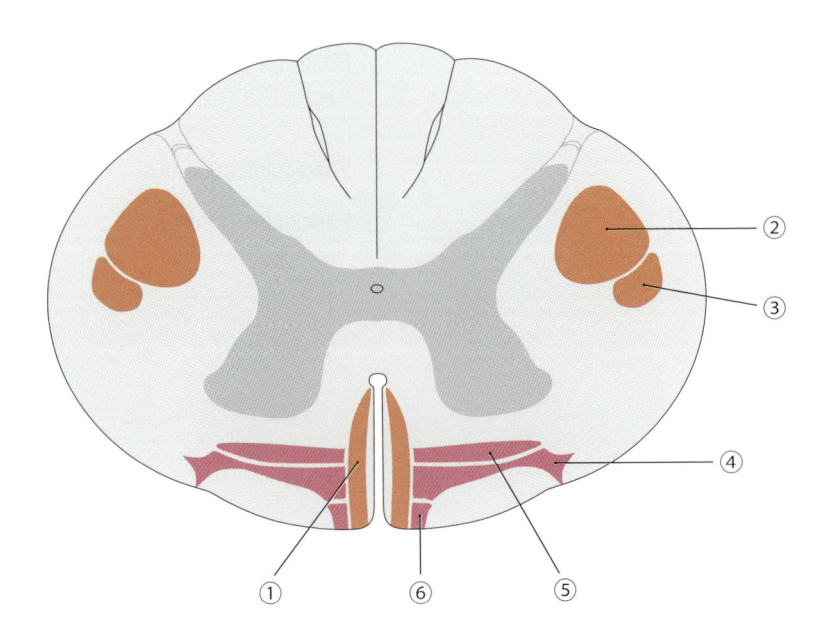

Q 脊髄に損傷を受け，障害側に痙性麻痺が出現した場合には，どの伝導路の障害が考えられるか？

脊髄の下行路

上面

① □ 前皮質脊髄路　　　　□ Anterior corticospinal tract
② □ 外側皮質脊髄路　　　□ Lateral corticospinal tract
③ □ 赤核脊髄路　　　　　□ Rubrospinal tract
④ □ 網様体脊髄路　　　　□ Reticulospinal tract
⑤ □ 前庭脊髄路　　　　　□ Vestibulospinal tract
⑥ □ 視蓋脊髄路　　　　　□ Tectospinal tract

A 　脊髄において錐体路(前・外側皮質脊髄路)が損傷されると，障害側に痙性麻痺が出現する．

1 表41.2. p.615　　2 表42.2. p.641

Visual System

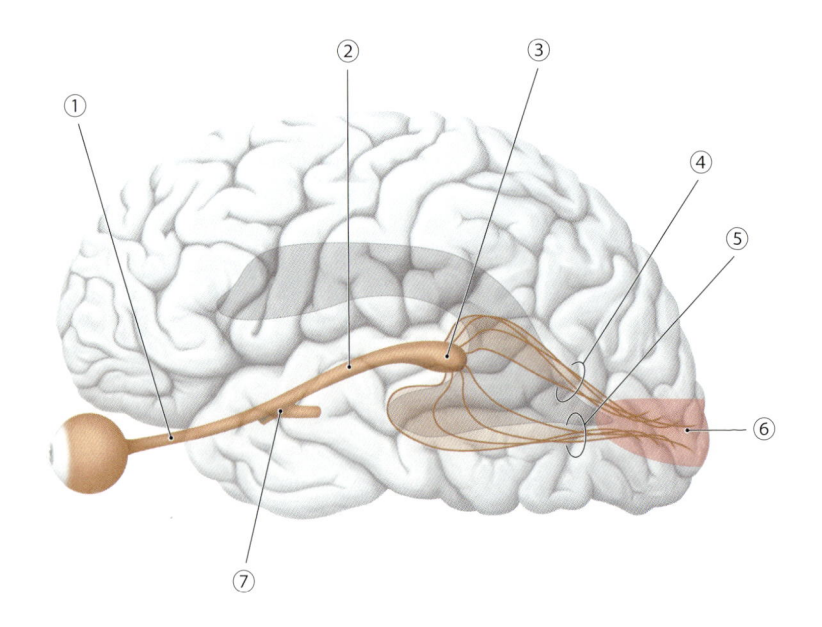

① ② ③ ④ ⑤ ⑥ ⑦

Q 視放線の線維のうち，視野の上半からの情報を伝達する線維はどの葉を通過するか？

視覚系

左外側面

① □ 視神経 　　　　　　　　□ Optic nerve（CN II）

② □ 視索 　　　　　　　　　□ Optic tract

③ □ 外側膝状体 　　　　　　□ Lateral geniculate body

④ □ 視放線（右視野の下半から □ Optic radiation
　　の情報を伝える）　　　　　（lower visual field）

⑤ □ 視放線（右視野の上半から □ Optic radiation
　　の情報を伝える）　　　　　（upper visual field）

⑥ □ 有線野 　　　　　　　　□ Striate area

⑦ □ 視交叉 　　　　　　　　□ Optic chiasm

A 　視野の上半からの情報は，視放線のうち下方の線維（側頭葉を通る線維，図の⑤）を通過する．左の側頭葉においてこの線維が障害を受けると，両眼の右視野の上半が欠ける（1/4 盲が出現する）．

1 図 41.8A. p.616　2 図 42.8A. p.642

Autonomic Nervous System

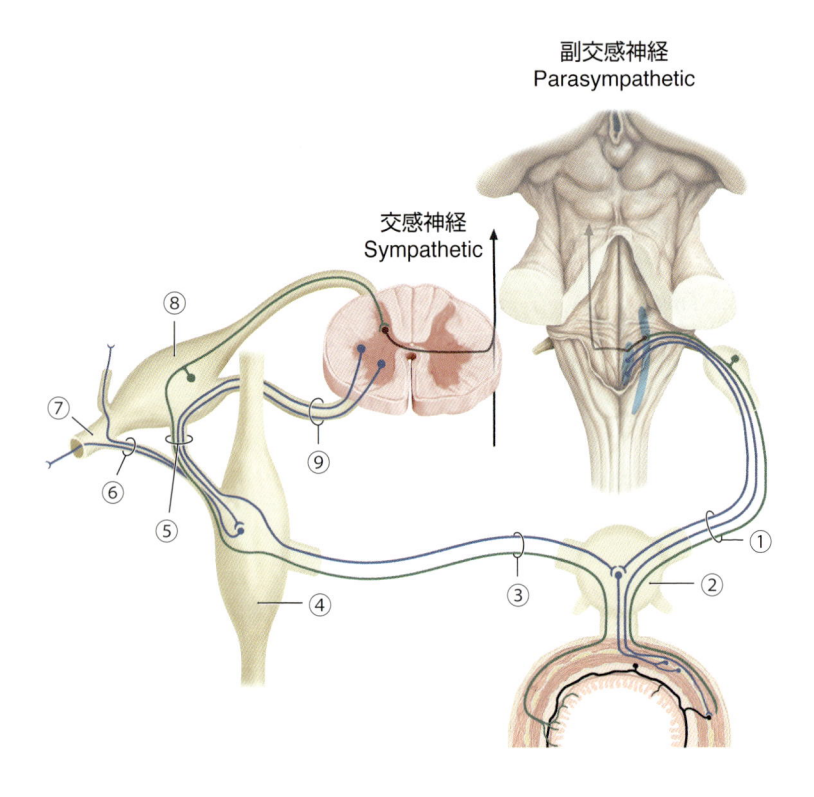

副交感神経
Parasympathetic

交感神経
Sympathetic

自律神経系

① □ 迷走神経　　　　　　　□ Vagus nerve (CN X)

② □ 椎前神経節　　　　　　□ Prevertebral ganglion

③ □ 内臓神経　　　　　　　□ Splanchnic nerve

④ □ 交感神経幹神経節　　　□ Sympathetic ganglion

⑤ □ 白交通枝　　　　　　　□ White ramus communicans

⑥ □ 灰色交通枝　　　　　　□ Gray ramus communicans

⑦ □ 前枝　　　　　　　　　□ Anterior ramus

⑧ □ 脊髄神経節　　　　　　□ Spinal ganglion

⑨ □ 前根　　　　　　　　　□ Anterior root

解説

自律神経系は平滑筋，心筋，腺に分布しており，交感神経系と副交感神経系に区分される．この2つの神経系は，血流(血圧)や分泌，臓器機能を調節する際に拮抗的な作用を示すことが多い．

1 図 42.1. p.622　　2 図 43.2. p.649

英文索引

- 項目の主要掲載ページは太字で示す.
- 英文中の a., aa. は artery, arteries を, l., ll. は ligament, ligaments を, n., nn. は nerve, nerves を, v., vv. は vein, veins を表す.

A

Abdominal
- aorta 腹大動脈 259, 263
- part of pectoralis major 腹部《大胸筋の》 319

Abducent n.(CN VI) 外転神経 557, **605**, 611, 713

Abductor
- digiti minimi
- -- 小指外転筋 357
- -- 小趾外転筋 487
- hallucis 母趾外転筋 485, 523, 531
- pollicis
- -- brevis 短母指外転筋 357
- -- longus 長母指外転筋 347, 363, 375
- --- tendon 長母指外転筋の腱 403

Accessory
- hemiazygos v. 副半奇静脈 97
- n.(CN XI) 副神経 55, **573**, 591, 687, 691, 713
- pancreatic duct 副膵管 227

Acetabular rim 寛骨臼縁《寛骨臼の》 423

Acetabulum 寛骨臼 419

Achilles tendon アキレス腱(踵骨腱) 461, 463, 523

Acromial
- articular surface 肩峰関節面 299
- end of clavicle 肩峰端《鎖骨の》 299

Acromioclavicular
- joint 肩鎖関節 309
- l. 肩鎖靱帯 309, 315

Acromion 肩峰 301, **303**, 313, 317

Adductor
- brevis 短内転筋 433, 435, 503
- canal 内転筋管 495
- hallucis 母趾内転筋 491
- hiatus [内転筋]腱裂孔 435, 497

- longus 長内転筋 433, 503, 537
- magnus 大内転筋 435, 437, **443**, 495, 503, 509, 533
- -- tendon 大内転筋の腱 497
- pollicis 母指内転筋 361
- tubercle 内転筋結節《大腿骨の》 421

Adenohypophysis 腺下垂体 705

Alveolar sac 肺胞嚢 159

Alveolus 肺胞 159

Ampulla 卵管膨大部 237

Amygdala 扁桃体 709

Anal
- canal 肛門管 217
- columns 肛門柱 217
- pecten(white zone) 肛門櫛(白帯) 217

Anatomical
- (anatomic) snuffbox 解剖学的嗅ぎタバコ入れ(橈骨窩) 403, 413
- neck of humerus 解剖頸《上腕骨の》 305

Anconeus 肘筋 345

Angular
- a. 眼角動脈 585
- v. 眼角静脈 583, 585

Ankle mortise 足関節窩 447

Annular l. of radius 橈骨輪状靱帯 335, 337

Anococcygeal raphe 肛門尾骨縫線 189

Ansa cervicalis 頸神経ワナ 669, 691

Anterior
- antebrachial interosseous n. 前[前腕]骨間神経 411
- arch of atlas 前弓《環椎の》 29
- belly of digastric muscle 前腹《顎二腹筋の》 659, 665
- cerebral a. 前大脳動脈 735
- chamber of eyeball 前眼房 617
- circumflex humeral aa. 前上腕回旋動脈 365
- clinoid process 前床突起 551

- commissure　前交連　705, 707
- corticospinal tract　前皮質脊髄路　743
- cranial fossa　前頭蓋窩　549
- cruciate l.　前十字靱帯　455, 457
- crural intermuscular septum　前下腿筋間中隔　525
- cusp of right atrioventricular valve　前尖《右房室弁の》　121, 127
- cutaneous branch of spinal n.　前皮枝《脊髄神経の》　79
- ethmoidal a.　前篩骨動脈　625, 627
- external vertebral venous plexus　前外椎骨静脈叢　49
- horn of spinal cord　前角《脊髄の》　737
- inferior iliac spine　下前腸骨棘　173
- intercostal
-- aa. branches of internal thoracic a.　前肋間枝《内胸動脈の》　75
-- vv.　前肋間静脈　49, 77
- internal vertebral venous plexus　前内椎骨静脈叢　49
- internodal bundles　前結節間束　133
- interosseous
-- a.　前骨間動脈　401, 411
-- v.　前骨間静脈　411
- interventricular
-- sulcus　前室間溝　117
-- (left anterior descending) branch of left coronary a.　前室間枝（前下行枝）《左冠状動脈の》　129
- jugular v.　前頸静脈　581
- lobe of adenohypophysis　前葉《腺下垂体の》　705
- longitudinal l.　前縦靱帯　31, **33**, 35, 173, 427
- mediastinum　前縦隔　91
- papillary muscle　前乳頭筋　121, 125
- rami of lumber nn.　前枝《腰神経の》　289
- ramus
-- of spinal n.　前枝《脊髄神経の》　51, 79, 747
-- of thoracic aorta　前枝《胸大動脈の》　47
- rectus sheath　前葉《腹直筋鞘の》　179, 181, 183
- root of spinal n.　前根《脊髄神経の》　747
- sacral foramina　前仙骨孔　23
- sacroiliac ll.　前仙腸靱帯　173, 427
- scalene　前斜角筋　67, 371, 687
- spinal a.　前脊髄動脈　735, 737
- spinocerebellar tract　前脊髄小脳路　741
- spinothalamic tract　前脊髄視床路　741
- sternoclavicular l.　前胸鎖靱帯　311
- superior
-- alveolar aa.　上前歯槽動脈　579
-- iliac spine　上前腸骨棘　**169**, 179, 293, 419, 423, 445, 515
-- segmental a. of kidney　上前区動脈《腎臓の》　261
- talofibular l.　前距腓靱帯　481
- thalamic nuclei　視床前核群　711
- tibial
-- a.　前脛骨動脈　**495**, 497, 527, 529, 535
-- v.　前脛骨静脈　527, 535
- tibiofibular l.　前脛腓靱帯　481
- tubercle of atlas　前結節《環椎の》　13
- vagal trunk　前迷走神経幹　101, 287
Antihelix　対輪　631
Anulus fibrosus of intervertebral disk　線維輪　33
Aortic
- aperture of diaphragm　大動脈裂孔《横隔膜の》　71
- arch　大動脈弓　**105**, 115, 137, 139
- valve　大動脈弁　127
Aorticorenal ganglia　大動脈腎動脈神経節　287
Apex
- of lung　肺尖　149, 151, 153
- of sacrum　仙骨尖　23
Apical axillary lymph node　上腋窩リンパ節　87
Arachnoid
- granulations　クモ膜顆粒　721, 727
- villi　クモ膜絨毛　721
Arcuate
- a.　弓状動脈　529
- a. of kidney　弓状動脈《腎臓の》　261
- line of pubis　弓状線《恥骨の》　169
Arm　上腕　297
Articular
- branch of spinal n.　関節枝《脊髄神経の》　51

―disk of sternoclavicular joint 関節円板《胸鎖関節の》 311
Aryepiglottic fold 披裂喉頭蓋ヒダ 677
Ascending
―aorta 上行大動脈 93, **95**, 111, 113, 117, 137, 161
―branch of lateral circumflex femoral a. 上行枝《外側大腿回旋動脈の》 517
―colon 上行結腸 195, 201, 213
―lumbar v. 上行腰静脈 271
―pharyngeal a. 上行咽頭動脈 667
Atlanto-occipital joint 環椎後頭関節 27
Atlas(C1) 環椎 **5**, 13, 29, 41
Atrioventricular
―bundle 房室束 133
―(AV) node 房室結節 133
Auricle 耳介 631
Auricular surface of sacrum 耳状面《仙骨の》 25
Auriculotemporal n. 耳介側頭神経 561, 587, **597**, 641
Axillary
―a. 腋窩動脈 85, 369, 373, **389**
―lymphatic plexus 腋窩リンパ叢 87
―n. 腋窩神経 369, **373**, 385, 391
―recess 腋窩陥凹 315
―v. 腋窩静脈 85, 389
Axis(C2) 軸椎(第2頸椎) 5, 11, 15, 41
Azygos v. 奇静脈 49, 83, **97**, 99, 107, 271

B

Bare area of liver 無漿膜野《肝臓の》 219
Base of metacarpal 底《中手骨の》 351
Basilar a. 脳底動脈 735
Basilic v. 尺側皮静脈 367
Biceps
―brachii 上腕二頭筋 319, **323**, 325, 339, 377, 393, 409
―femoris 大腿二頭筋 521
――tendon 大腿二頭筋の腱 461, 463
Bicipital aponeurosis 上腕二頭筋腱膜 323
Bile duct 総胆管 221, 223, 225
Bladder trigone 膀胱三角 233
Bochdalek's triangle (lumbocostal triangle) ボクダレク三角(腰肋三角) 71
Body
―of (urinary) bladder 膀胱体 255
―of epididymis 精巣上体体 249
―of fornix 脳弓体 703
―of pancreas 膵体 227
―of sternum 胸骨体 65, 139
Brachial
―a. 上腕動脈 365, 391, **393**, 395, 409
―plexus 腕神経叢 **369**, 371, 389, 685
―v. 上腕静脈 409
Brachialis 上腕筋 **325**, 341, 377, 409
Brachiocephalic
―trunk 腕頭動脈 115, 119
―v. 腕頭静脈 115
Brachioradialis 腕橈骨筋 339, 395, 411
Brainstem 脳幹 713, 715
Branch to sinoatrial node 洞房結節枝 129
Bridging v. 架橋静脈 723
Bronchial tree 気管支樹 157, 159
Bronchiole 細気管支 157
Bronchomediastinal trunk 気管支縦隔リンパ本幹 99
Bronchopulmonary lymph node 気管支肺リンパ節 163
Buccal
―a. 頬動脈 579, 593
―branches of facial n. 頬筋枝《顔面神経の》 563, 589
―n. 頬神経 561, 593, 641
Buccinator 頬筋 655, 659
Bulb of penis 尿道球 247
Bulbospongiosus 球海綿体筋 187, 241, 247, 257
Bulbourethral gland 尿道球腺 253, 257
Bundle of His ヒス束 133

C

C1 vertebra (Atlas) 第1頸椎(環椎) 5
C2 vertebra (Axis) 第2頸椎(軸椎) 5, 11
C5 spinal n. 第5頸神経《頸神経の》 369
C6 spinal n. 第6頸神経《頸神経の》 369
C7 spinal n. 第7頸神経《頸神経の》 369
C7 vertebra 第7頸椎 5, 7, 11
Calcaneal tuberosity 踵骨隆起 485
Calcaneofibular l. 踵腓靱帯 483
Calcaneus 踵骨 471, 463, 477

Capite 有頭骨 351
Capitellum of humerus 上腕骨小頭《上腕骨の》 305, 337
Cardia 噴門 209
Cardiac
 - apex 心尖 115, 139
 - conduction system 心臓刺激伝導系 133
 - impression 心圧痕 153
 - plexus 心臓神経叢 135
Carotid
 - canal 頸動脈管 547
 - sinus 頸動脈洞 569
 - triangle 頸動脈三角 683
Carpal
 - bones 手根骨 297
 - tunnel 手根管 397
Cartilaginous part of pharyngotympanic tube 軟骨部《耳管の》 633
Cauda equina 馬尾 717
Caudate
 - lobe of liver 尾状葉《肝臓の》 221
 - nucleus 尾状核 707, 711
Caval aperture of diaphragm 大静脈孔《横隔膜の》 69, 71, 105
Cavernous sinus 海綿静脈洞 583, 607, 733
Cecum 盲腸 213
Celiac
 - ganglion 腹腔神経節 287
 - lymph node 腹腔リンパ節 285
 - trunk 腹腔動脈 193, 225, 259, 263, **265**, 277
Central
 - axillary lymph node 中心腋窩リンパ節 87
 - canal of spinal cord 中心管《脊髄の》 729
 - sulcus 中心溝 697, 739
 - tendon of diaphragm 腱中心《横隔膜の》 69
Cephalic v. 橈側皮静脈 367, 387
Cerebellomedullary cistern 小脳延髄槽 727
Cerebellum 小脳 697, 699
Cerebral
 - aqueduct 中脳水道 729
 - arcuate fibers (U fibers) 大脳弓状線維 701
 - peduncle 大脳脚 701
Cervical
 - branch of facial n. 頸枝《顔面神経の》 563
 - canal 子宮頸管 237
 - cardiac branches of vagus n. 頸心臓枝《迷走神経の》 571
 - enlargement 頸膨大 717
 - fascia 頸筋膜 673
 - plexus 頸神経叢 589
 - vertebrae 頸椎 3, 11
Choana 後鼻孔 619
Chorda tympani 鼓索神経 565, 635
Chordae tendineae 腱索 125
Choroid
 - plexus 脈絡叢 705
 -- of fourth ventricle 第四脳室脈絡叢 727
 -- of third ventricle 第三脳室脈絡叢 727
Ciliary
 - body 毛様体 617
 - ganglion 毛様体神経節 559, 605
 - muscle 毛様体筋 617
Circumflex
 - a. of left coronary a. 回旋枝《左冠状動脈の》 129
 - scapular a. 肩甲回旋動脈 385, 391
Cisterna
 - chyli 乳ビ槽 99, 285
 - magna 大槽 727
Clavicle 鎖骨 165, **299**, 311, 313
Clavicular
 - head of sternocleidomastoid 鎖骨頭《胸鎖乳突筋の》 693
 - notch 鎖骨切痕 61, 65
 - part of pectoralis major 鎖骨部《大胸筋の》 319, 387
Clavipectoral fascia 鎖骨胸筋筋膜 387
Clitoris 陰核 239, 241
Clivus 斜台 551
Coccygeus 尾骨筋 189, 191
Coccyx 尾骨 3, 25
Cochlea 蝸牛 567, 629, 637
Cochlear root (n.) (CN Ⅷ) 蝸牛神経 567
Common
 - carotid a. 総頸動脈 75, 95, 663, **667**, 685

(Deep dorsal penile v.) *753*

- fibular n. 総腓骨神経 499, **507**, 521, 525
- hepatic
-- a. 総肝動脈 225, 265
-- duct 総肝管 223
- iliac
-- a. 総腸骨動脈 259, 281
-- lymph node 総腸骨リンパ節 285
-- v. 総腸骨静脈 271, 281
- palmar digital aa. 総掌側指動脈 399
- tendinous ring 総腱輪 603
Concha 耳甲介 631
Condylar process of mandibular 関節突起《下顎骨の》 639
Confluence of sinuses 静脈洞交会 725, 727, 731
Conjunctiva 結膜 613
Conoid tubercle 円錐靱帯結節 299
Conus
- arteriosus 動脈円錐 121
- medullaris of spinal cord 脊髄円錐 717
Cooper's (suspensory) ll. of breast クーパー靱帯(乳房提靱帯) 89
Coracoacromial l. 烏口肩峰靱帯 309, 315
Coracobrachialis 烏口腕筋 325, 377
Coracoclavicular l. 烏口鎖骨靱帯 315
Coracoid process 烏口突起 301, 313, 321
Cornea 角膜 617
Corona
- of glans 亀頭冠 247
- radiata 放線冠 701
Coronal suture 冠状縫合 541
Coronary
- l. of liver 肝冠状間膜 219
- sinus 冠状静脈洞 119, 131
Coronoid
- fossa of humerus 鈎突窩《上腕骨の》 337
- process
-- of mandible 筋突起《下顎骨の》 591, 639
-- of ulna 鈎状突起《尺骨の》 333
Corpus
- callosum 脳梁 701, 703, 707
- cavernosum of penis 陰茎海綿体 245, 247, 255
- spongiosum 尿道海綿体 247

Costal
- angle of rib 肋骨角《肋骨の》 63
- cartilage 肋軟骨 **61**, 63, 67, 311
- facet on transverse process 横突肋骨窩 19
- groove 肋骨溝 81
- margin (arch) 肋骨弓 61
- part
-- of diaphragm 肋骨部《横隔膜の》 69
-- of parietal pleura 壁側胸膜の肋骨部(肋骨胸膜) 83, 147
- tubercle of rib 肋骨結節《肋骨の》 63
Costoclavicular ligament 肋鎖靱帯 311
Costodiaphragmatic recess 肋骨横隔洞 81, 149
Cranial root 延髄根 573
Cremaster
- fascia 精巣挙筋膜 249, 251
- muscle 精巣挙筋 249, 251
Cribriform plate 篩板 551, 555, 623
Cricoid cartilage 輪状軟骨 155, 675, 677
Cricothyroid 輪状甲状筋 571, 659, 679
- l. 輪状甲状靱帯 675
Crista
- galli 鶏冠 621
- terminalis 分界稜 123
Crus
- of fornix 脳弓脚 703
- of penis 陰茎脚 247
Cuboid 立方骨 469, 479
Cutaneous
- branch
-- of deep fibular n. 皮枝《深腓骨神経の》 529
-- of obturator n. 皮枝《閉鎖神経の》 503
Cymba conchae 耳甲介舟 631
Cystic duct 胆囊管 223, 225

D

Deep
- branch
-- of radial n. 深枝《橈骨神経の》 395
-- of ulnar n. 深枝《尺骨神経の》 381
- cervical a. 深頸動脈 53
- dorsal penile v. 深陰茎背静脈 245

- femoral v. 大腿深静脈 533
- fibular n. 深腓骨神経 **511**, 525, 527, 529, 535
- inguinal lymph node 深鼠径リンパ節 285
- lingual a. 舌深動脈 649
- palmar arch 深掌動脈弓 401
- part of external anal sphincter 深部《外肛門括約筋の》 217
- penile a. 陰茎深動脈 245
- petrosal n. 深錐体神経 599
- plantar arch 深足底動脈弓 531
- temporal
-- aa. 深側頭動脈 579, 593
-- nn. 深側頭神経 593
-- vv. 深側頭静脈 581
- transverse
-- metacarpal l. 深横中手靱帯 357
-- perineal 深会陰横筋 191, 241

Deltoid 三角筋 317, **319**, 325, 327, 373, 387
- l. 三角靱帯 483
- tuberosity of humerus 三角筋粗面《上腕骨の》 305

Dens of axis (C2) 歯突起《第2頸椎の》 15, 29, 651
Dentate gyrus 歯状回 703
Depressor anguli oris 口角下制筋 553
Descending
- aorta 下行大動脈 93, 109, 141
- colon 下行結腸 207
- palatine a. 下行口蓋動脈 627
- part
-- of duodenum 下行部《十二指腸の》 211
-- of trapezius 下行部《僧帽筋の》 327, 383

Detrusor vesicae 排尿筋 233
Diaphragm 横隔膜 **69**, 71, 73, 81, 91, 107
Diaphragmatic
- apertures 開口部《横隔膜の》 73
- part of parietal pleura 横隔胸膜(壁側胸膜の横隔部) 81, 147

Diencephalon 間脳 705
Digastric muscle 顎二腹筋 565, **659**, 661, 665
Diploë of cranial bone 板間層 723

Distal
- interphalangeal joint 遠位指節間(DIP)関節 353
- radioulnar joint 下橈尺関節 353
- wrist crease 遠位手根線 413

Dorsal
- branch
-- of palmar digital nn. 背側枝《掌側神経の》 407
-- of ulnar n. 背側枝《尺骨神経の》 407
- clitoral
-- a. 陰核背動脈 243
-- n. 陰核背神経 243
- digital
-- expansion 指背腱膜 345
-- nn. 背側指神経 405, 407
- interossei of foot 背側骨間筋《足の》 491
- metatarsal aa. 背側中足動脈 529
- pedal a. 足背動脈 495, 529
- penile
-- a. 陰茎背動脈 245
-- n. (dorsal n. of penis) 陰茎背神経 245, 257, 291
- root of spinal n. 後根《脊髄神経の》 79, 719
- tarsal ll. 背側足根靱帯 481
- tubercle of radius 背側結節《橈骨の》 345
- venous network of hand 手背静脈網 367

Dorsum
- of tongue 舌背 643
- sellae 鞍背 549

Ductus deferens 精管 229, 253, 283
Duodenojejunal flexure 十二指腸空腸曲 199
Duodenum 十二指腸 199, 201, 209, **211**, 269
Dura mater 硬膜 721, 723
Dural Sinus 硬膜静脈洞 733

E

Earlobe 耳垂 631
Ejaculatory duct 射精管 255
Elbow joint 肘関節 335, 337
Emissary v. 導出静脈 723

Endothoracic fascia　胸内筋膜　81，83
Epididymis　精巣上体　249
Epiglottis　喉頭蓋　643，651，675，**677**，681
Epiploic appendices　腹膜垂　213
Esophageal
 − aperture of diaphragm　食道裂孔　69，71
 − plexus　食道神経叢　101
 − v.　食道静脈　275
Esophagus　食道　83，91，95，101，**105**，107，141，209，661，679
Ethmoid
 − bone　篩骨　543，601，619
 − bulla　篩骨胞　623
Extensor
 − carpi
 − − radialis
 − − − brevis　短橈側手根伸筋　347
 − − − longus　長橈側手根伸筋　345，347
 − − − − tendon　長橈側手根伸筋の腱　363
 − − ulnaris　尺側手根伸筋　345，363
 − digitorum　［総］指伸筋　345，363，411
 − − brevis　短趾伸筋　493
 − − longus　長趾伸筋　**459**，493，507，527
 − − tendon　［総］指伸筋の腱　345，375
 − hallucis
 − − brevis　短母趾伸筋　459
 − − − tendon　短母趾伸筋の腱　529
 − − longus　長母趾伸筋　459，493
 − − − tendon　長母趾伸筋の腱　529，537
 − indicis　示指伸筋　347
 − − tendon　示指伸筋の腱　363
 − pollicis
 − − brevis tendon　短母指伸筋の腱　403
 − − longus　長母指伸筋　347
 − − − tendon　長母指伸筋の腱　363，403，413
 − retinaculum of hand　伸筋支帯　363
External
 − anal sphincter　外肛門括約筋　187，203，217
 − auditory canal　外耳道　629，631
 − branch
 − − of accessory n.　外枝《副神経の》　691
 − − of superior laryngeal n.　外枝《上喉頭神経の》　571，679
 − carotid a.　外頸動脈　577

 − ear　外耳　629
 − iliac
 − − a.　外腸骨動脈　215，495
 − − lymph node　外腸骨リンパ節　285
 − − v.　外腸骨静脈　215
 − intercostal muscles　外肋間筋　45，67，179
 − jugular v.　外頸静脈　387，**581**，587，689
 − oblique　外腹斜筋　57，**177**，183，185，293
 − − aponeurosis　外腹斜筋腱膜　**177**，183，185，513
 − occipital protuberance　外後頭隆起　545，731
 − os of uterus　外子宮口　237
 − spermatic fascia　外精筋膜　251
 − urethral orifice　外尿道口　239
 − vertebral venous plexus　外椎骨静脈叢　731
Eyeball　眼球　617
Eyelid　眼瞼　613

F

Facial
 − a.　顔面動脈　**577**，585，591，655，691
 − n.（CN VII）　顔面神経　563，**565**，589，635，637，647
 − v.　顔面静脈　**583**，585，591，655，691
Falciform l. of liver　肝鎌状間膜　219
Falx cerebri　大脳鎌　723，725
Fascia lata　大腿筋膜　185
Fasciculus
 − cuneatus　楔状束　741
 − gracilis　薄束　741
Female pelvis　女性骨盤　171
Femoral
 − a.　大腿動脈　183，259，283，**495**，513，517，533
 − n.　大腿神経　183，499，501，**505**，511，513，517
 − v.　大腿静脈　183，259，283，513，**517**，533
Femoropatellar joint　膝蓋大腿関節　453
Femur　大腿骨　417，421
Fibrous pericardium　線維性心膜　103，105，147

Fibula 腓骨 417, 447
Fibular
- a. 腓骨動脈 497, 521, 535
- v. 腓骨静脈 535
Fibularis
- brevis 短腓骨筋 461, 535
- longus 長腓骨筋 461, 507, 525
-- tendon 長腓骨筋の腱 465, 479, 491
- tertius 第3腓骨筋 461
Fifth metatarsal 第5中足骨《中足骨の》 479
First
- distal phalanx of foot 第1末節骨《足の》 469
- dorsal interosseus of hand 第1背側骨間筋《手の》 357, 363, 403
- lumbar v. 第1腰静脈《腰静脈の》 77
- lumbrical of hand 第1虫様筋《手の》 379
- metacarpal 第1中手骨《中手骨の》 349
- metatarsal 第1中足骨《中足骨の》 469, 471, 479
- proximal phalanx of foot 第1基節骨《足の》 471
- rib 第1肋骨《肋骨の》 311
Flexor
- carpi
-- radialis 橈側手根屈筋 339, 379
--- tendon 橈側手根屈筋の腱 397
-- ulnaris 尺側手根屈筋 339, **345**, 355, 381, 411
- digiti minimi brevis
-- 短小指屈筋 359
-- 短小趾屈筋 487
- digitorum
-- brevis 短趾屈筋 487
-- longus 長趾屈筋 467, 521, 523
--- tendon 長趾屈筋の腱 465, 489
-- profundus 深指屈筋 **343**, 359, 379, 381, 411
--- tendons 深指屈筋の腱 341, 361, 397
-- superficialis 浅指屈筋 341, 343, 379
--- tendons 浅指屈筋の腱 361, 397
- hallucis
-- brevis 短母趾屈筋 491
-- longus 長母趾屈筋 467

--- tendon 長母趾屈筋の腱 463, 487
- pollicis
-- longus 長母指屈筋 343, 379
--- tendon 長母指屈筋の腱 341, 359, 397
- retinaculum
-- of foot 屈筋支帯《足の》 523
-- of hand 屈筋支帯《手の》 355, **357**, 397, 399
Flexors of forearm 前腕屈筋 339
Foramen
- cecum 舌盲孔 643
- magnum 大後頭孔 547, 549
- ovale 卵円孔 143, 145, **547**, 551, 597
Forearm 前腕 297
Fornix 脳弓 705, 709
Fossa ovalis 卵円窩 123
Fourth ventricle 第四脳室 729
Frenulum of upper lip 上唇小帯 653
Frontal
- belly of occipitofrontalis 前頭筋《後頭前頭筋の》 553
- bone 前頭骨 541, 543
- lobe 前頭葉 697, 699
- n. 前頭神経 559, 605, 609
- process of maxilla 前頭突起《上顎骨の》 621
- sinus 前頭洞 551, 555, 601
Frontotemporal fasciculus 前頭側頭束 701
Fundus 胃底 209
- of gallbladder 胆嚢底 223

G

Galea aponeurotica 帽状腱膜 553
Gallbladder 胆嚢 207, 221, **223**, 225
Gastrocnemius 腓腹筋 509, 535, 537
Gastrocolic l. 胃結腸間膜 197
Gastroduodenal a. 胃十二指腸動脈 265
Gastrosplenic l. 胃脾間膜 197
Geniculate ganglion 膝神経節 565, 637
Genioglossus オトガイ舌筋 645, 651
Geniohyoid オトガイ舌骨筋 645, 657
Glans
- of clitoris 陰核亀頭《陰核の》 241
- penis 陰茎亀頭 247, 249

Glenohumeral
- joint　肩甲上腕関節　309, 313
- ll.　関節上腕靱帯　315

Glenoid cavity of scapula　関節窩《肩甲骨の》　301, 313, 317

Glossopharyngeal n.(CN IX)　舌咽神経　569, 647

Gluteus
- maximus　大殿筋　57, 187, **439**, 443, 445
- medius　中殿筋　57, 439, 443, **445**
- minimus　小殿筋　441, 519

Gracilis　薄筋　435, **437**, 443, 503

Gray ramus communicans　灰白交通枝　289, 747

Great
- auricular n.　大耳介神経　53, 575, 587, **669**, 689
- cardiac v.　大心臓静脈　129, 131

Greater
- curvature of stomach　大弯　209
- horn of hyoid bone　大角《舌骨の》　661
- occipital n.　大後頭神経　53, 575, 587
- omentum　大網　193, 195
- palatine
-- a.　大口蓋動脈　627
-- n.　大口蓋神経　599, 627
- petrosal n.　大錐体神経　565, 599, 637
- sciatic
-- foramen　大坐骨孔　175, 515
-- notch　大坐骨切痕《坐骨の》　419
- splanchnic n.　大内臓神経　107, 287
- trochanter　大転子　421, 425
- tuberosity of humerus　大結節《上腕骨の》　307, 323
- wing of sphenoid bone　大翼《蝶形骨の》　541, 601

Groove
- for fibularis longus tendon　長腓骨筋腱溝　471
- for sigmoid sinus　S状洞溝　551
- for subclavius muscle　鎖骨下筋溝　299
- for transverse sinus　横洞溝　551
- for vertebral a.　椎骨動脈溝　13

H

Hamate　有鈎骨　349

Hard palate　硬口蓋　653
Haustra of colon　結腸膨起　213
Head
- of femur　大腿骨頭　421, 423
- of fibula　腓骨頭　445, 447, 507, 525
- of humerus　上腕骨頭　307
- of metacarpal　頭《中手骨の》　351
- of pancreas　膵頭　227
- of radius　橈骨頭　333, 337
- of rib　肋骨頭《肋骨の》　63
- of talus　距骨頭　469
Helix　耳輪　631
Hemiazygos v.　半奇静脈　97, 109, 271
Hemorrhoidal plexus　直腸静脈叢　217
Hepatic vv.　肝静脈　225, 271
Hepatoduodenal l.　肝十二指腸間膜　201, 209
Hepatogastric l.　肝胃間膜　193, 209
Hepatopancreatic duct　胆膵管　225
Hilum of lung　肺門　153
Hip
- bone　寛骨　169, 419
- joint　股関節　423, 425
Hippocampus　海馬　703
Hook of hamate　有鈎骨鈎　351
Horizontal
- fissure of right lung　水平裂《右肺の》　139, 151
- part of duodenum　水平部《十二指腸の》　201, 211
- plate of palatine bone　水平板《口蓋骨の》　619
Humeral head of pronator teres　上腕頭《円回内筋の》　379
Humero-ulnar head of flexor digitorum superficialis　上腕尺骨頭《浅指屈筋の》　343
Humerus　上腕骨　297, 305, 307
Hyoepiglottic l.　舌骨喉頭蓋靱帯　677
Hyoglossus　舌骨舌筋　645
Hyoid bone　舌骨　**645**, 649, 651, 661, 665, 675, 681
Hypogastric n.　下腹神経　291
Hypoglossal n.(CN XII)　舌下神経　591, **649**, 669, 691, 713
Hypophyseal fossa(sella turcica) of sphenoid bone　下垂体窩《蝶形骨の》　551, 621
Hypophysis　下垂体　699, 705

Hypothalamus　視床下部　705
Hypothenar eminence　小指球　413

I

Ileal aa.　回腸動脈　267
Ileocecal orifice　回腸口　213
Ileocolic a.　回結腸動脈　267
Ileum　回腸　195, 199
Iliac
　- crest　腸骨稜　7, 169, 419
　- fossa　腸骨窩《腸骨の》　171
Iliacus　腸骨筋　435
Iliococcygeus　腸骨尾骨筋　189
Iliocostalis　腸肋筋　43
Iliofemoral l.　腸骨大腿靱帯　427, 429
Iliohypogastric n.　腸骨下腹神経　501
Ilioinguinal n.　腸骨鼡径神経　499, 501
Iliolumbar l.　腸腰靱帯　173, 427, 429
Iliopectineal arch　腸恥筋膜弓　513
Iliopsoas　腸腰筋　431, 505
Iliotibial tract　腸脛靱帯　439, 445, 525
Ilium　腸骨　171
Impression for costoclavicular l.　肋鎖靱帯圧痕　299
Incisive canal　切歯管　619
Incus　キヌタ骨　635
Inferior
　- alveolar
　　- a.　下歯槽動脈　579, 593
　　- n.　下歯槽神経　561, 593, 641
　- angle of scapula (inferior scapular angle)　肩甲骨下角　7, 303
　- articular process　下関節突起　9
　- belly of omohyoid　下腹《肩甲舌骨筋の》　665
　- cerebellar peduncle　下小脳脚　715
　- colliculus of quadrigeminal plate　下丘《四丘体板の》　715
　- epigastric
　　- a.　下腹壁動脈　283
　　- v.　下腹壁静脈　283
　- extensor retinaculum　下伸筋支帯　493
　- horn of lateral ventricle　下角《側脳室の》　729
　- hypogastric plexus　下下腹神経叢(骨盤神経叢)　289
　- lacrimal canaliculi　下涙小管　615
　- laryngeal n.　舌喉頭神経　681
　- lobar bronchi　下葉気管支　149
　- lobe of left lung　下葉《左肺の》　141, 153
　- meatus　下鼻道　623
　- mesenteric
　　- a.　下腸間膜動脈　259, 269, 281
　　- ganglion　下腸間膜動脈神経節　287
　　- v.　下腸間膜静脈　275, 277, 281
　- nasal concha　下鼻甲介　615, 621
　- oblique v.　下斜筋　557
　- ophthalmic v.　下眼静脈　611
　- orbital fissure　下眼窩裂　599, 601
　- pancreaticoduodenal a.　下膵十二指腸動脈　265
　- pharyngeal constrictor　下咽頭収縮筋　659, 661, 679
　- phrenic v.　下横隔動脈　259, 273
　- posterior nasal branches of greater palatine n.　下後鼻枝《大口蓋神経の》　627
　- puncta　下涙点　615
　- rectal
　　- a.　下直腸動脈　281
　　- nn.　下直腸神経　243, 257, 291
　　- plexus　下直腸動脈神経叢　291
　- rectus　下直筋　557
　- root of ansa cervicalis　下根《頸神経ワナの》　669
　- suprarenal a.　下副腎動脈　273
　- tarsus　下瞼板　613
　- thoracic aperture　胸郭下口　61
　- thyroid
　　- a.　下甲状腺動脈　663, 679, 691
　　- v.　下甲状腺静脈　103, 685
　- tracheobronchial lymph node　下気管気管支リンパ節　163
　- ulnar collateral a.　下尺側側副動脈　393
　- vena cava　下大静脈　77, 83, 105, 113, 117, 131, 161, 201, 207, 221, 225, **263**, 271, 277, 281
　- vertebral notch　下椎切痕　21
Infraglenoid tubercle　関節下結節《肩甲骨の》　301
Infraorbital
　- a.　眼窩下動脈　579, 585
　- foramen　眼窩下孔　543, 561, 641
　- n.　眼窩下神経　561, 585, **599**, 641
Infrapatellar branch of saphenous n.　膝蓋下枝　505

Infraspinatus 棘下筋 329, 331, 385
Infraspinous fossa of scapula 棘下窩《肩甲骨の》 303
Infratemporal fossa 側頭下窩 593, 595, 597
Infundibulum 卵管漏斗 237
Inguinal l. 鼠径靱帯 **173**, 177, 183, 185, 513
Inner ear 内耳 637
Innermost intercostals 最内肋間筋 67
Interatrial
- bundle 心房間束 133
- septum 心房中隔 123, 125
Intercondylar
- eminence of tibia 顆間隆起《脛骨の》 451
- notch of femur 顆間窩《大腿骨の》 421, 451
Intercostal nn. 肋間神経 55, 81, 101
Interlobar a. 葉間動脈 261
Intermesenteric plexus 腸間膜動脈間神経叢 287
Internal
- anal sphincter 内肛門括約筋 217
- branch of superior laryngeal n. 内枝《上喉頭神経の》 679, 681
- capsule 内包 701, 707
- carotid
-- a. 内頸動脈 591, 605, 607, 633, 635, **667**, 691, 735
-- plexus 内頸動脈神経叢 605
- iliac
-- a. 内腸骨動脈 259, 279, 283
-- lymph node 内腸骨リンパ節 285
-- v. 内腸骨静脈 283
- intercostals 内肋間筋 67, 179
- jugular v. 内頸静脈 77, 97, 99, 163, **581**, 583, 589, 663, 673, 685, 731
- oblique 内腹斜筋 39, 45, **179**, 183, 185
- os of uterus 内子宮口 237
- pudendal
-- a. 内陰部動脈 215, 243, 257, 279
-- v. 内陰部静脈 215, 243, 257, 279, **281**
- spermatic fascia 内精巣筋膜 249, 251
- thoracic
-- a. 内胸動脈 75, 85, 103
-- vv. 内胸静脈 49, **77**, 85, 103
Interossei 骨間筋 381
Interosseous
- membrane 前腕骨間膜 333
-- of leg 下腿骨間膜 447
- talocalcanean l. 骨間距踵靱帯 477
Interscalene space 斜角筋隙 691
Interspinous ll. 棘間靱帯 33
Intertransverse ll. 横突間靱帯 35
Intertrochanteric crest 転子間稜《大腿骨の》 421
Intertubercular
- groove of humerus 結節間溝《上腕骨の》 305, 313
- synovial sheath 結節間滑液鞘 315
Interureteral fold 尿管間ヒダ 233
Interventricular
- foramen 室間孔 729
- septum 心室中隔 125, 133, 141
Intervertebral
- disk 椎間円板 3, 5, 33, 37
- foramen 椎間孔 3, 37, 719
- joint 椎体間関節 27
Intrinsic muscles of the back 固有背筋 43, 45
Investing layer of cervical fascia 浅葉《頸筋膜の》 673
Iris 虹彩 617
Ischial
- ramus 坐骨枝 169
- spine 坐骨棘 **169**, 171, 175, 189, 191, 419, 425
- tuberosity 坐骨結節 169, 419, **425**, 441
Ischioanal fossa 坐骨肛門窩(坐骨直腸窩) 215
Ischiocavernosus 坐骨海綿体筋 187, 241, 247
Ischiofemoral l. 坐骨大腿靱帯 429
Ischium 坐骨 169, 419
Isthmus
- of thyroid gland 甲状腺峡部 671
- of uterine tube 卵管峡部 237

J

Jejunal aa. 空腸動脈 267

Joint capsule of glenohumeral joint　関節包
　　《肩関節の》　315
Jugular
− foramen　頸静脈孔　547，573，733
− notch　頸切痕　61，**65**，165，693

K

Kidney　腎臓　207，229
Kiesselbach's area　キーゼルバッハ部位
　　625
Knee joint　膝関節　449，451

L

L1 vertebra　第1腰椎　5，207，501
L4 vertebra　第4腰椎　7，503
L5 vertebra　第5腰椎　193，717
Labia
− majora　大陰唇　239
− minora　小陰唇　239
Lacrimal
− a.　涙腺動脈　609
− apparatus　涙器　615
− caruncle　涙丘　615
− gland　涙腺　609，615
− n.　涙腺神経　609
− sac　涙嚢　615
Lactiferous
− duct　乳管　89
− sinus　乳管洞　89
Lambdoid suture　ラムダ縫合　545
Lamina of vertebral arch　椎弓板　9，**17**，
　　19，35
Laryngeal prominence of thyroid cartilage
　　喉頭隆起　675
Lateral
− antebrachial cutaneous n.　外側前腕皮神
　　経　377，395
− aortic lymph node　外側大動脈リンパ節
　　285
− arcuate l.　外側弓状靱帯　71
− branches of supraorbital n.　外側枝《眼窩
　　上神経の》　585
− cervical region　外側頸三角部　689
− collateral l. of knee joint　外側側副靱帯
　　《膝関節の》　453，457
− condyle of femur　外側顆《大腿骨の》
　　421，449，451
− cord　外側神経束　369，371，377
− corticospinal tract　外側皮質脊髄路　743
− cricothyroid　外側輪状甲状筋　681
− crus of superficial inguinal ring　外側脚
　　《浅鼠径輪の》　513
− cuneiform　外側楔状骨　469
− cutaneous branch
−− of intercostal n.　外側皮枝《肋間神経
　　の》　55
−− of posterior intercostal
−−− aa.　外側皮枝《肋間動脈の》　55
−−− vv.　外側皮枝《肋間静脈の》　55
−− of spinal n.　外側皮枝《脊髄神経の》
　　79
−− of thoracic aorta　外側皮枝《胸大動脈
　　の》　47
− epicondyle
−− of femur　外側上顆《大腿骨の》　453
−− of humerus　外側上顆《上腕骨の》
　　307
− femoral cutaneous n.　外側大腿皮神経
　　501，**511**，513，517
− geniculate body　外側膝状体　745
− head
−− of flexor hallucis brevis　外側頭《短母
　　趾屈筋の》　491
−− of gastrocnemius　外側頭《腓腹筋の》
　　439，461，463
−− of triceps brachii　外側頭《上腕三頭筋
　　の》　331，385
− intermuscular
−− septum　外側大腿筋間中隔　533
−−− of arm　外側上腕筋間中隔　409
− lip of linea aspera　外側唇《大腿骨の》
　　421
− malleolus　外果　**447**，461，463，475，
　　481
− masses of atlas　外側塊《環椎の》　13
− meniscus　外側半月　455，457
− olfactory stria　外側嗅条　707
　part of vaginal fornix　外側部《腟円蓋
　　の》　237
− pectoral nn.　外側胸筋神経　387，389
− plantar
−− a.　外側足底動脈　523，531
−− n.　外側足底神経　499，523，531

――v. 外側足底静脈 531
- plate of pterygoid process 外側板《翼状突起の》 547
- pterygoid 外側翼突筋 593
- rectus 外側直筋 557, 603, 611
- segment of globus pallidus 外節《淡蒼球の》 709
- semicircular canal 外側骨半規管 629
- spinothalamic tract 外側脊髄視床路 741
- sulcus 外側溝 697
- supracondylar ridge of humerus 外側顆上稜《上腕骨の》 307
- sural cutaneous n. 外側腓腹皮神経 525
- tarsal a. 外側足根動脈 529
- thoracic
――a. 外側胸動脈 75, 85, 365, 391
――v. 外側胸静脈 85
- ventricle 側脳室 707, 729
Latissimus dorsi 広背筋 39, 57, 323, **327**, 393
Left
- and right diaphragm leaflets 左・右の横隔膜円蓋 139
- atrioventricular valve 左房室弁 125
- atrium 左心房 111, **119**, 125, 137, 141, 145
- auricle 左心耳 117
- brachiocephalic v. 左腕頭静脈 99, 115, 149, **581**
- broncho-mediastinal trunk 左気管支縦隔リンパ本幹 163
- colic
――a. 左結腸動脈 269
――flexure 左結腸曲 213
- common carotid a. 左総頸動脈 95, 117
- coronary a. 左冠状動脈 129
- cusp of aortic valve 左半月弁《大動脈弁の》 127
- gastric
――a. 左胃動脈 263, 277
――v. 左胃静脈 275, 277
- gastro-omental
――a. 左胃大網動脈 277
――v. 左胃大網静脈 275, 277
- hypogastric n. 左下腹神経 291
- inferior
――lobar bronchi 左下葉気管支 155

――phrenic a. 左下横隔動脈 259, 273
- internal pudendal
――a. 左内陰部動脈 279
――v. 左内陰部静脈 279, 281
- lateral aortic lymph node 左外側大動脈リンパ節 285
- lobe of liver 左葉《肝臓の》 195
- lumbar trunk 左腰リンパ本幹 99
- lung 左肺 141, 149, 153
- main bronchus 左主気管支 93, 95, 109, **155**
- ovarian a. 左卵巣動脈 259
- phrenic n. 左横隔神経 109
- pulmonary
――a. 左肺動脈 109, 119
――vv. 左肺静脈 105, 119
- recurrent laryngeal n. 左反回神経 101, 135, **571**, 663
- renal
――a. 左腎動脈 259, 261, 273
――v. 左腎静脈 267, 273
- subclavian
――a. 左鎖骨下動脈 95, 101, 105, 667
――v. 左鎖骨下静脈 105
- suprarenal v. 左副腎静脈 229, 273
- ventricle 左心室 105, 115, **119**, 137
Lens 水晶体 617
Lesser
- curvature of stomach 小弯 209
- occipital n. 小後頭神経 575, 669, 689
- palatine n. 小口蓋神経 627
- petrosal n. 小錐体神経 597, 637
- sciatic foramen 小坐骨孔 175, 515
- trochanter 小転子 421, 423
- tuberosity of humerus 小結節《上腕骨の》 305, 313
- wing of sphenoid bone 小翼《蝶形骨の》 549
Levator
- ani 肛門挙筋 187, 189, 205, **215**, 241
- palpebrae superioris 上眼瞼挙筋 557, **603**, 609, 613
- scapulae 肩甲挙筋 39, 329
- veli palatini 口蓋帆挙筋 633
Levatores costarum 肋骨挙筋 45
Ligamenta flava 黄色靱帯 33, 35

Ligamentum
- arteriosum 動脈管索 109, 113, **121**, 145
- teres of liver 肝円索 145, 219
- venosum 静脈管索 145

Linea
- alba 白線 177, 293
- aspera 粗線《大腿骨の》 421, 425

Lingual
- a. 舌動脈 577, 649, 657
- n.(CN V$_3$) 舌神経 561, 593, 597, 641, 647, **649**
- tonsil 舌扁桃 643

Lingula of lung 小舌《肺の》 153
Liver 肝臓 143, 195, **219**, 221
Long
- ciliary nn. 長毛様体神経 605, 611
- head
- - of biceps brachii 長頭《上腕二頭筋の》 323
- - of biceps femoris 長頭《大腿二頭筋の》 439, 445, 509
- - of triceps brachii 長頭《上腕三頭筋の》 327, 331
- plantar l. 長足底靭帯 479
- saphenous v. 大伏在静脈 511
- thoracic n. 長胸神経 371, 391

Longissimus 最長筋 43
Lower
- leg 下腿 417
- trunk 下神経幹 371

Lumbar
- ganglia 腰神経節 289
- nn. 腰神経 289
- splanchnic n. 腰内臓神経 289
- triangle 腰三角 39
- vertebrae 腰椎 3, 21
- vv. 腰静脈 97, 271

Lumbocostal triangle(Bochdalek's triangle) 腰肋三角(ボクダレク三角) 71
Lumbosacral
- enlargement 腰膨大 717
- trunk 腰仙骨神経幹 501

Lumbricals
- of foot 虫様筋《足の》 489
- of hand 虫様筋《手の》 359, 379

Lunate 月状骨 351
Lungs 肺 149

M

Major
- calix 大腎杯 261
- duodenal papilla 大十二指腸乳頭 211, 223

Male pelvis 男性骨盤 173
Malleus ツチ骨 629, 635
Mammary
- gland 乳腺 89
- lobes 乳腺葉 89

Mammillary
- body 乳頭体 703, 711
- process of lumbar vertebrae 乳頭突起《腰椎の》 21

Mandible 下顎骨 541, 639
Mandibular
- angle 下顎角 639, 693
- division(CN V$_3$) 下顎神経 561, 575, 595, **597**, 641
- foramen 下顎孔 639
- fossa 下顎窩 547
- notch 下顎切痕 639

Manubrium sterni 胸骨柄 65, 67, 311
Marginal
- a. 結腸辺縁動脈 267
- mandibular branch of facial n. 下顎縁枝《顔面神経の》 563, 589

Masseter 咬筋 **553**, 587, 595, 655
Mastoid process of temporal bone 乳様突起 545
Matatarsus(metatarsal) 中足骨 469, 471, 479
Maxilla 上顎骨 **541**, 543, 547, 619, 621
Maxillary
- a. 顎動脈 577, 579, 595
- division(n.)(CN V$_2$) 上顎神経 561, 575, **599**, 641
- hiatus 上顎洞裂孔 623
- sinus 上顎洞 601
- v. 顎静脈 583

Medial
- border of scapula 内側縁《肩甲骨の》 303, 329
- branch
- - of spinal n. 内側枝《脊髄神経の》 51

(Middle meningeal a.) 763

－－of supraorbital n. 内側枝《眼窩上神経の》 585
－circumflex femoral a. 内側大腿回旋動脈 495, 517
－collateral l. of knee joint 内側側副靱帯《膝関節の》 453, 455, 457
－condyle
－－of femur 内側顆《大腿骨の》 421, 449, 451
－－of tibia 内側顆《脛骨の》 447, 449, 451
－cord 内側神経束 369, 381
－crus of superficial inguinal ring 内側脚《浅鼠径輪の》 513
－cuneiform 内側楔状骨 **469**, 471, 477, 479
－cutaneous branch of thoracic aorta 内側皮枝《胸大動脈の》 47
－epicondyle
－－of femur 内側上顆《大腿骨の》 421, 449, 451
－－of humerus 内側上顆《上腕骨の》 **305**, 335, 337, 339
－head
－－of clavicle 内側頭《鎖骨の》 165
－－of flexor hallucis brevis 内側頭《短母趾屈筋の》 491
－－of gastrocnemius 内側頭《腓腹筋の》 439, 463, 467, 535
－－of triceps brachii 内側頭《上腕三頭筋の》 331, 409
－intermuscular septum of arm 内側上腕筋間中隔 393
－lip of linea aspera 内側唇《大腿骨の》 421
－malleolus of tibia 内果《脛骨の》 447, 459
－meniscus 内側半月 453, 455
－pectoral nn. 内側胸筋神経 387, 389
－plantar
－－a. 内側足底動脈 523, 531
－－n. 内側足底神経 499, 523, 531
－plate of pterygoid process 内側板《翼状突起の》 547, 621
－pterygoid 内側翼突筋 595
－rectus 内側直筋 557, 603
－segment of globus pallidus 内節《淡蒼球の》 709

－superior genicular a. 内側上膝動脈 497
－thalamic nuclei 視床内側核群 711
－umbilical ll. 内側臍索 145
Median
－aperture of fourth ventricle 第四脳室正中口 727
－arcuate l. 正中弓状靱帯 71
－cubital v. 肘正中皮静脈 367
－n. 正中神経 369, **379**, 393, 395, 397, 399, 405, 407, 409, 411
－sacral
－－a. 正中仙骨動脈 259
－－crest 正中仙骨稜 25
－umbilical fold 正中臍ヒダ 195
Mediastinal part of parietal pleura 壁側胸膜の縦隔部(縦隔胸膜) 103, 147
Mediastinum 縦隔 91, 103
Medulla oblongata 延髄 697, 699
Medullary pyramid 腎錐体 261
Meninges 髄膜 721
Mental
－foramen オトガイ孔 543, 561, 639
－n. オトガイ神経 561, 585
Mesenteric root 腸間膜根 201
Mesentery 腸間膜 199
Mesometrium 子宮間膜 235
Mesosalpinx 卵管間膜 235
Metacarpals 中手骨 297, 349, 351
Metacarpophalangeal(MCP) joint 中手指節(MCP)関節 353
Metatarsophalangeal joints 中足趾節関節 473
Midcarpal joint 手根中央関節 353
Midclavicular line(MCL) 鎖骨中線 165
Middle
－cerebellar peduncle 中小脳脚 715
－cerebral a. 中大脳動脈 735
－cervical ganglion 中頸神経節 101, 663
－cluneal nn. 中殿皮神経 55
－colic a. 中結腸動脈 267
－cranial fossa 中頭蓋窩 549, 607
－internodal bundles 中結節間束 133
－lobe of right lung 中葉《右肺の》 149, 151
－meatus 中鼻道 621
－mediastinum 中縦隔 91
－meningeal a. 中硬膜動脈 595

- pharyngeal constrictor　中咽頭収縮筋　659, 661
- rectal
-- a.　中直腸動脈　279, 281
-- v.　中直腸静脈　279
- scalene　中斜角筋　67, 691
- suprarenal aa.　中副腎動脈　273
- transverse rectal fold　中直腸横ヒダ　217

Minor duodenal papilla　小十二指腸乳頭　211
Mons pubis　恥丘　239
Muscles of facial expression　表情筋　553
Muscular triangle　筋三角　683
Musculocutaneous n.　筋皮神経　377, 395
Musculophrenic a.　筋横隔動脈　75
Mylohyoid　顎舌骨筋　665
- branch of inferior alveolar a.　顎舌骨筋枝《下歯槽動脈の》　579
- n.　顎舌骨筋神経　597
Myometrium　子宮筋層　237

N

Nasal
- bone　鼻骨　543
- cavity　鼻腔　619
- septum　鼻中隔　555
Nasion　鼻根点　543
Nasociliary n.　鼻毛様体神経　559, 611
Nasolacrimal duct　鼻涙管　615
Nasopalatine n.　鼻口蓋神経　625
Navicular　舟状骨《足の》　**469**, 471, 475, 477, 479
Neck
- of bladder　膀胱頸　233
- of femur　大腿骨頸　421, 423
- of rib　肋骨頸　63
Nerve
- of pterygoid canal　翼突管神経　599
- of tensor veli palatini　口蓋帆張筋神経　597
Nipple　乳頭　89
Nuchal l.　項靱帯　29, 31
Nucleus pulposus of intervertebral disk　髄核《椎間円板の》　33

O

Oblique
- fissure
-- of left lung　斜裂《左肺の》　153
-- of right lung　斜裂《右肺の》　139, 141, 151
- head of adductor
-- hallucis　斜頭《母趾内転筋の》　491
-- pollicis　斜頭《母指内転筋の》　361
- pericardial sinus　心膜斜洞　113
Obliquus
- capitis
-- inferior　下頭斜筋　41, 53
-- superior　上頭斜筋　41
Obturator
- a.　閉鎖動脈　279, 281
- canal　閉鎖管　189
- externus　外閉鎖筋　435, 503
- foramen　閉鎖孔　169, 419
- internus　内閉鎖筋　187, 215, **437**, 441
-- fascia　内閉鎖筋筋膜　191
- membrane　閉鎖膜　173, 175
- n.　閉鎖神経　501, 503, 517
- v.　閉鎖静脈　279
Occipital
- a.　後頭動脈　53, 577
- bone　後頭骨　545
- condyle　後頭顆　547
- lobe　後頭葉　697
- triangle　後頭三角　683
Occipitofrontalis　後頭前頭筋　553
Oculomotor n.(CN III)　動眼神経　557, **605**, 607, 713
Olecranon　肘頭　333
- fossa of humerus　肘頭窩《上腕骨の》　307
Olfactory
- bulb　嗅球　555, 627, 699
- fibers　嗅神経糸　555, 625
- tract　嗅索　555, 699
Omental
- bursa　網嚢　197, 207
- foramen　網嚢孔　197
Omoclavicular triangle　肩甲鎖骨三角　683
Omohyoid　肩甲舌骨筋　665
Ophthalmic division (CN V_1)　眼神経　559, 575, 605

(Pedicle of vertebral arch) *765*

Opponens
- digiti minimi　小指対立筋　361
- pollicis　母指対立筋　359
Optic
- canal　視神経管　551, 601
- chiasm　視交叉　559, 607, 707, **745**
- disk　視神経円板(視神経乳頭)　617
- n.(CN II)　視神経　559, **605**, 607, 611, 617, 699, 745
- radiation　視放線　701, 745
- tract　視索　709, 745
Orbicularis
- oculi　眼輪筋　553, 613
- oris　口輪筋　553
Orbit　眼窩　601
Orbital
- part of lacrimal gland　眼窩部《涙腺の》615
- plate of ethmoid bone　眼窩板《篩骨の》601
- septum　眼窩隔膜　613
- surface of zygomatic bone　眼窩面《頬骨の》601
Ossicular chain　耳小骨連鎖　635
Otic ganglion　耳神経節　597
Ovarian
- a.　卵巣動脈　235
- v.　卵巣静脈　235, 271
Ovary　卵巣　235

P

Palatine
- bone　口蓋骨　547, 619, 623
- process of maxilla　口蓋突起《上顎骨の》547, 619
- tonsil　口蓋扁桃　643
Palatoglossal arch　口蓋舌弓　643, 653
Palatoglossus　口蓋舌筋　645
Palatopharyngeal arch　口蓋咽頭弓　643, 653
Palatopharyngeus　口蓋咽頭筋　663
Palmar
- aponeurosis　手掌腱膜　355
- branch
-- of median n.　掌枝《正中神経の》　405
-- of ulnar n.　掌枝《尺骨神経の》　405
- carpal l.　掌側手根靱帯　397, 399
- digital nn.　掌側指神経　405
- metacarpal aa.　掌側中手動脈　401
Palmaris
- brevis　短掌筋　355
- longus　長掌筋　339
-- tendon　長掌筋の腱　355
Palpebral part of orbicularis oculi　眼瞼部《眼輪筋の》613
Pampiniform plexus　蔓状静脈叢　249, 283
Pancreas　膵臓　193, 197, 201, 207, 211, **227**, 263
Pancreatic duct　膵管　223, 227
Pancreaticoduodenal a.　膵十二指腸動脈　265
Paracolic gutter　結腸傍溝　201
Parasympathetic n.　副交感神経　747
Paratracheal lymph node　気管傍リンパ節　163
Paraventricular nuclei of thalamus　視床室傍核群　711
Parietal
- bone　頭頂骨　545
- layer
-- of the serous pericardium　壁側板《漿膜性心膜の》　111
-- of tunica vaginalis　壁側板《精巣鞘膜の》　249, 251
- peritoneum　壁側腹膜　185
- pleura　壁側胸膜　147
Parotid
- duct　耳下腺管　585, 587, 655
- gland　耳下腺　655
- plexus　耳下腺神経叢　589
Patella　膝蓋骨　417, 449, 455
Patellar l.　膝蓋靱帯　433, 453, 457
Pectinate muscles　櫛状筋　123
Pectineal line　恥骨筋線　169, 171
Pectineus　恥骨筋　433, 505
Pectoral
- axillary lymph node　胸筋腋窩リンパ節　87
- fascia　胸筋筋膜　89
Pectoralis
- major　大胸筋　89, **319**, 325, 387
- minor　小胸筋　321, 389
Pedicle of vertebral arch　椎弓根　9, 19, 37

Pelvic
- floor 骨盤底 187, 189, 191
- girdle 下肢帯 171, 417
- splanchnic nn. 骨盤内臓神経 291
Penis 陰茎 245, 247, 249
Perforating aa. 貫通動脈 495, 519
Pericardiacophrenic
- a. 心膜横隔動脈 83, 103, 107
- v. 心膜横隔静脈 83, 103, 107
Pericardial cavity 心膜腔 111
Pericardium 心膜 83, 113
Perineal
- membrane 会陰膜（下尿生殖隔膜筋膜） 187
- nn. 会陰神経 243
- raphe 会陰縫線 239
Perirenal fat capsule 脂肪被膜 229
Peritoneal cavity 腹膜腔 195, 201
Perpendicular plate
- of ethmoid bone 垂直板《篩骨の》 543, 601, 619
- of palatine bone 垂直板《口蓋骨の》 623
Petrous
- part of temporal bone 岩様部《側頭骨の》 551, 629, 637
- ridge 錐体上縁 549
Phalanges 指(節)骨 297
Pharyngeal
- constrictors 咽頭収縮筋 659, 661
- muscles 咽頭筋 659
- orifice 咽頭口 633
-- of pharyngotympanic tube 耳管咽頭口 651
- plexus 咽頭神経叢 569
Pharyngotympanic (auditory) tube 耳管 629, 633, 651
Philtrum 人中 693
Phrenic n. 横隔神経 **83**, 103, 107, 371, 669, 687
Pia mater 軟膜 721
Pineal gland 松果体 705
Piriform recess 梨状陥凹 677
Piriformis 梨状筋 189, **191**, 437, 441, 515
Pisiform 豆状骨 351
Plantar
- aponeurosis 足底腱膜 485
- calcaneonavicular l. 底側踵舟靱帯 477, 479
- interossei 底側骨間筋 491
- metatarsal aa. 底側中足動脈 531
Plantaris 足底筋 465
Pons 橋 699, 713
Popliteal
- a. 膝窩動脈 495, **497**, 519, 521
- fossa 膝窩 439
- v. 膝窩静脈 519, 521
Popliteus 膝窩筋 465, 467
Portal v. 〔肝〕門脈 221, 275, 277
Postcentral gyrus 中心後回 697, 739
Posterior
- (dorsal)
-- ramus
--- of spinal n. 後枝《脊髄神経の》 51, 55, 79
-- root
--- of spinal n. 後根《脊髄神経の》 79, 719
- antebrachial cutaneous n. 後前腕皮神経 375
- arch of atlas 後弓《環椎の》 11, 13
- auricular
-- a. 後耳介動脈 577
-- n. 後耳介神経 563, 565
- belly of digastric muscle 後腹《顎二腹筋の》 565, 659, 661
- cerebral a. 後大脳動脈 735
- circumflex humeral a. 後上腕回旋動脈 365, 385
- communicating a. 後交通動脈 735
- cord 後神経束 371, 373
- cranial fossa 後頭蓋窩 549
- cricoarytenoid 後輪状披裂筋 663, 681
- cruciate l. 後十字靱帯 455, 457
- cusp
-- of aortic valve 後半月弁《大動脈弁の》 127
-- of right atrioventricular valve 後尖《右房室弁の》 127
- descending (interventricular) a. 後下行枝 131
- ethmoid sinus 後篩骨洞 623
- ethmoidal n. 後篩骨神経 559, 609
- femoral cutaneous n. 後大腿皮神経 499, 511, 519

(Pulmonary aa.) *767*

- horn of spinal cord　後角《脊髄の》　737
- inferior iliac spine　下後腸骨棘　419, 425
- intercostal
-- aa.　肋間動脈　47, 55, **75**, 81, 83
-- vv.　肋間静脈　49, 55, **77**, 81, 83, 97
- internal vertebral venous plexus　後内椎骨静脈叢　49, 719
- internodal bundles　後結節間束　133
- interosseous
-- a.　後骨間動脈　365
-- n.　後[前腕]骨間神経　375
- interventricular
-- (descending) a.　後室間枝(後下行枝)　131
-- v.　後室間静脈(中心臓静脈)　131
- labial
-- commissure　後陰唇交連　239
-- nn.　後陰唇神経　243
- longitudinal l.　後縦靱帯　31, 33, 35, **37**
- mediastinum　後縦隔　91
- papillary muscle　後乳頭筋　125
- parietal cortex　後頭頂野　739
- ramus of thoracic aorta　後枝《胸大動脈の》　47
- sacroiliac ll.　後仙腸靱帯　429
- scrotal nn.　後陰嚢神経　257
- segmental medullary a.　後髄節動脈　737
- septal branches of sphenopalatine a.　中隔後鼻枝《蝶口蓋動脈の》　625
- spinal aa.　後脊髄動脈　737
- spinocerebellar tract　後脊髄小脳路　741
- superior
-- alveolar
--- aa.　後上歯槽動脈　579
--- branches of superior alveolar nn.　後上歯槽枝《上歯槽神経の》　561, 599
-- iliac spine　上後腸骨棘　425, 429, 515
- talofibular l.　後距腓靱帯　483
- tibial
-- a.　後脛骨動脈　**497**, 521, 523, 535
-- v.　後脛骨静脈　535
- tibiofibular l.　後脛腓靱帯　483
- tubercle of atlas　後結節《環椎の》　13
Precentral gyrus　中心前回　739
Prefrontal cortex　前頭前野　739

Premotor cortex　運動前野　739
Pretracheal layer of cervical fascia　気管前葉《頸筋膜の》　673
Prevertebral ganglion　椎前神経節　747
Profunda
- brachii a.　上腕深動脈　365, 385
- femoris a.　大腿深動脈　495, 517, 533
Promontory of sacrum　岬角《仙骨の》　3, **23**, 171, 175, 437
Pronator
- quadratus　方形回内筋　343
- teres　円回内筋　339, 341, 379
Proper
- hepatic a.　固有肝動脈　221, 265
- ovarian l.　固有卵巣索　235
- palmar
-- digital
--- aa.　固有掌側指動脈　399
--- nn.　固有掌側指神経　381, 399
- plantar
-- digital
--- aa.　固有底側趾動脈　531
--- nn.　固有底側趾神経　531
Prostate　前立腺　203, 253, 255
Proximal
- interphalangeal joint　近位指節間(PIP)関節　353
-- crease　近位指節間関節線　413
- radioulnar joint　上橈尺関節　333
Psoas major　大腰筋　71, 229, 431
Pterygoid
- plexus　翼突筋静脈叢　581, 583
- process of sphenoid bone　翼状突起《蝶形骨の》　547, 621
Pterygopalatine
- fossa　翼口蓋窩　599
- ganglion　翼口蓋神経節　561, 627, 641
Pubic
- symphysis　恥骨結合　173, 191, 231
- tubercle　恥骨結節　169, 419, 423
Pubis　恥骨　169, 171
Pubococcygeus　恥骨尾骨筋　189
Pubofemoral l.　恥骨大腿靱帯　427
Puborectalis　恥骨直腸筋　189
Pudendal n.　陰部神経　243, 291, **499**, 519
Pulmonary
- aa.　肺動脈　145

- l. 肺間膜 151
- plexus 肺神経叢 135
- trunk 肺動脈幹 95, 113, 117, 125, 137, 149, **161**

Putamen 被殻 709

Pyloric
- antrum 幽門洞 209
- part of stomach 幽門部《胃の》 207
- sphincter 幽門括約筋 211

Pyramid of medulla oblongata 延髄錐体 713

Pyramidal lobe of thyroid gland 錐体葉《甲状腺の》 671

Pyramidalis 錐体筋 181

Q

Quadrate lobe of liver 方形葉《肝臓の》 221

Quadratus
- femoris 大腿方形筋 441
- plantae 足底方形筋 489, 531

Quadriceps femoris tendon 大腿四頭筋の腱 431, 453

Quadrigeminal plate 四丘体板 705, 715

R

Radial
- a. 橈骨動脈 **365**, 395, 401, 403
- collateral l. of proximal radio-ulnar joint 外側側副靱帯《上橈尺関節の》 335, 337
- head of flexor digitorum superficialis 橈骨頭《浅指屈筋の》 343
- n. 橈骨神経 **375**, 385, 391, 395, 403, 405, 409
- tuberosity 橈骨粗面 333

Radiocarpal joint 橈骨手根関節 353

Radius 橈骨 297, 333

Ramus of mandible 下顎枝《下顎骨の》 639

Rectouterine pouch 直腸子宮窩 205

Rectovesical pouch 直腸膀胱窩 203, 255

Rectum 直腸 203, 213, **215**, 217, 231

Rectus
- abdominis 腹直筋 181, 183, 293
- capitis posterior major 大後頭直筋 41
- femoris 大腿直筋 **431**, 505, 533, 537
- sheath 腹直筋鞘 179, 181, 183

Recurrent laryngeal n. 反回神経 101, 135, 687

Renal
- a. 腎動脈 259, 261, 273
- v. 腎静脈 267, 271, 273

Respiratory bronchiole 呼吸細気管支 157, 159

Reticulospinal tract 網様体脊髄路 743

Retina 網膜 617

Retromandibular v. 下顎後静脈 581

Retropharyngeal space 咽頭後隙 673

Rhomboid
- (romboideus) major 大菱形筋 39, 329
- fossa 菱形窩 715
- minor 小菱形筋 329

Rib 肋骨 69

Right
- atrioventricular
- - orifice 右房室口 123
- - valve 右房室弁 121, 123, 127,
- atrium 右心房 **119**, 121, 137, 141
- auricle 右心耳 117
- brachiocephalic v. 右腕頭静脈 77
- bundle branch of atrioventricular bundle 右脚《房室束の》 133
- colic
- - a. 右結腸動脈 267
- - flexure 右結腸曲 197
- common
- - iliac
- - - a. 右総腸骨動脈 203, 229, **259**, 281
- - - v. 右総腸骨静脈 203, 281
- coronary a. 右冠状動脈 129, 131
- crus of diaphragm 右脚《横隔膜の》 71
- cusp of aortic valve 右半月弁《大動脈弁の》 127
- gastric a. 右胃動脈 263
- gastro-omental a. 右胃大網動脈 263
- hepatic duct 右肝管 223
- inferior
- - lobar bronchi 右下葉気管支 155
- - suprarenal a. 右下副腎動脈 273
- internal
- - iliac a. 右内腸骨動脈 259, 279
- - jugular v. 右内頸静脈 97, 163

(Short head of biceps brachii) 769

－lobe of thyroid gland　右葉《甲状腺の》　671
－lumbar trunk　右腰リンパ本幹　285
－lung　右肺　139, 141, 149, **151**
－main bronchus　右主気管支　93, 155
－marginal
－－a.　右縁枝(鋭角縁枝)　129
－－v.　右辺縁静脈　129
－middle suprarenal a.　右中副腎動脈　273
－phrenic n.　右横隔神経　115, 135
－pulmonary
－－a.　右肺動脈　107, 111, 121, 149, 151, **161**
－－vv.　右肺静脈　113, 149, 151
－recurrent laryngeal n.　右反回神経　135, 571
－renal a.　右腎動脈　207
－subclavian v.　右鎖骨下静脈　163
－superior
－－lobar bronchus　右上葉気管支　155
－－suprarenal a.　右上副腎動脈　273
－testicular
－－a.　右精巣動脈　229
－－v.　右精巣静脈　229
－ventricle　右心室　115, 129, 137
Rubrospinal tract　赤核脊髄路　743

S

Saccule　球形嚢　567
Sacral
－canal　仙骨管　25, 175
－cornua　仙骨角　25
－hiatus　仙骨裂孔　25
－plexus　仙骨神経叢　287, 289, 517
Sacrococcygeal joint　仙尾関節　23
Sacroiliac joint　仙腸関節　171
Sacrospinous l.　仙棘靱帯　**173**, 175, 427, 429, 515
Sacrotuberous l.　仙結節靱帯　**175**, 427, 429, 441, 515
Sacrum　仙骨　23, 25, 171, 175, 189
Sagittal suture　矢状縫合　545
Salpingopharyngeus　耳管咽頭筋　633
Saphenous n.　伏在神経　499, **505**, 511, 517
Sartorius　縫工筋　**431**, 437, 505, 533
Scalp　頭皮　723

Scaphoid　舟状骨《手の》　**349**, 353, 397, 403
－fossa　舟状窩　631
Scapula　肩甲骨　301, 303, 329
Scapular
－notch　肩甲切痕　303
－spine　肩甲棘　7, 39, 303, 383
Scapulothoracic joint　肩甲胸郭関節　309
Sciatic n.　坐骨神経　**499**, 501, 507, 519, 533
Sclera　強膜　617
Scrotum　陰嚢　251
Second
－lumbrical of hand　第2虫様筋《手の》　379
－middle phalanx of hand　第2中節骨《手の》　349
－palmar interossei　第2掌側骨間筋《掌側骨間筋の》　361
－perforating a.　第2貫通動脈《貫通動脈の》　519
Segmental bronchus　区域気管支　157
Sella turcica(hypophyseal fossa) of sphenoid bone　トルコ鞍(下垂体窩)《蝶形骨の》　551
Semicircular ducts　半規管　567
Semilunar line　半月線　293
Semimembranosus　半膜様筋　439, 463, 509
Seminal vesicle　精嚢　203, 253, 255
Semispinalis capitis　頭半棘筋　45
Semitendinosus　半腱様筋　439, 509, 533
Septal
－cartilage　鼻中隔軟骨　619
－cusp of right atrioventricular valve　中隔尖《右房室弁の》　127
Septomarginal trabecula　中隔縁柱　121
Serous pericardium　漿膜性心膜　111
Serratus
－anterior　前鋸筋　177, 319, **321**, 323, 329
－posterior inferior　下後鋸筋　39
Sesamoids　種子骨　471, 475
Shaft of clavicle　鎖骨体　299
Short
－head of biceps
－－brachii　短頭《上腕二頭筋の》　323

――femoris 短頭《大腿二頭筋の》 443, 507
―saphenous v. 小伏在静脈 511
Shoulder
―girdle 上肢帯 297, 309
―joint 肩関節 309, 313, 315
Sigmoid
―aa. S状結腸動脈 269
―colon S状結腸 205, 213
―sinus S状静脈洞 583, 731, 733
Sinoatrial(SA) node 洞房結節 133
Sixth rib 第6肋骨 63
Small cardiac v. 小心臓静脈 131
Soft palate 軟口蓋(口蓋帆) 651, 653
Soleus ヒラメ筋 461, **465**, 467, 509, 535
Spermatic cord 精索 183, 185
Sphenoid
―bone 蝶形骨 **541**, 547, 549, 601
―sinus 蝶形骨洞 623
Sphenopalatine
―a. 蝶口蓋動脈 579, 595, 625
―foramen 蝶口蓋孔 623
Spinal
―branch of thoracic aorta 脊髄枝《胸大動脈の》 47
―cord 脊髄 31, 51, 717
―ganglion 脊髄神経節 79, 747
―n. 脊髄神経 51, 55, 79, 719
―root 脊髄根 573
Spinalis 棘筋 43, 45
Spinous process 棘突起 5, 7, 9, **11**, 17, 19, 21, 41
Spiral ganglia ラセン神経節 567
Splanchnic n. 内臓神経 747
Spleen 脾臓 197, 207
Splenic
―a. 脾動脈 263, 277
―v. 脾静脈 275, 277
Splenius
―capitis 頭板状筋 45
―cervicis 頸板状筋 43
Spongy part of urethra 海綿体部《尿道の》 245, 255
Squamous
―part of temporal bone 鱗部《側頭骨の》 541
―suture 鱗状縫合 541

Stapedius アブミ骨筋 635
Stellate ganglion 星状神経節 663, 687
Sternal
―angle of sternum 胸骨角《胸骨の》 65, 165
―articular surface 胸骨関節面 299
―head of sternocleidomastoid 胸骨頭《胸鎖乳突筋の》 693
Sternoclavicular joint 胸鎖関節 309, 311
Sternocleidomastoid 胸鎖乳突筋 41, **319**, 573, 587, 655, 673, 689, 693
Sternocostal
―joint 胸肋関節 311
―part of pectoralis major 胸肋部《大胸筋の》 319
Sternohyoid 胸骨舌骨筋 665
Sternothyroid 胸骨甲状筋 665, 691
Sternum 胸骨 63, 65, 69
Stomach 胃 193, 195, 207, **209**
Straight sinus 直静脈洞 727, 733
Stria medullaris thalami 視床髄条 705
Striate area 有線野 745
Styloglossus 茎突舌筋 645
Stylohyoid 茎突舌骨筋 565, 659, 661
Styloid
―process
――of radius 茎状突起《橈骨の》 333, 351
――of temporal bone 茎状突起《側頭骨の》 629
――of ulna 茎状突起《尺骨の》 349, 413
Stylomastoid foramen 茎乳突孔 565
Stylopharyngeus 茎突咽頭筋 569, 661
Subacromial bursa 肩峰下包 317
Subarachnoid space クモ膜下腔 31, 719
Subclavian
―a. 鎖骨下動脈 75, 85, 95, **371**, 389, 571, 685, 687
―v. 鎖骨下静脈 85, 163, **389**, 687
Subclavius 鎖骨下筋 321
Subcutaneous part of external anal sphincter 皮下部《外肛門括約筋の》 217
Subdeltoid bursa 三角筋下包 317
Sublingual gland 舌下腺 657
Submandibular
―(digastric) triangle 顎下三角 683
―duct 顎下腺管 657
―ganglion 顎下神経節 649

(Superior root of ansa cervicalis) *771*

- gland　顎下腺　591，**655**，657，693
- Submental triangle　オトガイ下三角　683
- Suboccipital n.　後頭下神経　53
- Subscapular
 - a.　肩甲下動脈　391
 - fossa　肩甲下窩　301
- Subscapularis　肩甲下筋　321，323，325
- Substantia nigra　黒質　711
- Subtalar（talocalcaneal）joint　距骨下関節　473，475，477
- Subthalamic nucleus　視床下核　711
- Sulcal a.　溝動脈　737
- Sulcus
 - for spinal n.　脊髄神経溝　11，17
 - terminalis　分界溝　643
- Superficial
 - branch
  -- of radial n.　浅枝《橈骨神経の》　375，395，403，407，411
  -- of ulnar n.　浅枝《尺骨神経の》　399
 - dorsal penile v.　浅陰茎背静脈　245
 - fibular n.　浅腓骨神経　499，**507**，511，525，527
 - head of flexor pollicis brevis　浅頭《短母指屈筋の》　357
 - inguinal
  -- lymph node　浅鼠径リンパ節　285
  -- ring　浅鼠径輪　177，293
 - layer of thoracolumbar fascia　浅葉《胸腰筋膜の》　39，43
 - palmar arch　浅掌動脈弓　365，399
 - part of external anal sphincter　浅部《外肛門括約筋の》　217
 - temporal
  -- a.　浅側頭動脈　577，593
  -- v.　浅側頭静脈　581，593
 - transverse
  -- metacarpal l.　浅横中足靭帯　485
  -- perineal　浅会陰横筋　187，241
- Superior
 - alveolar nn.　上歯槽神経　561，599
 - angle of scapula　上角《肩甲骨の》　301
 - articular process　上関節突起　9，21
 - belly of omohyoid　上腹《肩甲舌骨筋の》　665
 - cerebellar
  -- a.　上小脳動脈　735
  -- peduncle　上小脳脚　715
 - cervical ganglion　上頸神経節　591，691
 - cluneal nn.　上殿皮神経　55
 - colliculus of quadrigeminal plate　上丘《四丘体板の》　715
 - costal facet　上肋骨窩　19
 - extensor retinaculum　上伸筋支帯　493
 - gluteal
  -- a.　上殿動脈　519
  -- n.　上殿神経　519
  -- v.　上殿静脈　519
 - hypogastric plexus　上下腹神経叢　287，291
 - lacrimal canaliculi　上涙小管　615
 - laryngeal
  -- a.　上喉頭動脈　667，681
  -- n.　上喉頭神経　571，679，681
  -- v.　上喉頭静脈　681
 - lateral brachial cutaneous n.　上外側上腕皮神経　383
 - lobar bronchi　上葉気管支　149，151
 - lobe of left lung　上葉《左肺の》　141，149，153
 - longitudinal fasciculus　上縦束　701
 - mediastinum　上縦隔　91
 - mesenteric
  -- a.　上腸間膜動脈　193，201，207，211，259，**267**，277
  -- v.　上腸間膜静脈　201，207，211，275，**277**
 - nasal concha　上鼻甲介　621
 - nuchal line　上項線　41
 - oblique　上斜筋　557，603
 - ophthalmic v.　上眼静脈　583，611，733
 - orbital fissure　上眼窩裂　601
 - part of duodenum　上部《十二指腸の》　199
 - petrosal sinus　上錐体静脈洞　733
 - pharyngeal constrictor　上咽頭収縮筋　659，661
 - puncta　上涙点　615
 - rectal
  -- a.　上直腸動脈　269，281
  -- v.　上直腸静脈　275，281
 - rectus　上直筋　557，603，609
 - right pulmonary v.　右上肺静脈　161
 - root of ansa cervicalis　上根《頸神経ワナの》　669

－sagittal sinus　上矢状静脈洞　721, 723, 725, 727, **731**
－suprarenal aa.　上副腎動脈　273
－tarsal muscle　上瞼板筋　613
－tarsus　上瞼板　613
－thoracic
－－a.　最上胸動脈　75, 391
－－aperture　胸郭上口　61
－thyroid
－－a.　上甲状腺動脈　667, 685, 691
－－v.　上甲状腺静脈　581
－tracheobronchial lymph node　上気管気管支リンパ節　163
－transverse scapular l.　上肩甲横靱帯　315
－vena cava　上大静脈　77, 93, **97**, 103, 105, 107, 113, 115, 119, 123, 135, 137
Supinator　回外筋　**341**, 343, 347, 375
Supraclavicular
－lymph node　鎖骨上リンパ節　87
－nn.　鎖骨上神経　**383**, 387, 575, 669, 689
Supraglenoid tubercle　関節上結節《肩甲骨の》　301
Supraorbital
－aa.　眼窩上動脈　609
－margin　眼窩上縁　543
－n.　眼窩上神経　559, 585, 609
Suprarenal gland　副腎　229
Suprascapular
－a.　肩甲上動脈　383, 385, 389
－n.　肩甲上神経　371, 383, 385
Supraspinatus　棘上筋　317, 325, 329, **331**, 383
Supraspinous
－fossa of scapula　棘上窩《肩甲骨の》　303
－l.　棘上靱帯　29, 31, 33
Supratrochlear n.　滑車上神経　559, 585
Sural n.　腓腹神経　511, 525
Surgical neck of humerus　外科頸《上腕骨の》　307
Suspensory(Cooper's) ll. of breast　乳房提靱帯(クーパー靱帯)　89
Sustentaculum tali　載距突起　471, 475, 479

Sympathetic
－ganglion　交感神経幹神経節　51, 79, 747
－n.　交感神経　747
－trunk　交感神経幹　101, 107, **109**, 289, 663, 687

T

T3 vertebra　第3胸椎　7
T7 vertebra　第7胸椎　7
Taeniae coli　自由ヒモ　213
Tail of pancreas　膵尾　227
Talocalcaneonavicular joint　距踵舟関節　477
Talocrural joint　距腿関節　473, 475
Talonavicular joint　距舟関節　473
Talus　距骨　475, 477, 483
Tarsal
－bones　足根骨　417
－glands　瞼板腺　613
－tunnel　足根管　523
Tarsometatarsal joints　足根中足関節　473
Tectospinal tract　視蓋脊髄路　743
Telencephalon　大脳　701
Temporal
－bone　側頭骨　541, 551, **629**, 637
－branches of facial n.　側頭枝《顔面神経の》　563, 589
－lobe　側頭葉　697, 699
Temporalis　側頭筋　593
Tendinous
－arch of levator ani　肛門挙筋腱弓　191
－intersections　腱画　181
Tendon sheath　腱鞘　493
Tensor
－fasciae latae　大腿筋膜張筋　431, 441, **445**, 537
－tympani　鼓膜張筋　629, 635
－veli palatini　口蓋帆張筋　597, 633
Tentorial notch　テント切痕　725
Tentorium cerebelli　小脳テント　725, 733
Teres
－major　大円筋　323, 327, **331**, 385
－minor　小円筋　331, 373, 385
Terminal bronchiole　終末細気管支　157
Testicular
－a.　精巣動脈　249, 259, 283

−v. 精巣静脈 249, 271, 283
Testis 精巣 249
Thalamus 視床 705, 709
Thenar
 −crease 母指球線 413
 −eminence 母指球 413
Thigh 大腿 417
Third
 −palmar interossei 第3掌側骨間筋《掌側骨間筋の》 361
 −ventricle 第三脳室 709, 729
Thoracic
 −aorta 胸大動脈 47, **95**, 109, 141
 −aortic plexus 胸大動脈神経叢 135
 −duct 胸管 99, 163, 687
 −ganglion 胸神経節 107
 −part of esophagus 胸部《食道の》 91, 101, 105
 −vertebrae 胸椎 3, 19
Thoracoacromial a. 胸肩峰動脈 387, 389
Thoracodorsal
 −a. 胸背動脈 365, 391
 −n. 胸背神経 391
Thoracolumbar fascia 胸腰筋膜 39, 43, 55
Thymus 胸腺 103
Thyroarytenoid 甲状披裂筋 681
Thyrocervical trunk 甲状頸動脈 389, **667**, 685, 687
Thyrohyoid 甲状舌骨筋 665, 679
 −l. 甲状舌骨靱帯 677
 −membrane 甲状舌骨膜 675
Thyroid
 −cartilage 甲状軟骨 155, 665, **671**, 675, 693
 −gland 甲状腺 671, 673
Tibia 脛骨 417, **447**, 459, 475, 537
Tibial
 −n. 脛骨神経 499, **509**, 521, 523, 535
 −plateau 上関節面《脛骨の》 447, 449
 −tuberosity 脛骨粗面 447, 449
Tibialis
 −anterior 前脛骨筋 **459**, 461, 507, 527, 535, 537
 −−tendon 前脛骨筋の腱 529
 −posterior 後脛骨筋 **467**, 521, 523, 535
 −−tendon 後脛骨筋の腱 465, 491

Tibiofibular joint 脛腓関節 447, 457
Tongue 舌 643
Torus tubarius 耳管隆起 651
Trabeculae carneae of interventricular septum 肉柱《心室中隔の》 125
Trachea 気管 103, 105, 139, **155**, 671, 673
Tracheal
 −bifurcation 気管分岐部 155
 −cartilages 気管軟骨 155
Tracheobronchial lymph node 気管気管支リンパ節 163
Tragus 耳珠 631
Transversalis fascia 横筋筋膜 185
Transverse
 −cervical
 −−a. 頸横動脈 687
 −−n. 頸横神経 575, 669, 689
 −colon 横行結腸 195
 −facial a. 顔面横動脈 585
 −foramen 横突孔 15, 17
 −head of adductor
 −−hallucis 横頭《母趾内転筋の》 491
 −−pollicis 横頭《母指内転筋の》 357, 361
 −mesocolon 横行結腸間膜 193, 197, 199
 −part of trapezius 横行部（水平部）《僧帽筋の》 39, 327
 −pericardial sinus 心膜横洞 113
 −process 横突起 **5**, 9, 17, 21, 35, 63
 −−of atlas 横突起《環椎の》 13, 41
 −sinus 横静脈洞 731, 733
Transversus
 −abdominis 腹横筋 45, 181, 185
 −thoracis 胸横筋 67
Trapezium 大菱形骨 349
Trapezius 僧帽筋 39, 41, 57, 319, **327**, 383, 573, 689, 693
Trapezoid 小菱形骨 349
Triceps brachii 上腕三頭筋 327, **331**, 345, 375, 385, 409
Trigeminal
 −ganglion 三叉神経節 607
 −n.(CN V) 三叉神経 561, 641, 713
Triquetrum 三角骨 349
Trochlea 滑車 603
 −of humerus 上腕骨滑車 305

Trochlear
- n.(CN IV)　滑車神経　557, **605**, 609, 715
- notch of ulna　滑車切痕《尺骨の》　333

Tuberosity of fifth metatarsal　第5中足骨粗面《中足骨の》　471

Tunica
- albuginea　白膜　251
-- of corpus cavernosum　陰茎海綿体白膜　245
- dartos　肉様膜　251
- vaginalis　精巣鞘膜　249, 251

Tympanic
- cavity　鼓室　633
- membrane　鼓膜　635

U

Ulna　尺骨　297, 333, 411

Ulnar
- a.　尺骨動脈　**365**, 395, 397, 401
- collateral l. of elbow joint　内側側副靱帯《肘関節の》　335, 337
- groove(for ulnar n.) of humerus　尺骨神経溝《上腕骨の》　307
- n.　尺骨神経　**381**, 393, 395, 397, 401, 405, 407, 409

Umbilical
- a.　臍動脈　143, 145, 279
- v.　臍静脈　143

Umbilicus　臍　143, 177

Uncinate
- process
-- of cervical vertebrae　鉤状突起《頚椎の》　11
-- of pancreas　鉤状突起《膵臓の》　227

Uncovertebral joint　鉤椎関節　27

Upper
- eyelid　上眼瞼　613
- limb　上肢　297
- subscapular n.　上肩甲下神経　391
- trunk(C5-C6)　上神経幹(第5・6頚神経)　369

Ureter　尿管　215, **229**, 233, 235, 253, 261

Ureteral orifice　尿管口　233

Urethra　尿道　231, **233**, 245, 253

Urinary bladder　膀胱　203, 205, 229, 231, **233**, 253

Uterine
- a.　子宮動脈　279
- cervix　子宮頚　231
- fundus　子宮底　231, 235
- tube　卵管　235, 237
- v.　子宮静脈　279
- venous plexus　子宮静脈叢　279

Uterosacral l.　直腸子宮靱帯　235

Uterovaginal plexus　子宮腟神経叢　289

Uterus　子宮　205, 235, 237

Utricle　卵形嚢　567

Uvula　口蓋垂　633, 653

V

Vagina　腟　205, 231

Vaginal
- fornix　腟円蓋　237
- venous plexus　腟静脈叢　279

Vagus n.(CN X)　迷走神経　101, 107, 109, 135, 569, **571**, 573, 647, 663, 673, 685, 713, 747

Valve
- of coronary sinus　冠状動脈弁　123
- of inferior vena cava　下大静脈弁　123
- of pulmonary trunk　肺動脈弁　121

Valved
- orifice
-- of coronary sinus　冠状静脈口　123
-- of inferior vena cava　下大静脈口　123

Vasa recta　直細動脈　267

Vasocorona　血管冠　737

Vastus
- intermedius　中間広筋　433, 435, 505
- lateralis　外側広筋　**431**, 445, 505, 533, 537
- medialis　内側広筋　431, 437, 505

Ventricle　脳室系　729

Ventrolateral thalamic nuclei　視床外側腹側核群　711

Vertebra　椎骨　9
- prominens(C7)　隆椎(第7頚椎)　5, 11

Vertebral
- arch　椎弓　9, **15**, 17, 19, 21
- a.　椎骨動脈　17, 53, **577**, 719
- body　椎体　5, 9, **19**, 37

-canal　脊柱管　37
-column　脊柱　5
-foramen　椎孔　9
-venous plexus　椎骨静脈叢　49
Vesical plexus　膀胱神経叢　291
Vesicouterine pouch　膀胱子宮窩　205
Vestibular
-bulb　前庭球　241
-fold　前庭ヒダ　677
-ganglian　前庭神経節　567
-root(CN Ⅷ)　前庭神経　567, 637
Vestibule of vagina(vaginal vestibule)　腟前庭　239
Vestibulospinal tract　前庭脊髄路　743
Visceral
-layer
--of the serous pericardium　臓側板《漿膜性心膜の》　111
--of tunica vaginalis　臓側板《精巣鞘膜の》　249, 251
-pleura　臓側胸膜　81
Vitreous body　硝子体　617

Vocal fold　声帯ヒダ　677
Vomer　鋤骨　619

W

White ramus communicans of spinal n.　白交通枝　747
Wing of sacrum　仙骨翼　23, 171

X Z

Xiphoid process of sternum　剣状突起《胸骨の》　65, 165, 179
Zygapophyseal joint　椎間関節　27
Zygomatic
-arch　頬骨弓　541, 547
-bone　頬骨　543, 601, 693
-branches of facial n.　頬骨枝《顔面神経の》　563
-n.　頬骨神経　561
Zygomaticus major　大頬骨筋　553

和文索引

- 五十音電話帳方式で配列している．項目の主要掲載ページは太字で示す．
- 派生語や関連語は — をつけて上位の用語の下にまとめている．
- 「右」は「う」，「左」は「さ」，「肩」は「けん」，「膝」は「しつ」に配列している．
- 英文中のa., aa. は artery, arteries を，l., ll. は ligament, ligaments を，n., nn. は nerve, nerves を，v., vv. は vein, veins を表す．

あ

アキレス腱（踵骨腱） Achilles' tendon 461, 463, 523
アブミ骨筋 Stapedius 635
鞍背 Dorsum sellae 549

い

胃 Stomach 193, 195, 207, **209**
— 胃底 Fundus of stomach 209
— 幽門部 Pyloric part of stomach 207
胃結腸間膜 Gastrocolic l. 197
胃十二指腸動脈 Gastroduodenal a. 265
胃脾間膜 Gastrosplenic l. 197
咽頭筋 Pharyngeal muscles 659
咽頭口 Pharyngeal orifice 633
咽頭後隙 Retropharyngeal space 673
咽頭収縮筋 Pharyngeal constrictors 659, 661
咽頭神経叢 Pharyngeal plexus 569
陰核 Clitoris 239, 241
— 陰核亀頭 Glans of clitoris 241
陰核背神経 Dorsal clitoral n. 243
陰核背動脈 Dorsal clitoral a. 243
陰茎 Penis 245, 247, 249
— 陰茎亀頭 Glans penis 247, 249
— 陰茎脚 Crus of penis 247
陰茎海綿体 Corpus cavernosum of penis 245, 247, 255
陰茎海綿体白膜 Tunica albuginea of corpus cavernosum 245
陰茎深動脈 Deep penile a. 245
陰茎背神経 Dorsal penile n. (dorsal n. of penis) 245, 257, 291
陰茎背動脈 Dorsal penile a. 245
陰囊 Scrotum 251
陰部神経 Pudendal n. 243, 291, **499**, 519

う

右胃大網動脈 Right gastro-omental a. 263
右胃動脈 Right gastric a. 263
右縁枝（鋭角縁枝） Right marginal a. 129
右下葉気管支 Right inferior lobar bronchi 155
右肝管 Right hepatic duct 223
右冠状動脈 Right coronary a. 129, 131
右結腸曲 Right colic flexure 197
右結腸動脈 Right colic a. 267
右主気管支 Right main bronchus 93, 155
右上肺静脈 Superior right pulmonary v. 161
右上葉気管支 Right superior lobar bronchus 155
右心耳 Right auricle 117
右心室 Right ventricle 115, 129, 137
右心房 Right atrium **119**, 121, 137, 141
右精巣静脈 Right testicular v. 229
右精巣動脈 Right testicular a. 229
右肺 Right lung 139, 141, 149, **151**
— 斜裂 Oblique fissure of right lung 139, 141, 151
— 水平裂 Horizontal fissure of right lung 139, 151
— 中葉 Middle lobe of right lung 149, 151
右肺静脈 Right pulmonary vv. 113, 149, 151
右肺動脈 Right pulmonary a. 107, 111, 121, 149, 151, **161**
右半月弁《大動脈弁の》 Right cusp of aortic valve 127
右辺縁静脈 Right marginal v. 129
右房室口 Right atrioventricular orifice 123
右房室弁 Right atrioventricular valve 121, 123, 127

(かがくこつ—かがくし) 777

― 後尖　Posterior cusp of right atrioventricular valve　127
― 前尖　Anterior cusp of right atrioventricular valve　121，127
― 中隔尖　Septal cusp of right atrioventricular valve　127
右腰リンパ本幹　Right lumbar trunk　285
右腕頭静脈　Right brachiocephalic v.　77
烏口肩峰靱帯　Coracoacromial l.　309，315
烏口鎖骨靱帯　Coracoclavicular l.　315
烏口突起　Coracoid process　301，313，321
烏口腕筋　Coracobrachialis　325，377
運動前野　Premotor cortex　739

え

会陰神経　Perineal nn.　243
会陰縫線　Perineal raphe　239
会陰膜（下尿生殖隔膜筋膜）　Perineal membrane　187
腋窩リンパ叢　Axillary lymphatic plexus　87
腋窩陥凹　Axillary recess　315
腋窩静脈　Axillary v.　85，389
腋窩神経　Axillary n.　369，**373**，385，391
腋窩動脈　Axillary a.　85，369，373，**389**
S状結腸　Sigmoid colon　205，213
S状結腸動脈　Sigmoid aa.　269
S状静脈洞　Sigmoid sinus　583，731，733
S状洞溝　Groove for sigmoid sinus　551
円回内筋　Pronator teres　339，341，379
― 上腕頭　Humeral head of pronator teres　379
円錐靱帯結節　Conoid tubercle　299
延髄　Medulla oblongata　697，699
延髄根　Cranial root　573
延髄錐体　Pyramid of medulla oblongata　713
遠位指節間（DIP）関節　Distal interphalangeal joint　353
遠位手根線　Distal wrist crease　413

お

オトガイ下三角　Submental triangle　683
オトガイ孔　Mental foramen　543，561，639
オトガイ神経　Mental n.　561，585
オトガイ舌筋　Genioglossus　645，651
オトガイ舌骨筋　Geniohyoid　645，657
黄色靱帯　Ligamenta flava　33，35
横隔胸膜（壁側胸膜の横隔部）　Diaphragmatic part of parietal pleura　147
横隔神経　Phrenic n.　**83**，103，107，371，669，687
― 右横隔神経　Right phrenic n.　115，135
― 左横隔神経　Left phrenic n.　109
横隔膜　Diaphragm　**69**，71，73，81，91，107
― 右脚　Right crus of diaphragm　71
― 開口部　Diaphragmatic apertures　73
― 腱中心　Central tendon of diaphragm　69
― 肋骨部　Costal part of diaphragm　69
横筋筋膜　Transversalis fascia　185
横行結腸　Transverse colon　195
横行結腸間膜　Transverse mesocolon　193，197，199
横静脈洞　Transverse sinus　731，733
横洞溝　Groove for transverse sinus　551
横突間靱帯　Intertransverse ll.　35
横突起　Transverse process　**5**，9，17，21，35，63
横突孔　Transverse foramen　15，17
横突肋骨窩　Costal facet on transverse process　19

か

下咽頭収縮筋　Inferior pharyngeal constrictor　659，661
下横隔動脈　Inferior phrenic v.　259，273
― 左下横隔動脈　Left inferior phrenic a.　259，273
下下腹神経叢（骨盤神経叢）　Inferior hypogastric plexus　289
下顎窩　Mandibular fossa　547
下顎角　Mandibular angle　639，693
下顎孔　Mandibular foramen　639
下顎後静脈　Retromandibular v.　581
下顎骨　Mandible　541，639
― 下顎枝　Ramus of mandible　639

― 関節突起　Condylar process of mandibular　639
― 筋突起　Coronoid process of mandible　591, 639
下顎神経　Mandibular division (CN V₃)　561, 575, 595, **597**, 641
下顎切痕　Mandibular notch　639
下関節突起　Inferior articular process　9
下眼窩裂　Inferior orbital fissure　599, 601
下眼静脈　Inferior ophthalmic v.　611
下気管気管支リンパ節　Inferior tracheobronchial lymph node　163
下瞼板　Inferior tarsus　613
下甲状腺静脈　Inferior thyroid v.　103, 685
下甲状腺動脈　Inferior thyroid a.　663, 679, 691
下行結腸　Descending colon　207
下行口蓋動脈　Descending palatine a.　627
下行大動脈　Descending aorta　93, 109, 141
下後鋸筋　Serratus posterior inferior　39
下後腸骨棘　Posterior inferior iliac spine　419, 425
下肢帯　Pelvic girdle　171, 417
下歯槽神経　Inferior alveolar n.　561, 593, 641
下歯槽動脈　Inferior alveolar a.　579, 593
― 顎舌骨筋枝　Mylohyoid branch of inferior alveolar a.　579
下斜筋　Inferior oblique　557
下尺側側副動脈　Inferior ulnar collateral a.　393
下小脳脚　Inferior cerebellar peduncle　715
下伸筋支帯　Inferior extensor retinaculum　493
下神経幹　Lower trunk　371
下垂体　Hypophysis　699, 705
下垂体窩《蝶形骨の》　Hypophyseal fossa (sella turcica) of sphenoid bone　551, 621
下膵十二指腸動脈　Inferior pancreaticoduodenal a.　265
下前腸骨棘　Anterior inferior iliac spine　173
下腿　Lower leg　417
下腿骨間膜　Interosseous membrane of leg　447

下大静脈　Inferior vena cava　77, 83, 105, 113, 117, 131, 161, 201, 207, 221, 225, **263**, 271, 277, 281
下大静脈口　Valved orifice of inferior vena cava　123
下大静脈弁　Valve of inferior vena cava　123
下腸間膜静脈　Inferior mesenteric v.　275, 277, 281
下腸間膜動脈　Inferior mesenteric a.　259, 269, 281
下腸間膜動脈神経節　Inferior mesenteric ganglion　287
下直筋　Inferior rectus　557
下直腸神経　Inferior rectal nn.　243, 257, 291
下直腸動脈　Inferior rectal a.　281
下直腸動脈神経叢　Inferior rectal plexus　291
下椎切痕　Inferior vertebral notch　21
下頭斜筋　Obliquus capitis inferior　41, 53
下橈尺関節　Distal radioulnar joint　353
下尿生殖隔膜筋膜(会陰膜)　Perineal membrane　187
下鼻甲介　Inferior nasal concha　615, 621
下鼻道　Inferior meatus　623
下副腎動脈　Inferior suprarenal a.　273
― 右下副腎動脈　Right inferior suprarenal a.　273
下腹神経　Hypogastric n.　291
― 左下腹神経　Left hypogastric n.　291
下腹壁静脈　Inferior epigastric v.　283
下腹壁動脈　Inferior epigastric a.　283
下葉気管支　Inferior lobar bronchi　149
下涙小管　Inferior lacrimal canaliculi　615
下涙点　Inferior puncta　615
架橋静脈　Bridging v.　723
蝸牛　Cochlea　567, 629, 637
蝸牛神経　Cochlear root (n.) (CN Ⅷ)　567
顆間窩《大腿骨の》　Intercondylar notch of femur　421, 451
顆間隆起《頸骨の》　Intercondylar eminence of tibia　451
灰白交通枝　Gray ramus communicans　289, 747
回外筋　Supinator　**341**, 343, 347, 375
回結腸動脈　Ileocolic a.　267

（がいついこつじょうみゃくそう） **779**

回旋枝《左冠状動脈の》 Circumflex a. of left coronary a. 129
回腸 Ileum 195, 199
回腸口 Ileocecal orifice 213
回腸動脈 Ileal aa. 267
海馬 Hippocampus 703
海綿静脈洞 Cavernous sinus 583, 607, 733
解剖学的嗅ぎタバコ入れ（橈骨窩） Anatomic（anatomical） snuffbox 403, 413
外果 Lateral malleolus 447, 461, 463, **475**, 481
外頸静脈 External jugular v. 387, **581**, 587, 689
外頸動脈 External carotid a. 577
外肛門括約筋 External anal sphincter 187, 203, 217
— 深部 Deep part of external anal sphincter 217
— 浅部 Superficial part of external anal sphincter 217
— 皮下部 Subcutaneous part of external anal sphincter 217
外後頭隆起 External occipital protuberance 545, 731
外子宮口 External os of uterus 237
外耳 External ear 629
外耳道 External auditory canal 629, 631
外精筋膜 External spermatic fascia 251
外側顆《大腿骨の》 Lateral condyle of femur 421, 449, 451
外側顆上稜《上腕骨の》 Lateral supracondylar ridge of humerus 307
外側弓状靱帯 Lateral arcuate l. 71
外側嗅条 Lateral olfactory stria 707
外側胸筋神経 Lateral pectoral nn. 387, 389
外側胸静脈 Lateral thoracic v. 85
外側胸動脈 Lateral thoracic a. 75, 85, 365, 391
外側頸三角部 Lateral cervical region 689
外側楔状骨 Lateral cuneiform 469
外側広筋 Vastus lateralis **431**, 445, 505, 533, 537
外側溝 Lateral sulcus 697
外側骨半規管 Lateral semicircular canal 629

外側膝状体 Lateral geniculate body 745
外側上顆《上腕骨の》 Lateral epicondyle of humerus 307
外側上顆《大腿骨の》 Lateral epicondyle of femur 453
外側上腕筋間中隔 Lateral intermuscular septum of arm 409
外側神経束 Lateral cord 369, 371, 377
外側脊髄視床路 Lateral spinothalamic tract 741
外側前腕皮神経 Lateral antebrachial cutaneous n. 377, 395
外側足根動脈 Lateral tarsal a. 529
外側足底静脈 Lateral plantar v. 531
外側足底神経 Lateral plantar n. 499, 523, 531
外側足底動脈 Lateral plantar a. 523, 531
外側側副靱帯《膝関節の》 Lateral collateral l. of knee joint 453, 457
外側側副靱帯《上橈尺関節の》 Radial collateral l. of proximal radio-ulnar joint 335, 337
外側大腿回旋動脈, 上行枝 Ascending branch of lateral circumflex femoral a. 517
外側大腿筋間中隔 Lateral intermuscular septum 533
外側大腿皮神経 Lateral femoral cutaneous n. 501, **511**, 513, 517
外側大動脈リンパ節 Lateral aortic lymph node 285
— 左外側大動脈リンパ節 Left lateral aortic lymph node 285
外側直筋 Lateral rectus 557, 603, 611
外側半月 Lateral meniscus 455, 457
外側皮質脊髄路 Lateral corticospinal tract 743
外側腓腹皮神経 Lateral sural cutaneous n. 525
外側翼突筋 Lateral pterygoid 593
外側輪状甲状筋 Lateral cricothyroid 681
外腸骨リンパ節 External iliac lymph node 285
外腸骨静脈 External iliac v. 215
外腸骨動脈 External iliac a. 215, 495
外椎骨静脈叢 External vertebral venous plexus 731

外転神経 Abducent n.(CN VI) 557, **605**, 611, 713
外尿道口 External urethral orifice 239
外腹斜筋 External oblique 57, **177**, 183, 185, 293
外腹斜筋腱膜 External oblique aponeurosis **177**, 183, 185, 513
外閉鎖筋 Obturator externus 435, 503
外肋間筋 External intercostal muscles 45, 67, 179
角膜 Cornea 617
顎下三角 Submandibular(digastric) triangle 683
顎下神経節 Submandibular ganglion 649
顎下腺 Submandibular gland 591, **655**, 657, 693
顎下腺管 Submandibular duct 657
顎静脈 Maxillary v. 583
顎舌骨筋 Mylohyoid 665
顎舌骨筋神経 Mylohyoid n. 597
顎動脈 Maxillary a. 577, 579, 595
顎二腹筋 Digastric muscle 565, **659**, 661, 665
― 後腹 Posterior belly of digastric muscle 565, 659, 661
― 前腹 Anterior belly of digastric muscle 659, 665
「肩-」 → 「けん-」の項をみよ
滑車 Trochlea 603
滑車上神経 Supratrochlear n. 559, 585
滑車神経 Trochlear n.(CN IV) 557, **605**, 609, 715
滑車切痕《尺骨の》 Trochlear notch of ulna 333
肝胃間膜 Hepatogastric l. 193, 209
肝円索 Ligamentum teres of liver 145, 219
肝鎌状間膜 Falciform l. of liver 219
肝冠状間膜 Coronary l. of liver 219
肝十二指腸間膜 Hepatoduodenal l. 201, 209
肝静脈 Hepatic vv. 225, 271
肝臓 Liver 143, 195, **219**, 221
― 左葉 Left lobe of liver 195
― 尾状葉 Caudate lobe of liver 221
― 方形葉 Quadrate lobe of liver 221
― 無漿膜野 Bare area of liver 219
〔肝〕門脈 Portal v. 221, 275, 277

冠状静脈口 Valved orifice of coronary sinus 123
冠状静脈洞 Coronary sinus 119, 131
冠状静脈弁 Valve of coronary sinus 123
冠状縫合 Coronal suture 541
貫通動脈 Perforating aa. 495, 519
― 第2貫通動脈 2nd perforating a. 519
間脳 Diencephalon 705
寛骨 Hip bone 169, 419
寛骨臼 Acetabulum 419
― 寛骨臼縁 Acetabular rim 423
関節円板《胸鎖関節の》 Articular disk of sternoclavicular joint 311
関節上腕靱帯 Glenohumeral ll. 315
関節包《肩関節の》 Joint capsule of glenohumeral joint 315
環椎(第1頚椎) Atlas(C1) **5**, 13, 29, 41
― 横突起 Transverse process of atlas 13, 41
― 外側塊 Lateral masses of atlas 13
― 後弓 Posterior arch of atlas 11, 13
― 後結節 Posterior tubercle of atlas 13
― 前弓 Anterior arch of atlas 29
― 前結節 Anterior tubercle of atlas 13
環椎後頭関節 Atlanto-occipital joint 27
眼窩 Orbit 601
眼窩下孔 Infraorbital foramen 543, 561, 641
眼窩下神経 Infraorbital n. 561, 585, **599**, 641
眼窩下動脈 Infraorbital a. 579, 585
眼窩隔膜 Orbital septum 613
眼窩上縁 Supraorbital margin 543
眼窩上神経 Supraorbital n. 559, 585, 609
― 外側枝 Lateral branches of supraorbital n. 585
― 内側枝 Medial branches of supraorbital n. 585
眼窩上動脈 Supraorbital aa. 609
眼窩板《篩骨の》 Orbital plate of ethmoid bone 601
眼角静脈 Angular v. 583, 585
眼角動脈 Angular a. 585
眼球 Eyeball 617
眼瞼 Eyelid 613
眼神経 Ophthalmic division(CN V_1) 559, 575, 605

(きょうだいどうみゃく—こうし) *781*

眼輪筋　Orbicularis oculi　553，613
— 眼瞼部　Palpebral part of orbicularis oculi　613
顔面横動脈　Transverse facial a.　585
顔面神経　Facial n.(CN VII)　563，**565**，589，635，637，647
— 下顎縁枝　Marginal mandibular branch of facial n.　563，589
— 頬筋枝　Buccal branches of facial n.　563，589
— 頬骨枝　Zygomatic branches of facial n.　563
— 頸枝　Cervical branch of facial n.　563
— 側頭枝　Temporal branches of facial n.　563，589
顔面静脈　Facial v.　**583**，585，591，655，691
顔面動脈　Facial a.　**577**，585，591，655，691

き

キーゼルバッハ部位　Kiesselbach's area　625
キヌタ骨　Incus　635
気管　Trachea　103，105，139，**155**，671，673
気管気管支リンパ節　Tracheobronchial lymph node　163
気管支樹　Bronchial tree　157，159
気管支縦隔リンパ本幹　Bronchomediastinal trunk　99
気管支肺リンパ節　Bronchopulmonary lymph node　163
気管軟骨　Tracheal cartilages　155
気管分岐部　Tracheal bifurcation　155
気管傍リンパ節　Paratracheal lymph node　163
奇静脈　Azygos v.　49，83，**97**，99，107，271
基節骨《足の》
— 第1基節骨　1st proximal phalanx of foot　471
亀頭冠　Corona of glans　247
弓状動脈　Arcuate a.　529
弓状動脈《腎臓の》　Arcuate a. of kidney　261

球海綿体筋　Bulbospongiosus　187，241，247，257
球形嚢　Saccule　567
嗅球　Olfactory bulb　555，627，699
嗅索　Olfactory tract　555，699
嗅神経糸　Olfactory fibers　555，625
距骨　Talus　475，477，483
— 距骨頭　Head of talus　469
距骨下関節　Subtalar(talocalcaneal) joint　473，475，477
距舟関節　Talonavicular joint　473
距踵舟関節　Talocalcaneonavicular joint　477
距腿関節　Talocrural joint　473，475
強膜　Sclera　617
胸横筋　Transversus thoracis　67
胸郭下口　Inferior thoracic aperture　61
胸郭上口　Superior thoracic aperture　61
胸管　Thoracic duct　99，163，687
胸筋腋窩リンパ節　Pectoral axillary lymph node　87
胸筋筋膜　Pectoral fascia　89
胸肩峰動脈　Thoracoacromial a.　387，389
胸骨　Sternum　63，65，69
— 胸骨角　Sternal angle of sternum　65，165
— 胸骨体　Body of sternum　65，139
— 剣状突起　Xiphoid process of sternum　65，165
胸骨関節面　Sternal articular surface　299
胸骨甲状筋　Sternothyroid　665，691
胸骨舌骨筋　Sternohyoid　665
胸骨柄　Manubrium sterni　65，67，311
胸鎖関節　Sternoclavicular joint　309，311
胸鎖乳突筋　Sternocleidomastoid　41，**319**，573，587，655，673，689，693
— 胸骨頭　Sternal head of sternocleidomastoid　693
— 鎖骨頭　Clavicular head of sternocleidomastoid　693
胸神経節　Thoracic ganglion　107
胸腺　Thymus　103
胸大動脈　Thoracic aorta　47，**95**，109，141
— 外側皮枝　Lateral cutaneous branch of thoracic aorta　47
— 後枝　Posterior ramus of thoracic aorta　47

― 脊髄枝　Spinal branch of thoracic aorta　47
― 前枝　Anterior ramus of thoracic aorta　47
― 内側皮枝　Medial cutaneous branch of thoracic aorta　47
胸大動脈神経叢　Thoracic aortic plexus　135
胸椎　Thoracic vertebrae　3，19
胸内筋膜　Endothoracic fascia　81，83
胸背神経　Thoracodorsal n.　391
胸背動脈　Thoracodorsal a.　365，391
胸腰筋膜　Thoracolumbar fascia　39，43，55
― 浅葉　Superficial layer of thoracolumbar fascia　39，43
胸肋関節　Sternocostal joint　311
頬筋　Buccinator　655，659
頬骨　Zygomatic bone　543，601，693
― 眼窩面　Orbital surface of zygomatic bone　601
頬骨弓　Zygomatic arch　541，547
頬骨神経　Zygomatic n.　561
頬神経　Buccal n.　561，593，641
頬動脈　Buccal a.　579，593
橋　Pons　699，713
棘下筋　Infraspinatus　329，331，385
棘間靱帯　Interspinous ll.　33
棘筋　Spinalis　43，45
棘上窩《肩甲骨の》　Supraspinous fossa of scapula　303
棘上筋　Supraspinatus　317，325，329，**331**，383
棘上靱帯　Supraspinous l.　29，31，33
棘突起　Spinous process　5，7，9，**11**，17，19，21，41
近位指節間(PIP)関節　Proximal interphalangeal joint　353
近位指節間関節線　Proximal interphalangeal(PIP) joint crease　413
筋横隔動脈　Musculophrenic a.　75
筋三角　Muscular triangle　683
筋皮神経　Musculocutaneous n.　377，395

く

クーパー靱帯（乳房提靱帯）　Cooper's (suspensory) ll. of breast　89

クモ膜下腔　Subarachnoid space　31，719
クモ膜顆粒　Arachnoid granulations　721，727
クモ膜絨毛　Arachnoid villi　721
区域気管支　Segmental bronchus　157
空腸動脈　Jejunal aa.　267
屈筋支帯《足の》　Flexor retinaculum of foot　523
屈筋支帯《手の》　Flexor retinaculum of hand　355，**357**，397，399

け

茎状突起《尺骨の》　Styloid process of ulna　349，413
茎状突起《側頭骨の》　Styloid process of temporal bone　629
茎状突起《橈骨の》　Styloid process of radius　333，351
茎突咽頭筋　Stylopharyngeus　569，661
茎突舌筋　Styloglossus　645
茎突舌骨筋　Stylohyoid　565，659，661
茎乳突孔　Stylomastoid foramen　565
脛骨　Tibia　417，**447**，459，475，537
― 顆間隆起　Intercondylar eminence of tibia　451
― 脛骨粗面　Tibial tuberosity　447，449
― 上関節面　Tibial plateau　447，449
― 内果　Medial malleolus of tibia　447，459
― 内側顆　Medial condyle of tibia　447，449，451
脛骨神経　Tibial n.　499，**509**，521，523，535
脛腓関節　Tibiofibular joint　447，457
頸横神経　Transverse cervical n.　575，669，689
頸横動脈　Transverse cervical a.　687
頸筋膜　Cervical fascia　673
― 気管前葉　Pretracheal layer of cervical fascia　673
― 浅葉　Investing layer of cervical fascia　673
頸静脈孔　Jugular foramen　547，573，733
頸神経
― 第5頸神経　C5 spinal n.　369
― 第6頸神経　C6 spinal n.　369
― 第7頸神経　C7 spinal n.　369

頸神経叢　Cervical plexus　589
頸神経ワナ　Ansa cervicalis　669，691
— 上根　Superior root of ansa cervicalis　669
— 下根　Inferior root of ansa cervicalis　669
頸切痕　Jugular notch　61，**65**，165，693
頸椎　Cervical vertebrae　3，11
頸動脈管　Carotid canal　547
頸動脈三角　Carotid triangle　683
頸動脈洞　Carotid sinus　569
頸板状筋　Splenius cervicis　43
頸膨大　Cervical enlargement　717
鶏冠　Crista galli　621
血管冠　Vasocorona　737
結節間滑液鞘　Intertubercular synovial sheath　315
結節間溝《上腕骨の》　Intertubercular groove of humerus　305，313
結腸辺縁動脈　Marginal a.　267
結腸傍溝　Paracolic gutter　201
結腸膨起　Haustra of colon　213
結膜　Conjunctiva　613
楔状束　Fasciculus cuneatus　741
月状骨　Lunate　351
肩関節　Shoulder joint　309，313，315
肩甲下窩　Subscapular fossa　301
肩甲下筋　Subscapularis　321，323，325
肩甲下動脈　Subscapular a.　391
肩甲回旋動脈　Circumflex scapular a.　385，391
肩甲挙筋　Levator scapulae　39，329
肩甲胸郭関節　Scapulothoracic joint　309
肩甲棘　Scapular spine　7，39，303，383
肩甲骨　Scapula　301，303，329
— 下角　Inferior angle of scapula(inferior scapular angle)　7，303
— 関節下結節　Infraglenoid tubercle　301
— 関節窩　Glenoid cavity of scapula　301，313，317
— 関節上結節　Supraglenoid tubercle　301
— 棘下窩　Infraspinous fossa of scapula　303
— 棘上窩　Supraspinous fossa of scapula　303
— 上角　Superior angle of scapula　301
— 内側縁　Medial border of scapula　303，329
肩甲鎖骨三角　Omoclavicular triangle　683
肩甲上神経　Suprascapular n.　371，383，385
肩甲上動脈　Suprascapular a.　383，385，389
肩甲上腕関節　Glenohumeral joint　309，313
肩甲切痕　Scapular notch　303
肩甲舌骨筋　Omohyoid　665
— 上腹　Superior belly of omohyoid　665
— 下腹　Inferior belly of omohyoid　665
肩鎖関節　Acromioclavicular joint　309
肩鎖靱帯　Acromioclavicular l.　309，315
肩峰　Acromion　301，**303**，313，317
肩峰下包　Subacromial bursa　317
肩峰関節面　Acromial articular surface　299
剣状突起《胸骨の》　Xiphoid process of sternum　165，179
腱画　Tendinous intersections　181
腱索　Chordae tendineae　125
腱鞘　Tendon sheath　493
腱中心《横隔膜の》　Central tendon of diaphragm　69
腱裂孔　→[内転筋]腱裂孔　Adductor hiatus　435，497
瞼板腺　Tarsal glands　613

こ

呼吸細気管支　Respiratory bronchiole　157，159
固有肝動脈　Proper hepatic a.　221，265
固有掌側指神経　Proper palmar digital nn.　381，399
固有掌側指動脈　Proper palmar digital aa.　399
固有底側趾神経　Proper plantar digital nn.　531
固有底側趾動脈　Proper plantar digital aa.　531
固有背筋　Intrinsic muscles of the back　43，45
固有卵巣索　Proper ovarian l.　235
股関節　Hip joint　423，425
鼓索神経　Chorda tympani　565，635

鼓室　Tympanic cavity　633
鼓膜　Tympanic membrane　635
鼓膜張筋　Tensor tympani　629, 635
口蓋咽頭弓　Palatopharyngeal arch　643, 653
口蓋咽頭筋　Palatopharyngeus　663
口蓋骨　Palatine bone　547, 619, 623
— 水平板　Horizontal plate of palatine bone　619
— 垂直板　Perpendicular plate of palatine bone　623
口蓋垂　Uvula　633, 653
口蓋舌弓　Palatoglossal arch　643, 653
口蓋舌筋　Palatoglossus　645
口蓋突起《上顎骨の》　Palatine process of maxilla　547
口蓋帆（軟口蓋）　Soft palate　651, 653
口蓋帆挙筋　Levator veli palatini　633
口蓋帆張筋　Tensor veli palatini　597, 633
口蓋帆張筋神経　N. of tensor veli palatini　597
口蓋扁桃　Palatine tonsil　643
口角下制筋　Depressor anguli oris　553
口輪筋　Orbicularis oris　553
広背筋　Latissimus dorsi　39, 57, 323, **327**, 393
甲状頸動脈　Thyrocervical trunk　389, **667**, 685, 687
甲状舌骨筋　Thyrohyoid　665, 679
甲状舌骨靱帯　Thyrohyoid l.　677
甲状舌骨膜　Thyrohyoid membrane　675
甲状腺　Thyroid gland　671, 673
— 右葉　Right lobe of thyroid gland　671
— 甲状腺峡部　Isthmus of thyroid gland　671
— 錐体葉　Pyramidal lobe of thyroid gland　671
甲状軟骨　Thyroid cartilage　155, 665, **671**, 675, 693
甲状披裂筋　Thyroarytenoid　681
交感神経　Sympathetic n.　747
交感神経幹　Sympathetic trunk　101, 107, **109**, 289, 663, 687
交感神経幹神経節　Sympathetic ganglion　51, 79, 747
肛門管　Anal canal　217
肛門挙筋　Levator ani　187, 189, 205, **215**, 241

肛門挙筋腱弓　Tendinous arch of levator ani　191
肛門櫛（白帯）　Anal pecten (white zone)　217
肛門柱　Anal columns　217
肛門尾骨縫線　Anococcygeal raphe　189
岬角《仙骨の》　Promontory of sacrum　3, **23**, 171, 175, 437
虹彩　Iris　617
咬筋　Masseter　**553**, 587, 595, 655
後陰唇交連　Posterior labial commissure　239
後陰唇神経　Posterior labial nn.　243
後陰嚢神経　Posterior scrotal nn.　257
後下行枝　Posterior descending (interventricular) a.　131
後角《脊髄の》　Posterior horn of spinal cord　737
後距腓靱帯　Posterior talofibular l.　483
後脛骨筋　Tibialis posterior　**467**, 521, 523, 535
後脛骨筋の腱　Tibialis posterior tendon　465, 491
後脛骨静脈　Posterior tibial v.　535
後脛骨動脈　Posterior tibial a.　**497**, 521, 523, 535
後脛腓靱帯　Posterior tibiofibular l.　483
後結節間束　Posterior internodal bundles　133
後交通動脈　Posterior communicating a.　735
後骨間動脈　Posterior interosseous a.　365
後根《脊髄神経の》　Posterior (dorsal) root of spinal n.　79, 719
後篩骨神経　Posterior ethmoidal n.　559, 609
後篩骨洞　Posterior ethmoid sinus　623
後耳介神経　Posterior auricular n.　563, 565
後耳介動脈　Posterior auricular a.　577
後室間枝（後下行枝）　Posterior interventricular (descending) a.　131
後室間静脈（中心臓静脈）　Posterior interventricular v.　131
後十字靱帯　Posterior cruciate l.　455, 457
後縦隔　Posterior mediastinum　91
後縦靱帯　Posterior longitudinal l.　31, 33, 35, **37**

後上歯槽動脈　Posterior superior alveolar aa.　579
後上腕回旋動脈　Posterior circumflex humeral a.　365，385
後神経束　Posterior cord　371，373
後髄節動脈　Posterior segmental medullary a.　737
後脊髄小脳路　Posterior spinocerebellar tract　741
後脊髄動脈　Posterior spinal aa.　737
後仙腸靱帯　Posterior sacroiliac ll.　429
後［前腕］骨間神経　Posterior interosseous n.　375
後前腕皮神経　Posterior antebrachial cutaneous n.　375
後大腿皮神経　Posterior femoral cutaneous n.　499，511，519
後大脳動脈　Posterior cerebral a.　735
後頭下神経　Suboccipital n.　53
後頭顆　Occipital condyle　547
後頭蓋窩　Posterior cranial fossa　549
後頭骨　Occipital bone　545
後頭三角　Occipital triangle　683
後頭前頭筋　Occipitofrontalis　553
後頭頂野　Posterior parietal cortex　739
後頭動脈　Occipital a.　53，577
後頭葉　Occipital lobe　697
後内椎骨静脈叢　Posterior internal vertebral venous plexus　49，719
後乳頭筋　Posterior papillary muscle　125
後半月弁《大動脈弁の》　Posterior cusp of aortic valve　127
後鼻孔　Choana　619
後輪状披裂筋　Posterior cricoarytenoid　663，681
鉤状突起《頸椎の》　Uncinate process of cervical vertebrae　11
鉤状突起《尺骨の》　Coronoid process of ulna　333
鉤椎関節　Uncovertebral joint　27
鉤突窩《上腕骨の》　Coronoid fossa of humerus　337
喉頭蓋　Epiglottis　643，651，675，**677**，681
喉頭隆起　Laryngeal prominence of thyroid cartilage　675
硬口蓋　Hard palate　653
硬膜　Dura mater　721，723

硬膜静脈洞　Dural Sinus　733
項靱帯　Nuchal l.　29，31
溝動脈　Sulcal a.　737
黒質　Substantia nigra　711
骨間距踵靱帯　Interosseous talocalcanean l.　477
骨間筋　Interossei　381
骨盤底　Pelvic floor　187，189，191
骨盤内臓神経　Pelvic splanchnic nn.　291

さ

左胃静脈　Left gastric v.　275，277
左胃大網静脈　Left gastro-omental v.　275，277
左胃大網動脈　Left gastro-omental a.　277
左胃動脈　Left gastric a.　263，277
左下葉気管支　Left inferior lobar bronchi　155
左冠状動脈　Left coronary a.　129
— 回旋枝　Circumflex a. of left coronary a.　129
— 前室間枝（前下行枝）　Anterior interventricular(left anterior descending) branch of left coronary a.　129
左気管支縦隔リンパ本幹　Left bronchomediastinal trunk　163
左結腸曲　Left colic flexure　213
左結腸動脈　Left colic a.　269
左鎖骨下動脈　Left subclavian a.　667
左主気管支　Left main bronchus　93，95，109，**155**
左心耳　Left auricle　117
左心室　Left ventricle　105，115，**119**，137
左心房　Left atrium　111，**119**，125，137，141，145
左肺　Left lung　141，149，153
— 下葉　Inferior lobe of left lung　141，153
— 斜裂　Oblique fissure of left lung　153
— 上葉　Superior lobe of left lung　141，149，153
左肺静脈　Left pulmonary vv.　105，119
左肺動脈　Left pulmonary a.　109，119
左半月弁《大動脈弁の》　Left cusp of aortic valve　127
左副腎静脈　Left suprarenal v.　229，273

左房室弁　Left atrioventricular valve　125
左・右の横隔膜脚円蓋　Left and right diaphragm leaflets　139
左腰リンパ本幹　Left lumbar trunk　99
左卵巣動脈　Left ovarian a.　259
左腕頭静脈　Left brachiocephalic v.　99, 115, 149, **581**
鎖骨　Clavicle　165, **299**, 311, 313
— 肩峰端　Acromial end of clavicle　299
— 鎖骨体　Shaft of clavicle　299
— 内側頭　Medial head of clavicle　165
鎖骨下筋　Subclavius　321
鎖骨下筋溝　Groove for subclavius muscle　299
鎖骨下静脈　Subclavian v.　85, 163, **389**, 687
— 右鎖骨下静脈　Right subclavian v.　163
— 左鎖骨下静脈　Left subclavian v.　105
鎖骨下動脈　Subclavian a.　75, 85, 95, **371**, 389, 571, 685, 687
— 左鎖骨下動脈　Left subclavian a.　95, 101, 105
鎖骨胸筋筋膜　Clavipectoral fascia　387
鎖骨上リンパ節　Supraclavicular lymph node　87
鎖骨上神経　Supraclavicular nn.　**383**, 387, 575, 669, 689
鎖骨切痕　Clavicular notch　61, 65
鎖骨中線　Midclavicular line (MCL)　165
坐骨　Ischium　169, 419
— 坐骨枝　Ischial ramus　169
— 大坐骨切痕　Greater sciatic notch　419
坐骨海綿体筋　Ischiocavernosus　187, 241, 247
坐骨棘　Ischial spine　**169**, 171, 175, 189, 191, 419, 425
坐骨結節　Ischial tuberosity　169, 419, **425**, 441
坐骨肛門窩（坐骨直腸窩）　Ischioanal fossa　215
坐骨神経　Sciatic n.　**499**, 501, 507, 519, 533
坐骨大腿靱帯　Ischiofemoral l.　429
坐骨直腸窩（坐骨肛門窩）　Ischioanal fossa　215
細気管支　Bronchiole　157
最上胸動脈　Superior thoracic a.　75, 391

最長筋　Longissimus　43
最内肋間筋　Innermost intercostals　67
載距突起　Sustentaculum tali　471, 475, 479
臍　Umbilicus　143, 177
臍静脈　Umbilical v.　143
臍動脈　Umbilical a.　143, 145, 279
三角筋　Deltoid　317, **319**, 325, 327, 373, 387
三角筋下包　Subdeltoid bursa　317
三角筋粗面《上腕骨の》　Deltoid tuberosity of humerus　305
三角骨　Triquetrum　349
三角靱帯　Deltoid l.　483
三叉神経　Trigeminal n. (CN V)　561, 641, 713
三叉神経節　Trigeminal ganglion　607

し

子宮　Uterus　205, 235, 237
— 子宮底　Uterine fundus　235
子宮間膜　Mesometrium　235
子宮筋層　Myometrium　237
子宮頸　Uterine cervix　231
子宮頸管　Cervical canal　237
子宮静脈　Uterine v.　279
子宮静脈叢　Uterine venous plexus　279
子宮腟神経叢　Uterovaginal plexus　289
子宮底　Uterine fundus　231
子宮動脈　Uterine a.　279
四丘体板　Quadrigeminal plate　705, 715
— 上丘　Superior colliculus of quadrigeminal plate　715
— 下丘　Inferior colliculus of quadrigeminal plate　715
矢状縫合　Sagittal suture　545
指（節）骨　Phalanges　297
指背腱膜　Dorsal digital expansion　345
脂肪被膜　Perirenal fat capsule　229
視蓋脊髄路　Tectospinal tract　743
視交叉　Optic chiasm　559, 607, 707, **745**
視索　Optic tract　709, 745
視床　Thalamus　705, 709
視床下核　Subthalamic nucleus　711
視床下部　Hypothalamus　705

（しゅうじょうか） *787*

視床外側腹側核群　Ventrolateral thalamic nuclei　711
視床室傍核群　Paraventricular nuclei of thalamus　711
視床髄条　Stria medullaris thalami　705
視床前核群　Anterior thalamic nuclei　711
視床内側核群　Medial thalamic nuclei　711
視神経　Optic n.(CN II)　559，**605**，607，611，617，699，745
視神経円板(視神経乳頭)　Optic disk　617
視神経管　Optic canal　551，601
視神経乳頭(視神経円板)　Optic disk　617
視放線　Optic radiation　701，745
歯状回　Dentate gyrus　703
歯突起《第 2 頸椎の》　Dens of axis(C2)　15，29，651
篩骨　Ethmoid bone　543，601，619
― 眼窩板　Orbital plate of ethmoid bone　601
― 垂直板　Perpendicular plate of ethmoid bone　543，601，619
篩骨胞　Ethmoid bulla　623
篩板　Cribriform plate　551，555，623
示指伸筋　Extensor indicis　347
示指伸筋の腱　Extensor indicis tendon　363
耳下腺　Parotid gland　655
耳下腺管　Parotid duct　585，587，655
耳下腺神経叢　Parotid plexus　589
耳介　Auricle　631
耳介側頭神経　Auriculotemporal n.　561，587，**597**，641
耳管　Pharyngotympanic(auditory) tube　629，633，651
― 耳管咽頭口　Pharyngeal orifice of pharyngotympanic tube　651
― 軟骨部　Cartilaginous part of pharyngotympanic tube　633
耳管咽頭筋　Salpingopharyngeus　633
耳管隆起　Torus tubarius　651
耳甲介　Concha　631
耳甲介舟　Cymba conchae　631
耳珠　Tragus　631
耳小骨連鎖　Ossicular chain　635
耳神経節　Otic ganglion　597
耳垂　Earlobe　631
耳輪　Helix　631
自由ヒモ　Taeniae coli　213

軸椎(第 2 頸椎)　Axis(C2)　5，11，15，41
室間孔　Interventricular foramen　729
膝窩　Popliteal fossa　439
膝窩筋　Popliteus　465，467
膝窩静脈　Popliteal v.　519，521
膝窩動脈　Popliteal a.　495，**497**，519，521
膝蓋骨　Patella　417，449，455
膝蓋靱帯　Patellar l.　433，453，457
膝蓋大腿関節　Femoropatellar joint　453
膝関節　Knee joint　449，451
膝神経節　Geniculate ganglion　565，637
櫛状筋　Pectinate muscles　123
射精管　Ejaculatory duct　255
斜角筋隙　Interscalene space　691
斜台　Clivus　551
尺骨　Ulna　297，333，411
― 滑車切痕　Trochlear notch of ulna　333
― 茎状突起　Styloid process of ulna　349，413
― 鈎状突起　Coronoid process of ulna　333
尺骨神経　Ulnar n.　**381**，393，395，397，401，405，407，409
― 掌枝　Palmar branch of ulnar n.　405
― 深枝　Deep branch of ulnar n.　381
― 浅枝　Superficial branch of ulnar n.　399
― 背側枝　Dorsal branch of ulnar n.　407
尺骨神経溝《上腕骨の》　Ulnar groove(for ulnar nerve) of humerus　307
尺骨動脈　Ulnar a.　**365**，395，397，401
尺側手根屈筋　Flexor carpi ulnaris　339，**345**，355，381，411
尺側手根伸筋　Extensor carpi ulnaris　345，363
尺側皮静脈　Basilic v.　367
手根管　Carpal tunnel　397
手根骨　Carpal bones　297
手根中央関節　Midcarpal joint　353
手掌腱膜　Palmar aponeurosis　355
手背静脈網　Dorsal venous network of hand　367
種子骨　Sesamoids　471，475
終末細気管支　Terminal bronchiole　157
舟状窩　Scaphoid fossa　631

舟状骨《足の》 Navicular **469**, 471, 475, 477, 479
舟状骨《手の》 Scaphoid **349**, 353, 397, 403
十二指腸 Duodenum 199, 201, 209, **211**, 269
— 下行部 Descending part of duodenum 211
— 上部 Superior part of duodenum 199
— 水平部 Horizontal part of duodenum 201, 211
十二指腸空腸曲 Duodenojejunal flexure 199
縦隔 Mediastinum 91, 103
縦隔胸膜(壁側胸膜の縦隔部) Mediastinal part of parietal pleura 103, 147
女性骨盤 Female pelvis 171
鋤骨 Vomer 619
小陰唇 Labia minora 239
小円筋 Teres minor 331, 373, 385
小胸筋 Pectoralis minor 321, 389
小結節《上腕骨の》 Lesser tuberosity of humerus 305, 313
小口蓋神経 Lesser palatine n. 627
小後頭神経 Lesser occipital n. 575, 669, 689
小坐骨孔 Lesser sciatic foramen 175, 515
小指外転筋 Abductor digiti minimi 357
小指球 Hypothenar eminence 413
小指対立筋 Opponens digiti minimi 361
小趾外転筋 Abductor digiti minimi 487
小十二指腸乳頭 Minor duodenal papilla 211
小心臓静脈 Small cardiac v. 131
小錐体神経 Lesser petrosal n. 597, 637
小転子 Lesser trochanter 421, 423
小殿筋 Gluteus minimus 441, 519
小脳 Cerebellum 697, 699
小脳テント Tentorium cerebelli 725, 733
小脳延髄槽 Cerebellomedullary cistern 727
小伏在静脈 Short saphenous v. 511
小菱形筋 Rhomboid minor 329
小菱形骨 Trapezoid 349
小弯 Lesser curvature of stomach 209
松果体 Pineal gland 705

掌側骨間筋
— 第2掌側骨間筋 2nd palmar interossei 361
— 第3掌側骨間筋 3rd palmar interossei 361
掌側指神経 Palmar digital nn. 405
— 背側枝 Dorsal branches of palmar digital nn. 407
掌側手根靱帯 Palmar carpal l. 397, 399
掌側中手動脈 Palmar metacarpal aa. 401
硝子体 Vitreous body 617
漿膜性心膜 Serous pericardium 111
— 臓側板 Visceral layer of the serous pericardium 111
— 壁側板 Parietal layer of the serous pericardium 111
踵骨 Calcaneus 463, 471, 477
踵骨腱(アキレス腱) Achilles' tendon 461, 463, 523
踵骨隆起 Calcaneal tuberosity 485
踵腓靱帯 Calcaneofibular l. 483
上咽頭収縮筋 Superior pharyngeal constrictor 659, 661
上腋窩リンパ節 Apical axillary lymph node 87
上下腹神経叢 Superior hypogastric plexus 287, 291
上外側上腕皮神経 Superior lateral brachial cutaneous n. 383
上顎骨 Maxilla **541**, 543, 547, 619, 621
— 口蓋突起 Palatine process of maxilla 619
— 前頭突起 Frontal process of maxilla 621
上顎神経 Maxillary division (n.) (CN V_2) 561, 575, 599, 641
上顎洞 Maxillary sinus 601
上顎洞裂孔 Maxillary hiatus 623
上関節突起 Superior articular process 9, 21
上関節面《脛骨の》 Tibial plateau 447
上眼窩裂 Superior orbital fissure 601
上眼瞼 Upper eyelid 613
上眼瞼挙筋 Levator palpebrae superioris 557, **603**, 609, 613
上眼静脈 Superior ophthalmic v. 583, 611, 733

上気管気管支リンパ節　Superior tracheobronchial lymph node　163
上頸神経節　Superior cervical ganglion　591, 691
上肩甲横靱帯　Superior transverse scapular l.　315
上肩甲下神経　Upper subscapular n.　391
上瞼板　Superior tarsus　613
上瞼板筋　Superior tarsal muscle　613
上甲状腺静脈　Superior thyroid v.　581
上甲状腺動脈　Superior thyroid a.　667, 685, 691
上行咽頭動脈　Ascending pharyngeal a.　667
上行結腸　Ascending colon　195, 201, 213
上行大動脈　Ascending aorta　93, **95**, 111, 113, 117, 137, 161
上行腰静脈　Ascending lumbar v.　271
上後腸骨棘　Posterior superior iliac spine　425, 429, 515
上喉頭静脈　Superior laryngeal v.　681
上喉頭神経　Superior laryngeal n.　571, 679, 681
― 外枝　External branch of superior laryngeal n.　571, 679
― 内枝　Internal branch of superior laryngeal n.　679, 681
上喉頭動脈　Superior laryngeal a.　667, 681
上項線　Superior nuchal line　41
上矢状静脈洞　Superior sagittal sinus　721, 723, 725, 727, **731**
上肢　Upper limb　297
上肢帯　Shoulder girdle　297, 309
上歯槽神経　Superior alveolar nn.　561, 599
― 後上歯槽枝　Posterior superior alveolar branches of superior alveolar nn.　561, 599
上斜筋　Superior oblique　557, 603
上縦隔　Superior mediastinum　91
上縦束　Superior longitudinal fasciculus　701
上小脳脚　Superior cerebellar peduncle　715
上小脳動脈　Superior cerebellar a.　735

上伸筋支帯　Superior extensor retinaculum　493
上神経幹(第5・6頸神経)　Upper trunk (C5-C6)　369
上唇小帯　Frenulum of upper lip　653
上錐体静脈洞　Superior petrosal sinus　733
上前区動脈《腎臓の》　Anterior superior segmental a. of kidney　261
上前腸骨棘　Anterior superior iliac spine　**169**, 179, 293, 419, 423, 445, 515
上大静脈　Superior vena cava　77, 93, **97**, 103, 105, 107, 113, 115, 119, 123, 135, 137
上腸間膜静脈　Superior mesenteric v.　201, 207, 211, 275, **277**
上腸間膜動脈　Superior mesenteric a.　193, 201, 207, 211, 259, **267**, 277
上直筋　Superior rectus　557, 603, 609
上直腸静脈　Superior rectal v.　275, 281
上直腸動脈　Superior rectal a.　269, 281
上殿静脈　Superior gluteal v.　519
上殿神経　Superior gluteal n.　519
上殿動脈　Superior gluteal a.　519
上殿皮神経　Superior cluneal nn.　55
上頭斜筋　Obliquus capitis superior　41
上橈尺関節　Proximal radioulnar joint　333
上鼻甲介　Superior nasal concha　621
上副腎動脈　Superior suprarenal aa.　273
― 右上副腎動脈　Right superior suprarenal a.　273
上葉気管支　Superior lobar bronchi　149, 151
上涙小管　Superior lacrimal canaliculi　615
上涙点　Superior puncta　615
上肋骨窩　Superior costal facet　19
上腕　Arm　297
上腕筋　Brachialis　**325**, 341, 377, 409
上腕骨　Humerus　297, 305, 307
― 解剖頸　Anatomical neck of humerus　305
― 外側顆上稜　Lateral supracondylar ridge of humerus　307
― 外側上顆　Lateral epicondyle of humerus　307
― 外科頸　Surgical neck of humerus　307
― 結節間溝　Intertubercular groove of humerus　305, 313

— 鈎突窩 Coronoid fossa of humerus 337
— 三角筋粗面 Deltoid tuberosity of humerus 305
— 尺骨神経溝 Ulnar groove (for ulnar n.) of humerus 307
— 小結節 Lesser tuberosity of humerus 305, 313
— 上腕骨小頭 Capitellum of humerus 305, 337
— 上腕骨頭 Head of humerus 307
— 大結節 Greater tuberosity of humerus 307, 313
— 肘頭窩 Olecranon fossa of humerus 307
— 内側上顆 Medial epicondyle of humerus 305, **335**, 337, 339
上腕骨滑車 Trochlea of humerus 305
上腕三頭筋 Triceps brachii 327, **331**, 345, 375, 385, 409
— 外側頭 Lateral head of triceps brachii 331, 385
— 長頭 Long head of triceps brachii 327, 331
— 内側頭 Medial head of triceps brachii 331, 409
上腕静脈 Brachial v. 409
上腕深動脈 Profunda brachii a. 365, 385
上腕動脈 Brachial a. 365, 391, **393**, 395, 409
上腕二頭筋 Biceps brachii 319, **323**, 325, 339, 377, 393, 409
— 短頭 Short head of biceps brachii 323
— 長頭 Long head of biceps brachii 323
上腕二頭筋腱膜 Bicipital aponeurosis 323
静脈管索 Ligamentum venosum 145
静脈洞交会 Confluence of sinuses 725, 727, 731
食道 Esophagus 83, 91, 95, 101, **105**, 107, 141, 209, 661, 679
— 胸部 Thoracic part of esophagus 91, 101, 105
食道神経叢 Esophageal plexus 101
食道静脈 Esophageal v. 275
食道裂孔 Esophageal aperture of diaphragm 69, 71
心圧痕 Cardiac impression 153

心室中隔 Interventricular septum 125, 133, 141
— 肉柱 Trabeculae carneae of interventricular septum 125
心尖 Cardiac apex 115, 139
心臓刺激伝導系 Cardiac conduction system 133
心臓神経叢 Cardiac plexus 135
心房間束 Interatrial bundle 133
心房中隔 Interatrial septum 123, 125
心膜 Pericardium 83, 113
心膜横隔静脈 Pericardiacophrenic v. 83, 103, 107
心膜横隔動脈 Pericardiacophrenic a. 83, 103, 107
心膜横洞 Transverse pericardial sinus 113
心膜腔 Pericardial cavity 111
心膜斜洞 Oblique pericardial sinus 113
伸筋支帯《手の》 Extensor retinaculum of hand 363
深陰茎背静脈 Deep dorsal penile v. 245
深会陰横筋 Deep transverse perineal 191, 241
深横中手靱帯 Deep transverse metacarpal l. 357
深頸動脈 Deep cervical a. 53
深指屈筋 Flexor digitorum profundus **343**, 359, 379, 381, 411
深指屈筋の腱 Flexor digitorum profundus tendons 341, 361, 397
深掌動脈弓 Deep palmar arch 401
深錐体神経 Deep petrosal n. 599
深鼠径リンパ節 Deep inguinal lymph node 285
深足底動脈弓 Deep plantar arch 531
深側頭静脈 Deep temporal vv. 581
深側頭神経 Deep temporal nn. 593
深側頭動脈 Deep temporal aa. 579, 593
深腓骨神経 Deep fibular n. **511**, 525, 527, 529, 535
— 皮枝 Cutaneous branch of deep fibular n. 529
人中 Philtrum 693
腎静脈 Renal v. 267, 271, 273
— 左腎静脈 Left renal v. 267, 273
腎錐体 Medullary pyramid 261
腎臓 Kidney 207, 229
腎動脈 Renal a. 259, 261, 273

(ぜつへんとう) *791*

— 右腎動脈　Right renal a.　207
— 左腎動脈　Left renal a.　259, 261, 273

す

水晶体　Lens　617
膵管　Pancreatic duct　223, 227
膵十二指腸動脈　Pancreaticoduodenal a.　265
膵臓　Pancreas　193, 197, 201, 207, 211, **227**, 263
— 鉤状突起　Uncinate process of pancreas　227
— 膵体　Body of pancreas　227
— 膵頭　Head of pancreas　227
— 膵尾　Tail of pancreas　227
錐体筋　Pyramidalis　181
錐体上縁　Petrous ridge　549
髄核　Nucleus pulposus of intervertebral disk　33
髄膜　Meninges　721

せ

正中弓状靱帯　Median arcuate l.　71
正中臍ヒダ　Median umbilical fold　195
正中神経　Median n.　369, **379**, 393, 395, 397, 399, 405, 407, 409, 411
— 掌枝　Palmar branch of median n.　405
正中仙骨動脈　Median sacral a.　259
正中仙骨稜　Median sacral crest　25
声帯ヒダ　Vocal fold　677
星状神経節　Stellate ganglion　663, 687
精管　Ductus deferens　229, 253, 283
精索　Spermatic cord　183, 185
精巣　Testis　249
精巣挙筋　Cremaster muscle　249, 251
精巣挙筋膜　Cremaster fascia　249, 251
精巣鞘膜　Tunica vaginalis　249, 251
— 臓側板　Visceral layer of tunica vaginalis　249, 251
— 壁側板　Parietal layer of tunica vaginalis　249, 251
精巣上体　Epididymis　249
— 精巣上体体　Body of epididymis　249
精巣静脈　Testicular v.　249, 271, 283
精巣動脈　Testicular a.　249, 259, 283

精嚢　Seminal vesicle　203, 253, 255
赤核脊髄路　Rubrospinal tract　743
脊髄　Spinal cord　31, 51, 717
脊髄円錐　Conus medullaris of spinal cord　717
脊髄根　Spinal root　573
脊髄神経　Spinal n.　51, 55, 79, 719
— 外側皮枝　Lateral cutaneous branch of spinal n.　79
— 関節枝　Articular branch of spinal n.　51
— 後根　Dorsal root of spinal n.　79, 719
— 後枝　Posterior(dorsal) ramus of spinal n.　51, 55, 79
— 前根　Anterior root of spinal n.　747
— 前枝　Anterior(ventral) ramus of spinal n.　51, 79, 747
— 前皮枝　Anterior cutaneous branch of spinal n.　79
— 内側枝　Medial branch of spinal n.　51
— 白交通枝　White ramus communicans of spinal n.　747
脊髄神経溝　Sulcus for spinal n.　11, 17
脊髄神経節　Spinal ganglion　79, 747
脊柱　Vertebral column　5
脊柱管　Vertebral canal　37
切歯管　Incisive canal　619
舌　Tongue　643
— 舌背　Dorsum of tongue　643
舌咽神経　Glossopharyngeal n.(CN IX)　569, 647
舌咽頭収縮筋　Inferior pharyngeal constrictor　679
舌下神経　Hypoglossal n.(CN XII)　591, **649**, 669, 691, 713
舌下腺　Sublingual gland　657
舌喉頭神経　Inferior laryngeal n.　681
舌骨　Hyoid bone　**645**, 649, 651, 661, 665, 675, 681
— 舌骨体　Hyoid bone　675
— 大角　Greater horn of hyoid bone　661
舌骨喉頭蓋靱帯　Hyoepiglottic l.　677
舌骨舌筋　Hyoglossus　645
舌神経　Lingual n.(CN V$_3$)　561, 593, 597, 641, 647, **649**
舌深動脈　Deep lingual a.　649
舌動脈　Lingual a.　577, 649, 657
舌扁桃　Lingual tonsil　643

舌盲孔　Foramen cecum　643
仙棘靱帯　Sacrospinous l.　**173**, 175, 427, 429, 515
仙結節靱帯　Sacrotuberous l.　**175**, 427, 429, 441, 515
仙骨　Sacrum　**23**, 25, 171, 175, 189
― 岬角　Promontory of sacrum　3, 23, 171
― 耳状面　Auricular surface of sacrum　25
― 正中仙骨稜　Median sacral crest　25
― 仙骨角　Sacral cornua　25
― 仙骨管　Sacral canal　25, 175
― 仙骨尖　Apex of sacrum　23
― 仙骨翼　Wing of sacrum　23, 171
― 仙骨裂孔　Sacral hiatus　25
― 前仙骨孔　Anterior sacral foramina　23
仙骨神経叢　Sacral plexus　287, 289, 517
仙腸関節　Sacroiliac joint　171
仙尾関節　Sacrococcygeal joint　23
浅陰茎背静脈　Superficial dorsal penile v.　245
浅会陰横筋　Superficial transverse perineal　187, 241
浅横中足靱帯　Superficial transverse metacarpal l.　485
浅指屈筋　Flexor digitorum superficialis　341, 343, 379
― 上腕尺骨頭　Humero-ulnar head of flexor digitorum superficialis　343
― 橈骨頭　Radial head of flexor digitorum superficialis　343
浅指屈筋の腱　Flexor digitorum superficialis tendons　361, 397
浅掌動脈弓　Superficial palmar arch　365, 399
浅鼠径リンパ節　Superficial inguinal lymph node　285
浅鼠径輪　Superficial inguinal ring　177, 293
― 外側脚　Lateral crus of superficial inguinal ring　513
― 内側脚　Medial crus of superficial inguinal ring　513
浅側頭静脈　Superficial temporal v.　581, 593
浅側頭動脈　Superficial temporal a.　577, 593

浅腓骨神経　Superficial fibular n.　499, **507**, 511, 525, 527
腺下垂体　Adenohypophysis　705
― 前葉　Anterior lobe of adenohypophysis　705
線維性心膜　Fibrous pericardium　103, 105, 147
線維輪　Anulus fibrosus of intervertebral disk　33
前下腿筋間中隔　Anterior crural intermuscular septum　525
前外椎骨静脈叢　Anterior external vertebral venous plexus　49
前角《脊髄》　Anterior horn of spinal cord　737
前眼房　Anterior chamber of eyeball　617
前弓《環椎の》　Anterior arch of atlas　29
前距腓靱帯　Anterior talofibular l.　481
前鋸筋　Serratus anterior　177, 319, **321**, 323, 329
前胸鎖靱帯　Anterior sternoclavicular l.　311
前脛骨筋　Tibialis anterior　**459**, 461, 507, 527, 535, 537
前脛骨筋の腱　Tibialis anterior tendon　529
前脛骨静脈　Anterior tibial v.　527, 535
前脛骨動脈　Anterior tibial a.　**495**, 497, 527, 529, 535
前脛腓靱帯　Anterior tibiofibular l.　481
前頸静脈　Anterior jugular v.　581
前結節間束　Anterior internodal bundles　133
前交連　Anterior commissure　705, 707
前骨間静脈　Anterior interosseous v.　411
前骨間動脈　Anterior interosseous a.　401, 411
前根《脊髄神経の》　Anterior root of spinal n.　747
前室間溝　Anterior interventricular sulcus　117
前室間枝(前下行枝)《左冠状動脈の》　Anterior interventricular(left anterior descending) branch of left coronary a.　129
前斜角筋　Anterior scalene　67, 371, 687
前十字靱帯　Anterior cruciate l.　455, 457
前縦隔　Anterior mediastinum　91

(そくはいどうみゃく) **793**

前縦靱帯　Anterior longitudinal l.　31，**33**，35，173，427
前床突起　Anterior clinoid process　551
前上歯槽動脈　Anterior superior alveolar aa.　579
前上腕回旋動脈　Anterior circumflex humeral aa.　365
前脊髄視床路　Anterior spinothalamic tract　741
前脊髄小脳路　Anterior spinocerebellar tract　741
前脊髄動脈　Anterior spinal a.　735，737
前仙骨孔　Anterior sacral foramina　23
前仙腸靱帯　Anterior sacroiliac ll.　173，427
前［前腕］骨間神経　Anterior antebrachial interosseous n.　411
前大脳動脈　Anterior cerebral a.　735
前庭ヒダ　Vestibular fold　677
前庭球　Vestibular bulb　241
前庭神経　Vestibular root（CN Ⅷ）　567，637
前庭神経節　Vestibular ganglian　567
前庭脊髄路　Vestibulospinal tract　743
前頭蓋窩　Anterior cranial fossa　549
前頭筋《後頭前頭筋の》　Frontal belly of occipitofrontalis　553
前頭骨　Frontal bone　541，543
前頭神経　Frontal n.　559，605，609
前頭前野　Prefrontal cortex　739
前頭側頭束　Frontotemporal fasciculus　701
前頭洞　Frontal sinus　551，555，601
前頭葉　Frontal lobe　697，699
前内椎骨静脈叢　Anterior internal vertebral venous plexus　49
前乳頭筋　Anterior papillary muscle　121，125
前皮質脊髄路　Anterior corticospinal tract　743
前迷走神経幹　Anterior vagal trunk　101，287
前立腺　Prostate　203，253，255
前肋間静脈　Anterior intercostal vv.　49，77
前腕　Forearm　297
前腕屈筋　Flexors of forearm　339
前腕骨間膜　Interosseous membrane　333

前篩骨動脈　Anterior ethmoidal a.　625，627

そ

鼠径靱帯　Inguinal l.　**173**，177，183，185，513
粗線《大腿骨の》　Linea aspera　421
僧帽筋　Trapezius　39，41，57，319，**327**，383，573，689，693
— 横行部（水平部）　Transverse part of trapezius　39，327
— 下行部　Descending part of trapezius　327，383
総肝管　Common hepatic duct　223
総肝動脈　Common hepatic a.　225，265
総頸動脈　Common carotid a.　75，95，663，**667**，685
— 左総頸動脈　Left common carotid a.　95，117
総腱輪　Common tendinous ring　603
［総］指伸筋　Extensor digitorum　345，363，411
［総］指伸筋の腱　Extensor digitorum tendon　345，375
総掌側指動脈　Common palmar digital aa.　399
総胆管　Bile duct　221，223，225
総腸骨リンパ節　Common iliac lymph node　285
総腸骨静脈　Common iliac v.　271，281
— 右総腸骨静脈　Right common iliac v.　203，281
総腸骨動脈　Common iliac a.　259，281
— 右総腸骨動脈　Right common iliac a.　203，229，**259**，281
総腓骨神経　Common fibular n.　499，**507**，521，525
臓側胸膜　Visceral pleura　81
足関節窩　Ankle mortise　447
足根管　Tarsal tunnel　523
足根骨　Tarsal bones　417
足根中足関節　Tarsometatarsal joints　473
足底筋　Plantaris　465
足底腱膜　Plantar aponeurosis　485
足底方形筋　Quadratus plantae　489，531
足背動脈　Dorsal pedal a.　495，529

側頭下窩 Infratemporal fossa 593, 595, 597
側頭筋 Temporalis 593
側頭骨 Temporal bone 541, 551, **629**, 637
― 岩様部 Petrous part of temporal bone 551, 629, 637
― 茎状突起 Styloid process of temporal bone 629
― 鱗部 Squamous part of temporal bone 541
側頭葉 Temporal lobe 697, 699
側脳室 Lateral ventricle 707, 729
― 下角 Inferior horn of lateral ventricle 729

た

対輪 Antihelix 631
大陰唇 Labia majora 239
大円筋 Teres major 323, 327, **331**, 385
大胸筋 Pectoralis major 89, **319**, 325, 387
― 胸肋部 Sternocostal part of pectoralis major 319
― 鎖骨部 Clavicular part of pectoralis major 319, 387
― 腹部 Abdominal part of pectoralis major 319
大頰骨筋 Zygomaticus major 553
大結節《上腕骨の》 Greater tuberosity of humerus 307, 313
大口蓋神経 Greater palatine n. 599, 627
― 下後鼻枝 Inferior posterior nasal branches of greater palatine n. 627
大口蓋動脈 Greater palatine a. 627
大後頭孔 Foramen magnum 547, 549
大後頭神経 Greater occipital n. 53, 575, 587
大後頭直筋 Rectus capitis posterior major 41
大坐骨孔 Greater sciatic foramen 175, 515
大坐骨切痕 Greater sciatic notch 419
大耳介神経 Great auricular n. 53, 575, 587, **669**, 689
大十二指腸乳頭 Major duodenal papilla 211, 223

大静脈孔《横隔膜の》 Caval aperture of diaphragm 69, 71, 105
大心臓静脈 Great cardiac v. 129, 131
大腎杯 Major calix 261
大錐体神経 Greater petrosal n. 565, 599, 637
大槽 Cisterna magna 727
大腿 Thigh 417
大腿筋膜 Fascia lata 185
大腿筋膜張筋 Tensor fasciae latae 431, 441, **445**, 537
大腿骨 Femur 417, 421
― 顆間窩 Intercondylar notch of femur 421, 451
― 外側顆 Lateral condyle of femur 421, 449, 451
― 外側上顆 Lateral epicondyle of femur 453
― 外側唇 Lateral lip of linea aspera 421
― 小転子 Lesser trochanter 421, 423
― 粗線 Linea aspera 421, 425
― 大腿骨頸 Neck of femur 421, 423
― 大腿骨頭 Head of femur 421, 423
― 大転子 Greater trochanter 421, 425
― 転子間稜 Intertrochanteric crest 421
― 内側顆 Medial condyle of femur 421, 449, 451
― 内側上顆 Medial epicondyle of femur 421, 449, 451
― 内側唇 Medial lip of linea aspera 421
― 内転筋結節 Adductor tubercle 421
大腿四頭筋の腱 Quadriceps femoris tendon 431, 453
大腿静脈 Femoral v. 183, 259, 283, 513, **517**, 533
大腿神経 Femoral n. 183, 499, 501, **505**, 511, 513, 517
大腿深静脈 Deep femoral v. 533
大腿深動脈 Profunda femoris a. 495, 517, 533
大腿直筋 Rectus femoris **431**, 505, 533, 537
大腿動脈 Femoral a. 183, 259, 283, **495**, 513, 517, 533
大腿二頭筋 Biceps femoris 521
― 短頭 Short head of biceps femoris 443, 507

— 長頭　Long head of biceps femoris　439，445，509
大腿二頭筋の腱　Biceps femoris tendon　461，463
大腿方形筋　Quadratus femoris　441
大転子　Greater trochanter　421，425
大殿筋　Gluteus maximus　57，187，**439**，443，445
大動脈弓　Aortic arch　**105**，115，137，139
大動脈腎動脈神経節　Aorticorenal ganglia　287
大動脈弁　Aortic valve　127
— 右半月弁　Right cusp of aortic valve　127
— 後半月弁　Posterior cusp of aortic valve　127
— 左半月弁　Left cusp of aortic valve　127
大動脈裂孔《横隔膜の》　Aortic aperture of diaphragm　71
大内臓神経　Greater splanchnic n.　107，287
大内転筋　Adductor magnus　435，437，**443**，495，503，509，533
大内転筋の腱　Adductor magnus tendon　497
大脳　Telencephalon　701
大脳鎌　Falx cerebri　723，725
大脳脚　Cerebral peduncle　701
大脳弓状線維　Cerebral arcuate fibers（U fibers）　701
大伏在静脈　Long saphenous v.　511
大網　Greater omentum　193，195
大腰筋　Psoas major　71，229，431
大菱形筋　Rhomboid（romboideus）major　39，329
大菱形骨　Trapezium　349
大弯　Greater curvature of stomach　209
第1頸椎（環椎）　C1 vertebra（Atlas）　5
第1腰椎　L1 vertebra　5，207
第2頸椎（軸椎）　C2 vertebra（Axis）　5，11
第3胸椎　T3 vertebra　7
第3腓骨筋　Fibularis tertius　461
第三脳室　3rd ventricle　709，729
第三脳室脈絡叢　Choroid plexus of 3rd ventricle　727
第四脳室　4th ventricle　729
第四脳室正中口　Median aperture of 4th ventricle　727
第四脳室脈絡叢　Choroid plexus of 4th ventricle　727
第7胸椎　T7 vertebra　7
第7頸椎　C7 vertebra　5，7，11
胆膵管　Hepatopancreatic duct　225
胆囊　Gallbladder　207，221，**223**，225
— 胆囊底　Fundus of gallbladder　223
胆囊管　Cystic duct　223，225
淡蒼球
— 外節　Lateral segment of globus pallidus　709
— 内節　Medial segment of globus pallidus　709
短趾屈筋　Flexor digitorum brevis　487
短趾伸筋　Extensor digitorum brevis　493
短小指屈筋　Flexor digiti minimi brevis　359
短小趾屈筋　Flexor digiti minimi brevis　487
短掌筋　Palmaris brevis　355
短橈側手根伸筋　Extensor carpi radialis brevis　347
短内転筋　Adductor brevis　433，435，503
短腓骨筋　Fibularis brevis　461，535
短母指外転筋　Abductor pollicis brevis　357
短母指屈筋
— 浅頭　Superficial head of flexor pollicis brevis　357
短母指伸筋の腱　Extensor pollicis brevis tendon　403
短母趾屈筋　Flexor hallucis brevis　491
— 外側頭　Lateral head of flexor hallucis brevis　491
— 内側頭　Medial head of flexor hallucis brevis　491
短母趾伸筋　Extensor hallucis brevis　459
短母趾伸筋の腱　Extensor hallucis brevis tendon　529
男性骨盤　Male pelvis　173

ち

恥丘　Mons pubis　239
恥骨　Pubis　169，171
— 弓状線　Arcuate line of pubis　169

― 恥骨筋線　Pectineal line　169, 171
恥骨筋　Pectineus　433, 505
恥骨結合　Pubic symphysis　173, 191, 231
恥骨結節　Pubic tubercle　169, 419, 423
恥骨大腿靱帯　Pubofemoral l.　427
恥骨直腸筋　Puborectalis　189
恥骨尾骨筋　Pubococcygeus　189
腟　Vagina　205, 231
腟円蓋　Vaginal fornix　237
― 外側部　Lateral part of vaginal fornix　237
腟静脈叢　Vaginal venous plexus　279
腟前庭　Vestibule of vagina(vaginal vestibule)　239
中咽頭収縮筋　Middle pharyngeal constrictor　659, 661
中隔縁柱　Septomarginal trabecula　121
中間広筋　Vastus intermedius　433, 435, 505
中頸神経節　Middle cervical ganglion　101, 663
中結節間束　middle internodal bundles　133
中結腸動脈　Middle colic a.　267
中硬膜動脈　Middle meningeal a.　595
中斜角筋　Middle scalene　67, 691
中手骨　Metacarpals　297, 349, 351
― 第1中手骨　1st metacarpal　349
― 底　Base of metacarpal　351
― 頭　Head of metacarpal　351
中手指節(MCP)関節　Metacarpophalangeal (MCP) joint　353
中縦隔　Middle mediastinum　91
中小脳脚　Middle cerebellar peduncle　715
中心腋窩リンパ節　Central axillary lymph node　87
中心管《脊髄の》　Central canal of spinal cord　729
中心後回　Postcentral gyrus　697, 739
中心溝　Central sulcus　697, 739
中心前回　Precentral gyrus　739
中心臓静脈(後室間静脈)　Posterior interventricular v.　131
中節骨《手の》
― 第2中節骨　2nd middle phalanx of hand　349
中足骨　Matatarsus(metatarsal)　469, 471, 479

― 第1中足骨　1st metatarsal　469, 471, 479
― 第5中足骨　5th metatarsal　479
― 第5中足骨粗面　Tuberosity of 5th metatarsal　471
中足趾節関節　Metatarsophalangeal joints　473
中大脳動脈　Middle cerebral a.　735
中直腸横ヒダ　Middle transverse rectal fold　217
中直腸静脈　Middle rectal v.　279
中直腸動脈　Middle rectal a.　279, 281
中殿筋　Gluteus medius　57, 439, 443, **445**
中殿皮神経　Middle cluneal nn.　55
中頭蓋窩　Middle cranial fossa　549, 607
中脳水道　Cerebral aqueduct　729
中鼻道　Middle meatus　621
中副腎動脈　Middle suprarenal aa.　273
― 右中副腎動脈　Right middle suprarenal a.　273
虫様筋《足の》　Lumbricals of foot　489
虫様筋《手の》　Lumbricals of hand　359, 379
― 第1虫様筋　1st lumbrical of hand　379
― 第2虫様筋　2nd lumbrical of hand　379
肘関節　Elbow joint　335, 337
肘筋　Anconeus　345
肘正中皮静脈　Median cubital v.　367
肘頭　Olecranon　333
肘頭窩《上腕骨の》　Olecranon fossa of humerus　307
長胸神経　Long thoracic n.　371, 391
長趾屈筋　Flexor digitorum longus　467, 521, 523
長趾屈筋の腱　Flexor digitorum longus tendon　465, 489
長趾伸筋　Extensor digitorum longus　**459**, 493, 507, 527
長掌筋　Palmaris longus　339
長掌筋の腱　Palmaris longus tendon　355
長足底靱帯　Long plantar l.　479
長橈側手根伸筋　Extensor carpi radialis longus　345, 347
長橈側手根伸筋の腱　Extensor carpi radialis longus tendon　363

長内転筋　Adductor longus　433, 503, 537
長腓骨筋　Fibularis longus　461, 507, 525
長腓骨筋の腱　Fibularis longus tendon　465, 479, 491
長腓骨筋腱溝　Groove for fibularis longus tendon　471
長母指外転筋　Abductor pollicis longus　347, 363, 375
長母指外転筋の腱　Abductor pollicis longus tendon　403
長母指屈筋　Flexor pollicis longus　343, 379
長母指屈筋の腱　Flexor pollicis longus tendon　341, 359, 397
長母指伸筋　Extensor pollicis longus　347
長母指伸筋の腱　Extensor pollicis longus tendon　363, 403, 413
長母趾屈筋　Flexor hallucis longus　467
長母趾屈筋の腱　Flexor hallucis longus tendon　463, 487
長母趾伸筋　Extensor hallucis longus　459, 493
長母趾伸筋の腱　Extensor hallucis longus tendon　529, 537
長毛様体神経　Long ciliary nn.　605, 611
腸間膜　Mesentery　199
腸間膜根　Mesenteric root　201
腸間膜動脈間神経叢　Intermesenteric plexus　287
腸脛靱帯　Iliotibial tract　439, 445, 525
腸骨　Ilium　171
― 腸骨窩　Iliac fossa　171
腸骨下腹神経　Iliohypogastric n.　501
腸骨筋　Iliacus　435
腸骨鼠径神経　Ilioinguinal n.　499, 501
腸骨大腿靱帯　Iliofemoral l.　427, 429
腸骨尾骨筋　Iliococcygeus　189
腸骨稜　Iliac crest　7, 169, 419
腸恥筋膜弓　Iliopectineal arch　513
腸腰筋　Iliopsoas　431, 505
腸腰靱帯　Iliolumbar l.　173, 427, 429
腸肋筋　Iliocostalis　43
蝶形骨　Sphenoid bone　**541**, 547, 549, 601
― 小翼　Lesser wing of sphenoid bone　549
― 大翼　Greater wing of sphenoid bone　541, 601
― 翼状突起　Pterygoid process of sphenoid bone　547
蝶形骨洞　Sphenoid sinus　623
蝶口蓋孔　Sphenopalatine foramen　623
蝶口蓋動脈　Sphenopalatine a.　579, 595, 625
― 中隔後鼻枝　Posterior septal branches of sphenopalatine a.　625
直細動脈　Vasa recta　267
直静脈洞　Straight sinus　727, 733
直腸　Rectum　203, 213, **215**, 217, 231
直腸子宮窩　Rectouterine pouch　205
直腸子宮靱帯　Uterosacral l.　235
直腸静脈叢　Hemorrhoidal plexus　217
直腸膀胱窩　Rectovesical pouch　203, 255

つ

ツチ骨　Malleus　629, 635
椎間円板　Intervertebral disk　3, 5, 33, 37
― 髄核　Nucleus pulposus of intervertebral disk　33
― 線維輪　Anulus fibrosus of intervertebral disk　33
椎間関節　Zygapophyseal joint　27
椎間孔　Intervertebral foramen　3, 37, 719
椎弓　Vertebral arch　9, **15**, 17, 19, 21
― 椎弓根　Pedicle of vertebral arch　9, 19, 37
― 椎弓板　Lamina of vertebral arch　9, **17**, 19, 35
椎孔　Vertebral foramen　9
椎骨　Vertebra　9
椎骨静脈叢　Vertebral venous plexus　49
椎骨動脈　Vertebral a.　17, 53, **577**, 719
椎骨動脈溝　Groove for vertebral a.　13
椎前神経節　Prevertebral ganglion　747
椎体　Vertebral body　5, 9, **19**, 37
椎体間関節　Intervertebral joint　27
蔓状静脈叢　Pampiniform plexus　249, 283

て

テント切痕　Tentorial notch　725
底側骨間筋　Plantar interossei　491
底側踵舟靱帯　Plantar calcaneonavicular l.　477, 479
底側中足動脈　Plantar metatarsal aa.　531
転子間稜　Intertrochanteric crest　421

と

トルコ鞍（下垂体窩）《蝶形骨の》　Sella turcica (hypophyseal fossa) of sphenoid bone　551
豆状骨　Pisiform　351
頭頂骨　Parietal bone　545
頭半棘筋　Semispinalis capitis　45
頭板状筋　Splenius capitis　45
頭皮　Scalp　723
橈骨　Radius　297, 333
— 茎状突起　Styloid process of radius　333, 351
— 橈骨粗面　Radial tuberosity　333
— 橈骨頭　Head of radius　333, 337
— 背側結節　Dorsal tubercle of radius　345
橈骨窩（解剖学的嗅ぎタバコ入れ）　Anatomic (anatomical) snuffbox　403, 413
橈骨手根関節　Radiocarpal joint　353
橈骨神経　Radial n.　**375**, 385, 391, 395, 403, 405, 409
— 深枝　Deep branch of radial n.　395
— 浅枝　Superficial branch of radial n.　375, 395, 403, 407, 411
橈骨動脈　Radial a.　**365**, 395, 401, 403
橈骨輪状靱帯　Annular l. of radius　335, 337
橈側手根屈筋　Flexor carpi radialis　339, 379
橈側手根屈筋の腱　Flexor carpi radialis tendon　397
橈側皮静脈　Cephalic v.　367, 387
洞房結節　Sinoatrial (SA) node　133
洞房結節枝　Branch to sinoatrial node　129
動眼神経　Oculomotor n. (CN III)　557, **605**, 607, 713
動脈円錐　Conus arteriosus　121

動脈管索　Ligamentum arteriosum　109, 113, **121**, 145
導出静脈　Emissary v.　723

な

内陰部静脈　Internal pudendal v.　215, 243, 257, 279, **281**
— 左内陰部静脈　Left internal pudendal v.　279, 281
内陰部動脈　Internal pudendal a.　215, 243, 257, 279
— 左内陰部動脈　Left internal pudendal a.　279
内果　Medial malleolus of tibia　447, 459
内胸静脈　Internal thoracic vv.　49, **77**, 85, 103
内胸動脈　Internal thoracic a.　75, 85, 103
— 前肋間枝　Anterior intercostal arteries branches of internal thoracic a.　75
内頸静脈　Internal jugular v.　77, 97, 99, 163, **581**, 583, 589, 663, 673, 685, 731
— 右内頸静脈　Right internal jugular v.　97, 163
内頸動脈　Internal carotid a.　591, 605, 607, 633, 635, **667**, 691, 735
内頸動脈神経叢　Internal carotid plexus　605
内肛門括約筋　Internal anal sphincter　217
内子宮口　Internal os of uterus　237
内耳　Inner ear　637
内精筋膜　Internal spermatic fascia　249, 251
内臓神経　Splanchnic n.　747
内側顆《脛骨の》　Medial condyle of tibia　447, 449, 451
内側顆《大腿骨の》　Medial condyle of femur　421, 449, 451
内側胸筋神経　Medial pectoral nn.　387, 389
内側楔状骨　Medial cuneiform　**469**, 471, 477, 479
内側広筋　Vastus medialis　431, 437, 505
内側臍索　Medial umbilical ll.　145
内側上顆《上腕骨の》　Medial epicondyle of humerus　**305**, 335, 337, 339

内側上顆《大腿骨の》 Medial epicondyle of femur 421, 449, 451
内側上膝動脈 Medial superior genicular a. 497
内側上腕筋間中隔 Medial intermuscular septum of arm 393
内側神経束 Medial cord 369, 381
内側足底神経 Medial plantar n. 499, 523, 531
内側足底動脈 Medial plantar a. 523, 531
内側側副靱帯《膝関節の》 Medial collateral l. of knee joint 453, 455, 457
内側側副靱帯《肘関節の》 Ulnar collateral l. of elbow joint 335, 337
内側大腿回旋動脈 Medial circumflex femoral a. 495, 517
内側直筋 Medial rectus 557, 603
内側半月 Medial meniscus 453, 455
内側翼突筋 Medial pterygoid 595
内腸骨リンパ節 Internal iliac lymph node 285
内腸骨静脈 Internal iliac v. 283
内腸骨動脈 Internal iliac a. 259, 279, 283
— 右内腸骨動脈 Right internal iliac a. 259, 279
内転筋管 Adductor canal 495
［内転筋］腱裂孔 Adductor hiatus 435, 497
内腹斜筋 Internal oblique 39, 45, **179**, 183, 185
内閉鎖筋 Obturator internus 187, 215, **437**, 441
内閉鎖筋筋膜 Obturator internus fascia 191
内包 Internal capsule 701, 707
内肋間筋 Internal intercostals 67, 179
軟口蓋(口蓋帆) Soft palate 651, 653
軟膜 Pia mater 721

に

肉様膜 Tunica dartos 251
乳腺 Mammary gland 89
— 乳管 Lactiferous duct 89
— 乳管洞 Lactiferous sinus 89
— 乳腺葉 Mammary lobes 89
乳頭 Nipple 89
乳頭体 Mammillary body 703, 711
乳ビ槽 Cisterna chyli 99, 285
乳房提靱帯(クーパー靱帯) Suspensory (Cooper's) ll. of breast 89
乳様突起 Mastoid process of temporal bone 545
尿管 Ureter 215, **229**, 233, 235, 253, 261
尿管間ヒダ Interureteral fold 233
尿管口 Ureteral orifice 233
尿道 Urethra 231, **233**, 245, 253
— 海綿体部 Spongy part of urethra 245, 255
尿道海綿体 Corpus spongiosum 247
尿道球 Bulb of penis 247
尿道球腺 Bulbourethral gland 253, 257
人中 Philtrum 693

の

脳幹 Brainstem 713, 715
脳弓 Fornix 705, 709
脳弓脚 Crus of fornix 703
脳弓体 Body of fornix 703
脳室系 Ventricle 729
脳底動脈 Basilar a. 735
脳梁 Corpus callosum 701, 703, 707

は

馬尾 Cauda equina 717
背側骨間筋《足の》 Dorsal interossei of foot 491
背側骨間筋《手の》
— 第1背側骨間筋 1st dorsal interosseus of hand 357, 363, 403
背側指神経 Dorsal digital nn. 405, 407
背側足根靱帯 Dorsal tarsal ll. 481
背側中足動脈 Dorsal metatarsal aa. 529
肺 Lungs 149
— 小舌 Lingula of lung 153
— 肺尖 Apex of lung 149, 151, 153
肺間膜 Pulmonary l. 151
肺神経叢 Pulmonary plexus 135
肺動脈 Pulmonary aa. 145
肺動脈幹 Pulmonary trunk 95, 113, 117, 125, 137, 149, **161**

肺動脈弁　Valve of pulmonary trunk　121
肺胞　Alveolus　159
肺胞囊　Alveolar sac　159
肺門　Hilum of lung　153
排尿筋　Detrusor vesicae　233
白線　Linea alba　177, 293
白膜　Tunica albuginea　251
薄筋　Gracilis　435, **437**, 443, 503
薄束　Fasciculus gracilis　741
反回神経　Recurrent laryngeal n.　101, 135, 687
― 右反回神経　Right recurrent laryngeal n.　135, 571
― 左反回神経　Left recurrent laryngeal n.　101, 135, **571**, 663
半奇静脈　Hemiazygos v.　97, 109, 271
半規管　Semicircular ducts　567
半月線　Semilunar line　293
半腱様筋　Semitendinosus　439, 509, 533
半膜様筋　Semimembranosus　439, 463, 509
板間層　Diploë of cranial bone　723

ひ

ヒス束　Bundle of His　133
ヒラメ筋　Soleus　461, **465**, 467, 509, 535
披裂喉頭蓋ヒダ　Aryepiglottic fold　677
被殻　Putamen　709
脾静脈　Splenic v.　275, 277
脾臓　Spleen　197, 207
脾動脈　Splenic a.　263, 277
腓骨　Fibula　417, 447
― 外果　Lateral malleolus　**447**, 461, 463, 475, 481
― 腓骨頭　Head of fibula　445, 447, 507, 525
腓骨静脈　Fibular v.　535
腓骨動脈　Fibular a.　497, 521, 535
腓腹筋　Gastrocnemius　509, 535, 537
― 外側頭　Lateral head of gastrocnemius　439, 461, 463
― 内側頭　Medial head of gastrocnemius　439, 463, 467, 535
腓腹神経　Sural n.　511, 525
尾骨　Coccyx　3, 25
尾骨筋　Coccygeus　189, 191

尾状核　Caudate nucleus　707, 711
鼻腔　Nasal cavity　619
鼻口蓋神経　Nasopalatine n.　625
鼻骨　Nasal bone　543
鼻根点　Nasion　543
鼻中隔　Nasal septum　555
鼻中隔軟骨　Septal cartilage　619
鼻毛様体神経　Nasociliary n.　559, 611
鼻涙管　Nasolacrimal duct　615
「膝-」→「しつ-」の項をみよ
「左-」→「さ-」の項をみよ
表情筋　Muscles of facial expression　553

ふ

伏在神経　Saphenous n.　499, **505**, 511, 517
― 膝蓋下枝　Infrapatellar branch of saphenous n.　505
副交感神経　Parasympathetic n.　747
副神経　Accessory n.(CN XI)　55, **573**, 591, 687, 691, 713
― 外枝　External branch of accessory n.　691
副腎　Suprarenal gland　229
副膵管　Accessory pancreatic duct　227
副半奇静脈　Accessory hemiazygos v.　97
腹横筋　Transversus abdominis　45, 181, 185
腹腔リンパ節　Celiac lymph node　285
腹腔神経節　Celiac ganglion　287
腹腔動脈　Celiac trunk　193, 225, 259, 263, **265**, 277
腹大動脈　Abdominal aorta　259, 263
腹直筋　Rectus abdominis　181, 183, 293
腹直筋鞘　Rectus sheath　179, 181, 183
― 前葉　Anterior rectus sheath　179, 181, 183
腹膜腔　Peritoneal cavity　195, 201
腹膜垂　Epiploic appendices　213
噴門　Cardia　209
分界溝　Sulcus terminalis　643
分界稜　Crista terminalis　123

へ

閉鎖管　Obturator canal　189
閉鎖孔　Obturator foramen　169, 419

(ようせんこつしんけいかん) *801*

閉鎖静脈　Obturator v.　279
閉鎖神経　Obturator n.　501, 503, 517
― 皮枝　Cutaneous branch of obturator n.　503
閉鎖動脈　Obturator a.　279, 281
閉鎖膜　Obturator membrane　173, 175
壁側胸膜　Parietal pleura　147
― 横隔部(横隔膜)　Diaphragmatic part of parietal pleura　81, 147
― 縦隔部(縦隔胸膜)　Mediastinal part of parietal pleura　103, 147
― 肋骨部(肋骨胸膜)　Costal part of parietal pleura　83, 147
壁側腹膜　Parietal peritoneum　185
扁桃体　Amygdala　709

ほ

ボクダレク三角(腰肋三角)　Bochdalek's triangle(lumbocostal triangle)　71
母指球　Thenar eminence　413
母指球線　Thenar crease　413
母指対立筋　Opponens pollicis　359
母指内転筋　Adductor pollicis　361
― 横頭　Transverse head of adductor pollicis　357, 361
― 斜頭　Oblique head of adductor pollicis　361
母趾外転筋　Abductor hallucis　485, 523, 531
母趾内転筋　Adductor hallucis　491
― 横頭　Transverse head of adductor hallucis　491
― 斜頭　Oblique head of adductor hallucis　491
方形回内筋　Pronator quadratus　343
放線冠　Corona radiata　701
縫工筋　Sartorius　**431**, 437, 505, 533
房室結節　Atrioventricular(AV) node　133
房室束　Atrioventricular bundle　133
― 右脚　Right bundle branch of atrioventricular bundle　133
帽状腱膜　Galea aponeurotica　553
膀胱　Urinary bladder　203, 205, 229, 231, **233**, 253
― 膀胱頚　Neck of bladder　233
― 膀胱体　Body of (urinary) bladder　255

膀胱三角　Bladder trigone　233
膀胱子宮窩　Vesicouterine pouch　205
膀胱神経叢　Vesical plexus　291

ま み め

末節骨《足の》
― 第1末節骨　1st distal phalanx of foot　469
「右-」→「う-」の項をみよ
脈絡叢　Choroid plexus　705
迷走神経　Vagus n.(CN X)　101, 107, 109, 135, 569, **571**, 573, 647, 663, 673, 685, 713, 747
― 頸心臓枝　Cervical cardiac branches of vagus n.　571

も

毛様体　Ciliary body　617
毛様体筋　Ciliary muscle　617
毛様体神経節　Ciliary ganglion　559, 605
盲腸　Cecum　213
網嚢　Omental bursa　197, 207
網嚢孔　Omental foramen　197
網膜　Retina　617
網様体脊髄路　Reticulospinal tract　743

ゆ

有鈎骨　Hamate　349
有鈎骨鈎　Hook of hamate　351
有線野　Striate area　745
有頭骨　Capitate　351
幽門括約筋　Pyloric sphincter　211
幽門洞　Pyloric antrum　209

よ

葉間動脈　Interlobar a.　261
腰三角　Lumbar triangle　39
腰静脈　Lumbar vv.　97, 271
― 第1腰静脈　1st lumbar v.　77
腰神経　Lumbar nn.　289
― 前枝　Anterior rami of lumber nn.　289
腰神経節　Lumbar ganglia　289
腰仙骨神経幹　Lumbosacral trunk　501

腰椎 Lumbar vertebrae 3, 21
— 第1腰椎 L1 vertebra 501
— 第4腰椎 L4 vertebra 7, 503
— 第5腰椎 L5 vertebra 193, 717
— 乳頭突起 Mammillary process of lumbar vertebrae 21
腰内臓神経 Lumbar splanchnic n. 289
腰膨大 Lumbosacral enlargement 717
腰肋三角(ボクダレク三角) Lumbocostal triangle(Bochdalek's triangle) 71
翼口蓋窩 Pterygopalatine fossa 599
翼口蓋神経節 Pterygopalatine ganglion 561, 627, 641
翼状突起 Pterygoid process of sphenoid bone 547, 621
— 外側板 Lateral plate of pterygoid process 547
— 内側板 Medial plate of pterygoid process 547, 621
翼突管神経 Nerve of pterygoid canal 599
翼突筋静脈叢 Pterygoid plexus 581, 583

ら

ラセン神経節 Spiral ganglia 567
ラムダ縫合 Lambdoid suture 545
卵円窩 Fossa ovalis 123
卵円孔 Foramen ovale 143, 145, **547**, 551, 597
卵管 Uterine tube 235, 237
— 卵管峡部 Isthmus of uterine tube 237
卵管間膜 Mesosalpinx 235
卵管膨大部 Ampulla 237
卵管漏斗 Infundibulum 237
卵形嚢 Utricle 567
卵巣 Ovary 235
卵巣静脈 Ovarian v. 235, 271
卵巣動脈 Ovarian a. 235

り

梨状陥凹 Piriform recess 677
梨状筋 Piriformis 189, **191**, 437, 441, 515
立方骨 Cuboid 469, 479
隆椎(第7頸椎) Vertebra prominens(C7) 5, 11
菱形窩 Rhomboid fossa 715

輪状甲状筋 Cricothyroid 571, 659, 679
輪状甲状靱帯 Cricothyroid l. 675
輪状軟骨 Cricoid cartilage 155, 675, 677
鱗状縫合 Squamous suture 541

る

涙器 Lacrimal apparatus 615
涙丘 Lacrimal caruncle 615
涙腺 Lacrimal gland 609, 615
— 眼窩部 Orbital part of lacrimal gland 615
涙腺神経 Lacrimal n. 609
涙腺動脈 Lacrimal a. 609
涙嚢 Lacrimal sac 615

ろ

肋間静脈 (Posterior)intercostal vv. 49, 55, **77**, 81, 83, 97
— 外側皮枝 Lateral cutaneous branches of posterior intercostal vv. 55
肋間神経 Intercostal nn. 55, 81, 101
— 外側皮枝 Lateral cutaneous branches of intercostal n. 55
肋間動脈 Posterior intercostal aa. 47, 55, **75**, 81, 83
— 外側皮枝 Lateral cutaneous branches of posterior intercostal aa. 55
肋骨 Rib 69
— 第1肋骨 1st rib 311
— 第6肋骨 6th rib 63
— 肋骨角 Costal angle of rib 63
— 肋骨頸 Neck of rib 63
— 肋骨結節 Costal tubercle of rib 63
— 肋骨頭 Head of rib 63
肋骨横隔洞 Costodiaphragmatic recess 81, 149
肋骨弓 Costal margin(arch) 61
肋骨挙筋 Levatores costarum 45
肋骨胸膜(壁側胸膜の肋骨部) Costal part of parietal pleura 83, 147
肋骨溝 Costal groove 81
肋鎖靱帯 Costoclavicular ligament 311
肋鎖靱帯圧痕 Impression for costoclavicular l. 299
肋軟骨 Costal cartilage **61**, 63, 67, 311

わ

腕神経叢　Brachial plexus　**369**, 371, 389, 685

腕頭静脈　Brachiocephalic v.　115
腕頭動脈　Brachiocephalic trunk　115, 119
腕橈骨筋　Brachioradialis　339, 395, 411